Canadian Reviewers

Sharon L. Andersen, RN, BSN, MSN, Med, EdD
Faculty of Nursing
Kwantlen University College
Surrey, British Columbia
Canada

P. H. Bailey, RN, BN, MHSc, PhD
Professor
Laurentian University
Sudbury, Ontario
Canada

Patricia Grainger, RN, BN, MN
Nurse Educator
Centre for Nursing Studies
St. John's, Newfoundland
Canada

Brad Hagen, RN, PhD
Associate Professor
The University of Lethbridge
Lethbridge, Alberta
Canada

Claudette Kelly, RN, BScN, MA, PhD
Nurse Educator
The University College of the Cariboo
Kamloops, British Columbia
Canada

Linda S. Nugent, BN, MScN, PhD(c)
Professor
University of New Brunswick
Saint John, New Brunswick
Canada

Lynne Parsons, RN, BN, MN
Nursing Instructor
North Island College
Courtenay, British Columbia
Canada

Darlene Steven, RN, BScN, MHSA, PhD
Professor
Lakehead University
Thunder Bay, Ontario
Canada

Lynne E. Young, RN, BSN, MSN, PhD
Assistant Professor
University of Victoria School of Nursing
Vancouver, British Columbia
Canada

Preface

This first edition of *Canadian Essentials of Nursing Research* features state-of-the-art research undertaken by Canadian nurse researchers, as well as Canadian content relating to the history of nursing research, ethical considerations, models of nursing, and models of research utilization. At the same time, this edition retains all of the features that have made the original award-winning text so popular. *Essentials of Nursing Research* is widely hailed by faculty and students alike for its up-to-date, clear, concise, and "user-friendly" presentation. To make concepts discussed in the textbook less abstract, and to encourage research utilization by soon-to-be practitioners, actual research examples are presented at the end of each chapter, followed by a discussion of clinical implications of findings.

Nursing research is the conduct of systematic studies to generate new knowledge pertaining to health and illness-related experiences. Nurse researchers are scientists who seek answers to pressing questions through the systematic observation and recording of phenomena relating to nursing practice. There is a growing expectation that nurses—especially those in clinical practice—will utilize the results of scientific studies as a basis for their practice. The need to apply new knowledge from research requires that we overcome the challenges related to accessing, reading, understanding, and translating research findings into practice. One main purpose of this book is to assist consumers of nursing research in evaluating the adequacy of research findings in terms of their scientific merit and potential for utilization.

The 21st century is a very exciting era for nursing research in Canada. The information age is revolutioning the ways nurses teach, practice, and conduct research. Current nursing research agendas are more dynamic, more responsive to social and health care delivery developments, and more accessible to other health researchers, research users, funding agencies, and the public. The explosion of information technology has enabled clinicians and researchers to readily transcend geographical distances so that they may work together to answer important nursing questions. In addition, an expanding critical mass of well-funded nurse researchers makes for a more visible, productive, and collaborative health-related research enterprise. The unprecedented availability of funding for nursing research originates from new and innovative partnerships among federal and provincial governments, professional nursing associations, and private industry. We are also witnessing more concerted efforts on the part of nurse researchers to involve key stakeholders (lay individuals, nurses involved in direct care, clinical nurse specialists, etc.) in the design, conduct, evaluation and dissemination of nursing research. One challenge for the future of Canadian nursing research, however, will be to augment the means through which research findings are more broadly disseminated—there are still too few academic and professional Canadian nursing journals.

Growing evidence indicates that the presentation of knowledge that is personally relevant to students contributes to optimal learning. By "Canadianizing" this textbook, we believe that we can influence students' early socialization process to the discipline of nursing and help them develop a passion for nursing research.

The material gathered for this first Canadian edition is a testimony to the breadth and high quality of research conducted by Canadian nurse researchers, published in both English and French. This edition likely will stimulate students to become well-informed consumers of research and to get more actively involved in the discovery of nursing knowledge. Research plays an increasingly pivotal role in shaping the profession and the discipline of nursing and continues to ensure better care and optimal health-related outcomes for Canadians. We are honored to have had the opportunity to undertake the production of *Canadian Essentials of Nursing Research* at this promising moment in the history of nursing research in Canada.

Organization of the Text

The content of this edition is organized into six main parts.

Part I—Overview of Nursing Research serves as the overall introduction to fundamental concepts in nursing research. Chapter 1 introduces and summarizes the history and future of nursing research both in Canada and elsewhere, discusses the philosophical underpinnings of qualitative research versus quantitative research, and describes the major purposes of nursing research. Chapter 2 presents an overview of the steps in the research process for both qualitative and quantitative studies and defines some key research terms. Chapter 3 provides an introduction to research reports—what they are and how to read them. Chapter 4 is devoted to a discussion of ethics in research studies.

Part II—Preliminary Steps in the Research Process includes three chapters and focuses on the steps that are taken in getting started on a research project. Chapter 5 focuses on the development of research questions and the formulation of research hypotheses. Chapter 6 discusses how to prepare and critique literature reviews. Chapter 7 presents information about theoretical and conceptual frameworks.

Part III—Designs for Nursing Research presents material relating to the design of qualitative and quantitative nursing research studies. Chapter 8 describes some fundamental principles of research design and discusses many specific aspects of quantitative research design. Chapter 9 addresses the various research traditions that have contributed to the growth of naturalistic inquiry and qualitative research, and also describes integrated qualitative/quantitative designs. Chapter 10 presents various designs for the sampling of study participants.

Part IV—Collection of Research Data deals with options for data collection and strategies to assess the quality of data. Chapter 11 discusses the full range of data collection options available to researchers, including both qualitative and quantitative approaches. The chapter focuses primarily on self-reports, observational techniques, and biophysiologic measures, but other techniques are also mentioned. Chapter 12 explains methods of assessing data quality.

Part V—Analysis of Research Data is devoted to the organization and analysis of research data. Chapter 13 reviews methods of quantitative analysis. The chapter assumes no prior instruction in statistics and focuses primarily on helping readers to understand why statistics are needed, what tests might be appropriate in a given research situation, and what statistical information in a research report means. Chapter 14 presents a discussion of qualitative analysis.

Part VI—Critical Appraisal and Utilization of Nursing Research is intended to sharpen the critical awareness of consumers with respect to several key issues. Chapter 15 discusses the interpretation and appraisal of research reports. Chapter 16, the final chapter, is a guide to utilization for clinical practitioners.

Key Features

Many of the features successfully used in previous editions of *Essentials of Nursing Research* have been retained.

Research Examples: Each chapter concludes with one or two actual research examples designed to sharpen the readers' critical skills. In most chapters, there is an example of both a quantitative and a qualitative study. Students are asked to evaluate features of these studies according to the chapter's critiquing guidelines. Then, the clinical relevance of each example is explored. In addition, many real or fictitious research examples are used to illustrate key points in the text. The use of relevant examples is crucial to the development of both an understanding of and an interest in the research process. We also hope that the inclusion of many research ideas will stimulate an interest in further reading or pursuit of a utilization project of one's own.

Tips for Consumers of Nursing Research: Each chapter contains numerous tips on what to expect in research reports vis-a-vis the topics that have been discussed in the chapter. In these tips, we have paid special attention to helping students *read* research reports, which are often daunting to those without specialized research training. This feature will enable students to translate the material presented in the textbook into meaningful concepts as they approach the research literature. In this edition, these tips are located directly near related instructional material, rather than being placed at the end of the chapter.

Guidelines for Critiquing Research Reports: Each chapter has a section devoted to guidelines for conducting a critique. These sections provide a list of questions that walk the consumer through a study, drawing attention to aspects of the study that are amenable to appraisal by research consumers.

Features for Student Learning

To enhance and reinforce learning, several features are used to help focus the student's attention on specific areas of text content:

Chapter Objectives: Learning objectives are identified on the chapter opener to focus the reader's attention on critical content.

New Terms: Each chapter begins with a list of new terms that are defined in context when used for the first time.

Chapter Summary Points: A succinct bulleted list of summary points that focus on salient chapter content is included in each chapter.

Suggested Readings: Two lists of suggested readings, methodologic and substantive resources, are provided in each chapter to direct the student's further inquiry.

Actual Research Examples: This edition includes two recent full-length examples of Canadian studies—one quantitative and the other qualitative—that students can read, analyze, and critique.

Critical Thinking Activities: Each chapter of the textbook includes two or three questions or activities designed to reinforce student learning. The questions often relate specifically to the full research reports that are included in the appendix.

Teaching-Learning Package

Essentials of Nursing Research: Methods, Appraisal, and Utilization, Fifth Edition has an ancillary package designed with both the student and the instructor in mind. This package can be easily adapted by faculty and students to meet their teaching and learning needs.

Study Guide: The study guide augments the text and provides the student with application exercises that correspond to each text chapter. This supports the learning of fundamental research terms that appear in research journals and provides the opportunity to practice the application of the concepts presented in the text and explore hundreds of research possibilities. This edition provides the answers to the selected exercises at the end of the study guide. Selected study guide chapters will appear on the "Connection" companion website to reflect the focus of the Canadian Essentials of Nursing Research, including chapters 1, 4, 7, and 16.

Free CD-ROM: The study guide also includes a CD-ROM providing 225 review questions to assist students in self-testing. This review program provides the rationale for both correct and incorrect answers, helping students to identify areas of strength and areas needing further study. Students using *Canadian Essentials of Nursing Research* may choose to omit certain questions in chapters 1, 4, 7 and 16.

The Instructor's Manual and Testbank includes a chapter that corresponds to every chapter in the textbook. Each chapter of the instructor's manual contains the following: Statement of Intent, Comments on the Actual Research Examples in the Textbook, Answers to Selected Study Guide Exercises, and Test Questions and Answers. Faculty will want to use the *Instructor's Manual and Testbank* as a guide to developing Canadian-specific research critiques and adapting test questions to reflect the Canadian adaptation of the textbook.

It is our hope and expectation that the content, style, and organization of this first edition of *Canadian Essentials of Nursing Research* will be helpful to those students desiring to become thoughtful readers and well-informed consumers of nursing research studies and to those wishing to improve their clinical performance based on research findings. We also hope that this textbook will help to develop an enthusiasm for the kinds of discoveries and knowledge that research can produce.

Carmen G. Loiselle, RN, PhD
Joanne Profetto-McGrath, RN, PhD
Denise F. Polit, PhD
Cheryl Tatano Beck, DNSc, CNM, FAAN

In Appreciation

While initially contemplating a Canadian adaptation of the fifth edition of *Essentials of Nursing Research: Methods, Appraisal, and Utilization,* we were encouraged by emails, letters, and comments from many colleagues, nurse clinicians, and students as well as by formal reviews from numerous Canadian nurse researchers who have either taught from or who were considering adopting this textbook. Many were thankful for a textbook that would contribute to a heightened visibility of research undertaken by our English and French nursing colleagues in Canada. They all shared the belief that this was a much needed and timely platform to feature the work of Canadian nurse researchers and to render it more accessible to students.

Were it not for the initiative and encouragement of Carol McGimpsey, Corey Wolfe, Barry Wight, and Margaret Zuccarini at Lippincott, it never would have occurred to us to dedicate ourselves, at this time in our career, to a Canadian adaptation of this nursing research textbook. Our managing editor, Joseph Morita, patiently oversaw the smooth sailing and the meeting of deadlines from manuscript to finished product. His encouraging phone calls, his capacity to listen and to hear, and his timely electronic messages always seemed to arrive at critical times and when we needed them most.

Two institutions deserve special mention. McGill University and the University of Alberta provided the authors a wonderfully supportive and stimulating intellectual environment that fostered interesting discussions about nursing research in Canada. For this, we thank our colleagues and students in nursing and related health disciplines: Mark Angle, Gerald Batist, Linda Edgar, Susan French, Lucy Lach, Margaret Purden, and Sonia Semenic at McGill and Kate Caelli, Carole Estabrooks, Paula Holinski, and Connie Winthers at University of Alberta.

We also wish to thank all the Canadian nurse researchers who so generously provided us with reprints, publication lists, and contact suggestions. Lesley Degner and Barbara Paterson were particularly instrumental in directing us to content pertaining to the status of nursing research in Canada.

Jocelyne Saint-Arnaud also provided much-appreciated feedback on critical issues pertaining to nursing research. We would also like to extend our appreciation to our research assistants, Sylvie Lambert, RN, BScN, doctoral student, Maggie Newing, MS(A) student, Karen A. Smith, RN, BScN, master of nursing student, and medical librarians Lorie Kloda, MLIS and Laura Cobus, MLIS, who helped with the selection of studies and who made sure that we quickly received the reprints we had requested while providing us with those they thought we should have requested. They were an inherent part of the "Canadianization" of this textbook.

Most credit, however, goes to the original authors of Essentials of Nursing Research. Denise Polit, a new-found colleague and friend who oversaw the process of the textbook's adaptation chapter by chapter, provided timely comments, and suggested alternative studies as appropriate exemplars of particular research designs. In addition, Dr. Polit sensitively nurtured two neophytes in the process of book production. Our warmest thanks also go to coauthor Cheryl Tatano Beck for her feedback, suggestions for improvement, and keen eye for methodologic details.

To each of the above individuals we are indebted. Collectively, they made the production of this textbook a most pleasant, stimulating, and gratifying experience.

Last, we wish to acknowledge our families, to whom this book is dedicated. They remained most supportive and understanding throughout the preparation of this book, from beginning to end.

To Oliver, Henry, and Christopher Coomes and to Larry, Ryan, and James McGrath
with much love

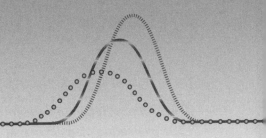

Contents

PART I
OVERVIEW OF NURSING RESEARCH

1 **Exploring Nursing Research**   *3*
2 **Comprehending the Research Process**   *29*
3 **Reading Research Reports**   *51*
4 **Understanding the Ethics of Nursing Research**   *71*

PART II
PRELIMINARY STEPS IN THE RESEARCH PROCESS

5 **Scrutinizing Research Problems, Research Questions, and Hypotheses**   *97*
6 **Reviewing the Research Literature**   *121*
7 **Examining Theoretical Frameworks**   *143*

PART III
DESIGNS FOR NURSING RESEARCH

8 **Understanding Quantitative Research Design**   *167*
9 **Understanding Qualitative Research Design**   *207*
10 **Examining Sampling Plans**   *233*

PART IV
COLLECTION OF RESEARCH DATA

11 **Scrutinizing Data Collection Methods**   *261*
12 **Evaluating Measurements and Data Quality**   *303*

PART V
ANALYSIS OF RESEARCH DATA

13 **Analyzing Quantitative Data**   *329*
14 **Analyzing Qualitative Data**   *381*

PART VI
CRITICAL APPRAISAL AND UTILIZATION OF NURSING RESEARCH

15 **Critiquing Research Reports**   *407*
16 **Using Research Findings in Nursing Practice**   *431*

Glossary   *465*

APPENDIX A

Quantitative Study—Preventing Smoking Relapse In Postpartum Women   *489*

APPENDIX B

Qualitative Study—Redefining Parental Identity: Caregiving and Schizophrenia   *505*

Index   *521*

Canadian Essentials of
Nursing Research

Canadian Essentials of
Nursing Research

CARMEN G. LOISELLE, PHD, RN
Assistant Professor
McGill University School of Nursing
Montreal, Quebec
Canada

JOANNE PROFETTO-MCGRATH, PHD, RN
Assistant Professor
University of Alberta Faculty of Nursing
Edmonton, Alberta
Canada

DENISE F. POLIT, PHD
President
Humanalysis, Inc.
Saratoga Springs, New York

CHERYL TATANO BECK, DNSC, CNM, FAAN
Professor
University of Connecticut School of Nursing
Storrs, Connecticut

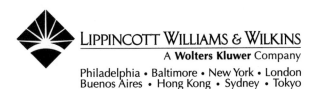

LIPPINCOTT WILLIAMS & WILKINS
A **Wolters Kluwer** Company
Philadelphia • Baltimore • New York • London
Buenos Aires • Hong Kong • Sydney • Tokyo

Acquisitions Editor: Margaret Zuccarini
Managing Editor: Joseph Morita
Senior Production Manager: Helen Ewan
Managing Editor / Production: Erika Kors
Design Coordinator: Brett MacNaughton
Cover Designer: Armen Kojoyian
Manufacturing Manager: William Alberti
Indexer: Angie Wiley
Compositor: Peirce Graphic Services
Printer: Maple-Vail

9 8 7 6 5 4 3 2 1

ISBN: 0-7817-4281-1
Library of Congress Cataloging-in-Publication Data is available upon request.

Care has been taken to confirm the accuracy of the information presented and to describe generally accepted practices. However, the authors, editors, and publisher are not responsible for errors or omissions or for any consequences from application of the information in this book and make no warranty, express or implied, with respect to the content of the publication.

The authors, editors, and publisher have exerted every effort to ensure that drug selection and dosage set forth in this text are in accordance with the current recommendations and practice at the time of publication. However, in view of ongoing research, changes in government regulations, and the constant flow of information relating to drug therapy and drug reactions, the reader is urged to check the package insert for each drug for any change in indications and dosage and for added warnings and precautions This is particularly important when the recommended agent is a new or infrequently employed drug.

Some drugs and medical devices presented in this publication have Food and Drug Administration (FDA) clearance for limited use in restricted research settings. It is the responsibility of the health care provider to ascertain the FDA status of each drug or device planned for use in his or her clinical practice.

LWW.com

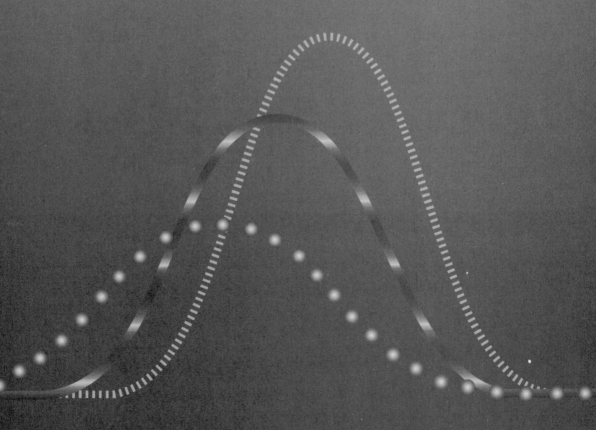

PART I

OVERVIEW OF NURSING RESEARCH

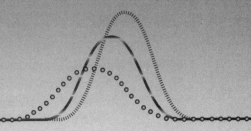

Exploring Nursing Research

AN INTRODUCTION TO NURSING RESEARCH
    What Is Nursing Research?
    The Importance of Research in Nursing
    Roles of Nurses in Nursing Research
NURSING RESEARCH: PAST, PRESENT, AND FUTURE
    The Early Years: From Nightingale to the
        1960s
    Nursing Research Since the 1970s
    Future Directions for Nursing Research
SOURCES OF KNOWLEDGE
PARADIGMS AND METHODS FOR NURSING RESEARCH
    The Positivist Paradigm
    The Naturalistic Paradigm
    Paradigms and Methods: Quantitative and
        Qualitative Research
    Multiple Paradigms and Nursing Research

PURPOSES OF NURSING RESEARCH
    Specific Purposes of Quantitative and
        Qualitative Research
    Basic and Applied Research
ASSISTANCE TO CONSUMERS OF NURSING RESEARCH
RESEARCH EXAMPLES
    Research Example of a Quantitative Study
    Research Example of a Qualitative Study
SUMMARY POINTS
CRITICAL THINKING ACTIVITIES
WORLD WIDE WEBSITES
SUGGESTED READINGS
    Methodologic and Theoretical References
    Substantive References

Student Objectives

On completion of this chapter, the student will be able to:

○ describe why research is important in the nursing profession and discuss why evidence-based practice is needed

○ describe historical trends in the evolution of nursing research and identify several areas of current priority for nurse researchers

○ describe alternative means of acquiring knowledge

○ describe the major characteristics and assumptions of the two alternative paradigms used by nurse researchers

○ identify similarities and differences between the traditional scientific method (quantitative research) and naturalistic methods (qualitative research)

○ identify several purposes of qualitative and quantitative research

○ define new terms in the chapter

New Terms

Applied research
Assumption
Basic research
Canadian Health Services Research
   Foundation (CHSRF)
Canadian Institutes of Health Research
   (CIHR)
Control
Deductive reasoning
Determinism
Empirical evidence
Evidence-based practice
Generalizability
Inductive reasoning
Journal club

National Institute of Nursing Research
   (NINR)
Naturalistic paradigm
Nursing research
Outcomes research
Paradigm
Positivist paradigm
Qualitative research
Quantitative research
Replication
Research methods
Research utilization
Scientific approach
Scientific research

AN INTRODUCTION TO NURSING RESEARCH

The purpose of this book is to provide you with the skills to read, understand, evaluate, and use nursing research. The goals of this introductory chapter are twofold: to highlight the important role of research in establishing a knowledge base for your nursing practice and to present an overview of approaches to nursing research.

What Is Nursing Research?

Research is systematic inquiry that uses disciplined methods to answer questions or solve problems. The ultimate goal of research is to develop, refine, and expand a body of knowledge. Researchers have searched for knowledge and have made discoveries that aid us in our daily lives.

Nurses are increasingly engaged in disciplined studies that benefit the profession and its patients. **Nursing research** is a systematic inquiry designed to develop knowledge about issues of importance to nurses, including nursing practice, nursing education, and nursing administration. In this book, we emphasize clinical nursing research, that is, research designed to generate knowledge to guide nursing practice and to improve the care and quality of life of patients.

Examples of nursing research questions:

Are nurses' empathic responses related to their patients' pain intensity after surgery? (Watt-Watson et al., 2000).

How satisfied are oncology patients with various aspects of the care they receive in an outpatient oncology centre? (Gourdji et al., 2003).

The Importance of Research in Nursing

The development and utilization of nursing knowledge is essential for continued improvement in patient care. Nurses increasingly are expected to adopt an **evidence-based practice (EBP),** which is broadly defined as the use of the best clinical evidence in making patient care decisions. Although there is no consensus about what types of "evidence" are appropriate for EBP (Goode, 2000), there is general agreement that research findings from rigorous studies constitute the best type of evidence for informing nurses' decisions, actions, and interactions with patients. Nurses are accepting of the need to base specific nursing actions and decisions on evidence indicating that the actions are clinically appropriate and cost-effective, and result in positive outcomes for their patients. Nurses who incorporate high-quality research evidence into their clinical decisions and clinical recommendations are being professionally accountable to their patients. They are also reinforcing the identity of nursing as a profession.

Another reason for nurses to engage in research involves the spiraling costs of health care and the cost-containment practices being instituted in health care facilities. Now, more than ever, nurses need to document the social relevance and the effectiveness of their practice not only to the profession but also to nursing care consumers, health care administrators, third-party payers (*e.g.,* insurance companies), and government agencies. Some research findings will help eliminate nursing actions that do not achieve desired outcomes. Other findings will help nurses identify the practices that alter health care outcomes and contain costs as well.

Nursing research is essential if nurses are to understand the varied dimensions of their profession. Research enables nurses to describe the characteristics of a particular nursing situation about which little is known, explain phenomena that must be considered in planning nursing care, predict the probable outcomes of certain nursing decisions, control the occurrence of undesired outcomes, and initiate activities to promote desired patient behaviour.

Roles of Nurses in Nursing Research

Undergraduate nursing students are sometimes puzzled by the requirement to take a course on nursing research. If you, too, are puzzled, you may be thinking that nursing research is not your responsibility. However, it is the responsibility of every nurse to engage in one or more roles along a continuum of research participation. At one end of the continuum are those nurses whose involvement in research is indirect. Consumers of nursing research read research reports to keep up-to-date on relevant findings that may affect their practice. At a minimum, nurses are expected to maintain this level of involvement with research. **Research utilization**—the use of the findings from research in a practice setting—depends on well-informed nursing research consumers.

At the other end of the continuum are the producers of nursing research, that is, nurses who actively participate in designing and implementing research studies. At one time, most nurse researchers were academics who taught in schools of nursing, but research is increasingly being conducted by practicing nurses who want to find what works best for their patients.

Between these two end points on the continuum lies a rich variety of research-related activities in which nurses engage as a way of improving their effectiveness and enhancing their professional lives. These activities include the following:

- Participating in a **journal club** in a practice setting, which involves regular meetings among nurses to discuss and critique research articles
- Attending research presentations at professional conferences
- Discussing the implications and relevance of research findings with patients
- Giving patients information and advice about participation in studies
- Assisting in the collection of research information (*e.g.*, distributing questionnaires to patients)
- Reviewing a proposed research plan with respect to its feasibility in a clinical setting and offering clinical expertise to improve the plan
- Assisting with the development of an idea for a clinical research project
- Participating on an institutional committee that reviews the ethical aspects of proposed research before it is undertaken
- Evaluating completed research for its possible use in practice, and using it when appropriate

In all these activities, nurses who have some research skills are in a better position to make a contribution to the nursing profession and to nursing knowledge; thus, most baccalaureate nursing programs include research methods as a requirement. A knowledge of nursing research can improve the depth and breadth of every nurse's professional practice. Learning about research methods allows you to evaluate and synthesize new information (*i.e.,* become a well-informed research consumer), develop knowledge that can be used in practice, and engage meaningfully in various research-related roles.

NURSING RESEARCH: PAST, PRESENT, AND FUTURE

Although nursing research has not always had the prominence and importance it enjoys today, its long and interesting history portends a distinguished future.

The Early Years: From Nightingale to the 1960s

Most people would agree that nursing research began with Florence Nightingale. Based on her skillful analyses of the factors affecting soldier mortality and morbidity during the Crimean War, she was successful in effecting some changes in nursing care—and, more generally, in public health. Her landmark publication, *Notes on Nursing* (1859), describes her early research interest in environmental factors that promote physical and emotional well-being— indeed, an interest of nurses that continues nearly 150 years later.

For many years after Nightingale's work, the nursing literature contained little nursing research. Some attribute this absence of research to the apprenticeship nature of nursing. The pattern of nursing research that eventually emerged at the turn of the century was closely aligned to the problems confronting nurses. For example, most studies conducted between 1900 and 1940 concerned nursing education. As more nurses received university-based education, studies concerning students—their problems, characteristics, and satisfactions—became more numerous. When the hospital staffing patterns changed, fewer students were available over a 24-hour period. As a consequence, researchers focused their investigations not only on the supply and demand of nurses but also on the amount of time required to perform certain nursing activities. During these years, nursing struggled with its professional identity, and nursing research took a twist toward studying nurses: who they were, what they did, how other groups perceived them, and what type of person entered the profession.

In the 1950s, a number of forces combined to put nursing research on the rapidly accelerating upswing it is on today. More nurses with baccalaureate and advanced academic preparation, the establishment of the *Nursing Research* journal in the United States, government funding to support nursing research, and upgraded faculty research skills are a few of the forces that propelled nursing research. In the late 1950s, the need for studies addressing clinical nursing problems was recognized, and in the 1960s, practice-oriented research on various clinical topics emerged in the literature. Nursing research advanced worldwide; the *International Journal of Nursing Studies* began publication in 1963, and the *Canadian Journal of Nursing Research* appeared in 1969.

Nursing Research Since the 1970s

By the 1970s, the growing number of studies and the increased discussion of theoretical and contextual issues relating to nursing research created the need for additional communication outlets. Several additional journals that focus on nursing research were established in the 1970s in the United States and in the United Kingdom, including *Advances in Nursing Science, Research in Nursing & Health,* the *Western Journal of Nursing Research,* and the *Journal of Advanced Nursing.* During that decade, there was a decided shift in emphasis from areas such as teaching, administration, and nurses themselves to the improvement of patient care. Nurses also began to pay more attention to the utilization of research findings in nursing practice. A seminal article by Stetler and Marram (1976) offered guidance on assessing research for application in practice settings.

Several events in the 1980s provided impetus for nursing research. For example, the first volume of the *Annual Review of Nursing Research* was published in 1983. These annual reviews include summaries of current research knowledge in selected areas of nursing practice and encourage utilization of research findings. The production of nursing knowledge and its dissemination in Canada have been invariably linked to the availability of federal funding (Degner, 2002). Federal funding for nursing research became available in Canada in the late 1980s through the National Health Research Development Program (NHRDP).

Funding was also important in the United States, where the National Center for Nursing Research (NCNR) was established within the National Institutes of Health (NIH) in 1986. The purpose of NCNR was to promote—and financially support—research training and clinical research focused on patient care. Also in the 1980s, nurses began to conduct formal research utilization projects, and an important new journal was established: *Applied Nursing Research.* This journal includes research reports on studies of special relevance to practicing nurses. Finally, several forces outside of the nursing profession in the late 1980s helped to shape today's nursing research landscape. A group from the McMaster Medical School designed a clinical learning strategy that was called evidence-based medicine (EBM). EBM, which promulgated the view that scientific research findings were far superior to the opinions of authorities as a basis for clinical decisions, constituted a profound shift for medical education and practice and has had a major effect on all health care professions.

After a long crusade by nursing organizations in the United States, nursing research was strengthened and given more visibility in 1993 when NCNR was promoted to full institute status within NIH. The birth of the **National Institute of Nursing Research (NINR)** helped put nursing research into the mainstream of research activities enjoyed by other health disciplines in the United States. Funding for nursing research is also growing. In 1986, the NCNR had a budget of $16.2 million, whereas in the fiscal year 2003, the budget for NINR was over $125 million. Funding opportunities for nursing research expanded in Canada as well during the 1990s. The **Canadian Health Services Research Foundation (CHSRF)** was established in 1997 with an endowment from federal funds, and plans for the **Canadian Institutes of Health Research (CIHR)** were underway. Beginning in 1999, the CHSRF allocated $25 million for nursing research through the establishment of a series of research chairs and related programs specific to nursing with a health services orientation. Likewise, CIHR, Canada's major federal funding agency for health research, is now becoming an important source of funding for nursing research. However, unlike the United States, the various institutes in the CIHR (13 to date) do not include a separate institute for nursing research, which means that Canadian nurse investigators must compete for funding with scientists from all disciplines within the CIHR designated fields of science (Degner, 2002). Several CHSRF/CIHR Chairs Awards were also recently granted to key investigators within the Canadian nursing research community. These 10-year awards are designed to promote knowledge generation and knowledge transfer in various nursing specialties (*e.g.,* oncology nursing, community health, nursing human resources). In addition to federal funding, most provincial governments increasingly have been providing funding to stimulate the development of specific programs of nursing research.

Several more research journals were inaugurated in the 1990s. They include *Qualitative Health Research* in 1990, *Clinical Nursing Research* in 1991, and *Clinical Effectiveness in Nursing* in 1996. These journals emerged in response to the growth in clinically oriented and in-depth research among nurses, and interest in evidence-based practice. Another major contribution to evidence-based practice was inaugurated in 1993: the Cochrane Collaboration—an international network of institutions and individuals—maintains and updates systematic reviews of hundreds of clinical interventions to guide EBP.

Some current nursing research is guided by priorities established by prominent nurse researchers, who were brought together by NCNR for two Conferences on Research Priorities (CORP). The priorities established by the first CORP for research through 1994 included low birth weight, HIV infection, long-term care, symptom management, nursing informatics, health promotion, and technology dependence.

In 1993, the second CORP established the following research emphases for a portion of NINR funding from 1995 through 1999: developing and testing community-based nursing models, assessing the effectiveness of nursing interventions in patients with HIV or AIDS, developing and testing approaches to remediating cognitive impairment, testing interventions for coping with chronic illness, and identifying biobehavioural factors and testing interventions to promote immunocompetence.

Future Directions for Nursing Research

Nursing research continues to develop at a rapid pace and will apparently flourish in the 21st century. Broadly speaking, the priority for nursing research in the future will be the promotion of excellence in nursing science. Toward this end, nurse researchers and practicing nurses will be sharpening their research skills and using those skills to address emerging issues of importance to the profession and its clientele.

Certain trends for the beginning of the 21st century are evident from developments taking shape in the late 1990s:

* *Increased focus on outcomes research.* **Outcomes research** is research designed to assess and document the effectiveness of health care services. The increasing number of studies that can be characterized as outcomes research has been stimulated by the need for cost-effective care that achieves positive outcomes without compromising quality. Nurses are increasingly engaging in outcomes research that is focused both on patients and on the overall health care delivery system.
* *Promotion of evidence-based practice.* Concerted efforts to translate research findings into practice will continue, and nurses at all levels will be encouraged to engage in evidence-based patient care. To support research findings dissemination and utilization in practice, the Canadian Nurses Foundation (CNF) has been allocated by the federal government some $5 million to promote clinical nursing research. An example at the provincial level is the funding by *the Fondation de recherche en sciences infirmières du Québec (FRESIQ)* of research dissemination-related activities proposed by clinical nurse specialists and their teams.
* *Development of a stronger knowledge base through multiple confirmatory strategies.* Practicing nurses cannot be expected to change a procedure or adopt an innovation on the basis of a single, isolated study. Confirmation is usually needed through deliberate **replication,** that is, the repeating of studies with different patients, in different clinical settings, and at different times to ensure that the findings are robust. Another strategy is the conduct of multiple-site investigations by a team of collaborating researchers in several locations.
* *Expanded dissemination of research findings.* The Internet and other modes of electronic communication have a great effect on the dissemination of research information, which in turn may help to promote research utilization. Through such technologic advances as online publishing (*e.g.,* the *Online Journal of Knowledge Synthesis for Nursing,* the *Online Journal of Clinical Innovation* and the new online *Canadian Journal of Nursing Research*), online resources such as Lippincott's NursingCenter.com, electronic document retrieval and delivery, e-mail, and electronic mailing lists, information about innovations can be communicated more widely and more quickly than ever before.

Priorities and goals for the future are also under discussion. NINR has established scientific goals and objectives for the 5-year period of 2000–2004.

The four broad goals are to: (1) identify and support research opportunities that will achieve scientific distinction and contribute significantly to health; (2) identify and support future areas of opportunity to advance research on high-quality, cost-effective care and to contribute to the scientific base for nursing practice; (3) communicate and disseminate research findings resulting from NINR-funded research; and (4) enhance the development of nurse researchers through training and career development opportunities. For the years 2000, 2001, and 2002, topics identified by NINR as special areas of research opportunity included:

- Chronic illnesses or conditions (*e.g.,* management of chronic pain, care of children with asthma, adherence to diabetes self-management)
- Behavioural changes and interventions (*e.g.,* research in informal caregiving; disparities of infant mortality, effective sleep in health and illness)
- Responding to compelling public health concerns (*e.g.,* reducing health disparities in cancer screening, end of life/palliative care)

SOURCES OF KNOWLEDGE

Think for a moment about a fact you have learned relating to the practice of nursing. Do you know the source of this information? Some facts are derived from research; some are not. Clinical knowledge used in nursing practice is a collage of sources that vary in their dependability and validity.

- *Tradition.* Within Western culture and within the nursing profession, certain beliefs are accepted as truths—and certain practices are accepted as effective—simply based on custom. However, tradition may undermine effective problem solving. That is, traditions may be so entrenched that their validity or usefulness is not challenged or evaluated.
- *Authorities.* An authority is a person with specialized expertise and recognition for that expertise. Reliance on nursing authorities (such as nursing faculty) is, to some degree, inevitable; however, like tradition, authorities as a source of information have limitations. Authorities are not infallible (particularly if their expertise is based primarily on personal experience), yet their knowledge often goes unchallenged.
- *Personal experience.* We all solve problems based on observations and experiences. The ability to recognize regularities, to generalize, and to make predictions based on observations is a hallmark of the human mind. Nevertheless, personal experience has limitations as a knowledge source because each person's experience may be too restricted to be useful in general terms, and personal experiences are often coloured by biases.
- *Trial and error.* Sometimes, we tackle problems by successively trying out alternative solutions. This approach may in some cases be practical, but it is often fallible and inefficient. The method tends to be haphazard, and the solutions are, in many instances, idiosyncratic.
- *Intuition.* Intuition is a type of knowledge that cannot be explained on the basis of reasoning or prior instruction. Although intuition and

hunches undoubtedly play a role in nursing practice—as they do in the conduct of research—it is difficult to develop policies and practices for nurses on the basis of intuition.

- *Logical reasoning.* Reasoning is the mental processing of ideas to solve problems. Two intellectual mechanisms are used in reasoning. **Inductive reasoning** is the process of developing conclusions and generalizations from specific observations. For example, a nurse may observe the anxious behaviour of (specific) hospitalized children and conclude that (in general) children's separation from their parents is very stressful. **Deductive reasoning** is the process of developing specific predictions from general principles. For example, if we assume that separation anxiety does occur in hospitalized children (in general), we might predict that the (specific) children in Memorial Hospital whose parents do not room-in would manifest symptoms of stress. Both systems of reasoning are useful as a means of understanding phenomena, and both play a role in research. However, reasoning in and of itself is limited because the validity of reasoning depends on the accuracy of the information (or premises) with which one starts, and reasoning may be an insufficient basis for evaluating accuracy.
- *Disciplined research.* Research conducted within a disciplined format is the most sophisticated method of acquiring knowledge that humans have developed. Nursing research combines aspects of logical reasoning with other features to create systems of problem solving that, although fallible, tend to be more reliable than other sources of knowledge.

The current emphasis on evidence-based health care requires nurses to base their clinical practice to the extent possible on research-based findings rather than on tradition, intuition, or personal experience—although nursing will always remain a rich blend of art and science.

PARADIGMS AND METHODS FOR NURSING RESEARCH

A **paradigm** is a world view, a general perspective on the complexities of the real world. Disciplined inquiry in the field of nursing is being conducted mainly within two broad paradigms, both of which have legitimacy for nursing research. This section describes the two paradigms and broadly outlines the research methods associated with them.

The Positivist Paradigm

The traditional scientific approach to conducting research has its underpinnings in the philosophical paradigm known as the **positivist paradigm.** Positivism is rooted in 19th-century thought, guided by such philosophers as Comte, Newton, and Locke. Although strict positivist thinking (sometimes referred to as *logical positivism*) has been challenged and undermined, a modified positivist position remains a dominant force in scientific research.

A fundamental assumption of positivists is that there is a reality out there that can be studied and known (an **assumption** is a basic principle that is believed to be true without proof or verification). Adherents of the scientific approach assume that nature is basically ordered and regular and that an objective reality exists independent of human observation. In other words, the world is assumed not to be merely a creation of the human mind. The related assumption of **determinism** refers to the positivists' belief that phenomena are not haphazard or random events, but rather have antecedent causes. If a person develops lung cancer, the scientist assumes that there must be one or more reasons that can be potentially identified and understood. Within the positivist paradigm, much of the scientific researcher's activity is directed at understanding the underlying causes of natural phenomena.

Because of their fundamental belief in an objective reality, positivists seek to be as objective as possible in their pursuit of knowledge. Positivists attempt to hold their personal beliefs and biases in check during their research. The positivists' scientific approach calls for orderly, disciplined procedures to test the researcher's ideas about the nature of the phenomena being studied and relationships among them.

The Naturalistic Paradigm

The **naturalistic paradigm** began as a countermovement to positivism with writers such as Weber and Kant. The naturalistic paradigm represents a major alternative system for conducting disciplined inquiry in the field of nursing. Table 1-1 compares four major assumptions of the positivist and naturalistic paradigms.

For the naturalistic inquirer, reality is not a fixed entity. Instead, it is a construction of the individuals participating in the research; reality exists within a context, and many constructions are possible. Naturalists thus take the position of relativism: if there are always multiple interpretations of reality that exist in people's minds, then there is no process by which the ultimate truth or falsity of the constructions can be determined.

The naturalistic paradigm assumes that knowledge is maximized when the distance between the inquirer and the participants in the study is minimized. The voices and interpretations of those under study are key to understanding the phenomenon of interest, and subjective interactions are the primary way to access them. The findings from a naturalistic inquiry are the product of the interaction between the inquirer and the participants.

Paradigms and Methods: Quantitative and Qualitative Research

The two perspectives on the nature of reality have implications for the methods used to acquire knowledge. (Broadly speaking, **research methods** are the techniques used by researchers to structure a study and to gather and analyze information relevant to the research question.) The most common methodologic distinction focuses on differences between **quantitative research,**

TABLE 1-1. Major Assumptions of the Positivist and Naturalistic Paradigms

PHILOSOPHICAL QUESTION	POSITIVIST PARADIGM ASSUMPTIONS	NATURALISTIC PARADIGM ASSUMPTIONS
Ontologic (What is the nature of reality?)	Reality exists; there is a real world driven by real natural causes.	Reality is multiple and subjective, mentally constructed by individuals.
Epistemologic (How is the inquirer related to those being researched?)	Inquirer is independent from those being researched; the findings are not influenced by the researcher.	The inquirer interacts with those being researched; findings are the creation of the interactive process.
Axiologic (What is the role of values in the inquiry?)	Values and biases are to be held in check; objectivity is sought.	Subjectivity and values are inevitable and desirable.
Methodologic (How is knowledge obtained?)	Deductive processes Emphasis on discrete, specific concepts Verification of researcher's hunches Fixed design Tight controls over context Emphasis on measured, quantitative information; statistical analysis Seeks generalizations	Inductive processes Emphasis on entirety of some phenomenon, holistic Emerging interpretations grounded in participants' experiences Flexible design Context bound Emphasis on narrative information; qualitative analysis Seeks patterns

which is most closely allied with the positivist tradition, and **qualitative research,** which is most often associated with naturalistic inquiry—although positivists sometimes undertake qualitative studies, and naturalistic researchers sometimes collect quantitative information.

The Scientific Approach and Quantitative Research

The traditional **scientific approach** refers to a general set of orderly, disciplined procedures used to acquire information. The traditional scientist uses deductive reasoning to generate hunches that are tested in the real world. In **scientific research**—the application of the scientific approach to the study of a question of interest—the researcher moves in a systematic fashion from the definition of a problem and the selection of concepts on which to focus, to the solution of the problem. Systematic means that the scientific investigator progresses logically through a series of steps, according to a prespecified plan of action. The researcher uses, to the extent possible, mechanisms designed to control the study. **Control** involves imposing conditions on the research situation so that biases are minimized and precision and validity are maximized.

In addressing research questions, the scientist gathers **empirical evidence**—evidence that is rooted in objective reality and gathered directly or indirectly through the senses rather than through personal beliefs or guesses. In a scientific study, formal instruments are used to collect the needed information. Usually (but not always) the information gathered is quantitative (*i.e.,* numeric information that results from formal measurement and that is analyzed with statistical procedures). Scientists strive to go beyond the specifics of the research situation; the degree to which research findings can be generalized (referred to as the **generalizability** of the research) is a widely used criterion for assessing the quality and importance of a traditional research study.

The scientific approach has enjoyed considerable stature as a method of inquiry, and it has been used productively by nurse researchers studying a wide range of nursing problems. This is not to say, however, that scientific research can solve all nursing problems or that the scientific method has been without criticism. One important limitation of the scientific method is its inadequacy for addressing moral or ethical questions. Many of our most persistent and intriguing questions about the human experience fall into this area (*e.g.,* Should euthanasia be practiced? Should abortion be legal?). Given the many moral issues that are linked to medicine and health care, it is inevitable that the nursing process will never rely exclusively on scientific information.

The scientific approach also must contend with problems of measurement. In studying a phenomenon, the scientist attempts to measure it. For example, if the phenomenon of interest was patient morale, a researcher may want to know if a patient's morale is high or low, or higher under certain conditions than under others. Although physiologic phenomena such as blood pressure, temperature, and cardiac activity can be measured with high accuracy, the same cannot be said of psychological phenomena, such as patient morale, pain, or self-image.

A final issue is that nursing research tends to focus on human beings, who are inherently complex and diverse. The scientific method typically focuses on a relatively small portion of the human experience (*e.g.,* weight gain, depression, chemical dependency) in a single study. Complexities tend to be controlled and, insofar as possible, eliminated in scientific studies rather than studied directly. Sometimes this narrow focus obscures insights.

Naturalistic Methods and Qualitative Research

Naturalistic methods of inquiry deal with the issue of human complexity by exploring it directly. Researchers in the naturalistic tradition stress the inherent complexity of humans, the ability of humans to shape and create their own experiences, and the idea that truth is a composite of realities. Consequently, naturalistic investigations emphasize understanding the human experience as it is lived by collecting and analyzing narrative, subjective (*i.e.,* qualitative) materials.

Some researchers reject the traditional scientific approach as reductionist (*i.e.,* it reduces human experience to the few concepts under investigation, with those concepts defined in advance by the researcher rather than emerging from the experience of those under study). Naturalistic researchers tend to focus on the dynamic, holistic, and individual aspects of phenomena and attempt to capture those aspects in their entirety, within the context of those who are experiencing them.

Flexible, evolving procedures are used to capitalize on findings that emerge in the course of the study. Naturalistic inquiry always takes place in the field (*i.e.,* in naturalistic settings), frequently over an extended period of time. The collection of information and its analysis typically progress concurrently. As the researcher sifts through the existing information and gains insight, new questions emerge, calling for additional evidence to amplify or confirm the insights. Through an inductive process, the researcher integrates the evidence to develop a theory or framework that helps explain the processes under observation.

Naturalistic studies result in rich, in-depth information that has the potential to clarify the multiple dimensions of a complicated phenomenon (*e.g.,* the process by which family caregivers adapt to their roles). The findings from in-depth qualitative research are typically grounded in the real-life experiences of people with first-hand knowledge of a phenomenon. However, the approach has several limitations. Human beings are the direct instruments through which qualitative information is gathered, and humans are intelligent and sensitive—but fallible—tools. The highly personal approach that enriches the analytic insights of a skillful researcher can sometimes result in petty and trivial "findings" among less competent ones.

Another potential limitation involves the subjective nature of the inquiry, which can raise questions about the idiosyncratic nature of the conclusions. Would two naturalistic researchers studying the same phenomenon in the same setting arrive at the same results? Moreover, most naturalistic studies involve a relatively small group of participants. Thus, the generalizability of findings from naturalistic inquiries can sometimes be challenged.

CONSUMER TIP

When a study is qualitative or conducted within the naturalistic paradigm, you are likely to find an explicit statement to this effect early in a research report. This is less characteristic of quantitative studies. Researchers rarely discuss their paradigmatic orientation explicitly, but they may explain their methodologic approach in relation to the research problem. ∎

Multiple Paradigms and Nursing Research

Paradigms are lenses that help us to sharpen our focus on a phenomenon of interest; they are not blinders that limit our intellectual curiosity. The emergence of alternative paradigms for studying nursing problems is, in our view, a healthy and desirable trend in the pursuit of new knowledge. The nursing knowledge base would be slim, indeed, without a rich array of approaches and methods available within the two paradigms—methods that are often complementary in their strengths and limitations and can be profitably used in tandem in a single investigation.

We have emphasized the differences between the positivist and naturalistic paradigms and their associated methods so that their distinctions would be easy to understand. Despite their differences, however, the alternative paradigms have many features in common. A few are mentioned below:

- *Ultimate goals.* The ultimate aim of disciplined inquiry, regardless of the paradigm, is knowledge. Both quantitative and qualitative researchers seek the truth about an aspect of the world in which they are interested, and both can make significant—and mutually beneficial—contributions.
- *External evidence.* Although the word *empiricism* is associated with the scientific approach, researchers in both traditions gather and analyze external evidence empirically, that is, through their senses. Neither qualitative nor quantitative researchers are "armchair" analysts, relying on their own beliefs and world views for their conclusions.
- *Reliance on human cooperation.* Because evidence for nursing research comes primarily from human study participants, the need for human cooperation is essential. To understand people's characteristics and experiences, researchers must persuade them to participate in the investigation and to act and speak candidly. In some areas of inquiry, the need for candor and cooperation is a challenging requirement—for researchers in either tradition.
- *Ethical constraints.* Research with human beings is guided by ethical principles that sometimes interfere with the researcher's ultimate goal. For example, if a researcher's aim is to test a potentially beneficial intervention, is it ethical to withhold the treatment from some people to see what happens? As discussed in Chapter 4, ethical dilemmas often confront researchers, regardless of paradigms or methods.
- *Fallibility of disciplined research.* Virtually all studies—in either paradigm—have limitations. Every research question can be addressed in many different ways, and inevitably there are tradeoffs. Financial constraints are universal, but limitations usually exist even when resources are abundant. This does not mean that small, simple studies have no value. It means that no single study can ever definitively answer a research question. Each completed study adds to a body of accumulated knowledge. If several researchers pose the same question and if each obtains the same or similar results, increased confidence can be placed in the answer to the question. The fallibility of any single study makes it important for you as a consumer of research to understand the tradeoffs and decisions that researchers make and to evaluate the adequacy of those decisions.

Despite philosophical and methodologic differences, researchers using the traditional scientific approach or more naturalistic methods usually share overall goals and face many similar constraints and challenges. The selection of an appropriate method depends to some degree on the researcher's personal taste and philosophy but largely on the nature of the research question. If a researcher asks, "What are the effects of surgery on circadian rhythms (biologic cycles)?" the researcher needs to express the effects through the careful quantitative measurement of various bodily processes subject to rhythmic variation. On the other hand, if a researcher asks, "What is the process by which parents learn to cope with the death of a child?" the researcher may be hard pressed to quantify the process. Researchers' personal world views help to shape the types of question they ask.

In reading about the alternative paradigms for nursing research, you were probably more attracted to one of the two paradigms—the paradigm that corresponds most closely to your view of the world and of reality. Learning about and respecting both approaches to disciplined inquiry, however, and recognizing the strengths and limitations of each are important. In this textbook, we provide an overview of the methods associated with both qualitative and quantitative research and offer guidance on how to understand, critique, and use findings from both.

PURPOSES OF NURSING RESEARCH

The general purpose of nursing research is to answer questions or solve problems of relevance to the nursing profession, but there are more specific purposes of disciplined inquiry.

Specific Purposes of Quantitative and Qualitative Research

The specific purposes of nursing research include identification, description, exploration, explanation, prediction, and control. Within each purpose, various types of questions are addressed by nurse researchers, and certain questions are more amenable to qualitative than to quantitative inquiry, and *vice versa*.

Identification

Many qualitative studies focus on phenomena about which little is known. In some cases, so little is known that the phenomenon has yet to be clearly identified or named—or has been inadequately defined or conceptualized. The in-depth, probing nature of qualitative research is well suited to the task of answering such questions as, "What is this phenomenon?" and "What is its name?" (Table 1-2). In quantitative research, by contrast, the researcher begins with a phenomenon that has been studied or defined previously, sometimes in a qualitative study. Thus, in quantitative research, identification typically precedes the inquiry.

Qualitative example of identification:

Olson et al. (2002) sought to understand why some individuals with cancer develop fatigue yet others do not. They identified an adaptive behavioural mode, which they labeled as *gliding,* among those who reported little or no fatigue.

Description

The main objective of many nursing research studies is the description and elucidation of phenomena relating to the nursing profession. The researcher

TABLE 1-2. Research Purposes and Research Questions

PURPOSE	TYPES OF QUESTIONS: QUANTITATIVE RESEARCH	TYPES OF QUESTIONS: QUALITATIVE RESEARCH
Identification		What is this phenomenon? What is its name?
Description	How prevalent is the phenomenon? How often does the phenomenon occur? What are the characteristics of the phenomenon?	What are the dimensions of the phenomenon? What variations exist? What is important about the phenomenon?
Exploration	What factors are related to the phenomenon? What are the antecedents of the phenomenon?	What is the full nature of the phenomenon? What is really going on here? What is the process by which the phenomenon evolves or is experienced?
Explanation	What are the measurable associations between phenomena? What factors caused the phenomenon? Does the theory explain the phenomenon?	How does the phenomenon work? Why does the phenomenon exist? What is the meaning of the phenomenon? How did the phenomenon occur?
Prediction and control	What will happen if we alter a phenomenon or introduce an intervention? If phenomenon X occurs, will phenomenon Y follow? How can we make the phenomenon happen, or alter its nature or prevalence? Can the occurrence of the phenomenon be controlled?	

who conducts a descriptive investigation observes, counts, describes, and classifies. Phenomena that nurse researchers have described vary. Examples include stress and coping, pain, health beliefs, rehabilitation success, and time patterns of temperature readings.

Description can be a major purpose for both qualitative and quantitative researchers. Quantitative description involves the prevalence, incidence, size, and measurable attributes of a phenomenon. Qualitative researchers, on the other hand, use in-depth methods to describe the dimensions, variations, importance, and meaning of phenomena. Table 1-2 compares some of the descriptive questions posed by quantitative and qualitative researchers.

⊞ *Quantitative example of description:*

Hesketh et al. (2003) conducted a study to describe nurses' experiences of violence in the workplace. Their report described the percentage of nurses who had experienced various types of violence (*e.g.,* physical assault, emotional abuse, sexual assault), by nursing specialty (*e.g.,* medical/surgical, critical care emergency).

Qualitative example of description:

Using information from individual and group interviews, Paterson and Thorne (2000) described how people with long-standing type 1 diabetes make everyday self-care decisions, particularly decisions pertaining to unanticipated blood glucose levels.

Exploration

Like descriptive research, exploratory research begins with some phenomenon of interest; however, rather than simply observing and describing the phenomenon, exploratory research investigates the full nature of the phenomenon and the other factors with which it is related. For example, a descriptive quantitative study of patients' preoperative stress might seek to document the degree of stress patients experience before surgery and the percentage of patients who actually experience it. An exploratory study might ask the following: "What factors are related to a patient's stress level?" "Is a patient's stress related to behaviours of the nursing staff?" "Does a patient's behaviour change in relation to the level of stress experienced?"

Exploratory studies are undertaken when a new area or topic is being investigated, and qualitative methods are especially useful for exploring a little-understood phenomenon. Exploratory qualitative research is designed to shed light on the various ways in which a phenomenon is manifested and on underlying processes.

Quantitative example of exploration:

Horsburgh et al. (2000) explored the relationship between personality traits on the one hand and self-care abilities and self-care actions on the other among adults awaiting renal transplant.

Qualitative example of exploration:

Ward-Griffin (2001) used in-depth interviews to explore both informal and formal caregiver's perceptions of their own caregiving and of each other's caregiving through interviews with 23 family caregivers and 15 nurses providing home care to the elderly.

Explanation

The goals of explanatory research include understanding the underpinnings of specific natural phenomena and explaining systematic relationships among phenomena. Explanatory research is often linked to a theory, which represents a method of deriving, organizing, and integrating ideas about the manner in which phenomena are interrelated. Whereas descriptive research provides new information, and exploratory research provides promising insights, explanatory research focuses on understanding the causes or full nature of a phenomenon.

In quantitative research, theories are used deductively as the basis for generating explanations that are then tested empirically. That is, based on previous theory or a body of evidence, the researcher makes specific explanatory predictions that, if upheld by the data, add further credibility to the theory. In qualitative studies, the researcher may search for explanations about how or why a phenomenon exists as a basis for developing a theory that is grounded in rich, in-depth, experiential evidence.

Quantitative example of explanation:

Harrisson et al. (2002) tested a model to explain psychological well-being among nursing assistants (NAs) based on a personality characteristic of the NAs (hardiness) and a characteristic of their work environment (work support).

Qualitative example of explanation:

Milliken and Northcott (2003) undertook a study that sought to explain how parents with an adult schizophrenic child redefined their identity and caregiving during the erratic course of their child's mental illness.

Prediction and Control

Many research problems defy absolute comprehension and explanation. Yet it is possible to predict and control phenomena based on research findings, even without complete understanding. For example, research has shown that the incidence of Down syndrome in infants increases with the age of the mother. Therefore, we can predict that a woman aged 40 years is at higher risk of bearing a child with Down syndrome than a woman aged 25 years. The incidence of Down syndrome may be partially controlled by educating women about the risks and offering amniocentesis to women older than 35 years of age. Note, however, that the ability to predict and control in this example does not depend on an explanation of *why* older women are at a higher risk for having a child with Down syndrome. There are many examples of nursing and health-related studies—typically, quantitative ones—in which prediction and control are key objectives.

Quantitative example of prediction:

Shamian et al. (2002) used a variety of work environment factors (*e.g.*, nurse–physician relationships, nurse autonomy) to predict health outcomes (*e.g.*, general health, emotional exhaustion) among registered nurses in Ontario's acute care hospitals.

CONSUMER TIP

Most nursing studies have multiple aims. Almost all studies have some descriptive intent. Some exploratory studies also have an expectation that the results will serve a predictive or control function. Truly explanatory studies are the least common in the nursing literature. ■

Basic and Applied Research

A study's purpose can also be characterized by the direct utility of the findings. **Basic research** is undertaken to accumulate information, extending the base of knowledge in a discipline to improve understanding, or to formulate or refine a theory. For example, a researcher may perform an in-depth study to understand better the normal process of grieving, without having an explicit nursing application in mind.

Applied research focuses on finding an immediate solution to an existing problem. The ultimate goal of applied research is the systematic planning of change in a problematic situation. For example, a study of the effectiveness of a specific nursing intervention to ease grieving would be applied research. Basic research is appropriate for discovering general principles of human behaviour and biophysiologic processes, but applied research is designed to indicate how these principles can be used to solve problems in nursing practice.

In nursing, as in medicine, the feedback process between basic and applied research operates more freely than in other disciplines. The findings from applied research almost immediately pose questions for basic research, whereas the results of basic research often suggest clinical applications.

> **CONSUMER TIP**
>
> Researchers rarely specify whether their intent is to address a pragmatic problem or to generate basic knowledge. The study's intent usually has to be inferred and, in some cases, may be ambiguous. ■

ASSISTANCE TO CONSUMERS OF NURSING RESEARCH

This book is designed to help you develop skills that will allow you to read, evaluate, and use nursing studies (*i.e.,* to become a well-informed consumer and user of nursing research). In each chapter of this book, we present information relating to the methods used by nurse researchers and provide specific guidance to consumers in two ways. First, interspersed throughout the chapters, we offer tips on what you can expect to find, with regard to the material discussed in the chapter, in actual research reports. These tips are identified with this icon: ✍ Second, we include guidelines for critiquing those aspects of a study covered in each chapter. The questions in Box 1-1 are designed to assist you in using the information in this chapter in an overall preliminary assessment of a research report.

RESEARCH EXAMPLES

Each chapter of this book presents brief descriptions of actual studies conducted by nurse researchers, followed by some comments on the study's clinical relevance. The descriptions focus on aspects of the study empha-

BOX 1-1

QUESTIONS FOR A PRELIMINARY OVERVIEW OF A RESEARCH REPORT

1. How relevant is the research to the actual practice of nursing? Can the study be described as *clinical* nursing research?

2. Does the study focus on a topic that is considered a priority area for nursing research?

3. Is the research qualitative or quantitative? What is the underlying paradigm?

4. What is the underlying purpose (or purposes) of the study—identification, description, exploration, explanation, or prediction and control?

5. Is the study fundamentally basic or applied in nature?

6. What might be the clinical applications of this research? To what type of people and settings is the research most relevant? How, if at all, can the results of this study be used by *me*?

---

sized in the chapter. In most cases, a review of the full research report in the nursing journal will enhance your assessment and will be a useful supplementary assignment. In this chapter, you can use the guidelines in Box 1-1 to do a brief preliminary assessment of some of the features of the two studies we describe next.

Research Example of a Quantitative Study

Côté and Pepler (2002) tested alternative interventions to improve the quality of life of men with HIV. Their report appeared in the journal *Nursing Research*.

Research Summary

Côté and Pepler noted that people who are HIV-positive are now living longer when they have contracted AIDS, and as a consequence often face prolonged periods of stress and depression. Earlier studies have found that psychological interventions during the early phases of HIV infection have beneficial effects, but there has been less research on interventions for people at more advanced, symptomatic stages of the disease.

The researchers developed and tested a nursing intervention that was specifically focused on developing and strengthening the cognitive coping skills of patients hospitalized for an exacerbation of HIV-related symptoms. The effect of this intervention on psychological well-being was compared with the effect of a more common nursing intervention that focuses on the expression of emotions.

A sample of 90 HIV-positive adult men were recruited at two tertiary care hospitals. The men were put into one of three groups, at random: (1) a cognitive coping skills (CCS) intervention group; (2) an expression of emotions (EE) intervention group; and (3) a group getting no special intervention. Both the CCS and EE interventions were administered on 3 consecutive days, in 20- to 30-minute daily sessions. The researchers assessed the mood, psychological distress, and anxiety of the men both before and after the intervention.

The researchers found that both the CCS and EE groups experienced reduced negative mood over time, but no change in positive mood was observed for either group. The CCS group also experienced a reduction in both distress and anxiety from immediately before to immediately after each session, whereas those in the EE group showed an increase in anxiety during the same period.

Clinical Relevance

In discussing their study, the researchers noted that further tests are needed to ascertain the efficacy of a cognitive coping skills intervention for acutely ill HIV-positive men. Nevertheless, this study offers fairly strong evidence of the feasibility and potential benefits of a nurse-initiated intervention for improving the quality of life of HIV-positive patients. The strength of the evidence lies in several factors—many of which you will appreciate more as you become familiar with research methods. First, the CCS intervention was based on a strong theoretical framework and on findings of previous research. Second, the study was scientifically rigorous. The researchers took care to ensure that the men in the study were treated in a comparable fashion during their hospitalization, so that any postintervention differences in psychological well-being reflected the interventions themselves and not some spurious factor. For example, the staff nurses who cared for the men were aware of the study, but they did not know which group the patients were in. Also, by putting the men into one of the three groups at random (and by taking other steps to equate the three groups), the researchers had some assurance that the postintervention differences were not the result of preexisting differences in the men's psychological state. Another strength of the research is that the study was conducted in two separate sites.

As the researchers themselves pointed out, one contribution of this study is the development of a theory-based nursing intervention that is sufficiently short for use in clinical settings. Despite advances in treatment, HIV-positive patients still need to cope with the unpredictable and chaotic nature of the disease. Although futher confirmatory research is desirable, the findings from this study suggest that the cognitive-based intervention had positive effects on the men's well-being. They also suggest that such beneficial interventions can be undertaken within a nursing environment.

Research Example of a Qualitative Study

Choudhry (2001) conducted an in-depth study of the immigration experiences of South Asian women. The study was published in the *Western Journal of Nursing Research*.

Research Summary

Choudhry sought to describe the challenges faced by elderly women from India who immigrated to Canada. She used an in-depth qualitative approach to explore the extent to which the women's beliefs, values, and culture mediated the stress experienced during immigration and resettlement.

In-depth interviews were conducted with 10 South Asian immigrant women who were between the ages of 59 and 78 years. The study participants were diverse in language, religion, family composition, and living arrangements. The interviews were conducted by a middle-aged woman from the same culture as the study participants, which helped in gaining their trust. The interviews, which averaged 1.5 to 2 hours in length, were conducted in the participants' homes and were audiotaped. The interviews included broad questions designed to elicit rich narrative responses. For example, the women were asked, "What is good about living in Canada?" and "What is not so good about living in Canada?"

The women's responses were analyzed to identify problems and challenges that they faced. Choudhry identified four recurring themes in the participants' narratives: (1) isolation and loneliness (*e.g.,* lack of informal support), (2) family conflict (*e.g.,* weakening of traditional family values), (3) economic dependence (*e.g.,* no personal source of income), and (4) settling in and coping (*e.g.,* attempts to build personal/social networks).

Clinical Relevance

Choudhry identified many stresses experienced by South Asian women since immigrating to Canada. The participants came to Canada with the prospect of enjoying the material comforts of an affluent society. However, they faced considerable uncertainty about their futures and struggled to cope with various stressors. For example, they experienced remorse and regret for having left their home country and they were emotionally challenged by the family conflict that resulted from abandoning long-held values. Being uprooted from their homeland and their changing family relationships were central to their feelings of isolation, loneliness, and loss of status.

Choudhry noted that these women, discontent with their present situation, tended to be more vulnerable to illness, abuse, and neglect. Health care professionals can therefore play a pivotal role in assisting older immigrant women in maintaining their health. Choudry's research highlights the need for awareness of the stress and conflict these women and their families face, and for timely interventions to promote their psychosocial adjustment to a new culture and environment.

The themes that emerged from this study suggest ways to improve clinical practice with this population. The clinical implications of the study are strengthened by the fact that Choudhry took steps to ensure the study's rigor. For example, Choudhry audiotaped her interviews and transcribed them verbatim to ensure accuracy. These, in turn, were reviewed, first independently and then jointly, by both a research assistant and the investigator. The emerging themes and subthemes were subsequently reviewed and validated by an independent researcher.

● ● ● ● ● *SUMMARY POINTS*

- **Nursing research** is systematic inquiry to develop knowledge about issues of importance to nurses and serves to establish a scientific base of knowledge for nursing practice.
- Nurses in various settings are adopting a **research-based** (or **evidence-based**) **practice** that incorporates research findings into their decisions and their interactions with patients.
- Knowledge of nursing research enhances the professional practice of all nurses, including both consumers of research (who read and evaluate studies) and producers of research (who design and undertake research studies).
- Nursing research began with Florence Nightingale but developed slowly until its rapid acceleration in the 1950s. Since the 1970s, nursing research has focused on problems relating to clinical practice.
- The **Canadian Health Services Research Foundation (CHSRF)** has been funding since 1999 a series of research chairs and related programs that are specific to nursing.
- **The National Institute of Nursing Research (NINR),** established at the U.S. National Institutes of Health in 1993, affirms the stature of nursing research.
- Future emphases of nursing research are likely to include **outcomes research,** research utilization projects, **replications** of research, multiple-site studies, and expanded dissemination efforts.
- Disciplined research stands in contrast to other sources of knowledge for nursing practice, such as tradition, voices of authority, personal experience, trial and error, intuition, and logical reasoning.
- Disciplined inquiry in nursing is conducted within two broad **paradigms,** or world views with underlying **assumptions** about the complexities of reality: the **positivist paradigm** and the **naturalistic paradigm**.
- In the positivist paradigm, it is assumed that there is an objective reality and that natural phenomena are regular and orderly. The related assumption of **determinism** refers to the belief that events are not haphazard but rather the result of prior causes.
- In the naturalistic paradigm, it is assumed that reality is not a fixed entity but is rather a construction of human minds, and thus "truth" is a composite of multiple constructions of reality.
- The positivist paradigm is associated with the traditional **scientific approach,** which is a systematic and controlled process. Scientists base their findings on **empirical evidence** (evidence collected by way of the human senses) and strive for **generalizability** of their findings beyond a single setting or situation. The scientific approach is associated with **quantitative research**—the collection and analysis of numeric information.
- Researchers within the naturalistic paradigm emphasize understanding the human experience as it is lived through the collection and analysis of subjective, narrative materials using flexible procedures that evolve in the field; this paradigm is associated with **qualitative research.**

- Research purposes include identification, description, exploration, explanation, prediction, and control.
- **Basic research** is designed to extend the base of information for the sake of knowledge.
- **Applied research** focuses on discovering solutions to immediate problems.

➤ ➤ ➤ ➤ CRITICAL THINKING ACTIVITIES

Chapter 1 of the accompanying *Study Guide to Accompany Essentials of Nursing Research,* 5th edition, offers various exercises and study suggestions for reinforcing the concepts presented in this chapter. In addition, you can consider the following:

1. Read the abstracts from one or both of the actual research studies in the Appendix of this book, and then answer questions 1, 2, 4, 5, and 6 in Box 1-1. Do the results of the study, as summarized in the abstract, seem to be consistent with any "facts" you have learned in your nursing studies, or do they have the potential to challenge what you have learned?

2. Is your world view closer to the positivist or the naturalistic paradigm? Explore the aspects of the two paradigms that are especially consistent with your world view.

WORLD WIDE WEBSITES

Canadian Institutes of Health Research (CIHR): http://www.irsc.ca

Canadian Health Services Research Foundation (CHSRF): http://www.chsrf.ca

The Canadian Association for Nursing Research: http://www.canr.ca

Canadian Association of Schools of Nursing: http://www.casn.ca

Canadian-International Nurse Researcher Database: http://nurseresearcher.com

Sigma Theta Tau International-Honor Society of Nursing: http://www.nursing society.org

Canadian Nurses Foundation: http://www.canadiannursesfoundation.com

Canadian Nurses Association: http://www.cna-nurses.ca

National Institute of Nursing Research: http://www.nih.gov/ninr

Nurse researcher mailing lists: http://www.springnet.com/np/nplstsrv/htm

SUGGESTED READINGS

Methodologic and Theoretical References

American Nurses Association Cabinet on Nursing Research. (1985). *Directions for nursing research: Toward the twenty-first century.* Kansas City, MO: American Nurses Association.

Goode, C. J. (2000). What constitutes "evidence" in evidence-based practice? *Applied Nursing Research, 13,* 222–225.

Guba, E. G. (Ed.). (1990). *The paradigm dialog.* Newbury Park, CA: Sage Publications.

Lincoln, Y. S., & Guba, E. G. (1985). *Naturalistic inquiry.* Beverly Hills: Sage Publications.

Nightingale, F. (1859). *Notes on nursing: What it is and what it is not.* Philadelphia: J.B. Lippincott.

Stetler, C. B., & Marram, G. (1976). Evaluating research findings for applicability in practice. *Nursing Outlook, 24,* 559–563.

Substantive References

Choudhry, U. K. (2001). Uprooting and resettlement experiences of South Asian Immigrant Women. *Western Journal of Nursing Research, 23,* 376–393.

Côté, J. K., & Pepler, C. (2002). A randomized trial of a cognitive coping intervention for acutely Ill HIV-Positive men. *Nursing Research, 51,* 237–244.

Degner, L. F. (2002). Pathfinding for Nursing Science in the 21st Century. Paper presented at the Think Tank Meeting of Canadian Nurse Scientists, Sponsored by the Nursing Policy Division of Health Canada, October 3. Toronto, Canada.

Gourdji, I., McVey, L., & Loiselle, C. (2003). Patients' satisfaction and importance ratings of quality in an outpatient oncology center. *Journal of Nursing Care Quality, 18,* 43–55.

Harrisson, M., Loiselle, C. G., Duquette, A., & Semenic, S. E. (2002). Hardiness, work support and psychological distress among nursing assistants and registered nurses in Quebec. *Journal of Advanced Nursing, 38,* 584–591.

Horsburgh, M. E., Beanlands, H., Locking-Cusolity, H., Howe, A., & Watson, D. (2000). Personality traits and self-care in adults awaiting renal transplant. *Western Journal of Nursing Research, 22,* 407–437.

Hesketh, K. L., Duncan, S. M., Estabrooks, C. A., Reimer, M., Giovanetti, P., Hyndman, K. et al. (2003). Workplace violence in Alberta and British Columbia hospitals. *Health Policy, 63,* 311–321.

Milliken, P. J., & Northcott, H. C. (2003). Redefining parental identity: Caregiving and schizophrenia. *Qualitative Health Research, 13,* 100–113.

Olson, K., Tom, B., Hewitt, J., Whittingham, J., Buchanan, L., & Ganton, G. (2002). Evolving routines: Preventing fatigue associated with lung and colorectal cancer. *Qualitative Health Research, 12,* 655–670.

Paterson, B. & Thorne, S. (2000). Expert decision making in relation to unanticipated blood glucose levels. *Research in Nursing & Health., 23,* 147–157.

Shamian, J., Kerr, M. S., Laschinger, H. K. S., & Thomson, D. (2002). A hospital-level analysis of the work environment and workforce health indicators for Registered Nurses in Ontario's acute-care hospitals. *Canadian Journal of Nursing Research, 33,* 35–50.

Ward-Griffin, C. (2001). Negotiating care of frail elders: Relationships between community nurses and family caregivers. *Canadian Journal of Nursing Research, 33,* 63–81.

Watt-Watson, J. Garfinkel, P., Gallop, R., Stevens, B., & Streiner, D. (2000). The impact of nurses' empathic responses on patients' pain management in acute care. *Nursing Research, 49,* 191–200.

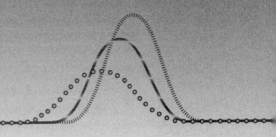

Comprehending the Research Process

BASIC RESEARCH TERMINOLOGY
  The Study
  Phenomena, Concepts, and Constructs
  Variables
  Data
  Relationships
MAJOR STEPS IN A QUANTITATIVE STUDY
  Phase 1: The Conceptual Phase
  Phase 2: The Design and Planning Phase
  Phase 3: The Empirical Phase
  Phase 4: The Analytic Phase
  Phase 5: The Dissemination Phase

ACTIVITIES IN A QUALITATIVE STUDY
  Conceptualizing and Planning a Qualitative
    Study
  Conducting the Qualitative Study
  Disseminating Qualitative Findings
GENERAL QUESTIONS IN REVIEWING A STUDY
RESEARCH EXAMPLES
  Research Example of a Quantitative Study
  Research Example of a Qualitative Study
SUMMARY POINTS
CRITICAL THINKING ACTIVITIES
SUGGESTED READINGS
  Methodologic References
  Substantive References

Student Objectives

On completion of this chapter, the student will be able to:

○ define new terms presented in the chapter
○ distinguish terms associated with quantitative and qualitative research
○ distinguish independent and dependent variables
○ describe the flow and sequence of activities in quantitative and qualitative research

New Terms

Associative relationship
Categorical variable
Cause-and-effect (causal) relationship
Coding
Concept
Conceptual model
Constant
Construct
Continuous variable
Data
Dependent variable
Functional relationship
Gaining entrée
Hypothesis
Independent variable
Informant
Interpretation
Investigator
Literature review
Operational definition
Outcome variable

Participants
Pilot study
Population
Qualitative data
Quantitative data
Raw data
Relationship
Representativeness
Research design
Research proposal
Research report
Researcher
Respondent
Sample
Sampling plan
Saturation
Site
Statistical analysis
Study participants
Theory
Variable

BASIC RESEARCH TERMINOLOGY

Research, like nursing or any other discipline, has its own language and terminology—its own *jargon*. Some terms are used by both qualitative and quantitative researchers, whereas others are used predominantly in connection with one or the other approach.

The Study

When researchers address a problem or answer a question through disciplined research—regardless of the underlying paradigm—they are doing a **study** (or an **investigation** or **research project**). Research studies with humans involve two sets of people: those who conduct the study and those who provide information. In a quantitative study, the people being studied are referred to as **study participants** or **subjects,** as shown in Table 2-1. (When the participants provide information to the researchers by answering questions, as in an interview, they may be called **respondents**). In a qualitative study, the individuals cooperating in the study play an active rather than a passive role and are therefore referred to as **informants** or study participants. The person who undertakes the research is called the **researcher** or **investigator** or **scientist**.

Phenomena, Concepts, and Constructs

Research focuses on abstract rather than tangible phenomena. For example, the terms *pain, patient care, coping,* and *grief* are all abstractions of particular aspects of human behaviour and characteristics. These abstractions are referred to as **concepts** (or, in qualitative research as **phenomena** or topics).

Researchers also use the term **construct.** Kerlinger and Lee (2000) distinguish concepts from constructs by noting that constructs are abstractions that are deliberately and systematically invented (or constructed) by researchers for a specific purpose. For example, *self-care* in Orem's model of health maintenance may be considered a construct. The terms *construct* and *concept* may

TABLE 2-1. Key Terms Used in Quantitative and Qualitative Research		
CONCEPT	**QUANTITATIVE TERM**	**QUALITATIVE TERM**
Person contributing information	Study participant Subject Respondent	Study participant — Informant
Person undertaking the study	Researcher Investigator Scientist	Researcher Investigator —
That which is being investigated	— Concepts Constructs Variables (independent, dependent)	Phenomena, topics Concepts — —
System of organizing concepts	Theory, theoretical framework Conceptual framework, conceptual model	Theory —
Information gathered	Data (numeric values)	Data (narrative descriptions)
Connections between concepts	Relationships (cause-and-effect, functional)	Patterns of association

be used interchangeably, although by convention, a construct often refers to a slightly more complex abstraction than a concept.

A **theory** is a systematic, abstract explanation of some aspect of reality. In a theory, concepts are knitted together into a coherent system to explain some aspect of the world. Theories play a role in both qualitative and quantitative research.

In a quantitative study, the researcher starts with a theory or a **conceptual model** (the distinction is discussed in Chap. 7), and, using deductive reasoning, makes predictions about how phenomena will behave *if the theory were true*. The researcher's specific predictions are then tested through research, and the results are used to reject, modify, or lend credence to the theory.

In qualitative research, information from the participants is the starting point from which the researcher begins to conceptualize, seeking to explain patterns emerging from the researcher–participant interactions. The goal is to arrive at a theory that explains phenomena as they occur, not as they are preconceived. Inductively generated theories from a qualitative study are sometimes subjected to more controlled confirmation through quantitative research.

Variables

In a quantitative study, concepts are usually referred to as **variables.** A variable, as the name implies, is something that varies. Weight, blood pressure readings, preoperative anxiety levels, and body temperature are all variables (*i.e.,* each of these properties varies or differs from one person to another). In fact, nearly all aspects of human beings and their environment are variables. For example, if everyone weighed 75 kilograms, weight would not be a variable; it would be a **constant.** But it is precisely because people and conditions *do* vary that most research is conducted. Most quantitative researchers seek to understand how or why things vary and to learn how differences in one variable are related to differences in another. For example, lung cancer research is concerned with the variable of lung cancer. It is a variable because not everybody has the disease. Researchers have studied what variables might be linked to lung cancer and have discovered that cigarette smoking is related to the disease. Again, smoking is a variable because not everyone smokes.

A variable, then, is any quality of a person, group, or situation that varies or takes on different values—typically, numeric values. Sometimes a variable can take on a range of different values (*e.g.,* height or weight); such variables are **continuous variables** because their values can be represented on a continuum. Other variables take on only a few discrete values (*e.g.,* pregnant/not pregnant, single/married/divorced/widowed). Variables of this type, which essentially place individuals into categories, are **categorical variables.**

Variables are often inherent characteristics, such as age, blood type, health beliefs, or grip strength. In some research situations, however, the investigator *creates* a variable. For example, if a researcher is interested in testing the effectiveness of patient-controlled analgesia as opposed to intramuscular analgesia in relieving pain after surgery, some patients would be given patient-controlled analgesia and others would receive intramuscular analgesia. In the context of this study, method of pain management has become a variable because different patients are given different analgesic methods.

 CONSUMER TIP

Every study focuses on one or more phenomenon, concept, or variable, but these terms *per se* are not necessarily used in research reports. For example, a report might say: "The purpose of this study is to examine the effect of primary nursing on patient satisfaction." Although the researcher has not explicitly labeled anything a concept, the concepts (variables) under study are *type of nursing* and *patient satisfaction.* ■

Dependent Variables and Independent Variables

Many quantitative studies are aimed at determining the causes of phenomena. Does a nursing intervention cause improved patient outcomes? Does a certain procedure cause stress? The presumed cause is referred to as the **independent variable,** and the presumed effect is referred to as the **dependent variable.**

Variation in the dependent variable is presumed to *depend on* variation in the independent variable. For example, the researcher investigates the extent to which lung cancer (the dependent variable) depends on smoking (the independent variable). In another study, a researcher might examine the effect of a special diet (the independent variable) on weight gain in premature infants (the dependent variable). The dependent variable (sometimes referred to as the **outcome variable**) is the variable the researcher is interested in understanding, explaining, or predicting. For example, in lung cancer and smoking research, it is the carcinoma that the researcher is trying to explain and predict, not smoking.

Frequently, the terms *independent variable* and *dependent variable* are used to designate the direction of influence between variables rather than cause and effect. For example, suppose a researcher studied urinary incontinence among community-dwelling older women and found that incontinence severity was greater among women with a slower gait. The researcher might be unwilling to take the position that the incontinence was caused by slower mobility. Yet the direction of influence clearly runs from gait to incontinence; it makes little sense to suggest that incontinence influenced the women's gait. Although in this example the researcher does not infer a cause-and-effect connection, it is appropriate to conceptualize incontinence as the dependent variable and gait as the independent variable.

Many of the dependent variables studied by researchers have multiple causes or antecedents. If we were interested in studying the factors that influence people's weight, for example, we might consider their age, height, physical activity, and eating habits as the independent variables. Two or more *dependent* variables also may be of interest to the researcher. For example, suppose we wanted to compare the effectiveness of two methods of nursing care for children with cystic fibrosis. Several dependent variables could be designated as measures of treatment effectiveness, such as length of stay in the hospital, number of recurrent respiratory infections, presence of cough, and so forth. In short, it is common to design studies with multiple independent and dependent variables.

It is important to understand that variables are not inherently dependent or independent. A dependent variable in one study may be an independent variable in another study. For example, a study might examine the effect of nurses' contraceptive counseling (the independent variable) on unwanted births (the dependent variable). Another study might investigate the effect of unwanted births (the independent variable) on the incidence of child abuse (the dependent variable). In short, whether a variable is independent or dependent is a function of the role that the variable plays in a particular study.

CONSUMER TIP

Almost no research report *explicitly* labels variables as dependent and independent, despite the importance of this distinction. Moreover, variables (especially independent variables) are sometimes not fully spelled out in research reports. Take the following research question: What is the effect of exercise on heart rate? In this example, heart rate is the dependent variable. Exercise, however, is not in itself a variable. Rather, exercise versus something else (*e.g.,* no exercise) is the variable; the "something else" is implied rather than stated in the research question. Note that, if exercise were not compared to something else, such as no exercise, then exercise would not be a variable. ■

Example of independent and dependent variables:

Research question: What is the effect of a public health nursing case management intervention (vs. self-directed care) on social adjustment among single parents on social assistance in a Canadian setting? (Markle-Reid et al., 2002)
Independent variable: Nursing care management intervention (vs. self-directed care)
Dependent variable: Social adjustment

Operational Definitions of Variables

In a quantitative study, the researcher clarifies and defines the research variables at the outset, indicating how the variable will be observed and measured in the actual research situation. Such a definition has a special name. An **operational definition** of a concept specifies the operations that the researcher must perform to collect the required information.

Variables differ in the ease with which they can be operationalized. The variable weight, for example, is easy to define and measure. We might operationally define weight as follows: the amount that an object weighs in terms of kilograms, to the nearest gram. Note that this definition designates that weight will be determined with one measuring system (metric) rather than another (pounds). The operational definition might also specify that the participants' weight will be measured to the nearest gram using a spring scale with participants fully undressed after 10 hours of fasting. This operational definition clearly indicates what is meant by the variable weight.

Unfortunately, few variables of interest in nursing research are operationalized as easily as weight. There are multiple methods of measuring most variables, and the researcher must choose the method that best captures the variables as he or she conceptualizes them. Take, for example, patient well-being, which can be defined in terms of either physiologic and psychological functioning. If the researcher chooses to emphasize the physiologic aspects of patient well-being, the operational definition might involve a measure such as heart rate, white blood cell count, blood pressure, or vital capacity. If, on the other hand, the researcher conceptualizes well-being as primarily a psychological phenomenon, the operational definition should identify the method by which emotional well-being will be assessed, such as the responses of the patient to certain questions or the behaviours of the patient as observed by the researcher. Readers of a research report may not agree with the way the investigator has conceptualized and operationalized the variables. Nevertheless, precision in defining the terms has the advantage of communicating exactly what the terms mean within the context of the study.

Example of an operational definition:

Research question: Were the benefits of a smoking relapse prevention intervention sustained at 12 months postpartum? (Ratner et al., 2000)?

Operational definition of maternal smoking abstinence: A mother's report of no smoking for the previous 12-month period and carbon monoxide level of less than 10 parts per million.

Qualitative researchers do not define the concepts in which they are interested in operational terms. This is because they seek to have the meaning of concepts defined by those being studied rather than having *a priori* definitions. Nevertheless, in summarizing the results of a study, all researchers should be careful in describing to readers the conceptual and methodologic bases of key research concepts.

CONSUMER TIP

A few research reports explicitly label the operational definitions, but most never use the term. Quantitative research reports do, however, provide information on how key variables were measured (*i.e.,* they specify the operational definitions even if they do not use this label). This information is generally included in a section of the research report called "Research Measures" or "Instruments." ■

Data

The research **data** (singular, datum) are the pieces of information obtained in a study. In a quantitative study, the researcher identifies the variables of interest, develops operational definitions of those variables, and then collects the relevant data from the participants. The variables, because they vary, take on different values. The actual values of the study variables are the data for a research project.

In quantitative studies, the researcher collects primarily **quantitative data** (*i.e.*, numeric information). For example, suppose we were conducting a quantitative study in which the dependent variable was *depression.* In such a study, we would try to measure how depressed different study participants were. We might ask the question, "Thinking about the past week, how depressed would you say you have been on a scale from 0 to 10, where 0 means 'not at all' and 10 means 'the most possible'?" Box 2-1 presents some quantitative data from three fictitious respondents. The participants have provided a number corresponding to their degree of depression: 9 for subject 1 (a high level of depression), 0 for subject 2 (no depression), and 4 for subject 3 (very mild depression). The numeric values for all participants in the study, collectively, would comprise the data on the variable depression.

In qualitative studies, the researcher collects primarily **qualitative data,** which are narrative descriptions. Narrative information can be obtained by having conversations with the participants, by making detailed notes about how participants behave in naturalistic settings, or by obtaining narrative records, such as diaries. As an example, suppose we were studying depression qualitatively. Box 2-2 presents some qualitative data from three participants responding conversationally to the question, Tell me about how you've been feeling lately—have you felt sad or depressed at all, or have you generally been in good spirits? Here, the data consist of narrative descriptions of the participants' emotional state.

In both qualitative and quantitative research, the collection and analysis of the research data are typically the most time-consuming aspects of a study. The analysis of qualitative data is a particularly labor-intensive process.

BOX 2-1 **EXAMPLE OF QUANTITATIVE DATA**

Question

Thinking about the past week, how depressed would you say you have been on a scale from 0 to 10, where 0 means "not at all" and 10 means "the most possible"?

Data

Subject 1: 9

Subject 2: 0

Subject 3: 4

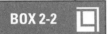

BOX 2-2

EXAMPLE OF QUALITATIVE DATA

Question

Tell me about how you've been feeling lately—have you felt sad or depressed at all, or have you generally been in good spirits?

Data

Participant 1: "I've been pretty depressed lately, to tell you the truth. I wake up each morning and I can't seem to think of anything to look forward to. I mope around the house all day, kind of in despair. I just can't seem to shake the blues, and I've begun to think I need to go see a shrink."

Participant 2: "I can't remember ever feeling better in my life. I just got promoted to a new job that makes me feel like I can really get ahead in my company. And I've just gotten engaged to a really great guy who is very special."

Participant 3: "I've had a few ups and downs the past week, but basically things are on a pretty even keel. I don't have too many complaints."

Relationships

Researchers usually study phenomena in relation to other phenomena—they explore or test relationships. A **relationship** is a bond or connection between phenomena; for example, researchers repeatedly have found that there is a relationship between cigarette smoking and lung cancer. Both qualitative and quantitative studies examine relationships.

In a quantitative study, the researcher is primarily interested in the relationship between the independent variables and dependent variables. Variation in the dependent variable is presumed to be systematically related to variation in the independent variable. Relationships are usually expressed in quantitative terms, such as *more than, less than,* and so on. For example, let us consider as a possible dependent variable a person's body weight. What variables are related to (associated with) a person's weight? Some possibilities include height, caloric intake, and exercise. For each of these three independent variables, we can make a prediction about the nature of the relationship to the dependent variable:

> *Height:* Taller people will weigh more than shorter people.
> *Caloric intake:* People with higher caloric intake will be heavier than those with lower caloric intake.
> *Exercise:* The lower the amount of exercise, the greater the person's weight.

Each of these statements expresses a presumed relationship between weight (the dependent variable) and a measurable independent variable.

Most quantitative research is conducted to determine whether relationships do or do not exist among variables, and often to quantify how strong the relationship is.

Variables can be related to one another in different ways. One type of relationship is referred to as a **cause-and-effect** (or **causal**) **relationship.** Within the positivist paradigm, natural phenomena are assumed not to be haphazard; they have antecedent causes that are presumably discoverable. In our example about a person's weight, we might speculate that there is a causal relationship between caloric intake and weight; all else being equal, eating more calories causes weight gain.

> *Example of a study focusing on a causal relationship:*
>
> Doran et al. (2002) studied whether training health care providers in continuous quality improvement strategies would improve problem solving, engagement in group interactions, and involvement in the quality improvement team.

Not all relationships between variables can be interpreted as cause-and-effect relationships. There is a relationship, for example, between a person's pulmonary artery and tympanic temperatures: people with high readings on one have high readings on the other. We cannot say, however, that pulmonary artery temperature caused tympanic temperature, nor that tympanic temperature caused pulmonary artery temperature, despite the relationship that exists between the two variables. This type of relationship is sometimes referred to as a **functional** (or **associative**) **relationship** rather than a causal one.

> *Example of a study focusing on a functional or associative relationship:*
>
> Bérubé and Loiselle (2003) studied the relationships among hope, uncertainty, and coping in a sample of individuals with a spinal cord injury.

Qualitative researchers are not concerned with quantifying relationships nor in testing and confirming causal relationships. Rather, qualitative researchers seek patterns of association as a way of illuminating the underlying meaning and dimensionality of phenomena of interest. Patterns of interconnected themes and processes are identified as a means of understanding the whole.

> *Example of a qualitative study of patterns:*
>
> Patterson and Thorne (2000) studied patterns of decision making related to self-care among individuals with long-standing type 1 diabetes in the specific context of unanticipated blood glucose levels. The investigators found that several contextual factors influenced the decision-making process and outcome. For instance, familiarity with the situation modified patterns of decision making about self-care activities.

MAJOR STEPS IN A QUANTITATIVE STUDY

One of the first decisions a researcher makes is whether to conduct a quantitative or qualitative study. Researchers generally work within a paradigm consistent with their world view—the paradigm that gives rise to questions that excite their curiosity. The maturity of the concept of interest also may lead to one or the other paradigm; when little is known about a topic, a qualitative approach is often more fruitful than a quantitative one. After the appropriate paradigm is identified, the progression of activities differs for the qualitative and quantitative researcher.

In a quantitative study, a researcher moves from the beginning point of a study (the posing of a question) to the end point (the obtaining of an answer) in a logical sequence of steps that is similar across studies. This section describes the flow of activities that is typical in a quantitative study; the next section describes how qualitative studies differ.

Phase 1: The Conceptual Phase

The early steps in a quantitative study typically involve activities with a strong conceptual or intellectual element. These activities include thinking, reading, rethinking, theorizing, and reviewing ideas with colleagues or advisors. During this phase, the researcher calls on such skills as creativity, deductive reasoning, insight, and grounding in previous research on the study topic.

Step 1: Formulating and Delimiting the Problem
The first step is to develop a significant, interesting research problem. In developing a research problem, nurse researchers need to consider its substantive dimensions (Is this research question of clinical or theoretical importance?); its methodologic dimensions (How can this question best be studied?); its practical dimensions (Are adequate resources available to conduct a study?); and its ethical dimensions (Can this question be studied in a manner consistent with guidelines for protecting participants?).

Step 2: Reviewing the Related Literature
Quantitative research is typically conducted within the context of previous knowledge. To build on existing theory or research, the quantitative researcher strives to understand what is already known about a topic. A thorough **literature review** provides a foundation on which to base new knowledge and generally is conducted well before any data are collected.

Step 3: Defining the Theoretical Framework
Theory is the ultimate aim of science: it transcends the specifics of a particular time, place, and group of people and aims to identify regularities in the relationships among variables. When quantitative research is performed within the context of a theoretical framework (*i.e.,* when previous theory is used as a

basis for generating predictions that can be tested), it is more likely that its findings will have broad significance and utility.

Step 4: Formulating Hypotheses

A **hypothesis** is the researcher's prediction of the relationship the researcher expects to find. The research question identifies the variables under investigation; a hypothesis predicts how those variables will be related. For example, the research question might be as follows: Is preeclamptic toxemia in pregnant women related to stress factors present during pregnancy? This might lead to the following hypothesis: Pregnant women with preeclamptic toxemia will report a higher incidence of stressful events during pregnancy than pregnant women who do not have symptoms. Most quantitative studies are designed to test research hypotheses.

Phase 2: The Design and Planning Phase

In the second major phase of a quantitative research project, the investigator makes decisions about the methods to be used to address the research question, and carefully plans for the collection of data. As a consumer, you should be aware that the methodologic decisions the researcher makes during this phase have implications for the integrity, interpretability, and clinical utility of the results. Thus, you must be able to evaluate the decisions so that you can determine how much faith can be put in the findings. A major objective of this book is to help you evaluate methodologic decisions.

Step 5: Selecting a Research Design

The **research design** is the overall plan for obtaining answers to the questions being studied. The design normally specifies which of the various research approaches will be adopted and how the researcher will implement controls to enhance the interpretability of the results. In quantitative studies, research designs tend to be highly structured and to include tight controls that reduce the effects of contaminating influences.

Step 6: Identifying the Population to Be Studied

During the design phase, quantitative researchers identify the population to be studied. A **population** is the aggregate of all the individuals or objects with some common, defining characteristic. For example, a researcher might specify that the study population consists of all licensed nurses residing in Canada. Quantitative researchers need to specify a population to indicate what characteristics the participants should possess and to clarify the group to which the results of the study can be generalized.

Step 7: Designing the Sampling Plan

Research studies generally collect data from a **sample,** which is a subset of the population. Using a sample is more practical than collecting data from the population, but the risk is that the sample will not adequately reflect the population's traits. In a quantitative study, a sample's adequacy is assessed by the criterion of **representativeness;** that is, the quality of the sample is a function of how typical, or representative, the sample is of the population. The **sampling plan** specifies in advance *how* the sample will be selected and *how many* participants there will be.

Step 8: Specifying Methods to Measure the Research Variables

Quantitative researchers develop or borrow methods to measure the research variables as accurately as possible. The first step is to clarify the conceptual meaning of the variables. The researcher then needs to select or design appropriate tools for operationalizing the variables (*i.e.*, for collecting the data). A variety of quantitative data collection approaches exist (*i.e.*, biophysiologic measurements, interviews, formal observations, and so on). The task of accurately measuring research variables is complex and challenging.

Step 9: Finalizing and Reviewing the Research Plan

Normally, researchers have their research plan reviewed before proceeding to the actual implementation of the plan. Students conducting a study as a requirement have their plans reviewed by faculty advisors. When a researcher needs financial support for the conduct of a study, the research plan is presented as a formal **research proposal** to a potential funder. Researchers also may need approval by a human subjects committee to ensure that the research plan does not violate ethical principles.

Step 10: Conducting a Pilot Study and Making Revisions

Unforeseen problems may arise in the course of a project. The effects of these problems may be sufficiently major that the study has to be stopped so that changes can be made. In a quantitative study, changes in the research design, the sampling plan, or the data collection instruments after the study is underway usually mean that data collected before the change must be discarded. Thus, some researchers carry out a **pilot study**—a small-scale trial run of the study—to obtain information for improving the project or assessing its feasibility.

Phase 3: The Empirical Phase

The empirical portion of a quantitative study involves the collection of research data and the preparation of those data for analysis. The empirical phase is usually the most time-consuming part of the investigation.

Step 11: Collecting the Data

The actual collection of data in a quantitative study normally proceeds according to a preestablished plan. The researcher's plan typically specifies procedures for recruiting the sample, describing the study to the participants, obtaining the necessary consents, training those who will be involved in the collection of the data, and collecting the data (*e.g.*, specifying where, when, and how the data will be gathered).

Step 12: Preparing the Data for Analysis

The data collected in a quantitative study are rarely amenable to direct analysis. Preliminary steps are needed before the analysis can proceed. One such step is known as **coding,** which is the process of translating data into numeric form. For example, patients' responses to a question about their gender might be coded (1) for females and (2) for males. Another preliminary step involves transferring the data from written documents to computer files for analysis.

Phase 4: The Analytic Phase

The quantitative data gathered in the empirical phase are not reported in raw form. They are subjected to analysis and interpretation, which occurs in the fourth major phase of the project.

Step 13: Analyzing the Data

To answer the research questions, the data must be processed and analyzed in an orderly, coherent fashion so that patterns and relationships can be discerned. Quantitative data are analyzed through statistical procedures. **Statistical analyses** cover a broad range of techniques, including some simple procedures as well as complex and sophisticated methods.

Step 14: Interpreting the Results

Interpretation is the process of making sense of the results and examining the implications of the findings within a broader context. Interpretation in quantitative studies is the researcher's attempt to explain the findings in light of what is known about theory and previous findings in the area and in light of the adequacy of the methods used in the investigation. Interpretation also involves determining how the findings can best be used in clinical practice, or what further research is needed before utilization can be recommended.

Phase 5: The Dissemination Phase

In the analytic phase, the researcher comes full circle: the questions posed in the first phase of the project are answered. The researcher's job is not completed, however, until the results of the study are disseminated.

Step 15: Communicating the Findings

The results of a research investigation are of little use if they are not communicated to others. Another—and often final—task of a research project, therefore, is the preparation of a **research report** that can be shared with others. We discuss research reports in the next chapter.

Step 16: Utilizing the Findings

Many nursing studies have little effect on nursing practice. Ideally, the concluding step of a high-quality study is to plan for its utilization in the real world. Although nurse researchers are not always in a position to implement a plan for utilizing research findings in clinical settings, they can contribute to the process by including recommendations in their research reports regarding how the results of the study could be incorporated into the practice of nursing.

ACTIVITIES IN A QUALITATIVE STUDY

Quantitative research involves a fairly linear progression of tasks (*i.e.*, the researcher lays out in advance the steps to be taken to maximize the integrity of the study and then follows those steps as faithfully as possible). In a qualitative study, by contrast, the progression is closer to a circle than to a straight line—the qualitative researcher is continually examining and interpreting data and making decisions about how to proceed based on what has already been discovered.

Because the qualitative researcher has a flexible approach to the collection and analysis of data, it is impossible to define the flow of activities precisely; the flow varies from one study to another, and researchers do not know ahead of time exactly how the study will proceed. We try to provide a sense of how a qualitative study is conducted, however, by describing some major activities and indicating how and when they might be performed.

Conceptualizing and Planning a Qualitative Study

Qualitative researchers are usually interested in an aspect of a topic that is poorly understood and about which little is known, and thus they do not develop hypotheses or pose refined research questions before going into the field. The topic area may be clarified on the basis of self-reflection and discussion with colleagues or clients, but usually the researcher proceeds with a broad research question that is sharpened and more clearly delineated after the study is underway.

There are conflicting ideas among qualitative researchers regarding the performance of a literature review at the outset of the study. At one extreme are those who believe that researchers should not consult the literature at all before collecting data. Their concern is that prior studies might unduly influence the researcher's conceptualization of the phenomena under study. According to this view, the phenomena should be elucidated based on participants' viewpoints rather than on prior information. Others believe that the researcher should conduct at least a cursory up-front literature review to obtain guidance, including guidance in identifying biases in previous studies. In any event, qualitative researchers typically find a relatively small body of relevant literature because of the type of questions they ask.

During the planning phase, the qualitative researcher must also identify a study **site** that is consistent with the research topic. For example, if the topic is the health care beliefs of the urban poor, an inner-city neighbourhood with a concentration of low-income residents must be identified. The researcher may have to further identify the types of **setting** within the site where data collection will occur (*e.g.,* in homes, clinics, the workplace, and so on). In many cases, the researcher needs to make preliminary contacts with key actors in the selected site to ensure cooperation and access to informants (*i.e.,* the researcher needs to **gain entrée** into the setting).

Conducting the Qualitative Study

In a qualitative study, the activities of sampling, data collection, data analysis, and interpretation take place iteratively. The qualitative researcher begins by talking with or observing people who have first-hand experience with the phenomenon under study. The discussions and observations are loosely structured, allowing for the expression of a full range of beliefs, feelings, and behaviours. Analysis and interpretation are ongoing and concurrent activities, used to guide the people to sample next and the questions to ask or observations to make. The actual process of data analysis, which is an intensive and time-consuming activity, involves clustering together related types of narrative information into a coherent scheme.

As analysis and interpretation progress, the researcher begins to identify themes and categories, which are used to build a descriptive theory of the phenomenon. The kinds of data obtained become increasingly focused and purposeful as a theory emerges. Theory development and verification shape the sampling process—as the theory develops, the researcher seeks participants who can confirm and enrich the theoretical understandings as well as participants who can potentially challenge them and lead to further theoretical development.

A quantitative researcher decides in advance how many participants to include in the study, but a qualitative researcher's sampling decisions are guided by the data. Many qualitative researchers use the principle of **saturation,** which occurs when themes and categories in the data become repetitive and redundant, such that no new information can be gleaned by further data collection.

Quantitative researchers seek to collect high-quality data by selecting measuring instruments that have been previously demonstrated to be accurate and rigorous. The qualitative researcher, by contrast, *is* the main data collection instrument and he or she takes steps to demonstrate the trustworthiness of the data while in the field. The central feature of these efforts is to confirm that the findings accurately reflect the experiences and viewpoints of the participants, rather than the perceptions of the researcher. For example, one confirmatory activity involves going back to participants and sharing preliminary interpretations with them so that they can evaluate whether the researcher's thematic analysis is consistent with their experiences.

Disseminating Qualitative Findings

Qualitative nursing researchers also strive to share their findings with other nurses and other health care specialists. Qualitative research reports are increasingly being published in the nursing literature.

Quantitative reports almost never contain any **raw data**—data exactly in the form they were collected, which are numeric values. Qualitative reports, by contrast, are generally filled with rich verbatim passages directly from the participants. The excerpts are used in an evidential fashion to support or illustrate the researcher's interpretations and theoretical formulations.

Example of raw data in a qualitative report:

Ward-Griffin and McKeever (2000) explored the nature of the relationship that develops between community nurses and family caregivers of the frail elderly. One participant described how nurses welcomed their participation in caring for their family member: "I think the nurses knew that I needed to be involved. I'm sure that was part of it, because if you're involved you feel as if you have some control over what's happening even if it's in a limited way" (p. 96).

Like quantitative researchers, qualitative nurse researchers want to see their findings used by other nurses. Qualitative findings often are used as the basis for the formulation of hypotheses that are tested by quantitative researchers. Qualitative findings are also useful in the development of assessment instruments used for both research and clinical purposes. Most important, qualitative studies can help to shape nurses' perceptions of a problem or situation, their conceptualization of potential solutions, and their understanding of patients' concerns and experiences.

GENERAL QUESTIONS IN REVIEWING A STUDY

The remaining chapters of this book contain guidelines to help you evaluate different aspects of a research report critically, focusing primarily on the methodologic decisions that the researcher made in conducting the study. Box 2-3 presents some further suggestions for performing a preliminary overview of a research report, drawing on the concepts explained in this chapter. These guidelines supplement those presented in Box 1-1 in Chapter 1.

RESEARCH EXAMPLES

This section presents brief overviews of a quantitative and a qualitative study. Our overviews deal primarily with the key concepts of the research. Use the questions in Box 2-3 as a guide to thinking about these studies. You may wish to consult the full research report in answering these questions and in think-

BOX 2-3

ADDITIONAL QUESTIONS FOR A PRELIMINARY OVERVIEW OF A STUDY

1. What is the study all about? What are the main phenomena, concepts, or constructs under investigation?

2. If the study is quantitative, what are the independent and dependent variables?

3. Are the key concepts clearly explained? Are operational definitions provided?

4. What is the nature of the relationship (if any) under study?

ing about the differences in style and content of qualitative and quantitative reports.

Research Example of a Quantitative Study

Dolinar, Kumar, Coutu-Wakulczyk, and Rowe (2000) examined the effect of a home-based asthma health education program on parental outcomes in terms of coping, perceptions of asthma change in their child, and quality of life. Despite the potential benefits of home-based educational interventions, rarely have they been systematically assessed.

Research Summary

Forty parents of children diagnosed with stable asthma were assigned to one of two groups. In one group, parents were provided with a booklet entitled "Childhood Asthma" as part of conventional educational practice. In the second group, parents received the same booklet in addition to a 2-hour one-to-one educational session by a trained individual in their own home. The independent variable was whether or not the family received the intervention. The dependent variables were improvement in coping, parental perception of child's asthma, and quality of life. Quality of life was assessed by the Pediatric Asthma Caregiver's Quality of Life Questionnaire detailing issues pertaining to caregiver well-being. Perception of asthma change was measured using the Caregiver Perception of Change in Asthma Severity scale. Coping was assessed using the 32-item Hymovich's Parent Perception Inventory. Data were collected at three points. At baseline, sociodemographic data, severity of the child's asthma, quality of life, and coping were measured (prior to the intervention). One month after the intervention, quality of life and parents' perceptions of change in the child's asthma severity were measured. Three months after the intervention, severity of the child's asthma, quality of life, perceptions of change in asthma severity, and coping were measured.

Parents in the second group demonstrated an improvement in several aspects of coping (*i.e.,* less need for information, reduced concerns, and increased utilization of coping) in comparison to the first group. Improvement was also noted in parents' perceptions of asthma severity. However, there was no detectable difference in quality of life between the two groups.

Clinical Relevance

Bronchial asthma is the most common chronic disease of childhood, resulting in frequent hospitalizations, visits to the emergency room, and missed school days. Over 150,000 Canadian children suffer from asthma resulting in frequent hospital admissions. Once a child with asthma is discharged from the hospital, responsibility for day-to-day asthma management rests with family caregivers. While parents strive to maintain acceptable levels of well-being and quality of life, they are also expected to monitor their child's respiratory status, administer medication, identify potential asthma triggers, seek assistance from health care professionals, ensure an outlet for release of emotional strain, and maintain financial stability to cover medication costs and equipment. Thus, a chronic illness such as asthma produces multiple challenges to normal daily living and parents must cope with their child's condition to minimize its effect on daily living. One way parents cope with their child's asthma is by accessing educational information. A home-based approach offers a promising avenue to provide asthma health education tailored to the needs of parents. Findings from this study support the use of home-based health educational interventions in assisting parents to cope with their child's asthma and reduce the stress and anxiety related to this chronic illness. Further research could compare the effectiveness of one-time home-based educational interventions with alternate formats (*e.g.,* more intensive, in other settings, using complementary educational strategies).

Research Example of a Qualitative Study

Dunn and Johnson (2001) sought to better understand the process of remaining a nonsmoker among adolescent girls. This is a first study that explored in-depth the thoughts and strategies involved in the process of deciding to remain smoke-free.

Research Summary

In-depth interviews were used to uncover processes that adolescent girls undertake to remain nonsmokers. Seventeen nonsmoking girls between the ages of 13 and 17 years were interviewed in their home using questions or opening statements developed by the researchers (*e.g.,* "Tell me about what it is like to be a nonsmoker."). These aimed at gaining a better understanding of a girl's experience of being a nonsmoker. Individual interviews lasted approximately 30 to 45 minutes. Six participants were later reinterviewed to clarify the meaning of emerging themes and to further inform the emerging theoretical propositions. The interviews were tape-recorded and then transcribed verbatim.

Data suggested that the process of remaining a nonsmoker is composed of three phases that evolve over time: (1) making sense of smoking (attitude change toward smoking), (2) rejecting smoking (deciding that smoking is pointless), and (3) declaring oneself smoke-free (accepting self and declaring self a nonsmoker). The core concept underpinning the process of remaining a nonsmoker was developing self-confidence. For example, while attempting to make sense out of smoking (phase 1), nonsmokers possessed a certain amount of self-confidence that enabled them to decide that they did not need to smoke to fit in. As one participant said: "I hang out with so many different groups of friends like more nonsmokers than smokers. All the smokers are basically the same but all my nonsmoking friends have like their own personalities. . .I think it's good to be more of an individual than it is to blend in."

Clinical Relevance

The study focused on the actual process that adolescent girls go through to remain nonsmokers. Findings suggest that several key strategies may be used to remain smoke-free throughout the process (*e.g.*, while trying to make sense of smoking many wanted to know more about the hazards of smoking and some even tried smoking). The themes and strategies that emerged from this study offer those who work in the field of health promotion new insights into ways to increase the ranks of nonsmokers. These findings also alert health promoters to the inherent complexity of the experience of adolescents who choose to remain nonsmokers. As such, the findings suggest that tobacco prevention programs focusing exclusively on educating adolescents about the harm of smoking may be limited. Interventions should also include consideration of the various strategies used by adolescents over time to remain nonsmokers. Further research is needed to determine optimal ways to teach these successful strategies to at-risk adolescents so that they also remain or become nonsmokers.

● ● ● ● ● SUMMARY POINTS

- A research study (or investigation or research project) is undertaken by one or more **researchers** (or **investigators** or scientists). The people who provide information to the researchers are referred to as **study participants, subjects,** or **respondents** (in quantitative research) or study participants or **informants** (in qualitative research).
- Researchers investigate **concepts** and phenomena (or **constructs**), which are abstractions or mental representations.
- Concepts are the building blocks of **theories,** which are systematic explanations of some aspect of the world.

- In quantitative studies, concepts are referred to as variables. A **variable** is a characteristic or quality that takes on different values (*i.e.*, a variable varies from one person or object to another).
- The **dependent variable** is the behaviour, characteristic, or outcome the researcher is interested in understanding, explaining, predicting, or affecting. The independent variable is the presumed cause of, antecedent to, or influence on the dependent variable.
- An **operational definition** is the specification of the elements (*e.g.*, observations, procedures or tools) required to measure a variable.
- **Data**—the information collected during the course of a study—may take the form of narrative information **(qualitative data)** or numeric values **(quantitative data).**
- Researchers often focus on the relationship between two or more concepts. A **relationship** is a link or a connection (or pattern of association) between two phenomena.
- In a quantitative study, the steps involved in conducting a study are fairly standard, and the researcher progresses in a linear fashion from posing a research question to answering it.
- The main phases and steps in a quantitative study are as follows:
  - The conceptual phase: defining the problem to be studied, doing a **literature review,** developing a theoretical framework, and formulating **hypotheses** to be tested.
  - The design and planning phase: selecting a **research design,** specifying the **population,** selecting a **sample,** specifying the methods to measure the research variables, finalizing the research plan, and, in some cases, conducting a **pilot study** and making revisions.
  - The empirical phase: collecting the data and preparing the data for analysis.
  - The analytic phase: analyzing the data through **statistical analysis** and interpreting the results.
  - The dissemination phase: communicating the findings and promoting their utilization.
- The flow of activities in a qualitative study is more flexible and less linear than in a quantitative study.
- Qualitative researchers begin with a broad question that is narrowed through the actual process of data collection and analysis. After selecting a **site** and **gaining entrée** into it, the researcher selects informants, collects data, and analyzes and interprets the data iteratively. Early analysis leads to refinements in sampling and data collection, until **saturation** (redundancy of information) is achieved.

▶ ▶ ▶ ▶ *CRITICAL THINKING ACTIVITIES*

Chapter 2 of the accompanying *Study Guide to Accompany Essentials of Nursing Research,* 5th edition, offers various exercises and study suggestions for reinforcing the concepts presented in this chapter. In addition, you can address the following:

1. Read the abstracts and the introduction from one or both of the actual research studies in the Appendix of this book, and then answer the questions in Box 2-3.

2. In describing the study, do either of the reports in the Appendix actually use the terms *operational definition, independent variable,* or *dependent variable?*

SUGGESTED READINGS

Methodologic References

Kerlinger, F. N., & Lee, H. B. (2000). *Foundations of behavioral research* (4th ed.). Fort Worth, TX: Harcourt College Publishers.

Morse, J. M., & Field, P. A. (1995). *Qualitative research methods for health professionals* (2nd ed.). Thousand Oaks, CA: Sage Publications.

Substantive References

Bérubé, M., & Loiselle, C. G. (2003). L'espoir, l'incertitude et le coping de personnes avec blessure médullaire [Hope, uncertainty, and coping among individuals with spinal cord injury]. *L'Infirmière du Québec, 10,* 16–23.

Dolinar, R. M., Kumar, V., Coutu-Wakulczyk, G., & Rowe, B. H. (2000). Pilot study of a home-based asthma health education program. *Patient Education & Counseling, 40,* 93–102.

Doran, D. I., Baker, G., Murray, M., Bohnen, J., Zahn, C., Sidani, S. et al. (2002). Achieving clinical improvement: An interdisciplinary intervention. *Health Care Management Review, 27,* 42–57.

Dunn, D. A., & Johnson, J. L. (2001). Choosing to remain smoke-free: The experiences of adolescent girls. *Journal of Adolescent Health, 29,* 289–297.

Markle-Reid, M., Browne, G., Roberts, J., Gafni, A., & Byrne, C. (2002). The 2-year costs and effects of a public health nursing case management intervention on mood-disordered single parents on social assistance. *Journal of Evaluation in Clinical Practice, 8,* 45–59.

Paterson, B., & Thorne, S. (2000). Expert decision making in relation to unanticipated blood glucose levels. *Research in Nursing & Health, 23,* 147–157.

Ratner, P. A., Johnson, J. L., Bottorff, J. L., Dahinten, S., & Hall, W. (2000). Twelve-month follow-up of a smoking relapse prevention intervention for postpartum women. *Addictive Behaviors, 25,* 81–92.

Ward-Griffin, C. & McKeever, P. (2000). Relationships between nurses and family caregivers: Partners in care? *Advances in Nursing Science, 22,* 89–103.

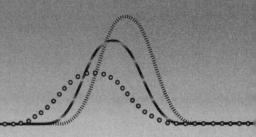

CHAPTER 3

Reading Research Reports

TYPES OF RESEARCH REPORTS
  Presentations at Professional Conferences
  Research Journal Articles
THE CONTENT OF RESEARCH JOURNAL ARTICLES
  The Abstract
  The Introduction
  The Method Section
  The Results Section
  The Discussion
  The References
THE STYLE OF RESEARCH JOURNAL ARTICLES

**READING, SUMMARIZING, AND CRITIQUING
  RESEARCH REPORTS**
  Reading and Summarizing Research Reports
  Critiquing Research Reports
RESEARCH EXAMPLES
  Research Example of a Quantitative Study
  Research Example of a Qualitative Study
SUMMARY POINTS
CRITICAL THINKING ACTIVITIES
SUGGESTED READINGS
  Methodologic References
  Substantive References

Student Objectives

On completion of this chapter, the student will be able to:

○ identify major types of research reports
○ identify and describe the major sections in a research journal article
○ characterize the style used in quantitative and qualitative research reports
○ describe tools for reading and comprehending research reports
○ distinguish research synopses and research critiques
○ define new terms presented in the chapter

New Terms

Abstract	Research critique
Blind review	Research findings
Journal article	Research report
Level of significance	Statistical analysis
Peer reviewer	Statistical significance
Poster session	Statistical test

TYPES OF RESEARCH REPORTS

Information about a nursing study is communicated to the nursing community through **research reports** that describe what was studied, how it was studied, and what was found. Research reports—especially reports for a quantitative study—are often daunting to those without research training. This chapter is designed to help make research reports more accessible even before you become familiar with research methods.

Researchers communicate information about their studies in various ways. The most common types of research reports are the following:

* *Theses and dissertations.* Most master's and doctoral degrees are granted on the successful completion of a study that is described in a thesis or dissertation.
* *Books.* Sometimes, research is reported in books or in a chapter in a book on a specific research topic.
* *Presentations at conferences.* Professional organizations (*e.g.,* Canadian Nurses Association, Sigma Theta Tau International) and institutions sponsor conferences that provide a forum for describing studies orally or in visual displays.
* *Journal articles.* Many nursing journals publish articles that summarize the results of a study.

Consumers of nursing research are most likely to encounter research results at professional conferences or in journals.

Presentations at Professional Conferences

The two main formats for presenting research findings at a conference are oral presentations and poster sessions. Oral presentations follow a format similar to that used in journal articles, which we discuss later in this chapter. The presenter of an oral report is typically allotted 10 to 20 minutes to describe the most important aspects of the study. In a **poster session,** many researchers simultaneously present visual displays summarizing their studies, and conference attendees circulate around the room perusing these displays.

Conference presentations are an important avenue for communicating research information. One attractive feature is that there is less time elapsed between the completion of a study and the dissemination of the findings than is the case with journal articles. Conferences also offer an opportunity for dialogue between the researcher and conference attendees. The listeners at oral presentations and viewers of poster displays can ask questions to help them better understand how the study was conducted or what the findings mean; moreover, they can offer the researchers suggestions relating to the clinical implications of the study. Thus, professional conferences offer a particularly valuable forum for a clinical audience.

Research Journal Articles

Research **journal articles** are reports in professional journals that summarize an investigation. Because the competition for journal space is keen, the typical research article is brief, generally only 10 to 15 double-spaced pages. This means that the researcher must condense a great deal of information about the study purpose, methods used, findings, interpretation, and clinical significance into a short report.

Journals accept research reports on a competitive basis. Usually, research articles are reviewed by several **peer reviewers** (other researchers doing work in the field) who make a recommendation about whether the article should be accepted, rejected, or revised and re-reviewed. These are usually **"blind" reviews**—the reviewers are not told the names of the researchers, and the researchers are not told the identity of the reviewers.

In major nursing research journals, the rate of acceptance is low—it can be as low as 5% of all submitted articles. Thus, consumers of research journal articles have some assurance that the reports have already been scrutinized for their merit and nursing relevance by other nurse researchers. Nevertheless, the publication of an article does not mean that the research findings can be accepted uncritically. The validity of the findings and their utility for clinical practice depend to a large degree on how the study was conducted. Research methods courses help consumers to understand the strengths and limitations of studies reported in professional journals.

THE CONTENT OF RESEARCH JOURNAL ARTICLES

Research reports in journals tend to follow a certain format and to be written in a particular style. Research reports begin with a title that succinctly conveys (typically in 15 or fewer words) the nature of the study. In qualitative studies, the title normally includes the central phenomenon and group under investigation; in quantitative studies, the title generally indicates the independent and dependent variables and the population under study. Research reports often consist of six major sections: an abstract, an introduction, a method section, a results section, a discussion, and references.

The Abstract

The **abstract** is a brief description of the study placed at the beginning of the journal article. The abstract answers, in about 100 to 200 words, the following questions: What were the research questions? What methods did the researcher use to address those questions? What did the researcher discover? What are the implications for nursing practice? Readers can readily review an abstract to assess whether the entire report is of interest.

Some journals have moved from having traditional abstracts, which are single paragraphs summarizing the main features of the study, to slightly longer and more informative abstracts with specific headings. For example, abstracts in *Nursing Research* after 1997 present information about the study organized under the following headings: Background, Objectives, Method, Results, Conclusions, and Key Words.

Box 3-1 presents abstracts from two studies. The first is a "new style" abstract for a quantitative study entitled "Does bathing newborns remove potentially harmful pathogens from the skin?" (Medves & O'Brien, 2001). The second is a more traditional abstract, for a qualititative study, entitled "Learning to live with early dementia" (Werezak & Stewart, 2002). These two studies are used as illustrations throughout this chapter.

The Introduction

The introduction acquaints readers with the research problem and with the context within which it was formulated. The introduction may or may not be specifically labeled "Introduction," but it nevertheless follows immediately after the abstract. The introduction usually describes the following:

- *The central phenomena, concepts, or variables under study.* The key topic under investigation is identified.
- *The statement of purpose, research questions, and/or hypotheses to be tested.*

| BOX 3-1 | **EXAMPLES OF ABSTRACTS FROM JOURNAL ARTICLES** |

Quantitative Study

Background: Newborn infants are routinely bathed after birth partly to reduce the possibility of transmitting potential pathogens to others. The extent to which a mild soap reduces the quantity and type of microbes found on the skin through normal colonization has not been reported. The objective of the study was to compare colonization rates between infants bathed in soap and water and infants bathed in plain water.

Method: One hundred and forty infants were randomly assigned to one group bathed in a mild pH neutral soap and water or to another group bathed in water alone. Microbiology swabs were taken on three occasions (before the first bath, 1 hour after the bath, and 24 hours after birth) from two sites (anterior fontanelle and umbilical area).

Results: No difference occurred between groups on type or quantity of organisms found at each time period. Skin colonization is a function of time, and the quantity of organisms identified increased over time (Friedman A^2 = 111.379, df = 5, p < 0.001).

Conclusions: Bathing with mild soap as opposed to bathing in water alone has minimal effect on skin bacterial colonization as colonization naturally increases over time. The findings did not support the efficacy of bathing with soap and water to reduce skin colonization of bacterial pathogens. Although the incidence of potential pathogens colonizing the skin during the first day of life is low and unlikely to pose a risk to healthy newborns, health care professionals may wish to wear gloves until the infant has been bathed (Medves & O'Brien, 2001).

Qualitative Study

Much of the literature on early dementia is focused on caregiver perspectives, whereas little is known about the perspective of persons with early-stage dementia, such as what it is like to live with this syndrome. This study was conducted to explore the process of learning to live with early-stage dementia. Interviews were conducted with 3 men and 3 women ranging in age from 61 to 79 years with early-stage dementia. Theory construction was facilitated using a qualitative approach and grounded theory. From the data a preliminary theoretical framework was developed, which outlines a 5-stage process of learning to live with dementia that begins with various antecedents and proceeds through the stages of anticipation, appearance, assimilation, and acceptance. This process evolved as participants' awareness of themselves and their outer world changed. Ultimately, the findings of this study have several implications for clinicians and researchers working with persons in early-stage dementia (Werezak & Stewart, 2002).

The reader is told what the researcher set out to accomplish by conducting the study.

- *A review of the related literature.* Current knowledge relating to the study problem is briefly described so that readers can understand how the study fits in with previous findings and can assess the contribution of the new study.

- *The theoretical framework.* In theoretically driven studies, the framework is usually presented in the introduction.
- *The significance of and need for the study.* The introduction to most research reports includes an explanation of why the study is important to nursing.

Thus, the introduction sets the stage for a description of what the researcher did and what was discovered.

Example of an introductory paragraph:

(. . .)Skin colonization is a normal process. Normal skin flora reduces colonization by means of potential pathogens and maintains the delicate pH balance between organisms required for normal skin integrity. The use of antibacterial solutions in newborn nurseries has declined because the incidence of skin infections has decreased and evidence supporting the efficacy of bathing infants with the solutions is lacking. A search of the literature revealed no reports on the effect of short maternity hospital stays on newborn skin colonization and the effects of other methods of cleaning such as mild soap and water or water alone (. . .). The objective of this study was to test the assumption that no difference would occur in the quantity of normal skin flora and potential pathogens found on newborn skin when infants were bathed in mild soap compared with infants bathed in water alone (Medves & O'Brien, 2001).

In this paragraph, the researchers indicated the independent variable (use of mild soap and water versus use of water alone), the dependent variable (skin colonization), the objective of the study, and the need for the study (the effect of the independent variable on the dependent variable is not known).

The Method Section

The method section communicates to readers what methods the researcher used to answer the research questions. The method section tells readers about major methodologic decisions and may offer rationales for those decisions. For example, a report for a qualitative study often explains why a qualitative approach was considered to be especially appropriate and fruitful.

In a quantitative study, the method section usually describes the following, which may be presented as labeled subsections:

- *The sample.* Quantitative research reports generally describe the population under study, specifying the criteria by which the researcher decided whether a person would be eligible for the study. The method section also describes the actual sample, indicating how people were selected and the number of participants in the sample.
- *The research design.* A description of the research design focuses on the overall plan for the collection of data, often including the steps the re-

searcher took to minimize biases and enhance the interpretability of the results by instituting various controls.

- *Measures and data collection.* In the method section, researchers describe the methods and procedures used to collect the data, including how the critical research variables were operationalized; they may also present information concerning the quality of the measuring tools.
- *Study procedures.* The method section contains a description of the procedures used to conduct the study, including a description of any intervention. The researcher's efforts to protect the rights of human subjects may also be documented in the method section.

Table 3-1 presents excerpts from the method section of the quantitative study by Medves and O'Brien (2001).

Qualitative researchers discuss many of the same issues, but with different emphases. For example, a qualitative study often provides more information about the research setting and the context of the study and less information on

TABLE 3-1. Excerpts from Method Section, Quantitative Report

METHODOLOGIC ELEMENT	EXCERPT FROM MEDVES & O'BRIEN (2001)
RESEARCH DESIGN	One hundred and forty infants were randomized to one of two groups: one group was bathed with mild soap and water and the other was bathed with water alone (p.162).
SAMPLE	The sample was recruited from infants born at a tertiary care centre in western Canada between February 8 and June 9, 1999. Infants born vaginally after at least 37 completed weeks' gestation who had Apgar scores of at least 7 by 5 minutes of age who were eligible for admission to the normal newborn nursery and who had no obvious physical abnormality were eligible for inclusion. Infants with planned discharge before 24 hours of life who lived outside the city limits were excluded. Infants born to mothers who were known to be HIV positive were also excluded because of institutional policies with respect to isolation of the mother and infant after birth (p. 162).
MEASUREMENT	The specimens were inoculated onto a 2.5-cm diameter area of blood agar beginning at the edge of the plate and using a rotary movement of the swab. The inoculated area was streaked with a sterile spreader in one movement. The agar plates were incubated at 37°C for 24–48 hours and aerobic microbe growth was assessed. The same research microbiology technologist who was blind to group assignment recorded all results (p. 163).
PROCEDURE	A sterile gauze template measuring 5×5 cm was used to guide the person obtaining the specimen. For umbilical swabs the gauze template was a square and for the anterior fontanelle site the gauze template was diamond shaped. The sterile swabs were placed in Stewart's medium and stored in a refrigerator until transfer to laboratory (p. 163).

sampling. Also, because formal instruments are not used to collect qualitative data, there is little discussion about data collection methods, but there may be more information on data collection procedures. Increasingly, reports of qualitative studies are including descriptions of the researchers' efforts to ensure high-quality data. Many qualitative reports also have a subsection on data analysis. There are fairly standard ways of analyzing quantitative data, but such standardization does not exist for qualitative data, so that qualitative researchers may describe their analytic approach. Table 3-2 presents excerpts from the method section of the qualitative study by Werezak and Stewart (2002).

The Results Section

The results section presents the **research findings** (*i.e.,* the results obtained in the analyses of the data). The text summarizes the findings, often accompanied by tables or figures that highlight the most noteworthy results.

Virtually all results sections contain basic descriptive information, including a description of the study participants (*e.g.,* their average age). In quantitative studies, the researcher provides basic descriptive information for

---

TABLE 3-2. Excerpts from Method Section, Qualitative Report

METHODOLOGIC ELEMENT	EXCERPT FROM WEREZAK & STEWART, 2002
SAMPLE	Theoretical sampling was carried out to obtain 6 participants (3 men and 3 women) with early-stage dementia (5 with Alzheimer's disease and 1 with vascular dementia). To recruit participants from various agencies, the researchers supplied the agency contact persons with a 1-page letter describing the study (pp. 69–70).
DATA COLLECTION	Data were initially collected from participants using a semistructured interview format based on previous research. Each participant was interviewed twice. Proxies were allowed to be present during the interview process but were informed that the purpose of the interview was to elicit the perspective of the person with dementia. A second interview was conducted with each participant for the purpose of verifying and clarifying the emerging theory. During this second interview, 1 to 3 months later, the interview process evolved and became more unstructured and open-ended as clarification was sought on issues that emerged in the previous interview (p. 71).
DATA ANALYSIS	Data were analyzed to identify core concepts that described the experience of living with dementia from the perspective of the person with early memory loss. Accounts from participants with different types of dementia were included and analyzed to capture variations in their experience. During the process of coding the first interviews, five preliminary categories emerged from the data, which the first author validated and expanded based on the second set of interviews (p. 72).

the key variables, using simple statistics. For example, in a study of the effect of prenatal drug exposure on the birth outcomes of infants, the results section might begin by describing the average birth weights and Apgar scores of the infants, or the percentage who were of low birth weight (< 2500 g).

In quantitative studies, the results section also reports the following information relating to the **statistical analyses** performed:

- *The name of statistical tests used.* A **statistical test** is a procedure for testing hypotheses and evaluating the believability of the findings. For example, if the percentage of low-birth-weight infants in the sample of drug-exposed infants is computed, how probable is it that the percentage is accurate? If the researcher finds that the average birth weight of drug-exposed infants in the sample is lower than the birth weight of infants who were not exposed to drugs, how probable is it that the same would be true for other infants not in the sample? That is, is the relationship between prenatal drug exposure and infant birth weight real and likely to be replicated with a new sample of infants? Statistical tests answer such questions. Dozens of statistical tests exist, but they are all based on common principles; readers do not have to know the names of all statistical tests to comprehend the findings.

- *The value of the calculated statistic.* Computers are used to compute a numeric value for the particular statistical test used. The value allows the researchers to draw conclusions about the meaning of the results. The actual numeric value of the statistic, however, is not inherently meaningful and need not concern readers of research reports.

- *The significance.* The most important information is whether the results of the statistical tests were significant (not to be confused with important or clinically relevant). If a researcher reports that the results have **statistical significance,** it means that, based on the statistical test, the findings are probably valid and replicable with a new sample of participants. Research reports also indicate the **level of significance,** which is an index of how probable it is that the findings are reliable. For example, if a report indicates that a finding was significant at the .05 level, this means that only 5 times out of 100 ($5/100 = .05$) would the obtained result be spurious or haphazard. In other words, 95 times out of 100, similar results would be obtained. Both the researcher and readers can therefore have a high degree of confidence—but not total assurance—that the findings are reliable.

⊞ **Example from the results section of a quantitative study:**

No difference occurred in skin colonization either in classification of microbes or in quantity of microbes between infants bathed in soap and water and infants bathed in water alone (*e.g.,* umbilicus 1 hour after bath: Friedman $A^2 = 0.381$, $df = 1$, $p = .537$). Skin colonization is a function of time (Friedman $A^2 = 111.379$, $df = 5$, $p < .001$) (Medves & O'Brien, 2001, pp. 163–164).

In this excerpt, the authors indicate that bathing with mild soap as opposed to bathing in water has no effect on skin bacterial colonization. The p value of .537 means that the small difference in skin colonization between the two groups could easily have happened by chance, that is, it could happen by chance alone 537 out of 1000 times. However, skin colonization significantly increased over time in both groups. The probability (p) that the latter finding is spurious is less than 1 in 1000 (1/1000 = .001). Thus, we have a high degree of confidence that this finding is reliable. Note that to comprehend this finding, it is not necessary for you to understand what the Friedman test is nor to concern yourself with the value of the statistics.

In qualitative reports, the researcher often organizes findings according to the major themes or processes that were identified in the data. The results section of qualitative reports sometimes has several subsections, the headings of which correspond to the researcher's labels for the themes. Excerpts from the raw data are presented to support and provide a rich description of the thematic analysis. The results section of qualitative studies may also present the researcher's emerging theory about the phenomenon under study, although this may appear in the concluding section of the report.

Example from the results section of a qualitative study:

The theory that emerged from the interviews can best be described as a continuous process of adjusting to early-stage dementia. The process consists of five core categories or stages that evolve over time, namely antecedents, anticipation, appearance, assimilation, and acceptance. The participants described a process of adjusting to early-stage dementia beginning with various antecedents and progressing through the next four stages of the model with differing levels of awareness connecting each stage to the next. (. . .) For instance, participants discussed various aspects of the process of acceptance as it related to having dementia. The following statement illustrates this point: "I think I am very fortunate. I have really managed to accept it and to say that I'm a lot luckier than a lot of other people. I could be a lot worse. I still can do my [lay ministry work], I still can see my kids, I can still do things that I like doing, and I think you have to sometimes just be grateful for what you have." (Werezak & Stewart, 2002, p. 78).

In this excerpt, through the use of a direct quote from one study participant, the researchers illustrate the finding that most participants found ways to accept and integrate their memory loss into their lives.

The Discussion

In the discussion, the researcher draws conclusions about the meaning and implications of the findings. This section tries to unravel what the results mean, why things turned out the way they did, and how the results can be used in practice. The discussion in both qualitative and quantitative reports may incorporate the following elements:

- *An interpretation of the results.* The interpretation involves the translation of findings into practical, conceptual, and/or theoretical meaning.
- *Implications.* Researchers often offer suggestions for how their findings could be used to improve nursing, and they may also make recommendations on how best to advance knowledge in the area through additional research.
- *Study limitations.* The researcher is in the best position possible to discuss study limitations, such as sample deficiencies, design problems, weaknesses in data collection, and so forth. A discussion section that presents these limitations demonstrates to readers that the author was aware of these limitations and probably took them into account in interpreting the findings.

> **Example from a discussion section of a qualitative report:**
>
> The findings suggest that nurse clinicans and researchers must become aware of the impact of their verbal and nonverbal communication on early-stage sufferers. Clinicians and researchers should adopt an individualized, unhurried approach in working with early-stage sufferers and should demonstrate their recognition of and respect for the unique difficulties and concerns of these persons (Werezak & Stewart, 2002, p. 81).

The References

Research journal articles conclude with a list of the books, reports, and journal articles that were cited in the text of the report. For those interested in pursuing additional reading on a substantive topic, the reference list of a current research study is an excellent place to begin.

THE STYLE OF RESEARCH JOURNAL ARTICLES

Research reports tell a story. However, the style in which many research journal articles are written—especially reports of quantitative studies—makes it difficult for beginning research consumers to become interested in the story. To unaccustomed audiences, research reports may seem stuffy, pedantic, and bewildering. Four factors contribute to this impression:

- *Compactness.* Journal space is limited; hence, authors try to compress many ideas and concepts into a short space. Interesting, personalized aspects of the investigation often cannot be reported. And, in qualitative studies, only a handful of supporting quotes can be included.
- *Jargon.* The authors of both qualitative and quantitative reports use research terms that are assumed to be part of the reader's vocabulary but that may seem esoteric.
- *Objectivity.* Quantitative researchers normally avoid any impression of

subjectivity; thus, research stories are told in a way that makes them sound impersonal. For example, most quantitative research reports are written in the passive voice (*i.e.,* personal pronouns are avoided). Use of the passive voice tends to make a report less inviting and lively than use of the active voice, and it tends to give the impression that the researcher did not play an active role in conducting the study. (Qualitative reports, by contrast, are more subjective and personal and are written in a more conversational style.)

- *Statistical information.* In quantitative reports, numbers and statistical symbols may intimidate readers who do not have strong mathematic interest or training. Most nursing studies are quantitative; thus, most research reports summarize the results of statistical analyses.

A major goal of this textbook is to assist nurses in understanding the content of research reports and in overcoming anxieties about their jargon, style, and statistical information.

READING, SUMMARIZING, AND CRITIQUING RESEARCH REPORTS

Nurses who seek to base their practice on research evidence must be able to read and critically appraise research reports. This section offers some general guidance on reading and evaluating nursing research reports.

Reading and Summarizing Research Reports

Beginning consumers of nursing research cannot be expected to critically appraise research immediately. The skills involved in critical appraisal must be developed over time. The first step in being able to use research findings in clinical practice is to read and comprehend research reports. In all likelihood, your first few attempts to read a research report will seem overwhelming, and you may wonder whether being able to comprehend, let alone appraise, research reports is a realistic goal. As you progress through this textbook, you will acquire skills to help you evaluate various aspects of research reports. Some preliminary tips on digesting research reports follow.

- Grow accustomed to the style of research reports by reading them frequently, even though you may not yet understand all the technical points. Try to keep the underlying rationale for the style of research reports in mind as you read.
- Read from a report that has been photocopied so that you can use a highlighter, underline portions of the article, write questions or notes in the margins, and so on.
- Read journal articles slowly. It may be useful to skim the article first to get the major points and then to read the article more carefully a second time.
- On the second or later reading of a journal article, train yourself to be-

come an active reader. Reading actively involves constantly monitoring yourself to determine whether you understand what you are reading. If you are having comprehension problems, go back and reread difficult passages or make notes about your confusion so that you can ask someone for clarification. In most cases, that "someone" will be your research instructor or another faculty member, but also consider contacting the researchers themselves. The postal and e-mail addresses of the researchers are usually included in the journal article, and researchers are generally more than willing to discuss their research with others.

- Keep this textbook with you as a reference while you are reading articles initially. This will enable you to look up unfamiliar terms in the glossary at the end of the book or in the index.
- Try not to get bogged down in (or scared away by) the statistical information. Try to grasp the gist of the story without letting formulas and numbers frustrate you.
- Until you become more accustomed to the style and jargon of research journal articles, you may want to translate, mentally or in writing, research articles. You can do this by translating compact paragraphs into looser constructions, by translating jargon into more familiar terms, by recasting the report into an active voice, and by summarizing the findings with words rather than with numbers. As an example, Box 3-2 presents a summary of a fictitious study, written in the style typically found in research journal articles. Terms that can be looked up in the glossary of this book are underlined, and the notes in the margins indicate the type of information the author is communicating. Box 3-3 presents a "translation" of this summary, recasting the research information into language that is more digestible. Note that it is not just the jargon specific to research methods that makes the original version complicated (*e.g.*, "sequelae" is more obscure than "consequences"). Thus, a dictionary may also be needed when reading research reports.

When you attain a reasonable level of comprehension of a research report, a useful next step is to write a brief, one- to two-page synopsis of the study. A synopsis summarizes the study's purpose, research questions, methods, findings, interpretation of the findings, and implications for practice. You do not need to be concerned at this point about critiquing the study's strengths and weaknesses, but rather about succinctly and objectively presenting a summary of what was done and what was learned. By preparing a synopsis, you will become more aware of aspects of the study that you did not comprehend.

Critiquing Research Reports

A written **research critique** is different from a research summary or synopsis. A research critique is a careful, critical appraisal of the strengths and limitations of a study. Critiques usually conclude with the reviewer's summary of

BOX 3-2	**SUMMARY OF FICTITIOUS STUDY FOR TRANSLATION**

Purpose of the study — The potentially negative sequelae of having an abortion on the psychological adjustment of adolescents have not been adequately studied. The present study sought to determine whether alternative pregnancy resolution decisions have different long-term effects on the psychological functioning of young women. — **Need for the study**

Research design — Three groups of low-income pregnant teenagers attending an inner-city clinic were the subjects in this study: those who delivered and kept the baby; those who delivered and relinquished the baby for adoption; and those who had an abortion. There were 25 subjects in each group. — **Study population** / **Research sample**

Research instruments — The study instruments included a self-administered questionnaire and a battery of psychological tests measuring depression, anxiety, and psychosomatic symptoms. The instruments were administered on entry into the study (when the participants first came to the clinic) and then 1 year after termination of the pregnancy or delivery. — **Research design & data collection procedures**

Data analysis procedure — The data were analyzed using analysis of variance (ANOVA). The ANOVA tests indicated that the three groups did not differ significantly in terms of depression, anxiety, or psychosomatic symptoms at the initial testing. At the posttest, however, the abortion group had significantly higher scores on the depression scale, and these girls were significantly more likely than the two delivery groups to report severe tension headaches. There were no significant differences on any of the dependent variables for the two delivery groups. — **Results**

Implications — The results of this study suggest that young women who elect to have an abortion may experience a number of long-term negative consequences. It would appear that appropriate efforts should be made to follow-up abortion patients to determine their need for suitable treatment. — **Interpretation**

BOX 3-3

TRANSLATED VERSION OF FICTITIOUS RESEARCH STUDY

As researchers, we wondered whether young women who had an abortion had any emotional problems in the long run. It seemed to us that not enough research had been done to know whether any psychological harm resulted from an abortion.

We decided to study this question ourselves by comparing the experiences of three types of teenagers who became pregnant—first, girls who delivered and kept their babies; second, those who delivered the babies but gave them up for adoption; and third, those who elected to have an abortion. All teenagers in the sample were poor, and all were patients at an inner-city clinic. Altogether, we studied 75 girls—25 in each of the three groups. We evaluated the teenagers' emotional states by asking them to fill out a questionnaire and to take several psychological tests. These tests allowed us to assess things such as the girls' degree of depression and anxiety and whether they had any complaints of a psychosomatic nature. We asked them to fill out the forms twice: once when they came into the clinic, and then again a year after the abortion or the delivery.

We learned that the three groups of teenagers looked pretty much alike in terms of their emotional states when they first filled out the forms. But when we compared how the three groups looked a year later, we found that the teenagers who had abortions were more depressed and were more likely to say they had severe tension headaches than teenagers in the other two groups. The teenagers who kept their babies and those who gave their babies up for adoption looked pretty similar a year after their babies were born, at least in terms of depression, anxiety, and psychosomatic complaints.

Thus, it seems that we might be right in having some concerns about the emotional effects of having an abortion. Nurses should be aware of these long-term emotional effects, and it even may be advisable to institute some type of follow-up procedure to find out if these young women need additional help.

the study's merits, recommendations regarding the utilization of the findings, and suggestions about improving the study or the report itself.

Research critiques of individual studies are prepared for various reasons, and they differ in scope, depending on their purpose. Peer reviewers who are asked to prepare a written critique for a journal considering publication of the report generally critique the following aspects of the study:

- *Substantive*—Was the research problem significant to nursing? Can the study make an important contribution?
- *Theoretical*—Were the theoretical underpinnings sound?
- *Methodologic*—Were the methods appropriate? Are the resulting findings believable?
- *Interpretive*—Did the researcher properly interpret data and develop reasonable conclusions?

- *Ethical*—Were the rights of the study participants protected?
- *Stylistic*—Is the report clearly written, grammatical, and well organized?

In short, the peer reviewer does a comprehensive review with the aim of providing feedback to the researchers and to journal editors about the merit of both the study and the report.

By contrast, a critique of a study that is designed to inform decisions about nursing practice need not be as comprehensive. For example, it is of little significance to practicing nurses that a research report is ungrammatical. A critique on the clinical utility of a study focuses on whether the findings are accurate, believable, and clinically meaningful. If the findings cannot be trusted, it makes little sense to incorporate them into nursing practice.

By understanding research methods, you will be in a position to critique the scientific merit of studies, and this is a primary aim of this book. Each chapter in this book offers guidelines for evaluating various research decisions that will help you come to an overall appraisal of a research study.

Nurses who are informed consumers of nursing research must be able to critique not only single, independent studies, but also a body of studies on a topic of clinical interest. We discuss literature reviews in Chapter 6, and we further explore the role of critical reviews in the final chapter of this book.

RESEARCH EXAMPLES

In this section, we present abstracts from two additional research studies. As we did in Box 3-2, we underline terms that can be looked up in the book's glossary or index to assist you in understanding unfamiliar terms. We also provide a "translated" version of the abstract.

Research Example of a Quantitative Study

Dennis, Hodnett, Gallop, and Chalmers (2002) conducted a study to evaluate the effect of peer support on breastfeeding duration among primiparous women.

Research Summary (Abstract)
Background: Most mothers stop breastfeeding before the recommended 6 months postpartum. A systematic review showed that breastfeeding support programs by health care professionals did not substantially improve breastfeeding outcomes beyond 2 months postpartum. The authors conducted a <u>randomized controlled trial</u> to evaluate the effect of peer (mother-to-mother) support on breastfeeding duration among first-time mothers. *Method:* 256 breastfeeding mothers from 2 semi-urban community hospitals near Toronto were <u>randomly assigned</u> to a <u>control</u> (conventional care) ($n=126$) or a peer support <u>group</u> (conventional care plus telephone-based support, initiated within 48 hours after

hospital discharge, from a woman experienced with breastfeeding who attended a 2.5-hour orientation session) ($n=132$). Follow-up of breastfeeding duration, maternal satisfaction with infant feeding methods, and perceptions of peer support received was conducted at 4, 8, and 12 weeks postpartum. *Results:* Significantly more mothers in the peer support group than in the control group continued to breastfeed at 3 months postpartum ($p=.01$) and did so exclusively ($p=.001$). Breastfeeding rates at 4, 8, and 12 weeks postpartum were 92.4%, 84.8%, and 81.1%, respectively, among the mothers in the peer support group, as compared to 83.9%, 75.0%, and 66.9% among those in the control group ($p \leq .05$ for all time periods). The corresponding relative risks were 1.10 (95% confidence interval [CI] 1.01–2.72) at 4 weeks, 1.13 (95% CI 1.00–1.28) at 8 weeks, and 1.21 (95% CI 1.04–1.41) at 12 weeks postpartum. In addition, when asked for an overall rating of their feeding experience, significantly fewer mothers in the peer support group than in the control were dissatisfied (1.5% vs. 10.5%) ($p=.02$). Of the 130 mothers who evaluated the peer support intervention, 81.6% were satisfied with their peer volunteer experience and 100% felt that all new breastfeeding mothers should be offered this peer support intervention. *Interpretation:* The telephone-based peer support intervention was effective in maintaining breastfeeding to 3 months postpartum and improving satisfaction with the infant feeding experience. The high satisfaction with and acceptance of the intervention indicates that breastfeeding peer support programs, in conjunction with professional health services, are effective.

Translated Version

We wanted to evaluate how effective peer support would be for first-time breastfeeding mothers. We wondered whether new mothers who received telephone-based support from women experienced with breastfeeding would breastfeed longer and be more satisfied with their infant feeding experience than new mothers who did not receive the additional support. A total of 256 new breastfeeding mothers took part in this study; 132 of them were put in a group that did not receive the special intervention. The other 124 mothers were put in the peer support group at random. These mothers, in addition to usual in-hospital and community postpartum support services, were paired with a peer volunteer. The peer volunteers were asked to contact the new mother within 48 hours after hospital discharge and as frequently thereafter as the mother thought necessary. The results indicated that more mothers in the group that received peer support were breastfeeding at 4, 8, and 12 weeks postpartum. The findings suggest that 21% more mothers would continue to breastfeed at 12 weeks postpartum if they were provided with peer support. Also important is the finding that more mothers in the peer support group than in the other group were exclusively breastfeeding at 12 weeks. Thus, peer volunteer support improved both breastfeeding duration and exclusivity.

Clinical Relevance

In Canada, national surveys indicate that about 79% of new mothers initiate breastfeeding. However, despite the well-documented health benefits of breastfeeding, the proportion of new mothers still breastfeeding at 8 weeks declines by up to 35%. One reason for the premature discontinuation is difficulties with breastfeeding. To address this issue, postpartum breastfeeding support programs have been developed by health care professionals. These programs, however, often do not show improvements in breastfeeding outcomes beyond 2 months postpartum. A growing trend in health care, and postpartum care in particular, is the use of lay support. Despite its potential to promote duration of breastfeeding among new mothers, few studies to date have documented the effect of peer support on breastfeeding duration. Moreover, findings from the few studies must be interpreted with caution because they often show limitations such as weak designs and small sample sizes. Here the authors used a strong design to ensure that their study would adequately document the potential contribution of peer support to knowledge and practices of breastfeeding first-time mothers. The findings suggested that the intervention was effective. The use of peer support helped new mothers reach their breastfeeding goal and added to their feelings of satisfaction with breastfeeding. Also, peer volunteers appear to be useful links between mothers in the community and health care professionals. Peer support may be particularly useful for socially disadvantaged breastfeeding mothers who may not have ready access to usual forms of support.

Research Example of a Qualitative Study

Friesen, Pepler, and Hunter (2002) conducted a qualitative study to describe the experience of families when a family member is diagnosed with cancer.

Research Summary

Patients recruited from an oncology outpatient clinic and a gynecologic inpatient unit of a teaching hospital were interviewed on one occasion with at least two immediate family members present in the patient's home (8 families, total 30 people). Semistructured interviews were tape-recorded and analyzed for themes and categories using the techniques of constant comparison. Overall, families described a learning process in which information was gathered, interpreted, and shared. Families learned together by reviewing the past, gathering and sharing information, and sharing their experience of living with someone undergoing treatment for cancer. By revealing their own personal perspectives, patients taught their families about their illness experiences and what constituted effective support. In sum, interactive family learning is a mode of learning and a form of support in which the whole family may participate early in the process of learning to live with cancer.

Translated Version

We conducted in-depth interviews with eight families to study their experience when a family member is diagnosed with cancer. Learning was the most striking element that arose when we asked patients and families general questions about their experience with cancer. Four emerging themes captured how family members learned to live with cancer: (1) reviewing the past (such as reflecting on past experiences with cancer and other major illnesses), (2) sharing the work and effort of gathering and interpreting illness-related information, (3) learning from each individual's experience while the illness experience and the treatment process unfold, and (4) learning through patients' disclosure of their own perspective.

Clinical Relevance

The findings of this study suggest that nurses can facilitate patient and family learning by considering the interactive manner by which they acquire illness-related information. Nurses also can support families in the learning process by exploring with them how they communicate to others their personal views on the illness experience. By acknowledging the expertise that families bring to the particular situation and the knowledge that they gained through their experience with cancer, nurses can promote open communication among family members so that optimal means to support each other are used.

● ● ● ● ● *SUMMARY POINTS*

- The most common types of research reports are theses and dissertations, books, conference presentations (including oral reports and **poster sessions**), and, especially, journal articles.
- Research **journal articles** provide brief descriptions of research studies and are designed to communicate the contribution the study has made to knowledge.
- Journal articles often consist of six major sections: the **abstract** (a brief synopsis of the study); introduction (explanation of the study problem and its context); method section (the strategies used to address the research problem); results (the actual study findings); discussion (the interpretation of the findings); and references.
- Research reports are often difficult to read because they are dense, concise, and contain jargon.
- Qualitative research reports are written in a more inviting and conversational style than quantitative ones, which are more impersonal and include statistical information.
- **Statistical tests** are procedures for testing research hypotheses and evaluating the believability of the findings. Findings that are **statistically significant** are ones that have a high probability of being valid.
- The ultimate goal of this book is to help students to prepare a **research critique,** which is a careful, critical appraisal of the strengths and limitations of a piece of research, often for the purpose of considering its utility for nursing practice.

➤ ➤ ➤ ➤ *CRITICAL THINKING ACTIVITIES*

Chapter 3 of the accompanying *Study Guide to Accompany Essentials of Nursing Research*, 5th edition, offers various exercises and study suggestions for reinforcing the concepts presented in this chapter. In addition, you can address the following:

1. Read the abstracts from one or both of the actual research studies in the Appendix of this book. Underline technical terms and look them up in the glossary. Then write a translated version of the abstract.

2. Make an outline of the major sections and subsections of one or both of the research studies in the Appendix. Compare this outline to the outline of sections described in this chapter.

3. Skim both of the research studies in the Appendix. Which story is more difficult to grasp? Why? Which parts of these research reports were especially problematic?

SUGGESTED READINGS

Methodologic References

Downs, F. S. (1999). How to cozy up to a research report. *Applied Nursing Research, 12,* 215–216.

Rankin, M., & Esteves, M. D. (1996). How to assess a research study. *American Journal of Nursing, 96,* 32–37.

Tornquist, E. M., Funk, S. G., Champagne, M. T., & Wiese, R. A. (1993). Advice on reading research: Overcoming the barriers. *Applied Nursing Research, 6,* 177–183.

Substantive References

Dennis, C-L., Hodnett, E., Gallop, R., & Chalmers, B. (2002). The effect of peer support on breast-feeding duration among primiparous women: A randomized controlled trial. *CMAJ-Canadian Medical Association Journal, 166,* 21–28.

Friesen, P., Pepler, C., & Hunter, P. (2002). Interactive family learning following a cancer diagnosis. *Oncology Nursing Forum, 29,* 981–987.

Medves, J. M., & O'Brien, B. (2001). Does bathing newborns remove potentially harmful pathogens from skin? *Birth, 28,* 161–165.

Werezak, L., & Stewart, N. (2002). Learning to live with early dementia. *Canadian Journal of Nursing Research, 34,* 67–85.

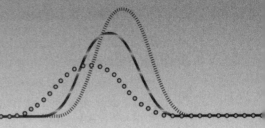

Understanding the Ethics of Nursing Research

THE NEED FOR ETHICAL GUIDELINES
Historical Background
Ethical Dilemmas in Conducting Research
Codes of Ethics
PRINCIPLE OF RESPECT FOR HUMAN DIGNITY
Free and Informed Consent
Issues Relating to the Principle of Respect
Respect for Vulnerable Persons
PRINCIPLE OF RESPECT FOR PRIVACY AND CONFIDENTIALITY
PRINCIPLE OF RESPECT FOR JUSTICE AND INCLUSIVENESS

PRINCIPLE OF BALANCING HARMS AND BENEFITS
Maximizing Benefits
Minimizing Harms
RESEARCH ETHICS BOARDS
CRITIQUING THE ETHICS OF RESEARCH STUDIES
RESEARCH EXAMPLES
Research Example of a Quantitative Study
Research Example of a Qualitative Study
SUMMARY POINTS
CRITICAL THINKING ACTIVITIES
WORLD WIDE WEBSITES
SUGGESTED READINGS
References on Research Ethics
Substantive References

Student Objectives

On completion of this chapter, the student will be able to:

○ discuss the historical background that led to the creation of various codes of ethics
○ understand the nature of the conflict, in certain situations, between ethics and research demands
○ identify the ethical principles articulated in the *Tri-Council Policy Statement* and the important dimensions encompassed by each
○ describe the concept of vulnerable persons and identify several relevant groups
○ describe the role of Research Ethics Boards in the review of research plans
○ given sufficient information, evaluate the ethical dimensions of a research report
○ define new terms in the chapter

New Terms

Anonymity	Identification number
Beneficence	Implied consent
Code of ethics	Informed consent
Coercion	Nonmaleficence
Confidentiality	Nuremberg Code
Consent form	Process consent
Covert data collection	Research Ethics Board (REB)
Debriefing	Risk–benefit ratio
Deception	Self-determination
Declaration of Helsinki	Stipend
Freedom from exploitation	*Tri-Council Policy*
Full disclosure	Vulnerable persons
Human subjects committees	

THE NEED FOR ETHICAL GUIDELINES

Nurses face many ethical dilemmas in their practice—the prolongation of life by artificial means, the institution of tube feedings when patients are unable to sustain oral nourishment, and the testing of new products to monitor care are but a few examples. Dilemmas such as these have led to numerous discussions and debates concerning ethical issues in nursing practice. Similarly, the increase of research with humans has led to ethical concerns about the rights of study participants, conflicts of interest, the balance of benefits and harms, and the consent of vulnerable participants. This chapter discusses some of the major ethical principles that should be considered in reviewing studies.

The requirement for ethical conduct in research may strike you as so self-evident as to require no further comment, but the fact is that ethical considerations have not always been given adequate attention.

Historical Background

As modern, civilized people, we might like to think that systematic violations of moral principles within a research context occurred centuries ago rather than in recent times, but this is not the case. The Nazi medical experiments of the 1930s and 1940s are the most famous example of recent disregard for ethical conduct. The Nazi program of research involved the use of prisoners of war and racial "enemies" in experiments designed to test the limits of human endurance and human reaction to diseases and untested drugs. The studies were unethical not only because they exposed these people to permanent physical harm and even death, but also because the participants could not refuse participation.

Some recent examples come from the United States. For instance, between 1932 and 1972, a study known as the Tuskegee Syphilis Study, sponsored by the U.S. Public Health Service, investigated the effects of syphilis on 400 men from a poor African-American community. Medical treatment was deliberately withheld to study the course of the untreated disease. Another well-known case of unethical research involved the injection of live cancer cells into elderly patients at the Jewish Chronic Disease Hospital in Brooklyn without the consent of those patients. Even more recently, it was revealed in 1993 that U.S. federal agencies had sponsored radiation experiments since the 1940s on hundreds of people, many of them prisoners or elderly hospital patients. Many other examples of studies with ethical transgressions—often much more subtle than these examples—have emerged to give ethical concerns the high visibility they have today.

Ethical Dilemmas in Conducting Research

Research that violates ethical principles is rarely done to be cruel but more typically occurs out of a conviction that knowledge is important and potentially beneficial in the long run. There are situations in which the rights of participants and the goals and demands of the research project are put in direct conflict. Here are some examples of research problems in which the desire for rigour conflicts with ethical considerations:

1. *Research question:* How empathic are nurses in their treatment of patients in intensive care units?
   Ethical dilemma: Ethics require that participants be cognizant of their role in a study. Yet if the researcher informs the nurses participating in this

study that their degree of empathy in treating patients will be scrutinized, will their behaviour be "normal"? If the nurses' behaviour is altered because of the known presence of research observers, the findings will not be valid.

2. *Research question:* What are the coping mechanisms of parents whose children have a terminal illness?
   Ethical dilemma: To answer this question, the researcher may need to probe into the psychological state of the parents at a vulnerable time in their lives; such probing could be painful and even traumatic. Yet knowledge of the parents' coping mechanisms might help to design more effective ways of dealing with parents' grief and anger.

3. *Research question:* Does a new medication prolong life in cancer patients?
   Ethical dilemma: The best way to test the effectiveness of an intervention is to administer the intervention to some participants but withhold it from others to see whether differences between the groups emerge. However, if the intervention is untested (*e.g.,* a new drug), the group receiving the intervention may be exposed to potentially hazardous side effects. On the other hand, the group not receiving the drug may be denied a beneficial treatment.

4. *Research question:* What is the process by which adult children adapt to the day-to-day stresses of caring for a terminally ill parent?
   Ethical dilemma: In a qualitative study, which would be appropriate for this research question, the researcher sometimes becomes so closely involved with the study participants that they become willing to share "secrets" and privileged information. Interviews can become confessions—sometimes of unseemly or even illegal or immoral behaviour. In this example, suppose a participant admitted to abusing an adult parent physically—how does the researcher respond to that information without undermining a pledge of confidentiality? And, if the researcher divulges the information to appropriate authorities, how can a pledge of confidentiality be given in good faith to other participants?

As these examples suggest, researchers are sometimes in a bind: their goal is to advance knowledge, using the best methods possible, but they must also adhere to the dictates of ethical rules that have been developed to protect the rights of study participants. It is precisely because of such conflicts that codes of ethics have been developed to guide the efforts of researchers and to help others evaluate their actions.

Codes of Ethics

Since the 1950s, largely in response to the human rights violations described earlier, various codes of ethics have been developed. One of the first internationally recognized set of ethical standards is referred to as the **Nuremberg Code,** developed after the Nazi atrocities were made public in the Nuremberg trials. Several other international standards have followed, the most notable of which is the **Declaration of Helsinki,** which was adopted in 1964 by the World Medical Assembly. It was revised in 1975 and amended in October 2000.

Most disciplines have established their own **code of ethics.** The Canadian Nurses Association (CNA) first published a document entitled *Ethical Guidelines for Nurses in Research Involving Human Participants* in 1983. It was revised in 1994 and again in 2002. The goal of this document is to provide nurses in all areas of professional practice with guidelines pertinent to research activities. The 2002 guidelines have been revised to complement the CNA Code of Ethics (CNA, 2002a). In Canada, Health Canada adopted the *Good Clinical Practice: Consolidated Guidelines* (GCP, 1997) as the guidelines for all clinical trial research involving human subjects. Health Canada specified the *Tri-Council Policy Statement: Ethical Conduct for Research Involving Humans* (*TCPS,* 1998) as the guideline to protect human subjects in all types of research. The *TCPS* was jointly prepared by the Medical Research Council (MRC), the Natural Sciences and Engineering Research Council (NSERC), and the Social Sciences and Humanities Research Council (SSHRC).

The *TCPS* (1998) articulates eight guiding ethical principles on which standards of ethical conduct in research are based: respect for human dignity, respect for free and informed consent, respect for vulnerable persons, respect for privacy and confidentiality, respect of justice and inclusiveness, balancing harms and benefits, minimizing harm, and maximizing benefit. According to the *TCPS* (1998) these principles are based on several sources, past guidelines of the councils, statements by other Canadian agencies such as the National Research Council of Canada, and statements from the international community. An essential component of the *GCP* and the *TCPS* is that a research ethics committee, formally known in Canada as a Research Ethics Board (REB), should first review and approve research studies that involve human subjects (CNA, 2002b).

PRINCIPLE OF RESPECT FOR HUMAN DIGNITY

The cardinal principle of modern research ethics is respect for human dignity. This principle aspires to protect the multiple and interdependent interests of the person from bodily to psychological and to cultural integrity. This principle forms the basis of the ethical obligations that are listed below. In certain situations, conflicts may arise from application of these principles in isolation from one another. Researchers and ethical review boards must carefully weigh all the principles and circumstances involved to reach a reasoned and defensible conclusion (*TCPS,* 1998, p. i.5).

This principle includes the right to self-determination and the right to full disclosure. Humans should be treated as autonomous agents, capable of controlling their own activities. The right to **self-determination** means that prospective participants have the right to decide voluntarily whether to participate in a study, without the risk of incurring any penalty or prejudicial treatment. It also means that participants have the right to ask questions, to refuse to give information, or to terminate their participation.

A person's right to self-determination includes freedom from coercion of any type. **Coercion** involves explicit or implicit threats of penalty for failing to participate in a study or excessive rewards from agreeing to participate. The obligation to protect potential participants from coercion requires careful consideration when the researcher is in a position of authority, control, or influence over potential participants, as might be the case in a nurse–patient relationship. The issue of coercion may also require scrutiny even when there is not a preestablished relationship. For example, a generous monetary incentive (or **stipend**) offered to encourage the participation of an economically disadvantaged group (*e.g.*, the homeless) might be mildly coercive because such incentives could place undue pressure on prospective participants.

The principle of respect for human dignity also includes people's right to make informed, voluntary decisions about study participation, which requires full disclosure. **Full disclosure** means that the researcher has fully described the nature of the study, the person's right to refuse participation, the researcher's responsibilities, and the likely risks and benefits that would be incurred. The right to self-determination and the right to full disclosure are the two major elements on which informed consent is based.

Free and Informed Consent

Individuals are usually presumed to have the capacity and right to make free and informed decisions. Respect for person thus means respecting the exercise of individual consent. In practical terms within the ethics review process, the principle of respect for persons translates into dialogue, process, rights, duties, and requirements for free and informed consent by the study participant (*TCPS*, 1998, p. i.5).

Informed consent means that participants have adequate information regarding the research, comprehend the information, and have the power of free choice, enabling them to consent voluntarily to participate in the research or decline participation. Researchers may document the informed consent process by having participants sign a **consent form,** an example of which is presented in Figure 4–1. This form includes information about the purpose of the study, the specific expectations regarding participation (*e.g.*, how much time will be involved), the voluntary nature of participation, and the potential costs and benefits.

Researchers rarely obtain written informed consent when the primary means of data collection is through a self-administered questionnaire. The researcher usually assumes **implied consent** (*i.e.*, that the return of the completed questionnaire reflects the respondent's voluntary consent to participate). This assumption, however, is not always warranted (*e.g.*, if patients feel that their treatment might be affected by failure to cooperate with the researcher).

I, _____ agree to take part in a nursing study about the use of research findings in postoperative pain management. I understand that participation in the study may involve one or two interviews with a researcher, which will be tape recorded, and that the recording will be typed into a written record. I will be answering questions about:

- My experiences with and beliefs about pain management
- My experiences using research evidence
- Factors that I believe make it easier or more difficult to use current research or to follow current pain management practices
- Factors that I think influence pain management practices in a unit and a hospital

I may also be completing short questions and scales (*e.g.,* answering questions using ratings of 1 to 5 or more) about research use and factors thought to influence it. Alternatively I may only be completing scales and questionnaires.

I have been told that the interviews will take about 30 to 60 minutes and occur at a convenient time and place in my off duty hours or with the unit manager's agreement during work hours.

I have been told that I may refuse to answer questions, stop the interview at any time or withdraw from the study. I do not have to answer any questions or discuss any subject in the interview if I do not want to. My name will not appear on the questionnaires and my specific answers will remain confidential. I will not be identified in any report or presentation that may arise from the study. Taking part in this study or dropping out will not affect my employment.

While I may not benefit directly from the study, the information gained may assist nurses with both research use and pain management for postoperative patients.

I have been told that the data (typed records of interviews, taped interviews, observations, results of questionnaires) will be preserved using record management standards that protect the privacy of the participants in the project and that guard against the disclosure of individual information. It has also been explained to me that the data may be used for other research studies in the future. If this is done, proper ethical review will be obtained to ensure the same practices of confidentiality are observed as within this study.

The above research procedures have been explained to me. Any questions have been answered to my satisfaction. I have been given a copy of this form to keep.

| _____ | _____ | _____ |
| (Signature of Participant) | (Date) | (Printed Name) |

| _____ | _____ | _____ |
| (Signature of Witness) | (Date) | (Printed Name) |

If you have any questions about this study please contact:

Dr. Carole Estabrooks (Principal Investigator) or **Telephone:** (780) 555-1234
Dr. Profetto-McGrath (Research Associate) **Telephone:** (780) 555-4321

FIGURE 4-1. Sample consent form.

In some qualitative studies, especially those requiring repeated contact with participants, it is difficult to obtain a meaningful informed consent at the outset. A qualitative researcher does not always know in advance how the study will evolve. Because the research design emerges during the data collection and analysis process, the researcher may not know the exact nature of the data to be collected, what the risks and benefits to participants will be, nor how much of a time commitment they will be expected to make. Thus, in a qualitative study, consent is often viewed as an ongoing, transactional process, referred to as **process consent.** In process consent, the researcher continuously renegotiates the consent, allowing participants to play a collaborative role in the decision-making process regarding their ongoing participation.

Example of informed consent:

Kalischuk and Davies (2001) undertook a grounded theory study focusing on individual family members' healing experiences in the aftermath of youth suicide. Before data collection, participants were given information about the study (*e.g.,* the time commitment involved, the voluntary nature of the research), and an assurance of confidentiality. Participants were informed of their right to withdraw from the study at any time without providing a reason. Each participant's informed consent was continually negotiated during the research process.

Issues Relating to the Principle of Respect

Certain circumstances make participants' right to self-determination and full disclosure problematic. One issue concerns some people's inability to make well-informed judgments about the costs and benefits of participation. Children, for example, may be unable to give truly informed consent. The issue of groups that are vulnerable within a research context is discussed later in this chapter.

Another issue is that full disclosure can sometimes result in two types of biases: (1) the bias resulting from distorted information and (2) the bias resulting from failure to recruit a good sample. Suppose a researcher were studying the relationship between high school students' substance abuse and their absenteeism from school; the researcher hypothesizes that students with a high rate of absenteeism are more likely to be substance abusers than students with a good attendance record. If the researcher approached potential participants and explained the purpose of the study, some students might refuse to participate, and nonparticipation would be selective; we would expect, in fact, that those least likely to volunteer for such a study would be students who are substance abusers—the very group of primary interest in the research. Moreover, by knowing the specific research question, those who do participate might be less inclined to give candid responses. The researcher in such a situation might argue that full disclosure would totally undermine the study.

One technique that researchers sometimes use in such situations is **covert data collection,** or *concealment*—the collection of information without the participants' knowledge and thus without their consent. This might happen, for example, if a researcher wanted to observe people's behaviour in a real-world setting and was concerned that doing so openly would result in changes in the very behaviour of interest. The researcher might choose to obtain the information through concealed methods, such as by observing through a one-way mirror, videotaping participants through hidden equipment, or observing while pretending to be engaged in other activities.

A second, and more controversial, technique is the researcher's use of deception. **Deception** can involve either deliberately withholding information about the study or providing participants with false information. For example, the researcher studying high school students' use of drugs might describe the research as a study of students' health practices, which is a mild form of misinformation.

Deception and concealment are problematic from an ethical standpoint because they interfere with the participants' right to make a truly informed decision regarding the personal costs and benefits of participation. Some people argue that the use of deception and concealment are never justified. Others, however, believe that, if the study involves minimal risk to participants and if there are anticipated benefits to science and society, deception or concealment may be justified to enhance the validity of the findings. Covert data collection and deception are least likely to be ethically acceptable if the research is focused on sensitive aspects of the participants' behaviour, such as drug use, sexual conduct, or illegal acts.

Respect for Vulnerable Persons

Respect for human dignity entails respect and high ethical obligations toward **vulnerable persons**—to those whose diminished competence or decision-making capacity make them vulnerable. Children, institutionalized persons, or others who are vulnerable are entitled, on grounds of human dignity, caring, solidarity, and fairness, to special protection against abuse, exploitation, or discrimination. Ethical obligations to vulnerable individuals in the research enterprise will often translate into special procedures to protect their interests (*TCPS*, 1998, p. i.5).

Adherence to ethical standards is often straightforward. The rights of special vulnerable groups, however, may need to be protected through additional procedures and heightened sensitivity on the part of the researcher. Vulnerable persons may be at high risk of unintended side effects because of their circumstances (*e.g.*, pregnant women). You should pay particular attention to the ethical dimensions of a study when people who are vulnerable are involved. Vulnerable groups include the following:

- *Children.* Legally and ethically, children do not have the competence to give their informed consent; therefore, the informed consent of children's parents or legal guardians is obtained. If the child is developmentally mature enough to understand the basic information involved in informed consent (*e.g.,* a 12-year-old child), the researcher should also obtain consent from the child as evidence of respect for the child's right to self-determination. With younger children, the study should be explained in simple terms and informal assent obtained.

- *Mentally or emotionally disabled people.* People whose disability makes it impossible for them to weigh the risks and benefits of participation and make an informed decision (*e.g.,* people affected by mental retardation, senility, mental illness, unconsciousness, and so on) also cannot legally or ethically provide informed consent. In such cases, the researcher obtains the written consent of the person's legal guardian. To the extent possible, informed consent from prospective participants should be sought as a supplement to consent from the guardian.

- *Physically disabled people.* For certain physical disabilities, special procedures for obtaining consent may be required. For example, with deaf people, the entire consent process may need to be in writing. For people who cannot read or write or who have a physical impairment preventing them from writing, alternative procedures for documenting informed consent (*e.g.,* videotaping the consent proceedings) can be used.

- *Institutionalized people.* Nurses often conduct studies with hospitalized or institutionalized people, and such people may feel pressured into participating or may believe that their treatment would be jeopardized by failure to cooperate. Inmates of prisons and other correctional facilities, who have lost their autonomy in many spheres of activity, may similarly feel constrained in their ability to give free consent. Researchers studying institutionalized groups need to emphasize the voluntary nature of participation.

- *Women and pregnant women.* According to Article 5.2 "Women shall not automatically be excluded from research solely on the basis of sex or reproductive capacity" (*TCPS,* 1998, p. A.9). The *TCPS* recommends that in considering research on pregnant women, researchers and ethical review groups must take into account potential harms and benefits for the pregnant woman and her embryo, fetus, or infant. The ethical duty to assess the harms and benefits of research thus extends to the special case of research involving pregnant or breastfeeding women.

⊞⊞ *Example of research with a vulnerable group:*

Peters (2001) studied the association between autonomic and motoric systems in preterm infants. Approval of the study plans was obtained from the Ethics Review Board at the University of Alberta (the researchers' affiliation) and from the ethics review committee of the hospital where the research was conducted. Parental consent was also obtained before the start of the study.

CONSUMER TIP

Many of the terms introduced in this chapter are rarely used explicitly in a research report. For example, a report almost never calls to the readers' attention that the participants in the study were members of a vulnerable group. Consumers need to be sensitive to the special needs of groups that may be unable to act as their own advocates or to assess adequately the costs and benefits of participating in a study. ■

PRINCIPLE OF RESPECT FOR PRIVACY AND CONFIDENTIALITY

Respect for human dignity also implies the principles of respect for privacy and confidentiality. In many cultures, privacy and confidentiality are considered fundamental to human dignity. Standards of privacy and confidentiality protect the access, control, and dissemination of personal information. In doing so, such standards help to protect mental or psychological integrity (*TCPS,* 1998, p. i.5).

Virtually all research with humans constitutes an intrusion into personal lives. Researchers should ensure that their research is not more intrusive than it needs to be and that the participants' privacy is maintained throughout the study.

Participants have the right to expect that any data they provide will be kept in strictest confidence. This can occur either through anonymity or through other confidentiality procedures. **Anonymity** occurs when even the researcher cannot link participants with their data. For example, if questionnaires were distributed to a group of nursing home residents and were returned without any identifying information on them, the responses would be anonymous. As another example, if a researcher reviewed hospital records from which all identifying information (*e.g.,* name, address, social insurance number, and so forth) had been expunged, anonymity would again protect people's right to privacy.

Example of anonymity:

Greenglass and Burke (2001) studied stress and the effects of hospital restructuring in nurses. Data were collected using an anonymous questionnaire mailed out to 3892 hospital nurses. The sample was chosen from 45,000 members of the nursing union using a computer-generated randomized program. Subjects were assured anonymity—the researchers did not know who received the questionnaires, which were returned to them by mail in the self-addressed, stamped envelope provided.

In situations in which anonymity is impossible, researchers implement other confidentiality procedures. A promise of **confidentiality** to participants is a pledge that any information the participant provides will not be publicly reported in such a way that the participant can be recognized or identified. As well, the information will not be made accessible to parties not involved in the research.

Researchers usually develop elaborate confidentiality procedures. These include securing individual confidentiality assurances from everyone involved in collecting or analyzing research data, maintaining identifying information in a locked file to which few people have access, substituting **identification numbers** for participants' names on study records and computer files to prevent any accidental breach of confidentiality, and reporting only aggregate data for groups of participants or taking steps to disguise a person's identity in a research report.

Extra precautions are often needed to safeguard the privacy of participants in qualitative studies. Anonymity is almost never possible in qualitative research because the researcher becomes thoroughly involved with participants. Moreover, because of the in-depth nature of many qualitative studies, there may be a greater invasion of privacy than is true in quantitative research. Researchers who spend time in the home of a study participant may, for example, have difficulty segregating the public behaviours the study participant is willing to share from the private behaviours that unfold unwittingly during the course of data collection. A final thorny issue many qualitative researchers face is adequately disguising study participants in their research reports. Because the number of respondents is small and because rich descriptive information is presented in a research report, qualitative researchers need to take extra precautions to safeguard participants' identity. This may mean more than simply using a fictitious name—it may also mean withholding information about the characteristics of the informant, such as age and occupation.

CONSUMER TIP

As a means of enhancing both personal and institutional privacy, research reports frequently avoid giving explicit information about the locale of the study. For example, the report might state that data were collected in a 150-bed nursing home without mentioning its name or location. ■

PRINCIPLE OF RESPECT FOR JUSTICE AND INCLUSIVENESS

Justice connotes fairness and equity. Procedural justice requires that the ethics review process have fair methods, standards, and procedures for reviewing research protocols, and that the process be effectively independent. Justice also concerns the distribution of benefits and burdens of research. On the one hand, distributive justice means that no segment of the population should be unfairly burdened with the demands of research. It thus imposes particular obligations toward individuals who are vulnerable and unable to protect their own interests to ensure that they are not exploited for the advancement of knowledge. History has many chapters of such exploitation. On the other hand, distributive justice also imposes duties neither to neglect nor discriminate against individuals and groups who may benefit from advances in research (*TCPS*, 1998, p. i.6).

Participants have the right to fair and equitable treatment before, during, and after their participation in the study. Fair treatment includes the following:

- The fair and nondiscriminatory selection of participants such that any risks or benefits will be equitably shared; selection should be based on research requirements and not on the vulnerability or compromised position of certain people
- The nonprejudicial treatment of people who decline to participate or who withdraw from the study after agreeing to participate
- The honouring of all agreements between the researcher and the participant, including adherence to the procedures described in advance and the payment of any promised stipends
- Participants' access to research personnel at any point in the study to clarify information
- Participants' access to appropriate professional assistance if there is physical or psychological damage
- Debriefing, if necessary, to divulge information withheld before the study or to clarify issues that arose during the study
- Sensitivity to and respect for the beliefs, habits, and lifestyles of people from different cultures
- Courteous and tactful treatment at all times
- Avoidance of conflicts of interests, particularly when the researcher is also a caregiver in nursing or in medicine

PRINCIPLE OF BALANCING HARMS AND BENEFITS

The analysis, balance, and distribution of harms and benefits are critical to the ethics of human research. Modern research ethics, for instance, require a favourable harms–benefit balance, that is, that the foreseeable harms should not outweigh anticipated benefits. Harms–benefits analysis thus affects the welfare and rights of research subjects, the informed assumption of harms and benefits, and the ethical justification for competing research paths. Because research involves advancing the frontiers of knowledge, its undertaking often involves uncertainty about the precise magnitude and kind of benefits or harms that attend proposed research. These realities and the principle of respect for human dignity impose ethical obligations on the design and conduct of research. These concerns are particularly evident in biomedical and health research (*TCPS*, 1998, p. i.6).

Box 4-1 summarizes major costs and benefits of research participation. Researchers can perhaps best evaluate the **risk–benefit ratio** by considering how comfortable they would feel having family members participate in

---

BOX 4-1 ☐ **POTENTIAL BENEFITS AND COSTS OF RESEARCH TO PARTICIPANTS**

Major Potential Benefits to Participants

Access to an intervention to which they otherwise may not have access

Gratification in being able to discuss their situation or problem with a nonjudgmental and friendly person

Increased knowledge about themselves or their conditions, either through opportunity for introspection and self-reflection or through direct interaction with the researcher

Escape from normal routine and excitement of being part of a study

Satisfaction that the information they provide may help others with similar problems or conditions

Direct monetary or material gains through stipends or other incentives

Major Potential Costs to Participants

Physical harm, including unanticipated side effects

Physical discomfort, fatigue, or boredom

Psychological or emotional distress resulting from self-disclosure, introspection, fear of the unknown or interacting with strangers, fear of eventual repercussions, anger or embarrassment at the type of questions being asked

Loss of privacy

Loss of time

Monetary costs (*e.g.,* for transportation, child care, or time lost from work)

---

the study. In your evaluation of the risk–benefit ratio of a study, you might consider whether you would have felt comfortable being a study participant.

The risk–benefit ratio should also be considered in terms of whether the risks to research participants are commensurate with the benefit to society and the nursing profession. The degree of risk to be taken by those participating in the research should never exceed the potential humanitarian benefits of the knowledge to be gained. Thus, an important question in assessing the overall risk–benefit ratio is whether the study focuses on a significant topic that has the potential to improve patient care.

Maximizing Benefits

One principle related to harms and benefits of research is **beneficence.** The principle of beneficence imposes a duty to benefit others and, in research ethics, a duty to maximize benefits. The principle has particular relevance for researchers in professions such as social work, education, health care, and applied psychology. As noted earlier, human research is intended to produce benefits for subjects themselves, for other individuals or society as a whole, or for the advancement of knowledge. In most research, the primary benefits produced are for society and for the advancement of knowledge (*TCPS*, 1998, p. i.6).

Minimizing Harms

Another principle directly related to harms–benefits analysis in **nonmaleficence,** or the duty to avoid, prevent, or minimize harms to others. Research participants must not be subjected to unecessary risks of harms, and their participation in research must be essential to achieving scientifically and societally important aims that cannot be realized without the participation of people. In addition, it should be kept in mind that the principle of minimizing harms requires that the research involve the smallest number of participants and smallest numbers of tests on these participants that will ensure scientifically valid data (*TCPS*, 1998, p. i.6).

Clearly, exposing study participants to experiences that result in serious or permanent harms is unacceptable. An ethical researcher must be prepared to terminate the research if there is reason to suspect that continuation would result in injury, death, disability, or undue distress to study participants. When a new medical procedure or drug is being tested, experimentation with animals or tissue cultures usually precedes tests with humans.

The psychological consequences of participating in a study are usually subtle and thus require close attention and sensitivity. For example, participants may be asked questions about their personal views, weaknesses, or fears. Such queries might lead people to reveal sensitive personal information. The point is not that researchers should refrain from asking questions but rather that they need to analyze the nature of the intrusion on people's psyches. Researchers strive to avoid inflicting psychological harm by tactfully phrasing questions, by providing **debriefing** sessions after the data collection is completed to permit participants to ask questions or air complaints, and, in some situations, by making referrals to appropriate health, social, or psychological services.

> **Example of risk reduction:**
>
> Varda and Behnke (2000) studied the effects of the timing of an infant bath (1 hour versus 2 hours after birth) on newborn temperature. To minimize risks, the researchers excluded all infants with conditions (*e.g.,* infection, fetal distress, hypoglycemia) that could predispose them to temperature instability.

Another aspect of minimizing harm to study participants involves ensuring **freedom from exploitation.** Involvement in a study should not place participants at a disadvantage or expose them to situations for which they have not been explicitly prepared. Participants need to be assured that their participation, or the information they might provide to the researcher, will not be used against them. For example, a person describing economic circumstances to a researcher should not be exposed to the risk of losing welfare benefits; the person reporting drug abuse should not fear exposure to criminal authorities.

Study participants enter into a special relationship with researchers, and it is crucial that this relationship not be exploited. Exploitation might be overt and malicious (*e.g.,* sexual exploitation, use of participants' identifying information to create a mailing list, and use of donated blood for the development of a commercial product), but it might also be more subtle. For example, suppose subjects have agreed to participate in a study requiring 30 minutes of their time and that the researcher decided 1 year later to go back to them, to follow their progress or circumstances. Unless the researcher had previously explained to the participants that there might be a follow-up study, the researcher could be accused of not adhering to the agreement previously reached with participants and of exploiting the researcher–participant relationship.

Because nurse researchers may have a nurse–patient (in addition to a researcher-participant) relationship, special care may be needed to avoid exploiting that bond. Patients' consent to participate in a study may result from their understanding of the researcher's role as *nurse,* not as *researcher.*

In qualitative research, the risk of exploitation may be especially acute because the psychological distance between the investigator and the participant typically declines as the study progresses. The emergence of a pseudotherapeutic relationship between the researcher and participant is not uncommon, and this imposes additional responsibilities on the researcher—and additional risks that exploitation could inadvertently occur. On the other hand, qualitative researchers are typically in a better position than quantitative researchers to do good, rather than just to avoid doing any harm, because of the close relationships they often develop with participants. Munhall (1988) has argued that qualitative nurse researchers have the responsibility of ensuring that the "therapeutic imperative of nursing (advocacy) takes precedent over the research imperative (advancing knowledge) if conflict develops" (p. 151).

RESEARCH ETHICS BOARDS

It is sometimes difficult for researchers to be objective in their assessment of the risk–benefit ratio or in the development of procedures to protect participants' rights. Biases may arise as a result of researchers' commitment to an area of knowledge and their desire to conduct a valid study. Because of the risk of a biased evaluation, the ethical dimensions of a study usually are subjected to external review.

Canada adheres to a model of ethics review that has emerged in the international community in recent decades. The model usually involves the application of national norms by multidisciplinary, independent local **Research Ethics Boards (REBs)** for reviewing the ethical standards of research projects developed within their institutions (*TCPS,* 1998, p. 8–9).

REBs are established to help ensure that ethical principles are applied to research involving human subjects. The REBs, therefore, have both educational and review roles. The boards serve the research communities as consultative bodies and thus contribute to education in research ethics; they are also charged with the responsibility for independent, multidisciplinary review of the ethics of research to determine whether the research should be permitted to start or to continue.

Example of REB approval:

Strang (2001) conducted an interpretive narrative study with eight women caregivers of persons with dementia to gain insight into how they as caregivers experienced respite. Approval of the study was obtained from the Research Ethics Board at the University of Alberta (the researcher's affiliation) and from the ethics committee of the local home care agency.

In Canada, research that involves living human subjects, human remains, cadavers, tissues, biologic fluids, embryos, or fetuses requires review and approval by an REB before it begins. Exceptions are listed in Appendix 2, Article 1.1 of the *TCPS* (1998). For example, research about individuals involved in the public arena that is based exclusively on information, documents, and records that are publicly available is exempt (p. A.2). Also, quality assurance studies, performance reviews, or testing within normal educational requirements need not be subject to REB review (p. A2). It is important to remember that even when research does not have to be reviewed by REBs or other formal committees, researchers have a responsibility to ensure that their research plans are ethically acceptable, and it is good practice for researchers to solicit external advice even when they are not required to do so.

CONSUMER TIP

Research reports do not always provide readers with information regarding adherence to ethical principles because space limitations in professional journals make it impossible to document all aspects of the study. The absence of any mention of procedures to safeguard participants' rights does not necessarily imply that no precautions were taken. When information about ethical considerations is presented, it almost always appears in the method section, typically in the subsection devoted to data collection procedures but sometimes in the subsection describing the sample. ■

CRITIQUING THE ETHICS OF RESEARCH STUDIES

Guidelines for critiquing the ethical aspects of a study are presented in Box 4-2. A person serving on a REB or **human subjects committee** should be provided with sufficient information to answer all these questions. As noted

GUIDELINES FOR CRITIQUING THE ETHICAL ASPECTS OF A STUDY

1. Was the study approved by an ethical review committee?

2. Is there evidence that informed consent was obtained from all participants or their representatives? How was it obtained?

3. Were the participants or their representatives informed about the purpose and nature of the study?

4. Were the participants or their representatives informed about any potential risks or discomfort that may result from participation in the study?

5. Were the participants protected from any harm or discomfort (physical, emotional, and psychological)?

6. Did the benefits to participants outweigh any potential risks or actual discomfort they might experience?

7. Were participants coerced or unduly influenced to participate in the study? Did they have the right to refuse to participate or withdraw without penalty? Were vulnerable participants involved?

8. Were appropriate steps taken to safeguard the privacy of the participants? How were data kept anonymous and/or confidential?

*Adapted from the work of Polit, Beck, & Hungler (2001) and Steven (2000)

earlier, however, it may not always be possible to critique the ethical aspects of a study based on a published research report. Nevertheless, we offer a few suggestions for considering the ethical aspects of a study.

Many research reports do acknowledge that the study procedures were reviewed by a REB or human subjects committee of the institution with which the researchers are affiliated. When a research report specifically mentions a formal external review, it is usually safe to assume that a panel of concerned people thoroughly reviewed the ethical issues raised by the study.

You can also come to some conclusions based on a description of the study methods. There is usually sufficient information to judge, for example, whether the study participants were subjected to any physical or psychological harm or discomfort. Reports do not always specifically state whether informed consent was secured, but you should be alert to situations in which the data could not have been gathered as described if participation were purely voluntary.

It is often especially difficult to determine by reading research reports whether the privacy of the participants was safeguarded unless the researcher specifically mentions pledges of confidentiality or anonymity. A situation requiring special scrutiny arises when data are collected from two people simultaneously (*e.g.,* a husband and wife who are jointly interviewed); in such situations, the absence of privacy raises not only ethical concerns but also questions regarding the participants' candor.

RESEARCH EXAMPLES

Two research examples that highlight ethical issues are presented below. Use the guidelines in Box 4-2 to evaluate the ethical aspects of the studies. You may need to review the actual research reports (cited at the end of the chapter) to assess more fully the adequacy of the steps the researchers took to safeguard the participants.

Research Example of a Quantitative Study

Gibbins, Stevens, Hodnett, Pinelli, Ohlsson, and Darlington (2002) conducted a study to compare the effectiveness and safety of three interventions to relieve pain linked to the lancing of heels in neonates.

Research Summary

Gibbins and her colleagues pointed out the need for high-quality evidence on effective pain-relieving strategies for neonates hospitalized in neonatal intensive care units (NICUs). Prior research had suggested that both the administration of sucrose and the provision of nonnutritive sucking (NNS) have beneficial effects. Gibbins and co-researchers used a rigourous research design to ascertain the efficacy of *combining* sucrose and NNS as a pain management intervention. However, the researchers noted that, given the existing evidence on the benefits of using NNS or sucrose, "it was considered unethical to deny neonates a form of treatment" (p. 378). Thus, their study compared the pain-relieving efficacy and safety of three interventions: (1) sucrose and NNS, (2) sucrose alone, or (3) sterile water and NNS. The study was approved by the Research Ethics Board of the university and the university-affiliated institution where the study was conducted.

The researchers recruited 190 preterm and term neonates who were scheduled for a heel lance procedure during the first week of life. The researchers were careful to include in their study only neonates whose health and safety could not be compromised by study participation. For example, only infants with an Apgar score of 7 or higher, those who had not been diagnosed with a major congenital disorder, and those who had not undergone surgery were eligible for the study.

Because neonates could not provide informed consent, consent for participation was obtained from the parents. Of 209 parents asked for consent, only 7 refused participation. Following parental consent, the infants were put into one of the three treatment groups by the research pharmacist using a lottery-type system. All solutions needed for the study were prepared under sterile conditions, were appropriately labelled, and were brought to the neonates immediately preceding the heel lance procedure. The pain response of the neonates in each of the three treatment groups was measured using the Premature Infant Pain Profile (PIPP), which is specifically designed to be used with neonates.

Gibbins and her colleagues found that the group of neonates who received the sucrose and NNS had significantly lower PIPP scores compared with the group that received sucrose alone or sterile water and NNS. The PIPP scores did not differ between neonates in the sucrose-only and sterile water plus NNS groups.

Clinical Relevance

Despite recent improvements in the pain management of neonates who are subjected to painful procedures such as heel lances, much work remains to be done in this area. Thus, the efforts of Gibbins and her colleagues to identify effective nonpharmacologic interventions has considerable significance for clinical settings. Their contribution to the evidence base is greatly enhanced by the care that the researchers took in designing and implementing a rigourous study. The strengths of their study include the use of a powerful research design, the recruitment of a sufficiently large sample of infants, the use of well-established data collection instruments, and the careful implementation of data collection procedures.

The information provided in the article also points to the researchers' adherence to ethical principles. For example, the researchers specifically avoided comparing the targeted treatment (sucrose plus NNS) with the absence of any pain-relieving treatment (*e.g.,* sterile water alone). The researchers also identified specific eligibility criteria that are consistent with the principal of nonmaleficence. They outlined in some detail the safety measures put into place to determine and record the nature and occurrence of any adverse events. A safety committee was established before the study began. This committee was charged with the responsibility of reviewing each undesirable episode and drawing on well-established rules to terminate the infant's participation in the study. The researchers noted that there were a few adverse events during the study, but they were benign in nature, resolved spontaneously, and did not require any special intervention.

Gibbins and her colleagues concluded that, of the three interventions they tested, the most effective and safe intervention was 0.5 mL 24% sucrose combined with NNS. They observed that this intervention is simple yet efficacious and that changes in pain practice for selective painful procedures "could easily be incorporated into standard NICU care" (p. 381). The researchers also recommended, however, that research on additional pain-relieving interventions be undertaken.

Research Example of a Qualitative Study

Werezak and Stewart (2002) undertook a study designed to explore the experiences of men and women living with dementia.

Research Summary

Werezak and Stewart's study sought to shed light on the adjustment process of individuals diagnosed with dementia. They noted that most research to date had focused on the perspectives of family members and formal caregivers, rather than on those directly affected by the disease.

The researchers provided a one-page letter describing the study to the contact person at a local Alzheimer agency. The contact person helped with recruitment by distributing the description to potential study participants, all of whom had previously undergone the clinical assessment for early-stage dementia.

Patients with Alzheimer disease who expressed a willingness to participate in the study were telephoned by one of the researchers, who offered to make a home visit to further explain the research. During the visit, the researcher carefully described the nature and requirements of the study and offered assurances of confidentiality to both propsective participants and their legal representatives (proxies). If the patients and the proxies signed a consent form, the researcher proceeded with the interview.

The sample included three men and three women with early-stage dementia. Werezak and Stewart noted that, according to the American Geriatrics Society Ethics Committee, individuals in the early stages of Alzheimer disease are capable of making decisions such as the one to participate in a research study. The research report explained in considerable detail the attention paid to protect participants' rights in this study. The researchers identified three ethical issues that investigators should consider when recruiting individuals with dementia for a study: their competence, their ability to provide informed consent, and the use of proxy consent. Werezak and Stewart described several specific procedures they used to address ethical considerations. First, each participant, and the proxy, provided informed consent. Second, all participants had been screened by the agency contact person before the initial interview. Following the interview, participants underwent additional testing to verify their degree of cognitive decline and stage of dementia. Third, as a precaution, proxies were allowed to be present during the interview, although they did not themselves participate. This enabled the proxies to ascertain that participants were being treated appropriately and that the interviews were not unduly stressful. Finally, participants were assigned pseudonyms in the report to protect their confidentiality.

On the basis of these interviews, the researchers developed a preliminary theory of learning to live with dementia. The evolving theory was confirmed and elucidated at a second interview conducted 1 to 3 months later.

Clinical Relevance

The number of Canadians being diagnosed with dementia is growing steadily as our population ages. Although there is a growing body of literature on certain aspects of the disease and its treatment, there is a paucity of studies that explore the experiences of those afflicted with dementia. Studies designed to better understand the perspectives of individuals diagnosed with dementia are crucial.

The study by Werezak and Stewart detailed the continous process of adjusting to early stage dementia, a stage when most individuals are still able to participate in planning the activities in their day-to-day lives. To help caregivers understand what the process was like for individuals in early-stage dementia, the researchers identified five central phases of adaptation: antecedents, anticipation, appearance, assimilation, and acceptance.

Werezak and Stewart appropriately chose a qualitative design to gain insight into the perspectives of individuals in early-stage dementia and were careful in handling ethical considerations. Werezak and Stewart verified and clarified their preliminary model with the participants who had been interviewed, thereby strengthening the credibility of the findings.

Werezak and Stewart's theory provides clinicians with an insider's perspective of the struggles and challenges that characterize the experiences of people diagnosed with dementia. This model could serve as a useful starting point in discussing with family members how to most effectively support, interact, and intervene with their loved one.

• • • • • *SUMMARY POINTS*

- Because research has not always been conducted ethically, and because of the genuine ethical dilemmas researchers often face in designing studies that are both ethical and methodologically rigourous, **codes of ethics** have been developed to guide researchers.
- The major ethical principles incorporated into most guidelines are respect for human dignity, respect for free and informed consent, respect for vulnerable persons, respect for privacy and confidentiality, respect for justice and inclusiveness, and balancing harms and benefits.
- Respect for human dignity includes the participants' right to **self-determination,** which means participants have the freedom to control their own activities, including their voluntary participation in the study.
- **Full disclosure** means the researcher has fully described to prospective participants their rights and the full nature of the study. When full disclosure poses the risk of biased results, researchers sometimes use **covert data collection** or concealment (the collection of information without the participants' knowledge or consent) or deception (either withholding information from participants or providing false information).
- **Informed consent** procedures, which provide prospective participants with information needed to make a reasoned decision about participation, normally would involve the signing of a **consent form** to document voluntary and informed participation. In qualitative studies, consent may need to be continually renegotiated with participants as the study evolves, through **process consent** procedures.

- **Vulnerable persons** require additional protection as study participants. These people may be vulnerable because they are not able to make a truly informed decision about study participation (*e.g.,* children); because their circumstances make them believe free choice is constrained (*e.g.,* inmates); or because their circumstances heighten the risk of physical or psychological harm (*e.g.,* pregnant women).
- Respect for human dignity implies the principles of respect for privacy and confidentiality. Privacy can be maintained through **anonymity** (wherein not even the researcher knows the identity of the participants) or through formal **confidentiality** procedures that safeguard the information participants provide.
- **Beneficence** involves doing good and the protection of participants from physical and psychological harm. **Nonmaleficence** involves reducing risks and protecting participants from exploitation.
- In evaluating the **risk–benefit ratio** of a study, consumers should weigh the benefits of participation against the costs to individual participants, as well as the risks to participants against the potential benefits to society.
- External review of the ethical aspects of a study by a human subjects committee or **Research Ethics Board (REB)** should be sought for research that involves living human subjects, human remains, cadavers, tissues, biologic fluids, embryos, or fetuses.

➤➤➤➤ *CRITICAL THINKING ACTIVITIES*

Chapter 4 of the accompanying *Study Guide to Accompany Essentials of Nursing Research,* 5th edition, offers various exercises and study suggestions for reinforcing the concepts presented in this chapter. In addition, you can address the following:

1. Read the introduction and method section from one or both of the actual research studies in the Appendix of this book, and then answer the questions in Box 4-2.

2. How comfortable would you have felt as a participant in the studies described in the Appendix? How likely is it that some of the participants in the study might have felt uncomfortable or anxious?

WORLD WIDE WEBSITES

The following websites are excellent sources for further information on ethics and research in Canada:

Canadian Institutes of Health Research (CIHR): http://www.cihr.ca

Canadian Health Services Research Foundation (CHSRF): http://www.chsrf.ca

Canadian Nurses Association: http://www.cna-nurses.ca

Health Canada (HC): http://www.hc-sc.gc.ca

National Council on Ethics in Human Research (NCEHR): http://www.ncehr-cnerh.org/english/mstr_frm.html

Inter-Agency Panel on Research Ethics (IPRE): http://www.nserc.ca/programs/ethics/english/index.htm

Solicitor General of Canada: http://www.sgc.gc.ca/index_e.asp (research on inmates)

SUGGESTED READINGS

References on Research Ethics

Canadian Nurses Association. (2002a). *Code of ethics for registered nurses.* Ottawa: Author.

Canadian Nurses Association. (2002b). *Ethical guidelines for nurses in research involving human subjects.* Ottawa: Author.

Medical Research Council of Canada, Natural Sciences and Engineering Research Council of Canada, and Social Sciences and Humanities Research Council of Canada. (1998). *Tri-council policy statement: ethical conduct for research involving humans.* Ottawa: Minister of Supply and Services.

Munhall, P. L. (2001). Ethical considerations in qualitative research. In P. L. Munhall (ed.). *Nursing research: A qualitative perspective* (pp. 537–549) Sudbury, MA: Jones & Bartlett Publishers.

National Commission for the Protection of Human Subjects of Biomedical and Behavioral Research. (1978). *Belmont Report: Ethical principles and guidelines for research involving human subjects.* Washington, DC: U.S. Government Printing Office.

Polit, D. F., Beck, C. T., & Hungler, B. P. (2001). *Essentials of Nursing Research* (5th ed.) Philadelphia: Lippincott Williams & Wilkins.

Silva, M. C. (1995). Ethical guidelines in the conduct, dissemination, and implementation of nursing research. Washington, DC: American Nurses Association.

Substantive References

Gibbins, S., Stevens, B., Hodnett, E., Pinelli, J., Ohlsson, A., & Darlington, G. (2002). Efficacy and safety of sucrose for procedural pain relief in preterm and term neonates. *Nursing Research, 51,* 375–382.

Greenglass, E. R., & Burke, R. J. (2001). Stress and the effects of hospital restructuring in nurses. *Canadian Journal of Nursing Research, 33,* 93–108.

Kalischuk, R. G., & Davies, B. (2001). A theory of healing in the aftermath of youth suicide. Implications for holistic nursing practice. *Journal of Holistic Nursing, 19,* 163–186.

Peters, K. L. (2001). Association between autonomic and motoric systems in the preterm infant. *Clinical Nursing Research, 10,* 82–90.

Steven, D. (2000). Nursing research: understanding the ethics of nursing research. Unpublished document. Laurentian University, Thunder Bay, Ontario, Canada.

Strang, V. R. (2001). Family caregiver respite and leisure: A feminist perspective. *Scandinavian Journal of Caring Sciences, 15,* 74–81.

Varda, K. E., & Behnke, R. S. (2000). The effect of timing of initial bath on newborn's temperature. *Journal of Obstetric, Gynecologic, and Neonatal Nursing, 29,* 27–32.

Werezak, L., & Stewart, N. (2002). Learning to live with dementia. *Canadian Journal of Nursing Research, 34,* 67–85.

PART II

PRELIMINARY STEPS IN THE RESEARCH PROCESS

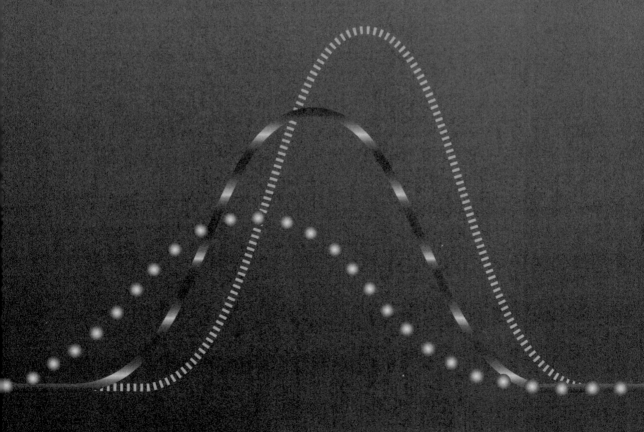

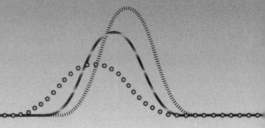

Scrutinizing Research Problems, Research Questions, and Hypotheses

RESEARCH PROBLEMS AND RESEARCH QUESTIONS
Basic Terms Relating to Research Problems
Research Problems and Paradigms
Sources of Research Problems
Development and Refinement of Research Problems
COMMUNICATING THE RESEARCH PROBLEM, PURPOSE, AND QUESTIONS
Problem Statements
Statements of Purpose
Research Questions
RESEARCH HYPOTHESES
Function of Hypotheses in Quantitative Research
Characteristics of Testable Hypotheses
Wording of the Hypothesis
Hypothesis Testing and Proof

CRITIQUING RESEARCH PROBLEMS, RESEARCH QUESTIONS, AND HYPOTHESES
Critiquing the Significance of a Research Problem
Critiquing Other Aspects of Research Problems
RESEARCH EXAMPLES
Research Example of a Quantitative Study
Research Example of a Qualitative Study
SUMMARY POINTS
CRITICAL THINKING ACTIVITIES
SUGGESTED READINGS
Methodologic References
Substantive References

Student Objectives

On completion of this chapter, the student will be able to:

○ evaluate the compatibility of a research problem and a paradigm
○ describe the process of developing and refining a research problem
○ distinguish the functions and forms of statements of purpose and research questions for quantitative and qualitative studies
○ describe the function and characteristics of research hypotheses and distinguish different types of hypotheses (*e.g.,* directional versus nondirectional, research versus null)
○ critique statements of purpose, research questions, and hypotheses in research reports with respect to their placement, clarity, wording, and significance to nursing
○ define new terms in the chapter

New Terms

Directional hypothesis	Research hypothesis
Hypothesis	Research problem
Nondirectional hypothesis	Research question
Null hypothesis	Statement of purpose
Problem statement	Statistical hypothesis
Research aim	

RESEARCH PROBLEMS AND RESEARCH QUESTIONS

A research study begins as a problem that a researcher would like to solve or as a question that a researcher would like to answer. This chapter discusses the formulation and evaluation of research problems, research questions, and hypotheses. We begin by clarifying some related terms.

Basic Terms Relating to Research Problems

At the most general level, a researcher is interested in a topic, which is sometimes referred to as the *focus* of the research. Patient compliance, coping with disability, and pain management are examples of research topics. Within these broad topic areas are many potential research questions or research problems. In this section, we illustrate various terms using the topic *side effects in chemotherapy patients.*

A **research problem** involves an enigmatic, perplexing, or troubling condition. The purpose of disciplined research is to "solve" the problem—or to contribute to its solution—by accumulating relevant information. A **problem statement** articulates the problem to be addressed. Table 5-1 presents a problem statement related to the topic of side effects in chemotherapy patients.

A **research question** is a statement of the specific query the researcher wants to answer, to address the research problem. The research question or questions guide the types of data to be collected in the study. A researcher who makes a prediction regarding answers to the research question poses a **hypothesis** that is tested empirically. Examples of both research questions and hypotheses are presented in Table 5-1.

In a research report, consumers might also encounter other related terms. For example, many reports include a **statement of purpose** (or purpose statement), which is the researcher's summary of the overall study goal. A researcher might also identify several specific **research aims** or *objectives*—the specific accomplishments the researcher hopes to achieve by conducting the study. The objectives include obtaining answers to the research questions but

TABLE 5-1. Example of Terms Relating to Research Problems	
TERM	**EXAMPLE**
Topic/focus	Side effects in chemotherapy patients
Problem statement	Nausea and vomiting are common side effects among chemotherapy patients, and interventions to date have been only moderately successful in reducing these effects. New interventions that can reduce or prevent these side effects need to be identified.
Research question	What is the relative effectiveness of patient-controlled antiemetic therapy versus nurse-controlled antiemetic therapy with regard to (1) medication consumption and (2) control of nausea and vomiting in chemotherapy patients?
Hypotheses	(1) Subjects receiving antiemetic therapy by way of a patient-controlled pump will report less nausea than subjects receiving the therapy by way of nurse administration. (2) Subjects receiving antiemetic therapy by way of a patient-controlled pump will vomit less than subjects receiving the therapy by way of nurse administration. (3) Subjects receiving antiemetic therapy by way of a patient-controlled pump will consume less medication than subjects receiving the therapy by way of nurse administration.
Statement of purpose	The purpose of the study is to test an intervention to reduce chemotherapy-induced side effects—specifically, to compare the effectiveness of patient-controlled and nurse-administered antiemetic therapy for controlling nausea and vomiting in chemotherapy patients.
Aims/objectives	This study seeks to accomplish the following objectives: (1) to develop and implement two alternative procedures for administering antiemetic therapy for patients receiving moderate emetogenic chemotherapy (patient-controlled versus nurse-controlled); (2) to test three hypotheses concerning the relative effectiveness of the alternative procedures on medication consumption and control of side effects; and (3) to use the findings to develop recommendations for possible changes to therapeutic procedures.

may also encompass some broader aims (*e.g.,* to develop recommendations for changes to nursing practice based on the study results), as illustrated in Table 5-1.

Research Problems and Paradigms

Some research problems are better suited for studies using qualitative versus quantitative methods. Quantitative studies usually involve concepts that are well developed and for which reliable measurement methods have been developed. For example, a quantitative study might be undertaken to determine whether postpartum depression is higher among women who return to work 6 months after delivery than among those who stay home with their babies. There are relatively accurate measures of depression that would yield quantitative information about the level of depression in a sample of employed and nonemployed postpartum women.

Qualitative studies are often undertaken because some aspect of a concept is poorly understood, and the researcher wants to develop a rich, comprehensive, and context-bound understanding of a phenomenon. In the example of postpartum depression, qualitative methods would not be well suited to comparing levels of depression among the two groups of women, but they would be ideal for exploring, for example, the *meaning* of postpartum depression among new mothers. In evaluating a research report, an important consideration is whether the research problem fits the chosen paradigm and its associated methods.

Sources of Research Problems

Where do ideas for research problems come from? At the most basic level, research topics originate with the researcher's interests. Because research is a time-consuming enterprise, curiosity about and interest in a topic are essential to the success of the project. Explicit sources that might fuel the researcher's curiosity include the following:

- *Clinical experience.* The nurse's everyday experience provides a rich supply of problems for investigation. Problems that are in need of immediate solution have high potential for clinical significance.
- *Nursing literature.* Ideas for studies often come from reading the nursing literature, including research reports, opinion articles, and summaries of clinical issues. Research reports may suggest problem areas indirectly by stimulating the reader's imagination and directly by explicitly stating what additional research is needed.
- *Social issues.* Topics are sometimes suggested by global social issues of relevance to the health care community. For example, the feminist movement has raised questions about such topics as gender equity and domestic violence.
- *Theories.* Another source of problems lies in theories from nursing and

other related disciplines. Beginning with a theory, the researcher asks, "If this theory is correct, what would I predict about people's behaviours, states, or feelings?" The predictions can then be tested through research.

- *Ideas from external sources.* External sources can sometimes provide the impetus for a research idea. For example, ideas for studies may emerge from reviewing research priorities or as a result of a brainstorming session with other nurses, researchers, or nursing faculty.

Development and Refinement of Research Problems

The development of a research problem is a creative process. Researchers often begin with an interest in a topic area, and then develop the topic into a more specific researchable problem. As an example, suppose a nurse working on a medical unit observed that some patients complained about having to wait for pain medication when certain nurses were assigned to them. The nurse wonders why this occurs. The general research problem is discrepancy in complaints from patients regarding pain medications administered by different nurses. The nurse might ask, "What accounts for this discrepancy?" or, "How could this situation be altered?" These questions are too broad to be research questions, but they may lead to other questions, such as, "How do the two groups of nurses differ?" or "What characteristics do the complaining patients share?" At this point, the nurse may observe that the cultural background of the patients and nurses appears to be a relevant factor. This may direct the nurse to a review of the literature for studies concerning ethnic groups and their relationship to nursing behaviours, or it may provoke a discussion of these observations with peers. These efforts may result in several research questions, such as:

- What is the essence of patient complaints among patients of different ethnic backgrounds?
- How do complaints by patients of different ethnic backgrounds get expressed by patients and perceived by nurses?
- Is the ethnic background of nurses related to the frequency with which they dispense pain medication?
- Is the ethnic background of patients related to the frequency and intensity of their complaints of having to wait for pain medication?
- Does the number of patient complaints increase when the patients are of dissimilar ethnic backgrounds as opposed to when they are of the same ethnic background as the nurse?
- Do nurses' dispensing behaviours change as a function of the similarity between their own ethnic background and that of the patients?

These questions stem from the same general problem, yet each would be studied differently; for example, some suggest a qualitative approach, and others suggest a quantitative one. A quantitative researcher might become curious about nurses' dispensing behaviours, based on some evidence in the literature regarding ethnic differences. Both ethnicity and nurses' dispensing behaviours are variables that can be reliably measured. A qualitative researcher who noticed differences in patient complaints would likely be more interested in understanding the essence of the complaints, the patients' experience of frustration, the process by which the problem was resolved, or the full nature of the nurse–patient interactions regarding the dispensing of medications. These are aspects of the research problem that would be difficult to measure quantitatively. Researchers choose the final problem to be studied based on several factors, including its inherent interest to them and its compatibility with a paradigm of preference.

COMMUNICATING THE RESEARCH PROBLEM, PURPOSE, AND QUESTIONS

Researchers communicate their research problems in various ways in research reports. This section discusses the wording and placement of problem statements, statements of purpose, and research questions, and the following major section discusses hypotheses.

Problem Statements

A problem statement is an expression of the dilemma or disturbing situation that needs investigation. A problem statement identifies the nature of the problem that is being addressed in the study and, typically, its context and significance. Generally, the problem statement should be broad enough to include central concerns but narrow enough in scope to serve as a guide to study design.

> *Example of a problem statement from a quantitative study:*
> Sucrose has been reported to have analgesic properties in newborns. (. . .) The American and Canadian pediatric societies have recommended the use of sucrose for such procedures as heel lances, injections, and intravenous line insertions. This is particularly important for preterm or ill infants in the neonatal intensive care unit (NICU) environment where they undergo multiple invasive, tissue-damaging, and presumably painful procedures daily. (. . .) There is mounting evidence that untreated procedural pain in newborn preterm infants can alter subsequent behaviour, specifically leading to less robust behavioural responses. Although the data on the effect of sucrose for a single painful procedure are strongly supportive of the use of sucrose for management of minor procedural pain, the effects of routine use of sucrose analgesia in preterm infants have not been evaluated (Johnston et al., 2002).

In this example, the general topic is the use of sucrose analgesia in newborns, but the investigators narrow the scope of their inquiry to studying the effect of sucrose analgesia among preterm infants. The problem statement underscores the nature of the health problem (procedural pain) and its significance for preterm care. In addition, this statement provides the rationale for conducting a new study in this area: the effect of routine use of sucrose analgesia in preterm infants has yet to be documented.

The problem statement for a qualitative study similarly expresses the nature of the problem, its context, and its significance.

Example of a problem statement from a qualitative study:

Members of cultural minority groups may find themselves surrounded by people whose values, beliefs, and interpretations differ from their own during hospitalization. This is often the case for Canada's aboriginal population because many live in culturally distinct communities (. . .). To promote healing among patients from minority cultural communities, it is important for nurses to understand the phenomenon of receiving care in an unfamiliar culture. This exploratory study examined how members of the Big Cove Mi'kmaq First Nation Community (. . .) subjectively experienced being cared for in a nonaboriginal institution (Baker & Daigle, 2000).

As in the previous example, the researchers clearly stated the nature of the problem and the justification for conducting a new study.

CONSUMER TIP

Problem statements generally appear in the introduction to a research report and are often interwoven with a review of the literature, which provides context by documenting knowledge gaps. They are rarely labeled "problem statement" and must therefore be ferreted out. ■

Statements of Purpose

Many researchers first articulate their goals as a broad statement of purpose, worded in the declarative form. The purpose statement captures, in one or two sentences, the essence of the study and establishes the general direction of the inquiry. The words *purpose* or *goal* usually appear in a purpose statement (*e.g.,* "The purpose of this study was. . ." or "The goal of this study was. . ."), but sometimes the words *intent, aim,* or *objective* are used instead.

In a quantitative study, a well-worded statement of purpose identifies the key study variables and their possible interrelationships as well as the nature of the population of interest.

Example of a statement of purpose from a quantitative study:

The purpose of this study was to determine the effectiveness of an information and support telephone intervention for reducing anxiety in patients who have undergone coronary artery bypass graft surgery, and their partners (Hartford et al., 2002).

This statement identified the populations of interest (patients who have undergone cardiac surgery and their partners), the independent variable (telephone intervention or no telephone intervention), and the dependent variable (anxiety).

In qualitative studies, the statement of purpose indicates the nature of the inquiry, the key concept or phenomenon under investigation, and the group, community, or setting under study.

Example of a statement of purpose from a qualitative study:

The purpose of this study is to describe Canadian South Asian women's use of traditional health practices, the factors affecting their use, and the importance of these practices in women's daily lives (Hilton et al., 2001).

This statement indicates the phenomenon of interest (use of traditional health practices) and the group under study (Canadian South Asian women).

The statement of purpose communicates more than just the nature of the problem. Through the researcher's selection of verbs, a purpose statement suggests the state of knowledge on the topic or the manner in which the researcher sought to solve the problem. A study whose purpose is to *explore* or *describe* a phenomenon is likely to focus on a little-researched topic; such a study often involves a qualitative approach. A statement of purpose for a qualitative study may also imply a flexible design through the use of verbs such as *understand, discover,* and *develop.* By contrast, a purpose statement indicating that the purpose is to *test* the effectiveness of some intervention or to *compare* two alternative nursing strategies suggests a study with a more established knowledge base, using a quantitative approach and perhaps a design with tight controls. Note that the researcher's choice of verbs in a statement of purpose should connote a certain degree of objectivity. A statement of purpose indicating that the intent of the study was to *prove, demonstrate,* or *show* something suggests a bias on the part of the researcher.

Research Questions

Research questions are, in some cases, direct rewordings of statements of purpose, phrased interrogatively rather than declaratively. The research questions for the examples cited earlier might be as follows:

- What is the effectiveness of an information and support telephone intervention for reducing anxiety in patients who have undergone coronary artery bypass graft surgery, and their partners?
- How do Canadian South Asian women use traditional health practices and how important are these in their lives?

Questions that are simple and direct invite an answer and help to focus attention on the kinds of data needed to provide that answer. Some research reports thus omit a statement of purpose and state only the research question. Other researchers use a set of research questions to clarify or amplify the purpose statement.

Example of research questions clarifying a statement of purpose:

Statement of purpose: The purpose of the present study was to examine women's interest in genetic testing for breast cancer risk to provide a basis for the development of community educational programs (Bottorff et al., 2002).

Research questions: What proportion of women are interested in genetic testing for breast cancer? Are there significant differences between women who have been diagnosed with breast cancer and those who have not with regard to interest in genetic testing for breast cancer risk? Are knowledge of genetic testing and sociodemographic factors associated with women's interest in genetic testing for breast cancer risk? What are the important gaps in women's knowledge of hereditary breast cancer risk and genetic testing?

In this example, the statement of purpose provides a global message about the researchers' goal. The research questions delineated more specifically the various aspects of genetic testing for breast cancer.

In a quantitative study, research questions identify the key variables (most often, the independent and dependent variable), the relationships among them, and the population under study.

Example of a research question from a quantitative study:

Does music modulate the physiologic and/or behavioural responses of preterm infants when it is played immediately following a stress-provoking event? (Butt & Kisilevsky, 2000).

In this example, the independent variable is music versus no music; the dependent variables are the physiologic and behavioural responses of preterm infants.

In qualitative studies, the research question may evolve over the course of the study. The researcher begins with a focus that defines the general boundaries of the inquiry. However, in a qualitative study the boundaries are not cast in stone; the boundaries "can be altered and, in the typical naturalistic inquiry, will be" (Lincoln & Guba, 1985, p. 228). The naturalist thus begins with a research question in mind but is sufficiently flexible that the question can be modified as new information makes it relevant to do so. As we will discuss in Chapter 9, several disciplines provide alternative traditions for qualitative research, and these traditions vary in their conceptualization of what types of questions are important and what type of methods should be used to answer them.

⊞ *Example of a research question from a qualitative study:*

How do First Nation women from a northern reserve community describe their encounters with local health care services? How are these encounters shaped by social, political, and economic factors? (Browne & Fiske, 2001).

🖉 **CONSUMER TIP**

Researchers most often state their purpose or research questions at the end of the introduction or immediately after the review of the literature. Sometimes, a separate section of a research report—typically located just before the method section—is devoted to stating the research problem formally and might be labeled "Purpose," "Statement of Purpose," or "Research Questions." ■

RESEARCH HYPOTHESES

In quantitative studies, researchers often present a statement of purpose and then one or more hypotheses. A hypothesis is a tentative prediction about the relationship between two or more variables in the population under study. In a qualitative study, the researcher does not begin with a hypothesis, in part because there is generally too little known about the topic to justify a hypothesis and in part because qualitative researchers want their inquiry to be guided by participants' viewpoints rather than by their own (although some qualitative studies may lead to the formulation of hypotheses). Thus, our discussion here focuses on hypotheses in quantitative research.

Function of Hypotheses in Quantitative Research

A hypothesis translates a research question into a prediction of expected outcomes. For instance, the research question might ask: "Does the temperature of normal saline used in endotracheal suctioning affect heart rate alterations?" The researcher might hypothesize as follows: Normal saline at room temperature used in endotracheal suctioning results in a greater decline in heart rate alterations than normal saline at body temperature.

Hypotheses sometimes emerge from a theoretical framework. The scientist reasons from theories to hypotheses and tests those hypotheses in the real world. The validity of a theory is never examined directly, but the worth of a theory can be evaluated through hypothesis testing. For example, the theory of reinforcement maintains that behaviour or activity that is positively reinforced (rewarded) tends to be learned or repeated. The theory is too abstract to test, but predictions (hypotheses) based on the theory can be tested. For instance, the following hypotheses have been deduced from reinforcement theory:

- Elderly patients who are praised (reinforced) by nursing personnel for self-feeding require less assistance in feeding than patients who are not praised.

- Pediatric patients who are given a reward (*e.g.*, a snack treat or permission to watch television) when they cooperate during nursing procedures are more compliant during those procedures than nonrewarded peers.

Both of these propositions can be tested in the real world. The theory gains support if the hypotheses are confirmed.

Even in the absence of a theoretical underpinning, well-conceived hypotheses can offer direction and suggest explanations. For example, suppose we hypothesized that nurses with a baccalaureate education are more likely to experience stress in their first nursing job than nurses with a diploma-school education. This prediction could be based on theory (*e.g.*, role conflict theory), earlier studies, or personal observations.

The development of predictions in and of itself forces the researcher to think logically, to exercise critical judgment, and to tie together earlier research findings.

Now let us suppose the above hypothesis is not confirmed by the evidence collected; that is, we find that baccalaureate and diploma nurses experience comparable stress in their first nursing assignment.

The failure of data to support a prediction forces the investigator to analyze theory or previous research critically, to review the limitations of the study's methods carefully, and to explore alternative explanations for the findings.

The use of hypotheses in quantitative studies tends to induce critical thinking and, hence, to facilitate interpretation of the data.

To further illustrate the utility of hypotheses, suppose the researcher conducted the study guided only by the research question, "Is there a relationship between a nurse's educational preparation and the degree of stress experienced on the first job?" The investigator without a hypothesis is, apparently, prepared to accept any results. The problem is that it is almost always possible to explain something superficially after the fact, no matter what the findings are. Hypotheses guard against superficiality and minimize the possibility that spurious results will be misconstrued.

CONSUMER TIP

Some quantitative research reports explicitly state the research hypotheses that guided the investigation, but most do not. In some cases, the absence of a hypothesis is appropriate, but often, the absence of a hypothesis is an indication that the researcher has failed to consider critically the implications of theory or the existing knowledge base or has failed to disclose the hunches that may have influenced the design of the study. ■

Characteristics of Testable Hypotheses

Testable research hypotheses state the expected relationship between the independent variable (the presumed cause or antecedent) and the dependent variable (the presumed effect) within a population.

Example of a research hypothesis:

Women diagnosed with preterm labour who receive relaxation therapy will have longer pregnancies than will women who do not receive relaxation therapy (Janke, 1999).

In this example, the independent variable is whether or not a woman with preterm labour received relaxation therapy, and the dependent variable is length of pregnancy. The hypothesis predicts that these two variables are related—longer pregnancies are expected among women who receive the therapy.

Unfortunately, researchers occasionally present hypotheses that fail to make a relational statement. For example, the following prediction is not a testable research hypothesis: Pregnant women who receive prenatal instruction by a nurse regarding the postpartum experience are not likely to experience postpartum depression. This statement expresses no anticipated relationship; in fact, there is only one variable (postpartum depression), and a relationship by definition requires at least two variables. This prediction, however, can be altered to make it a suitable hypothesis with an independent variable and dependent variable: Pregnant women who receive prenatal instruction are less likely to experience postpartum depression than pregnant women with no prenatal instruction. Here, the dependent variable is the women's depression and the independent variable is their receipt or nonreceipt of prenatal instruction.

The relational aspect of the prediction is embodied in the phrase "less . . . than." If a hypothesis lacks a phrase such as *more than, less than, greater than, different from, related to,* or something similar, it is not amenable to testing. As an example of why this is so, consider the original prediction: Pregnant women who receive prenatal instruction are not likely to experience postpartum depression. How would we know whether this hypothesis was supported—what absolute standard could be used to decide whether to accept or reject the hypothesis? To illustrate the problem more concretely, suppose we asked a group of mothers who received prenatal instructional the following question 1 month after delivery: "On the whole, how depressed have you been since you gave birth? Would you say:

1. Extremely depressed
2. Moderately depressed
3. Somewhat depressed
4. Not at all depressed

Based on this question, how could we compare the actual outcome with the predicted outcome? Would all the women in the sample have to say they were not at all depressed? Would the prediction be supported if 51% of the women said they were not at all depressed or only somewhat depressed? There is no adequate way of testing the accuracy of the prediction. A test is simple, however, if we modify the prediction, as suggested previously, to "Pregnant women who receive prenatal instruction are less likely to experience postpartum depression than those with no prenatal instruction." We would ask two groups of women with different prenatal instruction experiences to respond to the question and then compare the responses. The absolute degree of depression of either group would not be at issue.

Hypotheses, ideally, should be based on sound, justifiable rationales. The most defensible hypotheses follow from previous research findings or are deduced from a theory. When a relatively new area is being investigated, the researcher may have to turn to logical reasoning or personal experience to justify the predictions.

> ### CONSUMER TIP
>
> If a research report includes the researcher's hypotheses, they usually appear at the end of the introduction, just before the method section. Hypotheses are typically fairly easy to find and identify because the researcher makes a statement such as, "The study tested the following hypotheses . . ." or, "It was hypothesized that. . . ." ■

Wording of the Hypothesis

Hypotheses state the expected relationship between the independent variables and dependent variables. A hypothesis can predict the relationship between a single independent variable and a single dependent variable (a *simple hypothesis*), or it can predict a relationship between two or more independent variables or two or more dependent variables (a *complex hypothesis*). In the following examples, independent variables are indicated as IVs and dependent variables are identified as DVs:

> ### *Example of a simple hypothesis:*
>
> Parents who participated in a Stress Point Intervention by Nurses compared with those with usual care (IV) would have more satisfaction with family functioning (DV) after their children's hospitalization (Burke, Harrison, Kauffman, & Wong, 2001).

> ### *Example of a complex hypothesis—multiple independent variables:*
>
> Low-risk pregnant women who (1) value health highly, (2) believe that engaging in health-promoting behaviours will result in positive outcomes, and (3) perceive fewer barriers to health-promoting activities (IVs) are more likely to attend pregnancy-related educational programs (DV) than those women who do not show these characteristics (Serafine & Broom, 1999).

> **Example of a complex hypothesis—multiple dependent variables:**
> Chronically iron-loaded mice versus those in the placebo group (IV) would have dose-dependent increases in total heart iron concentrations, decreased antioxidant reserves as quantified by glutathione peroxidase activity, increases in oxygen free-radical production in the heart as quantified by cytotoxic aldehydes, and decreases in cardiac function (DVs) (Bartfay & Bartfay, 2000).

Hypotheses can be stated in various ways as long as the researcher specifies or implies the relationship that will be tested. Here is an example:

1. Lower levels of exercise postpartum are associated with greater weight retention.
2. There is a relationship between level of exercise postpartum and weight retention.
3. The greater the level of exercise postpartum, the lower the weight retention.
4. Women with different levels of exercise postpartum differ with regard to weight retention.
5. Weight retention postpartum decreases as the woman's level of exercise increases.
6. Women who exercise vigorously postpartum have lower weight retention than women who do not.

Other variations are also possible. The important point to remember is that the hypothesis specifies the independent variable (here, level of exercise), the dependent variable (weight retention), and the anticipated relationship between them.

Hypotheses, ideally, are worded in the present tense. The researcher makes a prediction about a relationship in the population—not just about a relationship that will be revealed in a particular sample of study participants.

Hypotheses can be either directional or nondirectional. A **directional hypothesis** is one that specifies the expected direction of the relationship between variables. That is, the researcher predicts not only the existence of a relationship but also its nature. In the six versions of the same hypothesis above, versions 1, 3, 5, and 6 are directional because there is an explicit prediction that women who do not exercise postpartum are at greater risk of weight retention than women who do. A **nondirectional hypothesis,** by contrast, does not stipulate the direction of the relationship, as illustrated in versions 2 and 4. These hypotheses predict that a woman's level of exercise and weight retention are related, but they do not stipulate whether the researcher thinks that exercise is related to more or less weight retention.

Hypotheses derived from theory are usually directional because theories provide a rationale for expecting variables to relate in certain ways. Existing studies also offer a basis for specifying directional hypotheses. When there is no theory or related research, when the findings of prior studies are contradictory, or when the researcher's own experience results in ambivalent expectations, the investigator may use nondirectional hypotheses. Some people argue, in fact, that nondirectional hypotheses are preferable because they connote a degree of impartiality. Directional hypotheses, it is said, imply that the researcher is intellectually committed to a certain outcome, and such a commitment might lead to bias. This argument fails to recognize that researchers typically do have hunches about the outcomes, whether they state those expectations explicitly or not. We prefer directional hypotheses—when there is a reasonable basis for them—because they demonstrate that the researcher has thought critically about the phenomena under investigation and because they clarify the study's framework.

Another distinction is the difference between research and null hypotheses. **Research hypotheses** (also referred to as *substantive, declarative,* or *scientific hypotheses*) are statements of expected relationships between variables. Such hypotheses indicate what the researcher expects to find as a result of conducting a study. The six hypotheses on page 110 are research hypotheses.

The logic of statistical inference, which is used in hypothesis testing, dictates that, for the purposes of the statistical analysis, hypotheses be expressed as though no relationship were expected. **Null hypotheses** (or **statistical hypotheses**) state that there is no relationship between the independent variables and dependent variables. The null form of the hypothesis used in our preceding examples would be: Weight retention is unrelated to exercise levels postpartum. The null hypothesis might be compared to the assumption of innocence of an accused criminal in the Canadian justice system; the variables are assumed to be "innocent" of any relationship until they can be shown to be "guilty" through statistical procedures. The null hypothesis is the formal statement of this presumed innocence.

Research reports typically present research rather than null hypotheses. When statistical tests are performed, the underlying null hypotheses are assumed without being explicitly stated. If the researcher's actual research hypothesis is that no relationship among variables exists, the hypothesis cannot be adequately tested using traditional statistical procedures. This issue is explained in Chapter 13.

 CONSUMER TIP

If the researcher used any statistical tests (and most quantitative studies do use them), it means that there are underlying hypotheses—whether the researcher explicitly stated them or not—because statistical tests are designed to test hypotheses. ■

Hypothesis Testing and Proof

Hypotheses are never *proved* through hypothesis testing; rather, they are *accepted* or *supported*. Findings are always tentative. Certainly, if the same results are replicated in numerous investigations, greater confidence can be placed in the conclusions. Hypotheses come to be increasingly supported with mounting evidence.

Let us look more closely at why this is so. Suppose we hypothesized that height and weight are related. We predict that, on average, tall people weigh more than short people. We would then obtain height and weight measurements from a sample and analyze the data. Now suppose we happened by chance to choose a sample that consisted of short, fat people, and tall, thin people. Our results might indicate that there is no relationship between a person's height and weight. Would we then be justified in stating that this study *supported* or *demonstrated* that height and weight in humans are unrelated?

As another example, suppose we hypothesize that tall people are better nurses than short people. This hypothesis is used here only to illustrate a point because, in reality, we would expect no relationship between height and a nurse's job performance. Now suppose that, by chance again, we draw a sample of nurses in which tall nurses received better job evaluations than short ones. Could we conclude definitively that height is related to a nurse's performance? These two examples illustrate the difficulty of using observations from a sample to generalize to the population from which the sample has been taken. Other problems, such as the accuracy of the measures, the validity of underlying assumptions, and the reasonableness of the logical deductions, prohibit researchers from concluding with finality that hypotheses are proved.

CRITIQUING RESEARCH PROBLEMS, RESEARCH QUESTIONS, AND HYPOTHESES

In critiquing research reports, you will need to evaluate the extent to which the researcher has adequately communicated the research problem. The researcher's description of the problem, the statement of the study purpose, the research questions, and the hypotheses set the stage for the description of what was done and what was learned by the researcher. Ideally, you should not have to dig too deeply to decipher the research problem or to discover the questions.

Critiquing the Significance of a Research Problem

A critique of the research problem involves multiple dimensions, including a substantive dimension. That is, you need to consider whether the problem has significance for nursing. The following issues are relevant in considering the significance of a study problem:

1. *Implications for nursing practice.* A primary consideration in evaluating the significance of a research problem for a nursing study is whether it has the potential to produce findings that can improve nursing

practice. The following questions should be posed: Are there practical applications that might stem from research on the problem? Will more knowledge about the problem make a difference that matters to practicing nurses? Will the findings challenge (or lend support to) untested assumptions about nursing or health status? If the answer to such questions is no, the significance of the problem is bound to be low. Numerous studies have focused on problems with strong implications for nursing practice. For example, researchers have studied (1) the effects of home visits to new mothers on breastfeeding frequency, infant weight gain, maternal anxiety, and satisfaction with services (Gagnon, Dougherty, Jimenez, & Leduc, 2002); (2) the effects of improving hospital-to-home transition on quality of life and health services utilization for individuals admitted to hospital with heart failure (Harrison, Browne, Roberts, Tugwell, Gafni, & Graham, 2002); and, (3) the effectiveness of individualized information about treatments to men newly diagnosed with prostate cancer on levels of psychological distress (Davison, Goldenberg, Gleave, & Degner, 2003). These studies yielded information that can be used to improve patient care.

2. *Extension of knowledge base.* A study that extends, refines, or corroborates previous knowledge has a better chance of being significant than a study on an isolated research problem. Studies that build in a meaningful way on the existing knowledge base are most likely to be immediately useful to nursing practice. For example, Harrison and colleagues (2002) tested the effect of reorganizing discharge planning of patients with congestive heart failure on hospital-to-home transition. Their study expanded previous knowledge on the positive effects of previously tested similar interventions by selecting different indicators of healthy outcomes. In addition, Harrison and colleagues focused on implementing their intervention using nurses already involved in patient care, whereas previous studies added a nurse to deliver the intervention. Researchers who develop a systematic program of research, building on their own earlier findings, are especially likely to make significant contributions. For example, Beck's series of studies relating to postpartum depression (e.g., Beck & Gable, 2000; Beck, 1995, 1996, 1998, 1999) have influenced women's health care worldwide.

3. *Promotion of theory development.* Studies that either test or develop a theory have a better chance of making a lasting contribution to knowledge than studies that do not have a conceptual context. For example, Doran, Sidani, Keatings, and Doidge (2002) investigated theoretical propositions provided by the Nursing Role Effectiveness Model.

4. *Correspondence to research priorities.* Research priorities have been established by research scholars, agencies that fund nursing research (such as the Canadian Institutes of Health Research and the National Institute of Nursing Research in the United States) and various professional nursing organizations. Clearly, research problems stemming from such

priorities have a high likelihood of yielding knowledge of importance to the nursing profession because they reflect expert opinion about areas of needed research. A research report typically indicates whether a study was based on a priority area. Loiselle, Semenic, Coté, Lapointe, and Gendron (2001), for instance, conducted a study on breastfeeding information and support offered by hospitals and community health centres in the Montreal region (Quebec), a research and public health priority previously identified by the Ministry of Health and Social Services.

When critiquing a study, you need to consider whether the research problem was meaningfully based on prior research, has a relationship to a theoretical context, addresses a current research priority, and, most important, can improve nursing practice.

Critiquing Other Aspects of Research Problems

Another dimension in critiquing the research problem concerns methodologic issues—in particular, whether the research problem is compatible with the chosen research paradigm and its associated methods. You should also evaluate whether the statement of purpose or research questions have been properly worded and lend themselves to empirical inquiry.

In a quantitative study, if the research report does not contain explicit hypotheses, you need to consider whether their absence is justified. If there are hypotheses, you should evaluate whether the hypotheses are logically connected to the research problem and whether they are consistent with available knowledge or relevant theory. The wording of the hypothesis should also be assessed. The hypothesis is a valid guidepost to scientific inquiry only if it is testable. To be testable, the hypothesis must contain a prediction about the relationship between two or more variables that can be measured. The hypothesis must imply the criteria by which it could be rejected or accepted through the collection of empirical data.

Specific guidelines for critiquing research problems, research questions, and hypotheses are presented in Box 5-1.

RESEARCH EXAMPLES

This section describes how the research problem and research questions were communicated in two nursing studies, one quantitative and one qualitative. The guidelines in Box 5-1 may be useful in evaluating these aspects of the study.

Research Example of a Quantitative Study

Van Servellen, Aguirre, Sarna, and Brecht (2002) tested four hypotheses in their study of emotional distress in HIV-infected men and women.

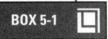

BOX 5-1

GUIDELINES FOR CRITIQUING RESEARCH PROBLEMS, RESEARCH QUESTIONS, AND HYPOTHESES

1. What is the research problem? Has the researcher appropriately delimited the scope of the problem?

2. Does the problem have significance for the nursing profession? How will the research contribute to nursing practice, nursing administration, or nursing education?

3. Is there a good match between the research problem and the paradigm within which the research was conducted?

4. Is the problem to be addressed formally stated as a statement of purpose, research question, or hypothesis to be tested? Is this information communicated clearly and concisely?

5. Are the purpose statements and research questions worded appropriately (*e.g.,* are key concepts or variables identified and the study group or population of interest specified)?

6. If the report does not formally state any hypotheses, is their absence justifiable?

7. Do the hypotheses (if any) flow from a theory or from previous research? If not, what is the basis for the researcher's predictions?

8. Are hypotheses (if any) properly worded (*i.e.,* do they state a predicted relationship between two or more variables)?

9. Are hypotheses directional or nondirectional? Is there a rationale for the manner in which they were stated?

10. Are hypotheses stated as research hypotheses or null hypotheses?

Research Summary

The researchers noted that, despite the fact that AIDS rates have been dropping for men but increasing for women, few studies have described the health experiences of HIV-infected women or compared them with those of men. This situation was viewed as especially troubling because of certain evidence indicating that, once HIV infected, women may be at greater risk than men for illness-related morbidity and adverse outcomes.

As stated by the researchers, the purpose of their study was "to describe and compare patterns of emotional distress in men and women with symptomatic HIV seeking care in community-based treatment centers" (p. 50). The conceptual framework for the study was attribution theory, which offers explanations of links between life stressors and emotional distress. This framework guided the development of the four study hypotheses, which were:

Hypothesis 1: Sociodemographic vulnerability (less than high school education, etc.) will be associated with emotional distress in both men and women.

Hypothesis 2: Poor physical and functional health status will be associated with emotional distress in both men and women.

Hypothesis 3: Optimism and social support will be associated with positive mental health outcomes (less emotional distress) in both men and women.

Hypothesis 4: Women will have higher levels of emotional distress than men (pp. 53–54).

Data for the study were collected from 82 men and 44 women with HIV disease in Los Angeles. The results indicated that women had greater disruptions in physical and psychosocial well-being than men, consistent with the fourth hypothesis. Physical health and optimism were the primary predictors of emotional distress in both men and women, supporting hypotheses 2 and 3. However, the first hypothesis was not supported in this low-income sample; there were no relationships between any sociodemographic vulnerability indicators and the participants' level of anxiety or depression.

Clinical Relevance

Current trends in the HIV/AIDS epidemic underscore the need for more attention devoted to understanding the experiences of women and the underserved who are affected by this disease. Documenting differences and similarities in the lives of men and women who have HIV/AIDS will guide the design of tailored intervention programs to improve quality of life and reduce emotional distress in this population.

Research Example of a Qualitative Study

McKeever, O'Neil, and Miller (2002) explored mothers' experiences of prolonged protective isolation with infants hospitalized for severe combined immunodeficiency.

Research Summary

In this study, mothers described their experience of prolonged protective isolation with infants treated in the protective isolation rooms for severe combined immunodeficiency. Mothers spent approximately 10 hours every day for 10.5 months in an 11-foot-square isolation room. Dressed in masks and surgical garb, they cared for their infants (no other family members were allowed in the room) but were prohibited from engaging in skin contact. In describing their research problem, the researchers stated that despite the documented deleterious physical, psychological, social, and sensory effects of even short periods of isolation among adult and child patients, very little is known about the experiences of parents who are not ill but who live through several months of isolation with extremely ill children. The objectives were to elicit women's accounts of mothering their infant in isolation and to explore the ways in which they managed the experience. The primary research questions that guided the study were:

What was it like for women to uproot themselves from their families, friends, and routine occupations to care for their infants in a segregated yet public space for up to a year's duration?

How did they manage their spatial and social relations?

How might such experiences be improved?

Five mothers participated in one to two structured, in-depth interviews lasting 1 to 1.5 hours. Mothers were asked to remember what it was like to enter the isolation room, stay with their infant, and leave the room for the last time on discharge. In analyzing the data, it became clear that all mothers experienced abrupt and profound changes in their daily routines and social relationships, and developed several strategies to manage time, space, self, and social relations.

Clinical Relevance

Information about the experiences of mothers secluded with their infants in a small protective isolation room has significant clinical and hospital policy implications. Interventions that include "sustained video links with the infant's home and family, audio-video communication with the parent residence to provide overnight reassurance for both mother and infant, and the teleprojection of family photographs, art, and other images onto the bare walls" provide important sources of pleasure and stimulation for those involved (McKeever, O'Neil, & Miller, 2002, p. 1030). In addition, encouraging the use of an additional caregiver to attend to the infant's needs is likely to reduce mothers' caregiving strain.

● ● ● ● ● *SUMMARY POINTS*

- A **research problem** is a perplexing or enigmatic situation that a researcher wants to address through disciplined inquiry. The most common sources of ideas for nursing research problems are experience, relevant literature, social issues, theory, and external sources.
- The researcher usually identifies a broad topic or focus and then narrows the scope of the problem and identifies questions consistent with a paradigm of choice.
- A **statement of purpose** summarizes the overall goal of the study; in both qualitative and quantitative studies, the purpose statement identifies the key concepts (variables) and the study group or population.
- A **research question** states the specific query the researcher wants to answer to address the research problem.
- A **hypothesis** is a statement of a predicted relationship between two or more variables. A testable hypothesis states the anticipated association between one or more independent and one or more dependent variables.
- A **directional hypothesis** specifies the expected direction or nature of a

hypothesized relationship; **nondirectional hypotheses** predict a relationship but do not stipulate the form that the relationship will take.
- **Research hypotheses** predict the existence of relationships; **statistical, or null,** hypotheses express the absence of any relationship.
- Hypotheses are never proved or disproved in an ultimate sense—they are accepted or rejected, supported or not supported by the data.

▶ ▶ ▶ ▶ *CRITICAL THINKING ACTIVITIES*

Chapter 5 of the accompanying *Study Guide to Accompany Essentials of Nursing Research*, 5th edition, offers various exercises and study suggestions for reinforcing the concepts presented in this chapter. In addition, you can address the following:

1. Read the introduction from one or both of the actual research studies in the Appendix of this book. Which of the following are explicitly stated in the research report: problem statement, statement of purpose, research questions, hypotheses, aim/objective? Where in the research report were these elements presented?

2. Respond to the questions in Box 5-1 with regard to one or both of the research reports in the Appendix.

SUGGESTED READINGS

Methodologic References

Kerlinger, F. N. (2000). *Foundations of behavioral research* (4th ed.). Fort Worth, TX: Harcourt College Publishers.

Lincoln, Y. S., & Guba, E. G. (1985). *Naturalistic inquiry.* Newbury Park, CA: Sage Publications.

Moody, L., Vera, H., Blanks, C., & Visscher, M. (1989). Developing questions of substance for nursing science. *Western Journal of Nursing Research, 11,* 393–505.

Polit, D. F., & Hungler, B. P. (2004). *Nursing research: Principles and methods* (7th ed.). Philadelphia: Lippincott, Williams & Wilkins.

Substantive References

Baker, C., & Daigle, M. C. (2000). Cross-cultural hospital care as experienced by Mi'kmaq clients. *Western Journal of Nursing Research, 22,* 8–28.

Bartfay, W. J., & Bartfay, E. B. (2000). Iron-overload cardiomyopathy: Evidence for free radical-mediated mechanisms of injury and dysfunction in a murine model. *Biological Research for Nursing, 2,* 1–11.

Beck, C. T. (1995). Perceptions of nurses' caring by mothers experiencing postpartum depression. *Journal of Obstetric, Gynecologic, and Neonatal Nursing, 24,* 819–825.

Beck, C. T. (1996). Postpartum depressed mothers' experiences interacting with their children. *Nursing Research, 45,* 98–104.

Beck, C. T. (1998). Effects of postpartum depression on child development: A meta-analysis. *Archives of Psychiatric Nursing, 12,* 12–20.

Beck, C. T. (1999). Maternal depression and child behavioral problems: A meta-analysis. *Journal of Advanced Nursing, 29,* 623–629.

Beck, C. T., & Gable, R. K. (2000). Postpartum Depression Screening Scale: Development and psychometric testing. *Nursing Research, 49*, 272–282.

Bottorff, J. L., et al. (2002). Women's interest in genetic testing for breast cancer risk: The influence of sociodemographics and knowledge. *Cancer Epidemiology, Biomarkers and Prevention, 11*, 89–95.

Browne, A. J., & Fiske, J. (2001). First Nations women's encounters with mainstream health care services. *Western Journal of Nursing Research, 23*(2), 126–147.

Burke, S. O., Harrison, M. B., Kauffmann, E., & Wong, C. (2001). Effects of stress-point intervention with families of repeatedly hospitalized children. *Journal of Family Nursing, 7*, 128–158.

Butt, M. L., & Kisilevsky, B. S. (2000). Music modulates behaviour of premature infants following heel lance. *Canadian Journal of Nursing Research, 31*, 17–39.

Davison, B. J., Goldenberg, L., Gleave, M. E., & Degner, L. F. (2003). Provision of individualized information to men and their partners to facilitate treatment decision making in prostate cancer. *Oncology Nursing Forum, 30*, 107–114.

Doran, D. I., Sidani, S., Keatings, M., & Doidge, D. (2002). An empirical test of the Nursing Role Effectiveness Model. *Journal of Advanced Nursing, 38*, 29–39.

Gagnon, A., Dougherty, G., Jimenez, V., & Leduc, N. (2002). Randomized trial of postpartum care after hospital discharge. *Pediatrics, 109*, 1074–1080.

Harrison, M. B., Browne, G. B., Roberts, J., Tugwell, P., Gafni, A., & Graham, I. D. (2002). Quality of life of individuals with heart failure: A randomized trial of the effectiveness of two models of hospital-to-home transition. [see comments]. *Medical Care, 40*, 271–282.

Hartford, K., Wong, C., & Zakaria, D. (2002). Randomized controlled trial of a telephone interaction by nurses to provide information and support to patients and their partners after elective coronary artery bypass graft surgery: Effects of anxiety. *Heart & Lung, 31*(3), 199–206.

Hilton, B. A., et al. (2001). The DESI ways: Traditional health practices of South Asian women in Canada. *Health Care for Women International, 22*, 553–567.

Janke, J. (1999). The effect of relaxation therapy on preterm labor outcomes. *Journal of Obstetric, Gynecologic, and Neonatal Nursing, 28*, 255–263.

Johnston, C. C., et al. (2002). Routine sucrose analgesia during the first week of life in neonates younger than 31 weeks' postconceptional age. *Pediatrics, 110*(3), 523–528.

Loiselle, C. G., Semenic, S. E., Côté, B., Lapointe, M., & Gendron, R. (2001). Impressions of breastfeeding information and support among first-time mothers within a multiethnic community. *Canadian Journal of Nursing Research, 33*(3), 31–46.

McKeever, P., O'Neill, S., & Miller, K-L. (2002). Managing space and marketing time: Mothering severely ill infants in hospital isolation. *Qualitative Health Research, 12*(8), 1020–1032.

Serafine, M., & Broom, B. L. (1999). Predicting low-risk women's attendance at a preterm birth prevention class. *Journal of Obstetric, Gynecologic, and Neonatal Nursing, 28*, 279–287.

van Servellen, G., Aguirre, M., Sarna, L., & Brecht, M-L. (2002). Differential predictors of emotional distress in HIV-infected men and women. *Western Journal of Nursing Research, 24*(1), 49–72.

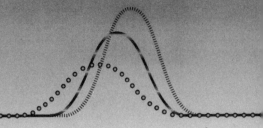

CHAPTER 6

Reviewing the Research Literature

PURPOSES AND USES OF LITERATURE REVIEWS
  Researchers and Literature Reviews
  Nonresearchers and Literature Reviews
LOCATING RELEVANT LITERATURE FOR A RESEARCH REVIEW
  Electronic Literature Searches
  The CINAHL Database
  Print Resources
PREPARING WRITTEN LITERATURE REVIEWS
  Screening References
  Abstracting and Recording Notes
  Organizing the Review
  Content of a Written Review
  Style of a Research Review
  Length of a Research Review

READING AND USING EXISTING RESEARCH REVIEWS
  Traditional Narrative Reviews
  Meta-analysis
  Qualitative Metasynthesis
  Critiquing Research Reviews
EXAMPLES OF RESEARCH LITERATURE REVIEWS
  Literature Review of a Quantitative Report
  Literature Review of a Qualitative Report
SUMMARY POINTS
CRITICAL THINKING ACTIVITIES
WORLD WIDE WEBSITES
SUGGESTED READINGS
  Methodologic References
  Substantive References

● ●

Student Objectives

On completion of this chapter, the student will be able to:

○ describe several purposes of a literature review
○ identify bibliographic aids for retrieving nursing research reports and locate references for a research topic
○ identify appropriate information to include in a review of the literature
○ understand the steps involved in writing a literature review
○ evaluate the adequacy of the types of information (*e.g.,* research findings versus anecdotes; primary versus secondary sources) included in a written literature review, and evaluate its organization and style
○ define new terms in the chapter

● ●

New Terms

Abstract journal	Online catalogue system
Author search	Online search
CINAHL database	Primary source
Electronic database	Print index
Key words	Secondary source
Literature review	Subject search
Mapping	Textword search
Meta-analysis	Unit of analysis
Metasynthesis	

PURPOSES AND USES OF LITERATURE REVIEWS

This chapter is different from other chapters in this book, which are aimed at helping nurses critically evaluate nursing research studies, rather than teaching them how to conduct research. The skills involved in reviewing the research literature and preparing a written review paper, however, are needed by both producers and consumers of nursing research. Thus, this chapter presents information on locating research reports, critiquing written literature reviews, and actually preparing a written research literature review.

The overall purpose of a research literature review is to assemble knowledge on a topic. The uses to which that knowledge are put are varied.

Researchers and Literature Reviews

For researchers, acquaintance with relevant research literature can help with the following:

- Identification of a research problem and development or refinement of research questions
- Orientation to what is known and not known about an area of inquiry, to ascertain what research can best make a contribution to knowledge
- Determination of any gaps or inconsistencies in a body of research
- Determination of a need to replicate a prior study in a different setting or with a different study population
- Identification or development of new or refined clinical interventions to test through empirical research
- Identification of relevant theoretical or conceptual frameworks for a research problem
- Development of hypotheses to be tested in a study
- Identification of suitable designs and data collection methods for a study
- Assistance in interpreting study findings and in developing implications and recommendations

Thus, a literature review helps to lay the foundation for a study with significance to nursing. A literature review is a crucial early task for most quantitative researchers. As previously noted, however, qualitative researchers sometimes deliberately avoid an in-depth literature search before entering the field to avoid having their inquiries guided by prior thought on the topic.

Researchers usually summarize relevant literature in the introduction to research reports, regardless of when they perform the literature search. The literature review provides readers with a background for understanding current knowledge on a topic and illuminates the significance of the new study. Written literature reviews thus serve an integrative function and facilitate the accumulation of knowledge. Written research reviews are also included in research proposals, documents that describe what a researcher is planning to study, how the study will be conducted, and, if funding is being sought, how much the study will cost to complete.

Nonresearchers and Literature Reviews

Research reviews are not prepared solely in the context of doing a research study. Nursing students, nursing faculty, clinical nurses, nurse administrators, and nurses involved in policy-making organizations also need to review and synthesize evidence-based information. The specific purpose of the review varies depending on the reviewer's role. Here are a few examples:

- Acquisition of knowledge on a topic (students, faculty, clinical nurses, administrators)
- Preparation of critiques of existing nursing practices and recommendations for innovations (faculty, clinical nurses, administrators, policy-oriented nurses)
- Development of research-based clinical protocols and interventions

to improve clinical practice (clinical nurses, administrators, graduate students)

- Development of a theory or conceptual framework (faculty)
- Development of and revisions to nursing curricula (faculty)
- Development of policy statements and practice guidelines (policy-oriented nurses)

Thus, both consumers and producers of nursing research need to acquire skills for preparing and reviewing written summaries of knowledge on a given problem.

LOCATING RELEVANT LITERATURE FOR A RESEARCH REVIEW

The ability to identify and locate documents on a research topic is an important skill. It is also a skill that requires adaptability; rapid technological changes, such as the expanding use of the Internet, are making manual methods of finding information from print resources obsolete, and more sophisticated methods of searching the literature are being introduced continuously. We urge you to consult with librarians at your institution or to search the Internet for updated information.

CONSUMER TIP

Locating all relevant information on a research question is a bit like being a detective. The various electronic and print literature retrieval tools are a tremendous aid, but there inevitably needs to be some digging for, and a lot of sifting and sorting of, the clues to knowledge on a topic. Be prepared for sleuthing! And do not hesitate to ask your reference librarians for help in your detective work. ∎

Electronic Literature Searches

Most college and university libraries offer students the capability of performing their own searches of **electronic databases**—huge bibliographic files that can be accessed by computer. Most of the electronic databases of interest to nurses can be accessed either through an **online search** (*i.e.,* by directly communicating with a host computer over telephone lines or the Internet) or by CD-ROM (compact discs that store the bibliographic information). Several competing commercial vendors (*e.g.,* Aries Knowledge Finder, Ovid, Paper-Chase, SilverPlatter) offer information retrieval services for bibliographic databases. Their programs are user-friendly—they are menu driven with on-screen support, so that retrieval usually can proceed with minimal instruction. Most of these service providers offer free trial services that allow you to test an online or CD-ROM system before subscribing.

The electronic databases that contain references on nursing research include the following:

- CINAHL (**C**umulative **I**ndex to **N**ursing and **A**llied **H**ealth **L**iterature)
- MEDLINE (**Med**ical Literature On-**Line**)
- PsycINFO (**Psyc**hology **Info**rmation)
- AIDSLINE (**AIDS** Information On-**Line**)
- CancerLit (**Cancer Lit**erature)
- HealthSTAR (**Health S**ervices, **T**echnology, **A**dministration, and **Re**search)
- CHID (**C**ombined **H**ealth **I**nformation **D**atabase)
- EMBASE (the **E**xcerpta **M**edica Data**base**)
- ETOH (Alcohol and Alcohol Problems Science Database)

Most libraries at institutions with nursing schools subscribe to CINAHL, one of the most useful databases for nurses. The CINAHL database is described more fully in the next section.

Several other types of electronic resources should be mentioned. First, the books and other holdings of libraries can almost always be scanned electronically using **online catalogue systems.** Moreover, through the Internet, the catalogue holdings of libraries across the country can be reviewed. Finally, it may be useful to search through Sigma Theta Tau International's Registry of Nursing Research on the Internet. This registry is an electronic research database with more than 16,000 studies that can be searched by key words, variables, and researchers' names. The registry provides access to studies that have not yet been published, which cuts down the publication lag time; however, caution is needed because these studies have not been subjected to peer review. Electronic publishing in general is expanding at a rapid pace; librarians and faculty should be consulted for the most useful websites.

CONSUMER TIP

It is rarely possible to identify all relevant studies exclusively through literature retrieval mechanisms. An excellent method of identifying additional references is to find recently published studies and examine their bibliography. Researchers are usually knowledgeable about other relevant studies and cite them to provide context for their own investigations. ■

The CINAHL Database

This section illustrates some of the features of an electronic search, through the use of the CINAHL database, the most important electronic database for nurses. Our illustrated example relied on the Ovid Search Software for CD-ROM, but similar features are available through other software programs or through direct online access.

The CINAHL database covers references to all English-language and many foreign-language nursing journals as well as to books, book chapters, nursing dissertations, and selected conference proceedings in nursing and allied health fields. The database covers materials dating from 1982 to the present. In addition to providing bibliographic information (*i.e.,* the author, title, journal, year of publication, volume, and page numbers of a reference), abstracts are available for more than 300 journals.

Most searches are likely to begin with a **subject search**—a search for references relating to a specific topic. After selecting the search command from the main menu, you would type in a word or phrase that captures the essence of the topic, and the computer would then proceed with the search. Fortunately, through **mapping** capabilities, the software translates (maps) the topic you type in to the most plausible CINAHL subject heading. An important alternative to a subject search is a **textword search** that looks for your specific words in text fields of each record, including the title and the abstract. (If you know the name of a researcher who has worked on a specific research topic, an **author search** might be productive.)

CONSUMER TIP

If you want to identify all major research reports on a topic, you need to be flexible and to think broadly about the key words and subject headings that could be related to your topic. For example, if you are interested in anorexia nervosa, you should look under anorexia, eating disorders, and weight loss, and perhaps under appetite, eating behaviour, nutrition, bulimia, body weight changes, and body image. ∎

After you have typed in your topic, the computer will tell you how many "hits" there are in the database (*i.e.*, matches against your topic). In most cases, the number of hits initially will be large, and you will want to constrain the search to ensure that you retrieve only the most relevant references. You can limit your search in a number of ways. For example, you can restrict the search to those entries for which your topic is the main focus of the document. You might also want only references published in nursing journals, only those that are for research studies, only those published in certain years (*e.g.*, after 1995), only those published in Canadian journals, or only those dealing with study participants in certain age groups (*e.g.*, infants).

To illustrate with a concrete example, suppose we were interested in recent research on treatments for postoperative pain, and we began our subject search by typing in "postoperative pain." In the CINAHL database, there are 11 subheadings for this topic, three of which (diet therapy, drug therapy, and therapy) relate to treatments. Here is an example of how many hits there were on successive restrictions to the search, using the CINAHL database current to November 2002:

Search Topic	*Restriction Hits*
Postoperative pain	1671
Restrict to main focus	1011
Restrict to therapy subheadings	710
Limit to core nursing journals	265
Limit to research reports	90
Limit to 1998–2002 publications	27

This narrowing of the search—from 1671 initial references on postoperative pain to 27 references for recent nursing research reports on treatments for postoperative pain—took less than a minute to perform. Next, we would review the 27 references on the monitor, and those references of interest could be printed or downloaded onto a disc. An example of one of the CINAHL record entries for a study identified through this search on postoperative pain treatments is presented in Figure 6-1. Each entry shows an accession number, which is the unique identifier for each record in the database. Then the authors and title of the study are displayed, followed by source information. The source indicates the following:

> Name of the journal (*Journal of Advanced Nursing*)
> Volume (36)
> Issue (4)
> Page numbers (535–545)
> Year and month of publication (2001 Nov.)
> Number of cited references (62 ref.)

The printout shows all the CINAHL subject headings for this entry, any one of which could have been used to retrieve this reference through a subject search. Note that the subject headings include both substantive/topical ones (*e.g.*, analgesics, clincial assessment tools) and methodologic ones (*e.g.*, convenience sample, correlational studies). Next, when formal, named instruments are used in the study, these are printed under Instrumentation. Finally, the abstract for the study is presented. Based on the abstract, you would decide whether this study was pertinent to your literature review; if so, the full research reports could be obtained and read. The reports in the CINAHL database can be ordered by mail or facsimile (fax); therefore, it is not necessary for your library to subscribe to the referenced journal.

☑ CONSUMER TIP

If your topic includes independent and dependent variables, you may need to do separate searches for each. For example, if you were interested in learning about the effect of stress on the health beliefs of AIDS patients, you might want to read about the effects of stress (in general) and about people's health beliefs (in general). Moreover, you might also want to learn something generally about AIDS patients and their problems. If you are searching for references electronically, you can also combine searches, so that the references for two independent searches can be linked (*e.g.*, the computer can identify those references that have both stress and health beliefs as subject headings). ■

Print Resources

Print-based resources that must be manually searched are being overshadowed by electronic databases, but their availability should not be ignored. Smaller libraries (such as hospital libraries) sometimes rely on these print resources. Moreover, it may be necessary to refer to print resources for early

Accession Number
> 2002023275.

Special Fields Contained
> Fields available in this record: abstract, cited references.

Authors
> Watt-Watson J. Stevens B. Garfinkel P. Streiner D. Gallop R.

Institution
> Associate Professor, Faculty of Nursing, University of Toronto, 50 St George Street, Toronto, Ontario, Canada M5S 3H4. E-mail: j.watt.watson@utoronto.ca.

Title
> Relationship between nurses' pain knowledge and pain management outcomes for their postoperative cardiac patients.

Source
> Journal of Advanced Nursing, 36(4):535–45, 2001 Nov. (62 ref)

Abbreviated Source
> J ADV NURS. 36(4):535–45, 2001 Nov. (62 ref)

Document Delivery
> NLM Serial Identifier: J10680000.

Journal Subset
> Core Nursing Journals. Nursing Journals. Peer Reviewed Journals. UK & Ireland Journals.

Special Interest Category
> Advanced Nursing Practice. Pain and Pain Management

Cinahl Subject Headings

Academic Medical Centers	Interviews
Adult	Male
Aged	McGill Pain Questionnaire
Aged, 80 and Over	Middle Age
Analgesics / ad[Administration and Dosage]	Multiple Regression
Cardiac Patients	Nursing Knowledge / ev[Evaluation]
Chi Square Test	*Nursing Knowledge
Clinical Assessment Tools	Ontario
Convenience Sample	Pain Measurement
Coronary Artery Bypass	Pearson's Correlation Coefficient
Correlational Studies	*Postoperative Pain / nu[Nursing]
Descriptive Research	*Postoperative Pain / dt[Drug Therapy]
Descriptive Statistics	Questionnaire
Female	T-Tests
Funding Source	Visual Analog Scaling

Instrumentation
> McGill Pain Questionnaire-Short Form (MPQ-SF). Social Desirability Scale (SDS).

Abstract
> Nurses' knowledge and perceived barriers related to pain management have been examined extensively. Nurses have evaluated their pain knowledge and management practices positively despite continuing evidence of inadequate pain management for patients. However, the relationship between nurses' stated knowledge and their pain management practices with their assigned surgical cardiac patients has not been reported. Therefore, nurses (n=94) from four cardiovascular units in three university-affiliated hospitals were interviewed along with 225 of their assigned patients. Data from patients, collected on the third day following their initial, uncomplicated coronary artery bypass graft (CABG) surgery, were aggregated and linked with their assigned nurse to form 80 nurse-patient combinations. Nurses' knowledge scores were not significantly related to their patients' pain ratings or analgesia administered. Critical deficits in knowledge and misbeliefs about pain management were evident for all nurses. Patients reported moderate to severe pain but received only 47% of their prescribed analgesia. Patients' perceptions of their nurses as resources with their pain were not positive. Nurses' knowledge items explained 7% of variance in analgesia administered. Hospital sites varied significantly in analgesic practices and pain education for nurses. In summary, nurses' stated pain knowledge was not associated with their assigned patients' pain ratings or the amount of analgesia they received.

FIGURE 6-1. Example of a printout from CINAHL search.

literature on a topic. For example, the CINAHL database does not include references to research reports published before 1982.

CONSUMER TIP

For students learning to do literature reviews, it may be useful to begin with a manual search of print resources and card catalogues before proceeding with a computer search. Manual searches can help to clarify and narrow the research topic and to identify key terms. ■

Print indexes are books used to locate research reports in journals and other documents. Indexes that are particularly useful to nurses are the *International Nursing Index, Cumulative Index to Nursing and Allied Health Literature* (the "red books"), *Nursing Studies Index, Index Medicus,* and *Hospital Literature Index*. Indexes are published periodically throughout the year (*e.g.,* quarterly), with an annual cumulative index. When using a print index, you need to first identify the appropriate subject heading. Subject headings can be located in the index's thesaurus, which lists commonly used terms, or **key words.** After the proper subject heading is determined, you can proceed to the subject section, which lists the actual references.

Abstract journals summarize articles that have appeared in other journals. Abstracting services are generally more useful than indexes because they provide a summary of a study rather than just a title. Two important abstract sources for the nursing literature are *Nursing Abstracts* and *Psychological Abstracts.*

CONSUMER TIP

If you are doing a completely manual search, it is a wise practice to begin the search for relevant references with the most recent issue of the index or abstract journal and then to proceed backward. (Most electronic databases are organized chronologically, with the most recent references appearing at the beginning of a listing.) ■

PREPARING WRITTEN LITERATURE REVIEWS

The task of identifying references for the literature review, using the guidelines and tools described in the previous section, is the first step in preparing a written review of research literature. Subsequent steps are summarized in Figure 6-2.

Screening References

As Figure 6–2 shows, after identifying potential references, you need to locate and screen them for relevance and appropriateness. In addition to obtaining reports through your library or through CINAHL and other electronic databases,

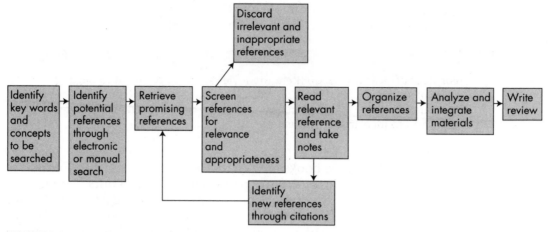

FIGURE 6-2. Flow of tasks in preparing a written research review.

many nursing journals (including *Nursing Research* and *Research in Nursing & Health*) are now available online.

The relevance of the references, which concerns whether the reference bears on the research topic, usually can be judged quickly by reading the report's abstract or introduction. Appropriateness concerns the nature of the information in the reference. The most important information for a research review comes from research reports that describe study findings. You should rely primarily on **primary source** research reports, which are descriptions of studies written by the researchers who conducted them. **Secondary source** research articles are descriptions of studies prepared by someone other than the original researcher. Literature review articles are secondary sources. Review articles, if they are recent, are an especially good place to begin a literature search because they summarize what is known and because the reference lists are helpful. However, secondary descriptions of studies should not be considered substitutes for primary sources.

Examples of primary and secondary sources relating ICU experiences:

Secondary source—a review of the literature on patient experiences in the ICU: Stein-Parbury, J., & McKinley, S. (2000). Patients' experiences of being in an intensive care unit: A select literature review. *American Journal of Critical Care, 9,* 20–27.

Primary source—an original qualitative study on patient experiences in the ICU: McKinley, S., Nagy, S., Stein-Parbury, J., Bramwell, M., & Hudson, J. (2002). Vulnerability and security in seriously ill patients in intensive care. *Intensive Critical Care Nursing, 18,* 27–36.

For some topics, it is also important to include references from the conceptual literature (*i.e.,* references on a theory or conceptual model) in a literature review. In the conceptual literature, a primary source is a description of a theory written by the developer of the theory, and a secondary source is a discussion or critique of the theory.

In addition to empirical and conceptual references, two other types of references may be identified through a literature search: opinion articles and articles describing anecdotes or clinical impressions. Opinion articles and anecdotal or other nonresearch articles may serve to broaden understanding of a research problem, illustrate a point, or demonstrate a need for research. They may thus play important roles in formulating research ideas, but they generally have limited utility in written research reviews because they are subjective and do not address the central question of written reviews: "What is the current state of knowledge on this research problem?"

Abstracting and Recording Notes

After a reference is judged to be relevant, the entire report should be read critically, using guidelines that are provided throughout this book. It is useful to photocopy an article, so that you can highlight or underline crucial information. Even with a copied article, taking notes or writing a summary of the report and its strengths and limitations is a good idea. A formal protocol is sometimes helpful for recording information in a systematic fashion. An example of such a protocol is presented in Figure 6-3. Although many of the terms on this protocol are probably unfamiliar to you at this point, you will learn their meaning as you progress through this book.

Organizing the Review

Organization of information is a crucial task in preparing a written review. When the literature on a topic is extensive, it is useful to prepare a summary table. The table could include columns with headings such as Author, Type of Study (Qualitative versus Quantitative), Sample, Design, Data Collection Approach, and Key Findings. Such a table provides a quick overview that allows the reviewer to make sense of a large mass of information.

> **⊞⊞**   ***Example of tabular organization:***
>
> Estabrooks et al. (2001) reviewed research to identify outcomes influenced by consumer decision aids (CDAs) and the particular effects of CDAs on the outcomes. Their article included four tables that summarized the research related to this topic. For example, their first table summarized 20 studies/22 reports related to CDAs. The headings in their column were: Reference (first author, date of publication, country, condition), Decision aid and Decision, Design, Subjects, Group assignment, and Control intervention.

Most writers find it helpful to work from an outline—a written one if the review is lengthy and complex, a mental one for short reviews. The important point is to sit back and work out a structure before writing so that the

Citation:
Authors: _____
Title: _____
Journal: _____
Year: _____ Volume _____ Issue _____ Pages: _____

Type of Study: ☐ Quantitative   ☐ Qualitative   ☐ Both

Location/setting: _____

**Key Concepts/
Variables:**
Concepts: _____
Intervention/Independent Variable: _____
Dependent Variable: _____
Controlled Variables: _____

Design Type: ☐ Experimental   ☐ Quasi-experimental   ☐ Pre-experimental ☐ Nonexperimental
Specific Design: _____
Descrip. of Intervention: _____
_____

☐ Longitudinal/prospective ☐ Cross-sectional   No. of data collection points: _____
Comparison group(s): _____

Qual. Tradition: ☐ Grounded theory   ☐ Phenomenology   ☐ Ethnography   ☐ Other: _____

Sample:
Size: _____ Sampling method: _____
Sample characteristics: _____

Data Sources:
Type: ☐ Self-report ☐ Observational   ☐ Biophysiologic ☐ Other: _____
Description of measures: _____
Data Quality: _____

Statistical Tests:
Bivariate: ☐ T test ☐ ANOVA ☐ Chi-square ☐ Pearson's r ☐ Other: _____
Multivariate: ☐ Multiple regression ☐ MANOVA ☐ Factor analysis ☐ Other: _____

Findings: _____
_____
_____

Recommendations: _____
_____

Strengths: _____
_____

Weaknesses: _____
_____

FIGURE 6-3. Example of a literature review protocol.

presentation has a meaningful flow. Lack of organization is a common weakness in early attempts to write a research review. Although the specifics of the organization differ from topic to topic, the overall goal is to structure the review in such a way that the presentation is logical, demonstrates meaningful integration, and leads to a conclusion of what is known and not known about the topic.

After organization of topics has been determined, a review of the notes (or the summary table) is in order. This not only helps refresh your memory about material read earlier but also lays the groundwork for decisions about where a particular reference fits in the outline. If certain references do not seem to fit anywhere, they may need to be discarded; the number of references is much less important than their relevance and the overall organization and quality of the review.

Content of a Written Review

A written research review should provide readers with an objective and thorough summary of the current state of knowledge on a topic. A literature review should be neither a series of quotes nor a series of abstracts. The central tasks are to summarize and evaluate the evidence to reveal the current state of knowledge on a topic. The review should point out both consistencies and contradictions in the literature and offer possible explanations for inconsistencies (*e.g.,* different conceptualizations or data collection methods).

Although important studies should be described in some detail, it is not necessary to provide extensive coverage for every reference. Reports of lesser significance that result in comparable findings can be summarized together.

Example of grouped studies:

Duncan et al. (2001) summarized several studies as follows: "Several authors concur that the study of workplace violence is usually limited to formal incident reports (Lippman, 1993; Lipscomb & Love, 1992; Pekrul, 1993)."

The literature should be summarized in your own words. The review should demonstrate that consideration has been given to the cumulative significance of the body of research. Stringing together quotes from various documents fails to show that previous research on the topic has been assimilated and understood.

Another point to bear in mind is that the review should be as objective as possible. Studies that conflict with personal values or hunches should not be omitted. In addition, the review should not deliberately ignore a study because its findings contradict other studies. Inconsistent results should be analyzed and the supporting evidence evaluated objectively.

The literature review should conclude with a summary of the state-of-the-art knowledge on the topic. The summary should recap study findings and indicate how credible they are; it should also make note of gaps or areas of research inactivity. The summary thus requires critical judgment about the extensiveness and dependability of the evidence on a topic.

As you progress through this book, you will become increasingly proficient in critically evaluating the research literature. We hope you will understand the mechanics of writing a research review when you have completed this chapter, but we do not expect that you will be in a position to write a state-of-the-art review until you have acquired more skills in research methods.

Style of a Research Review

Students preparing their first written research review often have trouble adjusting to the style of research reviews. Some students accept research results without criticism or reservation, reflecting a common misunderstanding about the conclusiveness of empirical research. You should keep in mind that no hypothesis or theory can be proved or disproved by empirical testing, and no research question can be definitely answered in a single study. The problem is partly a semantic one: hypotheses are not proved, they are supported by research findings; theories are not verified, but they may be tentatively accepted if a substantial body of evidence demonstrates their legitimacy. You should learn to adopt this language of tentativeness in writing a review of the literature.

A related stylistic problem is an inclination of novice reviewers to intersperse opinions (their own or someone else's) with the findings of research investigations. The review should include opinions sparingly and should be explicit about their source. The researcher's own opinions do not belong in a review, with the exception of an assessment of the quality of the studies.

The left-hand column of Table 6-1 presents several examples of stylistic flaws. The right-hand column offers recommendations for rewording the sentences to conform to a more acceptable form for a research literature review. Many alternative wordings are possible.

Length of a Research Review

There are no easy formulas for how long a review should be. The length depends on several factors, including the complexity of the research question, the extent of prior research, and the purpose for which the review is being prepared. Literature reviews prepared for proposals (*e.g.*, proposals to undertake a study, to test a clinical innovation, or to make a change in practice) tend to be comprehensive. Reviews in theses and dissertations are also lengthy. In these cases, the literature review serves both to summarize knowledge and to document the reviewer's thoroughness.

Because of space limitations in journal articles, literature reviews that appear within research reports are brief. Literature reviews in the introduction to research reports demonstrate the need for the new study and provide a context for the research questions. The literature review sections of qualitative reports tend to be especially brief.

TABLE 6-1. Examples of Stylistic Difficulties for Research Reviews

INAPPROPRIATE STYLE OR WORDING	RECOMMENDED CHANGE*
1. It is known that unmet expectations engender anxiety.	1. Several experts (Abraham, 2003; Lawrence, 2000) have asserted that unmet expectations engender anxiety.
2. The woman who does not participate in childbirth preparation classes tends to manifest a high degree of stress during labor.	2. Previous studies indicate that women who participate in preparation for childbirth classes manifest less stress during labor than those who do not (Klotz, 2000; McTygue, 2003).
3. Studies have proved that doctors and nurses do not fully understand the psychobiologic dynamics of recovery from a myocardial infarction.	3. The studies by Singleton (2003) and Fortune (2000) suggest that doctors and nurses do not fully understand the psychobiologic dynamics of recovery from a myocardial infarction.
4. Attitudes cannot be changed overnight.	4. Attitudes have been found to be relatively enduring attributes that cannot be changed overnight (O'Connell, 2003; Valentine, 2000).
5. Responsibility is an intrinsic stressor.	5. According to Dr. A. Cassard, an authority on stress, responsibility is an intrinsic stressor (Cassard, 2002, 2003).

*All references are fictious.

READING AND USING EXISTING RESEARCH REVIEWS

Most of this chapter provided guidance on how to conduct a literature review—how to locate and screen references, what type of information to seek, and how to organize and write a review. In some instances, however, a consumer may not need to conduct a full-fledged review if a recent literature review on the topic of interest has been published. For example, clinical nurses who want to develop a research-based intervention may be fortunate enough to find a relevant review that can offer them adequate direction—although they would probably also want to read the primary sources for the most pertinent studies.

Several different types of review that can be used to support evidence-based nursing practice are briefly described in this section.

Traditional Narrative Reviews

A traditional narrative literature review is one that synthesizes and summarizes, in narrative terms, a body of research literature. The information offered in this chapter has been designed to help you prepare such a review.

Narrative literature reviews are frequently published in nursing journals, especially in nursing specialty journals. These reviews may have a number of different purposes, including providing practitioners with state-of-the-art research-based information, providing a foundation for the development of innovations for clinical practice, and developing an agenda for further research.

> **Example of a narrative research review:**
>
> Buchanan et al. (2002) conducted a critical review of studies that examined reminiscing with older adults. Using CINAHL, MEDLINE, and PsycINFO databases, they identified 11 studies meeting specified criteria. Their review indicated four important components related to reminiscing with older adults: the material examined, the therapeutic goals, the process and the players, and the benefits. Their review concluded with a discussion of both research and practice implications.

Meta-analysis

Meta-analysis is a method of integrating quantitative research findings statistically. In essence, meta-analysis treats the findings from a study as one piece of data. The findings from multiple studies on the same topic are then combined to create a data set that can be analyzed in a manner similar to that obtained from individuals. Thus, instead of study participants being the **unit of analysis** (the most basic entity on which the analysis focuses), individual studies are the unit of analysis in a meta-analysis. Typically, the meta-analyst takes information about the strength of the relationship between the independent and dependent variables from each study, quantifies that information, and then essentially takes an average across all studies.

Traditional narrative research reviews can be handicapped by some factors that are uncharacteristic of meta-analysis. For example, if there are a large number of studies and the results are inconsistent, it may be difficult in a narrative review to draw conclusions. Furthermore, narrative reviews can be subject to reviewer biases; for example, the reviewer might ignore or minimize the validity of studies with certain findings. Another advantage of meta-analysis is that it can take into account the quality of the studies that are being combined. For example, studies with larger samples can be given more weight than studies with smaller samples. Meta-analysis provides a convenient and objective method of integrating a large body of findings and of observing patterns and relationships that might otherwise have gone undetected. Meta-analysis can thus serve as an important tool in research utilization.

> **Example of a meta-analysis:**
>
> Ratner et al. (2001) conducted a meta-analysis to identify factors that influenced the effectiveness of interventions in increasing women's use of mammography screening. The researchers integrated results from 69 studies promoting mammography. They found that more recent studies (those conducted from 1990 to 1996) were associated with higher screening rates. Conversely, those designed to target older women (minimum age, 50–65 years) and those set in clinics exhibited smaller screening rates. The aggregated evidence indicated that community-targeted interventions were more successful than clinic-targeted interventions. The meta-analysis also suggested methodologic issues that must be considered before the relative strength of various interventions can be assessed rigorously.

Qualitative Metasynthesis

There is an increasing awareness of the need for integrative reviews of qualitative studies so that there can be an accumulation of the understandings gained from such studies. Efforts are underway to develop techniques for qualitative metasynthesis, and several strategies have evolved. An interpretive metasynthesis is more than just a narrative integration and summary of qualitative findings (*i.e.,* a traditional literature review). **Metasynthesis** has been defined as "the theories, grand narratives, generalizations, or interpretive translations produced from the integration or comparison of findings from qualitative studies" (Sandelowski, Docherty, & Emden, 1997, p. 366). Although there are certain thorny issues that pose challenges to the conduct of a metasynthesis, there is little doubt that this is an important avenue for furthering nursing knowledge.

> *Example of a qualitative metasynthesis:*
>
> Beck (2001) conducted a metasynthesis of 14 qualitative studies on the meaning of caring within nursing education. The metasynthesis revealed five themes that permeated caring in nursing education, whether it was faculty caring for each other or their nursing students or nursing students caring for each other or their clients. These themes centred on reciprocal connecting, which consisted of presencing, sharing, supporting, competence, and the uplifting effects of caring.

Critiquing Research Reviews

Some nurses never prepare a written research review, and perhaps you will never be required to do one. Most nurses, however, do read research reviews (including the literature review sections of research reports) and they should be prepared to evaluate them critically. It may be difficult for you to critique a research review because you are likely to be less familiar with the topic than the writer. Therefore, you may not be able to judge whether the author has included all relevant literature and has adequately summarized knowledge on that topic. Many aspects of a research review, however, are amenable to evaluation by readers who are not experts on the topic. Some suggestions for evaluating written research reviews are presented in Box 6-1. Additionally, when a literature review—whether it be a traditional review, a meta-analysis, or a metasynthesis—is published as a stand-alone article, it should include information that will help you understand its scope and evaluate its thoroughness, such as the following:

- What were the criteria for selecting studies to be included in the review? For example, were studies published before a certain date excluded? Were studies involving subjects in a certain age group excluded? Were articles in a language other than English excluded?
- How were the studies identified? Was a computerized search performed, and if so, of what databases?
- What were the key words or terms used in the search?

BOX 6-1   **GUIDELINES FOR CRITIQUING RESEARCH LITERATURE REVIEWS**

1. Does the coverage of the literature seem thorough? Does it appear that the review includes all or most of the major studies that have been conducted on the topic of interest? Are recent research reports cited?

2. Does the review rely on appropriate materials (*e.g.,* mainly on research reports, using primary sources)?

3. Is the review organized in such a way that the development of ideas is clear?

4. If the review is part of a research report for a new study, does the review support the need for the new research? If the review is designed to guide clinical practice, does the review of the evidence support the need for (or lack of need for) changes in practice?

5. Does the review conclude with a synopsis of the state-to-the-art knowledge on the topic?

6. Is the style of the review appropriate? Does the reviewer paraphrase, or is there an overreliance on quotes? Does the review appear unbiased? Does the reviewer use appropriately tentative language?

In assessing a written literature review, the overarching question is whether the review summarizes the current state of research evidence. If the review is written as part of an original research report, an equally important question is whether the review lays a solid foundation for the new study.

EXAMPLES OF RESEARCH LITERATURE REVIEWS

The best way to learn about the style, content, and organization of research literature reviews is to read them. We present two excerpts from reviews here and urge you to read other reviews on a topic of interest to you.

Literature Review of a Quantitative Research Report

Ross, Carswell, and Dalziel (2001) conducted a study to investigate family caregiving following the admission of an elderly relative to a long-term care facility. These researchers wanted to know how frequently families visited their relative after admission to a long-term facility, the reasons they visited, the care they took part in while visiting their institutionalized relative, the level of satisfaction with the care provided by health care workers, and the needs and resources they require as family members. The study appeared in the journal of *Clinical Nursing Research*.

Excerpt From the Review

Research findings belie the notion of family abandonment following admission to a long-term care facility. Visiting occurs regularly (Evans & Scullion, 2000; Friedmann, Montgomery, Rice, & Farrell, 1999; Keefe & Fancey, 1996; Ross, Rosenthal, & Dawson, 1998). Families' feelings of responsibility for residents' physical and emotional well-being continue, as does the provision of care by family members (Duncan & Morgan, 1994; Hopp, 1999; Keefe & Fancey, 2000; Ross, Rosenthal, & Dawson, 1997).

Questions, however, remain about the visiting experience. Although there is evidence that families visit often, little is known about what the visiting experience is like for family members. There are reports that feelings of guilt, sadness, and depression are associated with visiting (Ross et al., 1998) and that visiting can be depressing and demoralizing for families (Grau, Teresi, & Chandler, 1993; Perris, Kinney, & Osgrocki, 1991). Motivation for visiting may lie in a long tradition of duty and obligation, with resultant feelings of duty and obligation (Ross et al., 1998). Questions also remain about task performance. The provision of care by families in an institutional setting frequently goes beyond the traditional list of tasks typically explored in research studies. Task performance has been conceptualized in many ways, including preservative, preventative, anticipatory, supervisory, and instrumental care (Bowers, 1998); technical and nontechnical care (Dempsey & Pruchno, 1993); personal, instrumental, relational, recreational and spiritual care (Ross et al., 1997); and direct and indirect care (Keefe & Fancey, 2000).

Clinical Relevance

Given the trend of an aging population in Canada, the increase in institutionalization of the elderly, and the potential need to increase resources in these settings, this study is particularly significant. The researchers report that 48% of the family members visited their relatives several times during the week. The other half of the families reported visiting once a week, daily, or less than weekly. Of these, 35% felt that they were not well prepared for the visits because they were unsure about their role during the visit. During the visits family members provided direct care (hands-on care such as bathing, grooming, toileting, feeding, etc.) and indirect care (activities related to the organization and management of care). Generally family members played a significant role in the care of their institutionalized relatives. Although the researchers reported that family caregivers were satisfied with the care received by their relatives, one third of the participants reported that the level of information shared and communication about health status was suboptimal. Sixty-one percent of family members were interested in learning how to better provide emotional support. Ross and her colleagues suggest that these findings can be used to enhance family learning to increase their contentment with the care provided to the institutionalized relatives.

Literature Review of a Qualitative Research Report

Olson, Tom, Hewitt, Whittingham, Buchanan, and Ganton (2002) conducted a study of the experiences of 29 individuals with lung and colerectal cancer before, during, and after treatment to develop a model that could explain why some individuals with cancer developed fatigue, whereas others did not. A portion of the literature review for their research report is presented below.

Excerpt From the Review

A number of investigators have documentd the presence of fatigue during and following cancer surgery (Rose & King, 1978), chemotherapy (Gianola, Sugarbaker, Barofsky, White, & Meyers, 1986; Pickard-Holley, 1991; Richardson, Ream, & Wilson-Barnett, 1998), radiotherapy (Baracos, Urtasun, Humen, & Haennel, 1994; Haylock, & Hart, 1979; King, Nail, Kreamer, Strohl, & Johnson, 1985), and both chemotherapy and radiotherapy (Irvine et al., 1994). Researchers have also shown that fatigue worsens when individuals being treated for cancer are also experiencing poor symptom control (Blesch et al., 1991; Osoba, Zee, Warr, Latreille, Kaiser, & Pater, 1997) and have documented a relationship between fatigue, symptom distress, and survival (Degner & Sloan, 1995).

Cancer treatment likely contributes to fatigue in many ways. Although we identified no studies reporting a relationship between absolute neutrophil count and fatigue, our clinical observations suggested that fatigue was associated with low absolute neutrophil counts; once patients' absolute neutrophil counts began to rise, they reported less fatigue. Several investigators have reported a relationship between fatigue, a reduction in quality of life, and a reduction in hemoglobin during cancer treatment (Abels, Larholt, Krantz, & Bryant, 1991; Ludwig et al., 1995).

Clinical Relevance

The researchers interviewed 29 men and women with lung and colerectal cancer to understand why some individuals with cancer developed fatigue, whereas others did not. The analysis of the data revealed that individuals receiving the same treatment seldom followed the same fatigue pattern. The researchers identified a 3-stage process, evolving routines, and an adaptive behavioural mode labeled gliding that characterized those who reported little or no fatigue, even when hemoglobin levels were low.

Olson and her colleagues discuss strategies for preventing fatigue and note than poor symptom control further reduces available energy. One important implication of their research was that if the side effects of treatment hypothesized to be causing sleep disturbance could be diminished, it might be possible to decrease sleep disturbances and in turn reduce fatigue, improve quality of life, and possibly increase survival.

● ● ● ● ● SUMMARY POINTS

- A research **literature review** is a written summary of the state of existing knowledge on a research problem.
- Researchers prepare literature reviews to determine knowledge on a topic of interest, to provide a context for a study, and to justify the need for a study; consumers review and synthesize evidence-based information to gain knowledge and improve nursing practice.
- An important bibliographic development for locating references is the various **electronic databases,** many of which can be accessed through an **online search** or by way of CD-ROM. For nurses, the **CINAHL database** is especially useful.
- Although electronic information retrieval is widespread, print resources such as **print indexes** and **abstract journals** are also available.
- In writing a research review, the reviewer should carefully organize the relevant materials, which should consist primarily of **primary source** research reports.
- The role of the reviewer is to point out what has been studied to date, how adequate and dependable those studies are, and what gaps exist in the body of research.
- Nurses also need to have skills in critiquing and using research reviews prepared by others, including traditional narrative reviews; **meta-analyses** (the integration of study findings using statistical procedures); and qualitative **metasyntheses** (interpretive translations produced from the integration of findings from qualitative studies).

➤ ➤ ➤ ➤ CRITICAL THINKING ACTIVITIES

Chapter 6 of the accompanying *Study Guide to Accompany Essentials of Nursing Research,* 5th edition, offers various exercises and study suggestions for reinforcing the concepts presented in this chapter. In addition, you can address the following:

1. Read the literature review sections from one or both of the actual research studies in the Appendix of this book, and then answer the questions in Box 6-1.

*For additional review, see questions 62–72 on the study CD provided with Polit: *Study Guide to Accompany Essentials of Nursing Research.*

WORLD WIDE WEBSITES

The websites for the literature retrieval service providers are:

Aries Knowledge Finder: http://www.ariessys.com

Ovid: http://www.ovid.com

PaperChase: http://www.paperchase.com

SilverPlatter: http://www.silverplatter.com

Sigma Theta Tau International Registry: http://www.nursingsociety.org

Online Journal of Issues in Nursing: http://ana.org/ojin

Information about direct online access to CINAHL can be obtained at the CINAHL website: http://www.cinahl.com

SUGGESTED READINGS

Methodologic References

Holmes, S. (1996). Systematic search offers a sound evidence base. *Nursing Times, 92,* 37–39.

Martin, P. S. (1997). Writing a useful literature review for a quantitative research project. *Applied Nursing Research, 10,* 159–162.

Sandelowski, M., Docherty, S., & Emden, C. (1997). Qualitative metasynthesis: Issues and techniques. *Research in Nursing & Health, 20,* 365–371.

Sparks, S. M. (1999). Electronic publishing and nursing research. *Nursing Research, 48,* 50–54.

Substantive References

Beck, C. T. (2001). Caring within nursing education. *Journal of Nursing Education, 40*(3), 101–109.

Buchanan, D., Moorhouse, A., Cabico, L., Krock, M., Campbell, H., & Spevakow, D. (2002). A critical review and synthesis of literature on reminiscing with older adults. *Canadian Journal of Nursing Research, 34,* 123–139.

Duncan, S. M., Hyndman, K., Estabrooks, C. A., Hesketh, K., Humphrey, C. K., Wong, J. S., Acorn, S., & Giovannetti, P. (2001). Nurses' experience of violence in Alberta and British Columbia Hospitals. *Canadian Journal of Nursing Research, 32,* 57–78.

Estabrooks, C., Goel, V., Thiel, E., Pinfold, P., Sawka, C., & Williams, I. (2001). Decision aids: Are they worth it? A systematic review. *Journal of Health Services Research & Policy, 6,* 170–182.

Olson, K., Tom, B., Hewitt, J., Whittingham, J., Buchanan, L., & Ganton, G. (2002). Evolving routines: Preventing fatigue associated with lung and colerectal cancer. *Qualitative Health Research, 12,* 655–670.

Ratner, P. A., Bottorff, J. L., Johnson, J. L., Cook, R., & Lovato, C. Y. (2001). A meta-analysis of mammography screening promotion. *Cancer Detection and Prevention, 25,* 147–160.

Ross, M. M., Carswell, A., & Dalziel, W. B. (2001). Family caregiving in long-term care facilities. *Clinical Nursing Research, 10,* 347–363.

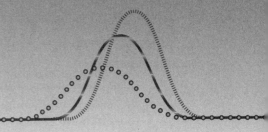

Examining Theoretical Frameworks

THEORIES, MODELS, AND FRAMEWORKS
    Theories
    Models
    Frameworks
DEVELOPING AND TESTING THEORY THROUGH RESEARCH
    Developing Theory Through Qualitative Research
    Testing Theory Through Quantitative Research
CONCEPTUAL MODELS AND THEORIES USED BY NURSE RESEARCHERS
    Conceptual Models of Nursing
    Other Models Used by Nurse Researchers

CRITIQUING CONCEPTUAL AND THEORETICAL FRAMEWORKS
RESEARCH EXAMPLES OF THEORETICAL CONTEXTS
    Research Example of a Quantitative Study
    Research Example of a Qualitative Study
SUMMARY POINTS
CRITICAL THINKING ACTIVITIES
SUGGESTED READINGS
    Methodologic References
    Substantive References

Student Objectives

On completion of this chapter, the student will be able to:

○ identify the major characteristics of theories, conceptual models, and frameworks
○ describe how theory and research are linked in quantitative and qualitative studies
○ identify several conceptual models of nursing and other conceptual models frequently used by nurse researchers
○ discuss the limitations of a study that does not have a theoretical basis or a study whose link to a theory or conceptual framework is contrived
○ define new terms in the chapter

New Terms

Borrowed theory
Conceptual definition
Conceptual framework
Conceptual map
Conceptual model
Descriptive theory
Framework
Grand theory

Grounded theory
Macro-theory
Middle-range theory
Model
Schematic model
Statistical model
Theoretical framework
Theory

THEORIES, MODELS, AND FRAMEWORKS

Theories and conceptual models are the primary mechanisms by which researchers organize findings into a broader conceptual context. Different terms are used in connection with conceptual contexts for research, including *theories, models, frameworks, schemes,* and *maps.* There is overlap in how these terms are used, partly because they are used differently by different writers. We offer guidance in distinguishing them but note that there is a blurring of these terms in the literature and that our definitions are not universal.

Theories

The term *theory* is used in many ways. For example, nursing instructors and students frequently use the term to refer to the content covered in classrooms, as opposed to the actual practice of nursing. In both lay and scientific language, the term *theory* connotes an abstraction.

Classically, scientists have used **theory** to refer to an abstract generalization that presents a systematic explanation about how phenomena are interrelated. Thus, the traditional definition requires a theory to embody at least two concepts that are related in a manner that the theory purports to explain.

Other researchers use the term *theory* less restrictively to refer to a broad characterization of a phenomenon. Some authors specifically refer to this type of theory as **descriptive theory**—a theory that accounts for (*i.e.*, thoroughly describes) a single phenomenon. Fawcett (1999) defines descriptive theories as empirically driven theories that "describe or classify specific dimensions or characteristics of individuals, groups, situations, or events by summarizing commonalities found in discrete observations" (p. 7). Descriptive theory plays an especially important role in qualitative studies.

Both classical and descriptive theory serve to make research findings meaningful and interpretable. Theories allow researchers to knit together observations into an orderly system. Theories also serve to explain research findings: theory guides the researcher's understanding not only of the "what" of natural phenomena but also of the "why" of their occurrence. Finally, theories help to stimulate research and the extension of knowledge by providing both direction and impetus.

As classically defined, theories consist of concepts and a set of propositions that form a logically interrelated deductive system. This means that the theory provides a mechanism for logically arriving at new statements from the original propositions. To illustrate, consider the theory of reinforcement, which posits that behaviour that is reinforced (*i.e.*, rewarded) tends to be repeated and learned. This theory consists of concepts (reinforcement and learning) and a proposition stating the relationship between them. The proposition readily lends itself to deductive hypothesis generation. For example, if the theory of reinforcement is valid, we could deduce that hyperactive children who are praised or rewarded when they are engaged in quiet play will exhibit less acting-out behaviours than similar children who are not praised. This prediction, as well as many others based on the theory of reinforcement, could then be tested in a study.

Theories are abstractions that are created and invented by humans. The building of a theory depends not only on observable facts but also on the theorist's ingenuity in pulling those facts together and making sense of them. Because theories are not just "out there" waiting to be discovered, it follows that theories are tentative. A theory can never be proved—a theory simply represents a theorist's best efforts to describe and explain phenomena. Through research, theories evolve and are sometimes discarded.

Theories are sometimes classified in terms of their level of generality. **Grand theories** (also known as **macro-theories**) purport to explain large segments of the human experience. Some learning theorists, such as Clark Hull, or sociologists, such as Talcott Parsons, developed general theoretical systems to account for broad classes of behaviour and social functioning. Within nursing, theories are more restricted in scope, focusing on a narrow range of phenomena. Theories that explain a portion of the human experience are sometimes referred to as **middle-range theories.** For example, there are middle-range theories that attempt to explain such phenomena as decision-making behaviour, infant attachment, and stress. This limited scope is consistent with the state of scientific developments in many fields concerned with human behaviour.

Models

A **conceptual model** deals with abstractions (concepts) that are assembled because of their relevance to a common theme. Conceptual models provide a conceptual perspective regarding interrelated phenomena, but they are more loosely structured than theories and do not link concepts in a logically derived deductive system. A conceptual model broadly presents an understanding of the phenomenon of interest and reflects the assumptions and philosophical views of the model's designer. There are many conceptual models of nursing that offer broad explanations of the nursing process. Conceptual models are not directly testable by researchers in the same way that theories are. However, conceptual models, like theories, can serve as important springboards for the generation of hypotheses to be tested.

Some writers use the term **model** to designate a mechanism for representing phenomena with a minimal use of words. Words that define a concept can convey different meanings to different people; thus, a visual or symbolic representation of a phenomenon can sometimes help to express abstract ideas in a more understandable or precise form. Two types of models referred to in the research literature are schematic models and statistical models.

Statistical models, not elaborated on here, are mathematic equations that express the nature and magnitude of relationships among a set of variables. These models are tested using sophisticated statistical methods. A **schematic model** (also referred to as a **conceptual map**) represents a phenomenon of interest in a diagram. Concepts and the linkages between them are represented through boxes, arrows, or other symbols. An example of a schematic model is presented in Figure 7–1. This model, known as *Pender's Health Promotion Model* (HPM), is described by its designer as "a multivariate paradigm for explaining and predicting the health-promotion component of lifestyle" (Pender, Walker, Sechrist, & Frank-Stromborg, 1990, p. 326). Schematic models of this type can be useful in clarifying concepts and their associations.

Frameworks

A **framework** is the conceptual underpinnings of a study. Not every study is based on a theory or conceptual model, but every study has a framework. In a study based on a theory, the framework is referred to as the **theoretical framework;** in a study that has its roots in a specified conceptual model, the framework is often called the **conceptual framework.** (However, the

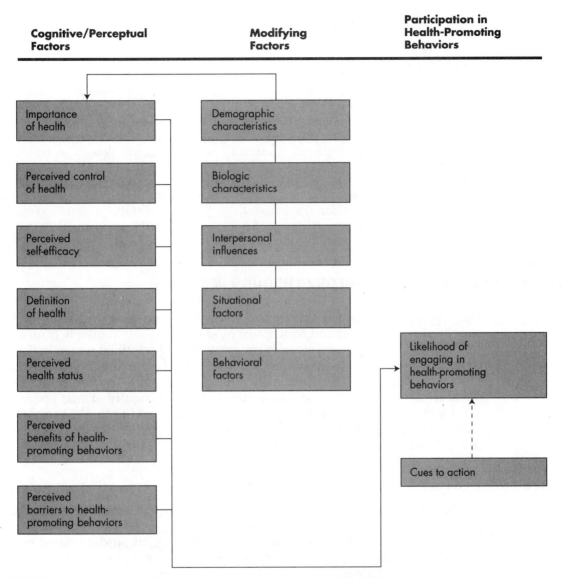

FIGURE 7-1. The health promotion model. (From Pender et al., 1990).

terms *conceptual framework, conceptual model,* and *theoretical framework* are often used interchangeably).

The framework for a study is often implicit (*i.e.,* not formally acknowledged or described by the researcher). World views (and views on nursing) shape how concepts are defined and operationalized; researchers frequently fail to clarify the conceptual underpinnings of their variables. Consider, for example, the concept of caring. Caring can be conceptualized as a human trait, a moral ideal, an affect, an interaction, or an intervention (Morse, Solberg,

Neander, Bottorff, & Johnson, 1990). Researchers undertaking studies concerned with caring should make clear what **conceptual definition** of caring they have adopted (*i.e.,* what the framework for the study is), just as the researchers must describe the operational definition.

Example of a conceptual definition:

In their study of the impact of nurses' empathic responses on patients' pain intensity, Watt-Watson et al. (2000) offered the following definitions of *empathic care.*

Conceptual definition: Empathic care is an interactive process in which health professionals wish to know and understand the subjective experience of the patient.

Operational definition: Empathic care was measured by an instrument called the Staff–Patient Interaction Response Scale (SPIRS). Nurses' verbal responses to hypothetical patient statements are scored for empathy according to instructions in a scoring manual for the scale.

DEVELOPING AND TESTING THEORY THROUGH RESEARCH

The relationship between theory and research is a reciprocal and mutually beneficial one. Theories and conceptual models are built inductively from observations, and one source of those observations is disciplined research. Concepts and relations that are validated empirically become the foundation for theory development. The theory, in turn, must be tested by subjecting deductions from it (hypotheses) to further scientific inquiry. Thus, research plays a dual and continuing role in theory building and testing. Theory can guide and generate ideas for research; research can assess the worth of the theory and provides a foundation for new ones.

Developing Theory Through Qualitative Research

Qualitative researchers often strive to develop a conceptualization of the phenomena under study that is grounded in actual observations. These researchers seek to develop a **grounded theory**—an empirically based conceptualization for integrating and making sense of a process or phenomenon.

Theory development in a qualitative study is an inductive process. The qualitative researcher seeks to identify patterns, commonalities, and relationships through the scrutiny of specific instances and events. During the ongoing analysis of data, the qualitative researcher moves from specific pieces of data to abstractions that synthesize and give structure to the observed phenomenon. The goal is to use the data, grounded in reality, to provide an explanation of events as they occur in reality—not as they have been conceptualized in preexisting theories.

Not all qualitative studies have theory development as a goal. Moreover, some qualitative researchers acknowledge an existing conceptual model as a framework for their study. For example, a number of qualitative nurse researchers acknowledge that the philosophical roots of their studies lie in such conceptual models of nursing as those developed by Rosemarie Parse (1995) or Martha Rogers (1994).

⊞ **Example of theory in a qualitative study:**

Fergus et al. (2002) examined the understudied topic of patient-provided support for spouse caregivers in the context of prostate cancer. Based on three rounds of interviews with 34 men with prostate cancer and their caregiving wives, the researchers identified a central process that they labeled *active consideration*. Active consideration encompassed four dimensions: easing spousal burden, keeping us up, maintaining connection, and considering spouse. The researchers used their findings as the basis for developing a theory expounding on the double bind of being both a patient and an agent.

Testing Theory Through Quantitative Research

There are several ways in which quantitative researchers link research to a theory, but the most common approach is to test hypotheses deduced from an existing theory. Usually, the theory (or conceptual model) was developed on the basis of cumulated research evidence, but sometimes the theory is the product of a theory-generating qualitative inquiry.

The process of theory testing begins when a researcher extrapolates the implications of the theory or conceptual framework for a problem of interest. The researcher asks: "If this theory or model is correct, what kinds of behaviour would I expect to find in specified situations?" and "What evidence could be found to support this theory?" Through such questioning, the researcher deduces implications of the theory in the form of research hypotheses. These hypotheses are predictions about how the variables would be related, if the theory were correct. For example, a researcher might deduce from reinforcement theory that verbal support and encouragement during primipara's attempts at breastfeeding would result in higher rates of successful continuation with breastfeeding. Theories are never tested directly; it is the hypotheses deduced from theories that are subjected to testing. Comparisons between the observed outcomes of research and the relationship predicted by the hypotheses are the major focus of the testing process.

⊞ **Example of theory testing in a quantitative study:**

Maurier and Northcutt (2000) used Lazarus and Folkman's (1984) Theory of Stress and Coping to examine nurses' coping strategies during the restructuring of health care in Alberta. According to the theory, the relationship between stress and a person's coping ability is mediated by primary appraisal—the *perception* of an experience as stressful or nonstressful. Maurier and Northcutt hypothesized that nurses who appraised the health care reform as threatening (high primary appraisal) would report higher levels of depression and lower levels of physical health than nurses who appraised the health care reform as a challenge with which they could cope (high secondary appraisal). Their hypothesis was supported.

Researchers sometimes base a new study on a theory or model in an effort to explain findings from previous research. For example, suppose that several researchers discovered that patients in nursing homes demonstrate greater levels of depression, anxiety, and noncompliance with nursing staff around bedtime than at other times. These descriptive findings are interesting, but they shed no light on the underlying cause of the problem and consequently suggest no way to ameliorate it. Several explanations, rooted in such theories as social learning theory, Lazarus and Folkman's stress and coping model, or one or more of the models of nursing, may be relevant in explaining the behaviour and moods of the nursing home patients. By directly testing the theory in a new study (*i.e.,* deducing hypotheses derived from the theory), a researcher could gain some understanding of why bedtime is a vulnerable period for the elderly in nursing homes.

CONSUMER TIP

When a quantitative study is based on a theory or conceptual model, the research report generally states this fact fairly early—often in the first paragraph, or even in the title. Many studies also have a subsection of the introduction called "Conceptual Framework" or "Theoretical Framework." The report usually includes a brief overview of the theory so that even readers with no theoretical background can understand, in a general way, the conceptual context of the study. ∎

A few nurse researchers have begun to adopt a useful strategy for furthering knowledge through the direct testing of two competing theories in a single study. Almost all phenomena can be explained in alternative ways. The researcher who directly tests alternative explanations, using a single sample of participants, is in a position to make powerful comparisons about the utility of the competing theories.

Example of testing competing theories:

Blythe et al. (2001) compared the utility of two alternative models for understanding the effects of hospital restructuring on nurses' lives: one pertaining to the survivor syndrome and one pertaining to empowerment. The findings suggested that the survivor syndrome may not be the most useful model to explain low morale following restructuring as it identifies nurses as "patients" in need of therapy. The empowerment model that takes into consideration nurses' concerns about uncertainty and integration appears to hold most promise for developing strategies to enhance nurses' experiences of hospital restructuring.

CONCEPTUAL MODELS AND THEORIES USED BY NURSE RESEARCHERS

Nurse researchers have used both nursing and nonnursing frameworks to provide a conceptual context for their studies. This section discusses some of the more prominent frameworks that have appeared in the nursing research literature.

Conceptual Models of Nursing

Nurses have formulated a number of conceptual models of nursing that constitute formal explanations of what nursing is. As Fawcett (1994) has noted, four concepts are central to models of nursing: person, environment, health, and nursing. The various nursing models define these concepts differently, link them in diverse ways, and give different emphasis to the relationships among them. Moreover, different models emphasize different processes as being central to nursing. For example, Sister Callista Roy's Adaptation Model identifies adaptation of patients as a critical phenomenon (Roy & Andrews, 1998). Martha Rogers and colleagues (1994), by contrast, emphasizes the centrality of the individual as a unified whole, and her model views nursing as a process in which individuals are aided in achieving maximum well-being within their potential. Nurse researchers increasingly are turning toward these conceptual models for their inspiration in formulating research questions and hypotheses. Other conceptual models of nursing that have been used in nursing studies include Allen's McGill Model of Nursing (Gottlieb & Rowat, 1987; Kravitz & Frey, 1989); King's (1981) Open System Model; Neuman's (1989) Health Care Systems Model; Orem's (1995) Model of Self-Care; and Parse's (1992, 1995) Theory of Human Becoming. Table 7-1 lists 11 conceptual models of nursing, together with a study for each that claimed the model as its framework.

Let us consider one conceptual model of nursing that has received particular attention among nurse researchers—Roy's Adaptation Model. In this model, human beings are biopsychosocial adaptive systems who cope with environmental change through the process of adaptation. Within the human system, there are four subsystems or response modes: physiologic needs, self-concept, role function, and interdependence. These subsystems constitute adaptive modes that provide mechanisms for coping with environmental stimuli and change. The goal of nursing, according to this model, is to promote patient adaptation during health and illness. Roy's Adaptation Model has been cited as the conceptual framework by many researchers.

> ***Example of a study using Roy's Adaptation Model:***
>
> Cook et al. (2001) explored the incidence and impact of physician verbal abuse on perioperative nurses, using the Roy Adaptation Model as their conceptual framework. The researchers examined how nurses used adaptive coping behaviours and problem-focused skills to deal with the abuse.

In addition to conceptual models that describe and characterize the entire nursing process, nurses have developed other models and theories that focus on specific phenomena of interest to nurses. An important example is Nola Pender's Health Promotion Model (Pender & Pender, 1996), for which a conceptual map is presented in Figure 7-1. Another example is Mishel's Uncertainty in Illness Theory (1988, 1990), which focuses on the concept of uncertainty—the inability of a person to determine the meaning of illness-related

TABLE 7-1. Conceptual Models of Nursing Used by Nurse Researchers

THEORIST AND REFERENCE	NAME OF MODEL/THEORY	KEY THESIS OF THE MODEL	RESEARCH EXAMPLE
Imogene King, 1981	Open Systems Model	Personal systems, interpersonal systems, and social systems are dynamic and interacting within which transactions occur.	Doornbos (2000) based her framework on King's model; she tested the prediction that family stressors, coping, and other factors affected family health with young adults with serious mental illness.
Madeline Leininger, 1991	Theory of Culture Care Diversity and Universality	Caring is a universal phenomenon but varies transculturally.	Gagnon and Vissandjee (2001) described how Innuit women perceived the care provided to them by family members to understand the transcultural meanings of family and care.
Myra Levine, 1973	Conservation Model	Conservation of integrity contributes to maintenance of a person's wholeness.	Deiriggi and Miles (1995) based their study of the effects of waterbeds on heart rate in preterm infants on Levine's concept of conservation.
F. Moyra Allen (In Gottlieb & Rowat, 1987 and Kravitz & Frey, 1989)	McGill Model of Nursing	Nursing is the science of health-promoting interactions. Health promotion is a process of helping individuals cope and develop; the goal of nursing is to work with and actively promote patient and family strengths toward achievement of life goals.	Edgar, Rosenberger, and Collet (2001) used concepts from the McGill model in the development of a psychoeducational coping skills training intervention, which they tested in a sample of individuals with newly diagnosed breast or colorectal cancer.
Betty Neuman, 1994	Health Care Systems Model	Each person is a complete system; the goal of nursing is to assist in maintaining patient system stability.	Skillen, Anderson, and Knight (2001) identified factors that were congruent with Neuman's concept of the created environment in their description of nurse case managers' reported use of physical assessment skills in their work with residents of continuing care facilities.
Margaret Newman, 1994	Health as Expanding Consciousness	Health is viewed as an expansion of consciousness with health and disease parts of the same whole; health is seen in an evolving pattern of the whole in time, space, and movement.	Endo and colleagues (2000) used Newman's theory to study pattern recognition as a caring partnership between Japanese nurses and families with a family member diagnosed with ovarian cancer.
Dorothy Orem, 1995	Self-Care Model	Self-care activities are what people do on their own behalf to maintain health and well-being; the goal of	Horsburgh, Beanlands, Locking-Cusolito, Howe, and Watson (2000) studied the relationship between personality factors and

(continued)

TABLE 7-1. Conceptual Models of Nursing Used by Nurse Researchers (*Continued*)

THEORIST AND REFERENCE	NAME OF MODEL/THEORY	KEY THESIS OF THE MODEL	RESEARCH EXAMPLE
		nursing is to help people meet their own therapeutic self-care demands.	the concepts of self-care agency and self-care as defined by Orem with a sample of patients with end-stage renal disease who were awaiting a kidney transplant.
Rosemarie Rizzo Parse, 1992, 1995	Theory of Human Becoming	Health and meaning are cocreated by indivisible humans and their environment; nursing involves having patients share views about meanings.	Using Parse's theory, Jonas-Simpson (2001) explored the lived experience of feeling understood among women living with a persisting health-related condition.
Martha Rogers, 1970, 1986	Science of Unitary Human Beings	The individual is a unified whole in constant interaction with the environment; nursing helps individuals achieve maximum well-being within their potential.	Using Rogers' framework, Bays (2001) explored the phenomenon of hope and associated factors in older patients who had experienced a stroke.
Sr. Callista Roy, 1984, 1991	Adaptation Model	Humans are adaptive systems that cope with change through adaptation; nursing helps to promote patient adaptation during health and illness	Roy's Adaptation Model provided the framework for John's (2001) study of whether perceptions of quality of life change over time in adults who receive curative radiation therapy.
Jean Watson, 1999	Theory of Caring	Caring is the moral ideal, and entails mind-body-soul engagement with one another.	Bourret, Bernick, Cott, and Kontos (2001) used the concepts of caring and interaction from Watson's theory as a basis from which to generate knowledge about nurses and residents' perceptions of mobility in long-term care facilities.

events. According to this theory, a situation appraised as uncertain will mobilize individuals to use their resources to adapt to the situation. Mishel's conceptualization of uncertainty has been used as a framework for both qualitative and quantitative studies.

Example of a study based on uncertainty theory:

Guided by Mishel's Uncertainty in Illness Theory, Bérubé and Loiselle (2003) studied the relationships among uncertainty, hope, and coping among individuals dealing with a spinal cord injury.

Other Models Used by Nurse Researchers

Some phenomena of interest to nurse researchers are not unique to nurses, and therefore nursing studies can be linked to frameworks that are not models of nursing. Three conceptual models that have been used frequently in nursing studies are:

- *Becker's Health Belief Model* (HBM). The HBM is a framework for explaining people's health-related behaviour, such as health care use and compliance with a medical regimen. According to the model, health-related behaviour is influenced by a person's perception of a threat posed by a health problem as well as by the value associated with actions aimed at reducing the threat (Becker, 1978). Nurse researchers have used the HBM extensively—for example, Black, Stein, and Loveland-Cherry (2001) used the HBM in their study of the contribution of the self-concept to older women's adherence to regular mammography screening behaviour.
- *Lazarus and Folkman's Theory of Stress and Coping.* This model, which explains people's methods of dealing with stress, posits that coping strategies are learned, deliberate responses to stressors that are used to adapt to or change the stressors. According to this model, people's perception of mental and physical health is related to the ways they evaluate and cope with the stresses of living (Lazarus & Folkman, 1984). An example of a nursing study based on this theory is Belleau, Hagan, and Masse's study (2001) on the effects of an educational intervention on preoperative anxiety in women awaiting a mastectomy.
- *Azjen and Fishbein's Theory of Reasoned Action* (TRA). The TRA provides a framework for understanding the relationships among a person's attitudes, intentions, and behaviours. According to the TRA, behavioural intentions are the best predictor of a person's behaviour, and behavioural intentions are a function of attitude toward performing the behaviour and subjective norms—the person's perception of whether others think the behaviour should be performed (Azjen & Fishbein, 1980). The TRA has been used in many nursing studies, including a study of the subjective norms and attitudes of female adolescents toward breastfeeding and the extent to which norms and attitudes are related to intention to breastfeed (Ross & Goulet, 2002).

The use of theories and conceptual models from other disciplines such as psychology (**borrowed theories**) has not been without controversy—some commentators advocate the development of unique nursing theories. However, nursing research is likely to continue on its current path of conducting studies within a multidisciplinary and multitheoretical perspective.

CONSUMER TIP

Among nursing studies that are linked to a conceptual model or theory, about half are based on borrowed theories. Among the models of nursing, those of Orem, Rogers, and Roy are especially likely to be used as the basis for research. ■

CRITIQUING CONCEPTUAL AND THEORETICAL FRAMEWORKS

You are likely to find references to theories and conceptual frameworks in some of the studies you read. It is often challenging to critique the theoretical context of a published research report.

In a qualitative study in which a grounded theory is presented, you will not be given enough information to refute the proposed descriptive theory; only evidence supporting the theory is presented. However, you can determine whether the theory seems logical, whether the conceptualization is truly insightful, and whether the evidence is solid and convincing.

Critiquing a theoretical framework in a quantitative report is also difficult. Most of you are not likely to be familiar with the range of relevant models in nursing and other related disciplines. Furthermore, the whole notion of theoretical frameworks, precisely because they are abstract, may provoke anxiety. Some suggestions for evaluating the conceptual basis of a quantitative study are offered in the following discussion and in Box 7-1 in the hope of lessening some of that anxiety.

The first task is to determine whether the study does, in fact, have a theoretical or conceptual framework. If there is no mention of a theory or conceptual model, you should consider whether the contribution that the study is

---

BOX 7-1 **GUIDELINES FOR CRITIQUING THEORETICAL OR CONCEPTUAL FRAMEWORKS**

1. Does the research report describe an explicit theoretical or conceptual framework for the study? If not, does the absence of an explicit framework detract from the usefulness or significance of the research?

2. Does the report adequately describe the major features of the framework so that readers can understand the conceptual basis of the study?

3. Is the framework consistent with the research paradigm?

4. Do the research problem and hypotheses naturally flow from the framework, or does the purported link between the problem and the framework seem contrived?

5. Are conceptual definitions of the concepts in the study provided? Are the conceptual definitions consistent with the framework? Are the definitions clear and sufficiently detailed?

6. Did the framework guide the study methods? For example, do the operational definitions correspond to the conceptual definitions? Were hypotheses tested statistically?

7. Does the researcher tie the findings of the study back to the framework at the end of the report? How do the findings support or undermine the framework? Are the findings interpreted within the context of the framework?

likely to make to knowledge is diminished by the absence of such a framework. Nursing has been criticized for producing many pieces of isolated research that are difficult to integrate because of the absence of a theoretical foundation, but in many cases, the research may be so pragmatic that it does not really need a theory to enhance its usefulness. For example, research designed to determine the optimal frequency of turning patients has a utilitarian goal; it is difficult to see how a theory would enhance the value of the findings.

 CONSUMER TIP

In most quantitative nursing studies, the research problem is *not* linked to a specific theory or conceptual model. Thus, you may read many studies before finding a study with an explicit theoretical underpinning. ■

If the study does involve an explicit framework, you must then ask whether this particular framework is appropriate. You may not be able to challenge the researcher's use of a particular theory or model or to recommend an alternative because that would require a solid theoretical grounding. However, you can evaluate the logic of using a particular framework and assess whether the link between the problem and the theory is genuine. Does the researcher present a convincing rationale for the framework used? Do the hypotheses flow from the theory? Will the findings contribute to the validation of the theory? Does the researcher interpret the findings within the context of the framework? If the answer to such questions is no, students may have grounds for criticizing the study's framework, even though they may not be in a position to articulate how the conceptual basis of the study could be improved.

 CONSUMER TIP

Some studies (in nursing as in any other discipline) claim theoretical linkages that are not justified. This is most likely to occur when researchers first formulate the research problem and then find a theoretical context to fit it. An after-the-fact linkage of theory to a research question *may* prove useful, but it is usually problematic because the researcher will not have taken the nuances of the theory into consideration in designing the study. If a research problem is truly linked to a conceptual framework, then the design of the study, the measurement of key constructs, and the analysis and interpretation of data will flow from that conceptualization. ■

RESEARCH EXAMPLES OF THEORETICAL CONTEXTS

This section presents two examples of the linkages between theory and research from the nursing research literature—one from a quantitative study and the other from a qualitative study.

Research Example of a Quantitative Study

The McGill Model of Nursing developed by Moyra Allen (Gottlieb & Rowat, 1987; Kravitz & Frey, 1989) has been used as the conceptual framework in numerous studies. For example, Besner (2000) used elements of the McGill Model as the conceptual framework in her study of nursing practices in relation to patient outcomes among a group of public health nurses delivering care to mothers and newborns as part of a community postpartum program. Feeley and Gottlieb (2000) examined how individual and family strengths (strengths being a key concept of the McGill Model) can best be used in identifying and making use of health-related resources. Here we describe in some detail another study based on the McGill Model of Nursing.

Research Summary

The McGill Model of Nursing views health and illness as separate entities coexisting within a person. Two key dimensions of health that promote a sense of meaning are coping, defined as problem solving, and development directed toward the achievement of life goals. In the McGill model, the goal of nursing is to acknowledge the capabilities and strengths that patients and their family possess and to actively work with them to maintain, strengthen, and develop their health potential.

Grossman and colleagues (2000) used the McGill model and theoretical underpinnings of cognitive processing to study the psychological adjustment of 51 critically injured patients 3 months after an unexpected, potentially life-threatening accident. Because the McGill model suggests that both health and illness can coexist within the person, psychological adjustment was conceptualized in terms of both psychological well-being and depressive symptomatology. The researchers administered a subscale of the Brief Symptom Inventory (as a measure of depressive symptoms) and Bradburn's Psychological Well-being Scale during face-to-face interviews with study participants.

Grossman and colleagues hypothesized that psychological adjustment would be related to patients' cognitive processing, sense of meaning, and use of coping strategies. The relationships among patients' ability to cognitively integrate the traumatizing event, to restore a sense of meaning, and to use the various coping strategies had not been previously documented. The main finding of their research was that restoring a sense of meaning in life was central to psychological adjustment following a critical injury.

Clinical Relevance

A particular strength of the study by Grossman and coworkers is that it adds to the conceptualization of personal and family strengths, key concepts of the McGill model. The significant relationship between perceived personal capabilities and psychological well-being following a traumatizing experience is consistent with a proposition of the McGill model that people often have the personal strengths to overcome adversity. Nurses' acknowledgement of personal strengths appears to be key in assisting patients and family in the process of recovery. In addition, their findings highlight the importance, for nurses, to explore individuals' perceptions of the traumatic event and how this event has an impact on their perceived strengths, coping strategies, and goals. The authors indicate that the knowledge gained from this study is one step toward the development of sensitive nursing intervention programs that would be tailored to the needs and strengths of individuals and their families facing the acute phase of recovery following a potentially life-threatening accident.

Research Example of a Qualitative Study

As noted earlier in this chapter, many qualitative studies have theory development as an explicit goal. Here we describe the efforts of Bournes and Mitchell (2002), qualitative researchers who developed a conceptual model of waiting. These researchers acknowledged Parse's Theory of Human Becoming (1992, 1995) as the theory underlying their work on the concept of waiting.

Research Summary

In Parse's theory, health is the way people go on and live what is important to them. The goal of nursing guided by Parse's human becoming theory is to participate with people in ways that make a difference to their quality of life from their own perspective.

Bournes and Mitchell (2002) noted that research guided by such theory focuses seeks to enhance our understanding of people's perspectives of universal lived experiences, such as waiting. They conducted a qualitative study to explore the experience of waiting among individuals who had a family member or friend hospitalized in a critical care unit. Parse's (1992) research method of discovering the essence of human experience was used to answer the research question: What is the structure of the lived experience of waiting?

The researchers studied waiting in a sample of 12 family members and friends of patients admitted to an adult medical-surgical critical care unit for a variety of reasons (*e.g.*, traumatic injuries, complicated surgical procedures). Data were gathered through in-depth dialogues with study participants. The researchers initiated the dialogues by saying, "Please tell me about your experience of waiting" (p. 60). The dialogues were then analyzed using the method Parse calls extraction–synthesis. This is a process of moving from the language of the participants to a level of abstraction that generates an answer to the research question. This process includes synthesizing stories and essences (core ideas) from the transcribed dialogues, conceptualizing the essences in the language of the researcher, synthesizing propositions from the essences of the participants' descriptions, extracting and synthesizing ideas that capture the central meaning of the propositions, and synthesizing a structure of the lived experience by making statements that join the core concepts. These core concepts are central ideas described by all study participants, and when joined together, form a structure that answers the research question. Bournes and Mitchell's main finding can be summarized as follows: "The lived experience of waiting is a vigilant attentiveness surfacing amid an ambiguous turbulent lull as contentment emerges with uplifting engagements" (p. 62).

According to Bournes and Mitchell the three core concepts of the structure of waiting are:

Vigilant attentiveness: waiting as a focused, persistent, and diligent watchfulness

Ambiguous turbulent lull: waiting as a grueling experience of unsure stillness

Contentment with uplifting engagements: calming and comforting experiences of helpful associations with others and activities while waiting

In presenting their model, Bournes and Mitchell described these three core concepts with rich excerpts from their in-depth interviews. Here is an example of the excerpt illustrating the core concept of "ambiguous turbulent lull":

The big thing about waiting is not knowing. Sometimes we just sat there for days, and it seemed we were getting no information at all. Your mind does all kinds of things—it's a real whirlwind. Generally, I have no concept of time—it absolutely stands still and yet it goes fast. It goes slow in that I am waiting to see progress, and that's slow. It goes fast in that it's supper time already, and I've been here all day (p. 63).

In their discussion, Bournes and Mitchell describe how their findings contribute to the knowledge base of nursing by adding to Parse's Theory of Human Becoming. The core concepts that comprise the experience of waiting are conceptually integrated with Parse's theory. For example, the ideas captured by the core concept of vigilant attentiveness relates to Parse's construct called *imaging.* In Parse's theory, imaging refers to knowing at both explicit and tacit levels. Imaging is apparent in such comments by the participants as "all kinds of things were going on" in their heads as they tried to imagine what was happening (p. 64). Bournes and Mitchell suggest that further research on any of these phenomena would add to our understanding of the experience of waiting and contribute new knowledge pertaining to human becoming.

Clinical Relevance

Because waiting is a common experience among individuals dealing with health-related situations, Bournes and Mitchell's conceptual development of waiting is clearly relevant to nursing. This qualitatively based model has immediate clinical implications for various health-related situations. Taken together, the three core concepts of vigilant attentiveness, ambiguous turbulent lull, and contentment with uplifting engagements enhance nurses' understanding of the experience of people waiting and which, in turn, can assist them in developing nursing interventions that optimize outcomes related to waiting. An increased understanding of the experience of waiting may also lead nurses to reevaluate current practices, policies, and procedures that would reduce the potentially negative impacts of waiting.

● ● ● ● ● *SUMMARY POINTS*

- A **theory** is a broad and abstract characterization of phenomena. As classically defined, a theory is an abstract generalization that systematically explains the relationships among phenomena. **Descriptive theory** thoroughly describes a phenomenon.
- The overall objective of theory is to make scientific findings meaningful, summarize existing knowledge into coherent systems, stimulate new research by providing direction and impetus, and explain the nature of relationships among variables.
- The basic components of a theory are concepts; classically defined theories consist of a set of propositions about the interrelationships among concepts, arranged in a logically interrelated system that permits new statements to be derived from them.
- Concepts are also the basic elements of **conceptual models,** but the concepts are not linked to one another in a logically ordered, deductive system.
- **Schematic models** (sometimes referred to as **conceptual maps**) are symbolic representations of phenomena that depict a conceptual model through the use of symbols or diagrams.
- A **framework** is the conceptual underpinning of a study. In many studies, the framework is implicit and not fully explicated.
- Qualitative studies are often used to develop inductively derived theories. Some qualitative researchers specifically seek to develop **grounded theories**—data-driven explanations to account for phenomena under study.
- Quantitative studies test hypotheses developed on the basis of an existing theory or conceptual model.
- Several conceptual models of nursing have been developed and have been used in nursing research (*e.g.,* Orem's Self-Care Model). The concepts central to models of nursing are person, environment, health, and nursing.
- Nonnursing models used by nurse researchers (*e.g.,* Lazarus and Folkman's Theory of Stress and Coping) are referred to as **borrowed theories.**
- Researchers sometimes develop a problem, design a study, and then look for a conceptual framework; such an after-the-fact selection of a framework is less compelling than the systematic testing of a particular theory.

➤➤➤➤ *CRITICAL THINKING ACTIVITIES*

Chapter 7 of the accompanying *Study Guide to Accompany Essentials of Nursing Research,* 5th edition, offers various exercises and study suggestions for reinforcing the concepts presented in this chapter. In addition, you can address the following:

1. Read the introduction to one or both of the actual research studies in the Appendix of this book, and then answer the questions in Box 7-1.

2. Select one of the conceptual models of nursing cited in Table 7-1 and read a primary or secondary source description of the model. Prepare a one-page summary of the model.

3. Read a study linked to the model selected for exercise 2. Answer the questions in Box 7-1 regarding this study.

SUGGESTED READINGS

Methodologic References

Azjen, I., & Fishbein, M. (1980). *Understanding attitudes and predicting social behavior.* Englewood Cliffs, NJ: Prentice-Hall.

Becker, M. (1978). The Health Belief Model and sick role behavior. *Nursing Digest, 6,* 35–40.

Fawcett, J. (1994). *Analysis and evaluation of conceptual models of nursing* (3rd ed.). Philadelphia: F. A. Davis.

Fawcett, J. (1999). *The relationship between theory and research* (3rd ed.). Philadelphia: F. A. Davis.

Gottlieb, L. N. , & Rowat, K. (1987). The McGill Model of Nursing: A practice-derived model. *Advances in Nursing Science, 9,* 51–61.

King, I. M. (1981). *A theory for nursing: Systems, concept, and process.* New York: John Wiley & Sons.

Kravitz, M., & Frey, M. A. (1989). The Allen Nursing Model. In J. Fitzpatrick & A. Whall (Eds.), *Conceptual models of nursing-analysis and application* (2nd ed., pp. 313–329). Norwalk CT: Appleton & Lange.

Lazarus, R. S., & Folkman, S. (1984). *Stress, appraisal, and coping.* New York: Springer.

Leininger, M. (1991). *Culture care diversity and universality: A theory of nursing.* New York: National League for Nursing.

Levine, M. E. (1973). *Introduction to clinical nursing* (2nd ed.). Philadelphia: F. A. Davis.

Mishel, M. H. (1988). Uncertainty in illness. *Image: The Journal of Nursing Scholarship, 20,* 225–232.

Mishel, M. H. (1990). Reconceptualization of the uncertainty in illness theory. *Image: The Journal of Nursing Scholarship, 22,* 256–262.

Morse, J. M., Solberg, S. M., Neander, W. L., Bottorff, J. L., & Johnson, J. L. (1990). Concepts of caring and caring as a concept. *Advances in Nursing Science, 13,* 1–14.

Neuman, B. (1989). *The Neuman systems model* (2nd ed.). Norwalk, CT: Appleton & Lange.

Newman, M. (1994). *Health as expanding consciousness.* New York: National League for Nursing.

Orem, D. E. (1995). *Concepts of practice* (5th ed.). New York: McGraw-Hill.

Parse, R. R. (1992). Human becoming: Parse's theory. *Nursing Science Quarterly, 5,* 35–42.

Parse, R. R. (1995). *Illuminations: The human becoming theory in practice and research.* New York: National League for Nursing.

Pender, N., & Pender, A. R. (1996). *Health promotion in nursing practice* (3rd ed.). Norwalk, CT: Appleton & Lange.

Rogers, M. E. (1970). *An introduction to the theoretical basis of nursing.* Philadelphia: F. A. Davis.

Rogers, M. E. (1986). Science of unitary human beings. In V. Malinski (Ed.), *Explorations on Martha Rogers' science of unitary human beings.* Norwalk, CT: Appleton-Century-Crofts.

Rogers, M. E., Malinski, V. M., & Barrett, E. A. (1994). *Martha E. Rogers: Her life and her work.* Philadelphia: F. A. Davis.

Roy, C. (1984). *Introduction to nursing: An adaptation model* (2nd ed.). Englewood Cliffs, NJ: Prentice-Hall.

Roy, C. Sr., & Andrews, H. (1991). *The Roy Adaptation Model: The definitive statement.* Norwalk, CT: Appleton & Lange.

Roy, C. Sr., & Andrews, H. A. (1998). *The Roy Adaptation Model.* Norwalk, CT: Appleton & Lange.

Watson, J. (1999). *Postmodern nursing and beyond.* New York: Churchill Livingston.

Substantive References

Bays, C. L. (2001). Older adults' descriptions of hope after stroke. *Rehabilitation Nursing, 26,* 18–20.

Belleau, F. P., Hagan, L., & Masse, B. (2001). Effects of an educational intervention on the anxiety of women awaiting mastectomies. *Canadian Oncology Nursing Journal, 11,* 176–180.

Berubé, M., & Loiselle, C. G. (2003). L'incertitude, le coping et l'espoir chez les blessés médullaires. Uncertainty, coping and hope among individuals with a spinal cord injury. *L'Infirmière du Québec, 10,* 16–23.

Besner, J. (2000). Public health nursing: A comparison of theoretical and actual practice. *Primary Health Care Research and Development, 1,* 91–102.

Black, M. E. C., Stein, K. F., & Loveland-Cherry, C. J. (2001). Older women and mammography screening behaviour: Do possible selves contribute? *Health Education and Behavior, 28,* 200–216.

Blythe, J., Baumann, A., & Giovannetti, P. (2001). Nurses' experiences of restructuring in three Ontario hospitals. *Journal of Nursing Scholarship, 33,* 61–68.

Bourret, E. M., Bernick, L. G., Cott, C. A., & Kontos, P. C. (2001) The meaning of mobility for residents and staff in long-term care facilities. *Journal of Advanced Nursing, 37,* 338–345.

Bournes, D. A., & Mitchel, G. J. (2002). Waiting: The experience of persons in a critical care waiting room. *Research in Nursing & Health, 25,* 58–67.

Cook, J. K., Green, M., & Topp, R. V. (2001). Exploring the impact of physician abuse on perioperative nurses. *AORN Journal, 74,* 317–327.

Deiriggi, P. M., & Miles, K. E. (1995). The effects of waterbeds on heart rate in preterm infants. *Scholarly Inquiry for Nursing Practice, 9,* 245–262.

Doornbos, M. M. (2000). King's systems framework and family health: The derivation and testing of a theory. *Journal of Theory Construction and Testing, 4,* 20–26.

Edgar, L., Rosenberger, Z., & Collet, J. (2001). Lessons learned: Outcomes and methodology of a coping skills interventional trial comparing individual to group formats for patients with cancer. *International Journal of Psychiatry in Medicine, 31,* 289–304.

Endo, E., Nitta., N., Inayoshi, M., Saito, R., Takemura, K., Minegishi, H., Kubo, S., & Kondo, M. (2000). Pattern recognition as a caring partnership in families with cancer. *Journal of Advanced Nursing, 32,* 603–610.

Feeley, N., & Gottlieb, L. (2000). Nursing approaches for working with family strengths and resources. *Journal of Family Nursing, 6,* 9–24.

Fergus, K. D., Gray, R. E., Fitch, M. I., Labreque, M., & Phillips, C. (2002). Active consideration: Conceptualizing patient-provided support for spouse caregivers in the context of prostate cancer. *Qualitative Health Reseach, 12,* 492–514.

Gagnon, L., & Vissandjee, B. (2001) Que signifie pour les ainés inuites le soin offert par leurs proches? *L'Infirmière du Québec, 8*(4), 44–47.

Grossman, M., Lee, V., Van Neste Kenny, J., Godin, M., & Chambers-Evans, J. (2000). Psychological adjustment of critically injured patients three months after an unexpected, potentially life-threatening accident. *Journal of Clinical Nursing, 9,* 801–815.

Horsburgh, M. E., Beanlands, H., Locking-Cusolito, H., Howe, A., & Watson, D. (2000). Personality traits and self-care in adults awaiting renal transplant. *Western Journal of Nursing Research, 22*(4), 407–437.

Jonas-Simpson, C. M. (2001). Feeling understood: A melody of human becoming. *Nursing Science Quarterly, 14*(3), 222–230.

John, L. D. (2001). Quality of life in patients receiving radiation therapy for non-small cell lung cancer. *Oncology Nursing Forum, 28,* 807–813.

Maurier, W. L., & Northcott, H. C. (2000). Job uncertainty and health status for nurses during restructuring of health care in Alberta. *Western Journal of Nursing Research, 22,* 623–641.

Pender, N. J., Walker, S. N., Sechrist, K. R., & Frank-Stromborg, M. (1990). Predicting health-promoting lifestyles in the workplace. *Nursing Research, 39,* 326–332.

Ross, L., & Goulet, C. (2002). Attitudes et normes subjectives d'adolescentes québécoises face à l'allaitement maternel. Breastfeeding-related atttitudes and subjective norms of Quebec female teenagers. *Revue Canadienne de Santé Publique, 93,* 198–202.

Skillen, D. L., Anderson, M. C., & Knight, C. L. (2001). The created environment for physical assessment by case managers. *Western Journal of Nursing Research, 23*(1), 72–89.

Watt-Watson, J., Garfinkel, P., Gallop, R., Stevens, B., & Streiner, D. (2000). The impact of nurses' empathic responses on patients' pain management in acute care. *Nursing Research, 49,* 191–200.

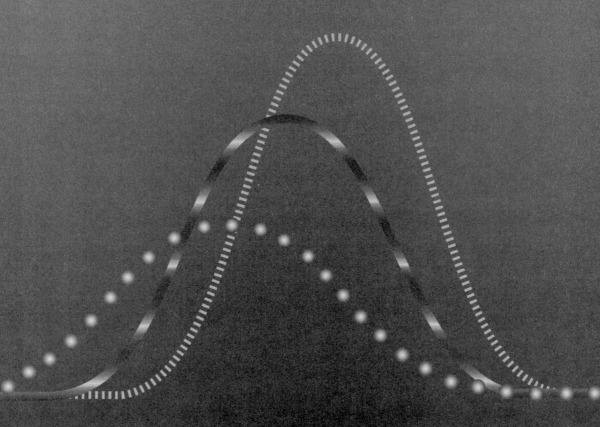

PART III

DESIGNS FOR NURSING RESEARCH

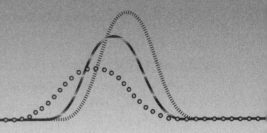

Understanding Quantitative Research Design

PURPOSES AND DIMENSIONS OF RESEARCH DESIGN
IN QUANTITATIVE STUDIES
EXPERIMENTAL, QUASI-EXPERIMENTAL, AND
NONEXPERIMENTAL DESIGNS
  Experimental Research
  Quasi-Experimental Research
  Nonexperimental Research
RESEARCH DESIGN AND THE TIME DIMENSION
  Cross-Sectional Designs
  Longitudinal Designs
SPECIFIC TYPES OF QUANTITATIVE RESEARCH
  Surveys
  Evaluations
TECHNIQUES OF RESEARCH CONTROL
  Research Control
  Controlling External Factors
  Controlling Intrinsic Factors

INTERNAL AND EXTERNAL VALIDITY
  Internal Validity
  External Validity
CRITIQUING QUANTITATIVE RESEARCH DESIGNS
RESEARCH EXAMPLES
  Research Example of an Experimental
    Evaluation
  Research Example of a Quasi-Experimental
    Study
  Research Example of a Nonexperimental
    Survey
SUMMARY POINTS
CRITICAL THINKING ACTIVITIES
SUGGESTED READINGS
  Methodologic References
  Substantive References

Student Objectives

On completion of this chapter, the student will be able to:

○ describe the decisions that are specified in a research design for a quantitative study

○ describe the characteristics of experimental, quasi-experimental, preexperimental, and nonexperimental designs and discuss their strengths and weaknesses

○ identify several specific designs (*e.g.*, repeated-measures design, nonequivalent control-group design, retrospective design) and describe some of their advantages and disadvantages

○ distinguish between and evaluate cross-sectional and longitudinal designs

○ identify the purposes and some of the distinguishing features of surveys, evaluations, and outcomes research

○ identify and evaluate alternative methods of controlling external and intrinsic extraneous variables

○ describe various threats to the internal and external validity of quantitative studies

○ evaluate a quantitative study in terms of its overall research design and methods of controlling extraneous variables, including the resulting internal and external validity of the design

○ define new terms in the chapter

New Terms

After-only design
Analysis of covariance
Attrition
Baseline data
Before–after design
Between-subjects design
Case-control design
Cell
Clinical trial
Comparison group
Constancy of conditions
Control group
Correlational research
Cost–benefit analysis
Crossover design
Cross-sectional study
Descriptive correlational study
Descriptive research
Double-blind experiment
Evaluation
Ex post facto research

Experimental research
Experimental group
External validity
Extraneous variable
Factor
Factorial design
Follow-up study
Hawthorne effect
History threat
Homogeneity
Impact analysis
Implementation analysis
Interaction effects
Internal validity
Intervention
Level
Longitudinal study
Main effects
Manipulation
Matching
Maturation threat

Mediating variable
Mortality threat
Net effects
Nonequivalent control-group after-only design
Nonequivalent control-group before–after design
Nonexperimental research
One-group before–after design
Outcome analysis
Outcomes research
Panel study
Posttest data
Posttest-only design
Preexperimental design
Pretest data
Pretest–posttest design
Process analysis
Prospective study
Quasi-experimental research

Random assignment
Randomization
Repeated-measures design
Research control
Research design
Research protocol
Retrospective study
Rival hypothesis
Selection threat
Self-report
Self-selection
Survey
Systematic bias
Table of random numbers
Threats to internal validity
Time-series design
Treatment
Trend study
Within-subjects design

PURPOSES AND DIMENSIONS OF RESEARCH DESIGN IN QUANTITATIVE STUDIES

Research design refers to the researcher's overall plan for answering the research questions or testing the research hypotheses. In a quantitative study, the research design spells out the strategies the researcher plans to adopt to develop information that is accurate and interpretable. Typically, a quantitative research design involves decisions with regard to the following aspects of the study:

- *Will there be an intervention?* In some situations, nurse researchers study the effects of a specific intervention (*e.g.,* an innovative program to promote breast self-examination); in others, researchers gather information about phenomena as they currently exist. This is a distinction between experimental and nonexperimental research. When there is an intervention, the research design specifies its nature and how it is to be implemented.
- *What types of comparison will be made?* Researchers usually plan comparisons within their studies so that their results will be more clearly interpretable. Consider the example presented in Chapter 3, in which the researchers studied the emotional consequences of having an abortion by comparing women who had an abortion with women who delivered a baby. Without a comparison group, the researchers would not have known whether the abortion group members' emotional status was of

special concern. Sometimes, researchers use a before–after comparison (*e.g.,* preoperative and postoperative), and sometimes several comparisons are used.

- *What procedures will be used to control extraneous variables?* The complexity of relationships among variables makes it difficult to test hypotheses unambiguously unless efforts are made to control factors extraneous to the research question (*i.e.,* to control **extraneous variables**). This chapter discusses techniques for achieving control.
- *When and how many times will data be collected from study participants?* In many studies, data are collected from participants at a single point in time, but some studies include multiple contacts with participants, for example, to determine how things have changed over time. The research design designates how often and also when, relative to other events, the data will be collected (*e.g.,* 1 day after surgery).
- *In what setting will the study occur?* Sometimes, data for quantitative studies are collected in real-world settings, such as in clinics or people's homes. Other studies are conducted in laboratory settings (*i.e.,* in highly controlled environments established for research purposes).

The research design incorporates key methodologic decisions. Other aspects of the study—the data collection plan, the sampling plan, and the analysis plan—also involve important decisions, but the research design stipulates the fundamental form the research will take. For this reason, it is crucial for you to understand the implications of researchers' design decisions.

There is no single, easy-to-describe typology of research designs because they vary along a number of dimensions. As shown in Table 8-1, the dimensions involve whether the researcher has control over the independent variable, what type of comparison is made, how many times data are collected, whether the researcher looks forward or backward in time for the occurrence of the independent and dependent variables, and what setting is used for data collection. Each dimension is, with a few exceptions, independent of the others. For example, an experimental design can be a between-subjects or within-subjects design; experiments can also be cross-sectional or longitudinal, and so on (these terms are discussed later). Moreover, within any one category, there are a number of variants; for example, there are several alternative experimental designs. The sections that follow elaborate on different designs for quantitative nursing research. Qualitative research design is discussed in Chapter 9.

CONSUMER TIP

Research reports typically present information about the research design early in the method section. Complete information about the design is not always provided, however, and some researchers use terminology that is different from that used in this book. (Occasionally, researchers even misidentify the study design.) ■

TABLE 8-1. Dimensions of Quantitative Research Designs

DIMENSION	DESIGN	MAJOR FEATURES
Control over independent variable	Experimental	Manipulation of independent variable, control group, randomization
	Quasi-experimental	Manipulation of independent variable but no randomization or no control group
	Nonexperimental	No manipulation of independent variable
Type of group comparisons	Between-subjects	Participants in groups being compared are different people.
	Within-subjects	Participants in groups being compared are the same people.
Number of data collection points	Cross-sectional	Data collected at one point in time
	Longitudinal	Data collected at multiple points in time over extended period
Occurrence of independent and dependent variable	Retrospective	Study begins with dependent variable and looks backward for cause or influence.
	Prospective	Study begins with independent variable and looks forward for the effect.
Setting	Naturalistic	Data collected in a real-world setting
	Laboratory	Data collected in artificial, contrived setting

EXPERIMENTAL, QUASI-EXPERIMENTAL, AND NONEXPERIMENTAL DESIGNS

This section reviews designs that differ with regard to the amount of control the researcher has over the independent variable. We begin with research designs that offer the greatest amount of control: experimental designs.

Experimental Research

Experimental research differs from nonexperimental research in one important respect: The researcher using an experimental design is an active agent rather than a passive observer. Early physical scientists found that, although observation of natural phenomena is valuable, the complexity of naturally occurring events often obscures relationships. This problem was addressed by isolating phenomena in a laboratory setting and controlling the conditions under which they occurred. Procedures developed by physical scientists were adopted by biologists during the 19th century, resulting in many achievements in physiology and medicine. Researchers interested in human behaviour and psychological states began using experimental methods in the 20th century.

Characteristics of Experiments

Experiments are not necessarily performed in laboratories; they can be conducted in any setting. To qualify as an experiment, a research design need only possess the following three properties:

1. *Manipulation.* The experimenter does something to participants in the study.
2. *Control.* The experimenter introduces controls over the experimental situation, including the use of a control group.
3. *Randomization.* The experimenter assigns participants to control or experimental groups randomly.

Using **manipulation,** the experimenter controls and consciously varies the independent variable and then observes its effect on the dependent variable. The investigator manipulates the independent variable by administering an experimental **treatment** (or **intervention**) to some participants while withholding it from others (or administering an alternative treatment, such as a placebo). As an illustration, suppose we were investigating the effect of physical restraint with a Posey belt on heart rate, using rats as subjects. One experimental design for this research problem is a **before–after design** (also known as a **pretest–posttest design**). This design involves the observation of the dependent variable (heart rate) at two points in time: before and after the treatment. Each of the rats in the experimental group is restrained with a Posey belt, whereas those in the control group are not. This design permits us to examine what changes in heart rate were *caused* by the restraint because only some rats were restrained, providing an important comparison. In this example, we met the first criterion of a true experiment by manipulating physical restraint of the rats, the independent variable.

This example also meets the second requirement for experiments, the use of a control group. Campbell and Stanley (1963), in a classic monograph on research design, noted that scientific evidence requires at least one comparison. But not all comparisons provide equally persuasive evidence. Let us look at an example. If we were to supplement the diet of a sample of premature neonates with special nutrients for 2 weeks, the infants' weight at the end of the 2-week period would give us no information about the effectiveness of the treatment. At a bare minimum, we would need to compare their posttreatment weight with their pretreatment weight to determine whether, at least, their weights had increased. But suppose we find an average weight gain of half a pound. Does this finding indicate that there is a causal relationship between the nutritional supplements (the independent variable) and weight gain (the dependent variable)? No, it does not. Infants normally gain weight as they mature. Without a control group—a group that does not receive the supplements—it is impossible to separate the effects of maturation from those of the treatment. The term **control group** refers to a group of participants whose performance on a dependent variable is used as a basis for evaluating the performance of the **experimental group** (the group that receives the treatment of interest to the researcher) on the same dependent variable.

To qualify as an experiment, the design must also involve the assignment of participants to groups randomly. Through **randomization** (or **random assignment**), every participant has an equal chance of being included in any group. If people are randomly assigned, there is no **systematic bias** in the groups with respect to attributes that may affect the dependent variable. *Randomly assigned groups are expected to be comparable, on average, with respect to an infinite number of biologic, psychological, and social traits at the outset of the study.* Any group differences that emerge after random assignment can therefore be attributed to the treatment.

Random assignment can be accomplished by flipping a coin or pulling names from a hat. Researchers typically either use computers to perform the randomization or rely on a **table of random numbers,** a table displaying hundreds of digits arranged in a random order.

Experimental Designs

Basic Designs.   The most basic experimental design involves the random assignment of participants to two groups and the subsequent collection of data after the intervention. This design is sometimes called an **after-only** (or **posttest-only**) **design.** A more refined design, discussed previously, is the pretest–posttest or before–after design, which involves the collection of **pretest data** (also known as **baseline data**) before the experimental manipulation and **posttest data** after it.

> *Example of an after-only design:*
>
> Milne (2000) used an after-only design to study the effect of an educational intervention pertaining to urinary incontinence on the subsequent help-seeking behaviours of older adults. One group was provided with both individualized instruction and written information, whereas the second group was provided with written information only. Two months later, Milne recorded how many participants within each group sought professional assistance for urinary incontinence.

Factorial Design.   Researchers sometimes manipulate two or more variables simultaneously. Suppose, for example, that we were interested in comparing the effects of tactile stimulation versus auditory stimulation on cardiac responsiveness in premature infants, and that we were also interested in learning whether the daily *amount* of stimulation had any effects. Figure 8–1 illustrates the structure of this experiment.

This type of study, which involves a **factorial design,** permits the testing of three hypotheses. Here, the three research questions are:

1. Does auditory stimulation have a different effect on cardiac responsiveness in premature infants than tactile stimulation?
2. Is the amount of stimulation (independent of modality) related to cardiac responsiveness?
3. Is auditory stimulation most effective when linked to a certain dose

Type of stimulation

		Auditory A1		Tactile A2	
Daily exposure	15 Min. B1	A1	B1	A2	B1
	30 Min. B2	A1	B2	A2	B2
	45 Min. B3	A1	B3	A2	B3

FIGURE 8-1. Schematic diagram of a factorial experiment.

and tactile stimulation most effective when coupled with a different dose?

The third question demonstrates a major strength of factorial designs: they permit us to evaluate not only **main effects** (effects resulting from the manipulated variables, as exemplified in questions 1 and 2) but also **interaction effects** (effects resulting from combining the treatment methods). Our results may indicate, for example, that 15 minutes of tactile stimulation and 45 minutes of auditory stimulation are the most beneficial treatments. We could not have learned this by conducting two separate experiments that manipulated one independent variable at a time.

In factorial experiments, participants are assigned at random to a combination of treatments. In our example, premature infants would be assigned randomly to one of the six cells. The term **cell** is used in experimental research to refer to a treatment condition and is represented in a schematic diagram as a box. In a factorial design, the independent variables are referred to as **factors.** Type of stimulation is factor A and amount of exposure is factor B. Each factor must have two or more **levels.** Level one of factor A is *auditory,* and level two of factor A is *tactile.* The research design in Figure 8–1 would be described as a 2 × 3 design: two levels of factor A times three levels of factor B.

Example of a factorial design:

Pridham et al. (1999) used a 2 × 2 design to study the effects of two factors—prescribed versus *ad libitum* infant feedings, and two caloric densities of the formula—on weight gain in premature infants. The 78 infants were randomly assigned to one of four treatment conditions, and weight change was then assessed over a 5-day period.

Repeated-Measures Design. Thus far, we have described experimental studies in which the participants who are randomly assigned to groups are different people. For instance, the infants given 15 minutes of auditory stimulation in the factorial experiment are not the same infants as those exposed to the other treatment conditions. This broad class of designs is referred to as **between-subjects designs** because the comparisons made are between different people. When the same participants are compared, the general class of designs is known as **within-subjects designs.**

A **repeated-measures design** (sometimes called a **crossover design**) involves the exposure of the same study participants to more than one treatment. Such studies are true experiments only if the participants are randomly assigned to different orderings of treatment. For example, if a repeated-measures design were used to compare the effects of auditory and tactile stimulation on infants, some participants would be randomly assigned to receive auditory stimulation first, and others would receive tactile stimulation first. In such a study, the three conditions for an experiment have been met: manipulation, randomization, and control, with *participants serving as their own control group.*

A repeated-measures design has the advantage of ensuring the highest possible equivalence among participants exposed to different conditions. Repeated-measures designs are inappropriate for certain research questions, however, because of possible carryover effects. When participants are exposed to two different treatments, they may be influenced in the second condition by their experience in the first. Drug studies rarely use a repeated-measures design because drug B administered after drug A is not the same treatment as drug B before drug A.

CONSUMER TIP

Some nonexperimental studies use a *statistical* repeated-measures feature for dealing with multiple points of data collection. A design is an experimental repeated-measures design only when the researcher introduces two or more treatments and randomizes the order of presentation of the treatments. ■

Example of a repeated-measures or crossover design:

Winkelman (2000) used a randomized crossover design to examine the effect of two alternative backrest positions (flat/horizontal or 30° elevation) on intracranial and cerebral profusion pressures in adults with brain injuries. The elevated backrest position contributed to significant and clinically important improvements in both intracranial and cerebral perfusion pressures.

Clinical Trials.   Medical researchers and epidemiologists often evaluate an innovative treatment through the use of a randomized clinical trial. **Clinical trials** involve the testing of a clinical treatment; random assignment of participants to experimental and control conditions; collection of outcome information, sometimes after a long period has elapsed; and, usually, use of a large, heterogeneous sample of participants, often from multiple, geographically dispersed sites to ensure that the findings are not unique to a single setting. Clinical trials typically use a before–after or after-only design and are thus not so much a specific design type as a distinctive application of experimental design.

> **Example of a clinical trial:**
> Goulet et al. (2001) conducted a clinical trial among women with preterm labour (N=250). Women were assigned randomly to either home care management (the experimental group) or hospital care management (the control group). The two groups subsequently were compared in terms of gestational age, birth weight, antenatal stress, satisfaction with social support, and family functioning.

Advantages and Disadvantages of Experiments

Experiments are the most powerful designs for testing hypotheses of cause-and-effect relationships. Because of its special controlling properties, an experiment offers greater corroboration than any other research approach that the independent variable (*e.g.*, diet, drug dosage, teaching approach) affects the dependent variable (*e.g.*, weight loss, recovery of health, learning).

Lazarsfeld (1955) identified three criteria for causality. First, a cause must precede an effect in time. To test the hypothesis that saccharin causes bladder cancer, it would be necessary to demonstrate that the participants had not developed cancer before exposure to saccharin. Second, there must be an empirical relationship between the presumed cause and the presumed effect. In the saccharin and cancer example, the researcher would have to demonstrate an association between the ingestion of saccharin and the presence of a carcinoma (*i.e.*, that people who used saccharin experienced a higher incidence of cancer than those who did not). The final criterion for causality is that the relationship cannot be due to the influence of a third variable. Suppose, for instance, that people who use saccharin tend also to drink more coffee than nonusers. Thus, a relationship between saccharin use and bladder cancer may reflect an underlying causal relationship between a substance in coffee and bladder cancer. It is particularly because of this third criterion that the experimental approach is so strong. Through the controlling properties of manipulation, control groups, and randomization, alternative explanations to a causal interpretation can often be ruled out or discredited.

Despite the advantages of experiments, they have some limitations. First, a number of interesting variables simply are not amenable to manipulation. A large number of human characteristics, such as disease or health habits, cannot be randomly conferred on people.

Second, there are many variables that could technically—but not ethically—be manipulated. For example, to date there have been no experiments to study the effect of cigarette smoking on lung cancer. Such an experiment would require us to assign people randomly to a smoking group (people forced to smoke) or a nonsmoking group (people prohibited from smoking). Experimentation with humans, therefore, is subject to a number of ethical constraints.

In many health care settings, experimentation may not be feasible because it is impractical. It may, for instance, be impossible to secure the necessary cooperation from administrators or other key people to conduct an experiment.

Another potential problem is the **Hawthorne effect,** a term derived from a series of experiments conducted at the Hawthorne plant of the Western Electric Corporation in which various environmental conditions (*e.g.,* light, working hours) were varied to determine their effect on worker productivity. Regardless of what change was introduced (*i.e.,* whether the light was made better or worse), productivity increased. Thus, knowledge of being in a study may cause people to change their behaviour, thereby obscuring the effect of the research variables.

In a hospital situation, the researcher might have to contend with a double Hawthorne effect. For example, if an experiment investigating the effect of a new postoperative patient routine were conducted, nurses as well as patients might be aware of participating in a study, and both groups could alter their actions accordingly. It is for this reason that **double-blind experiments,** in which neither the participants nor those administering the treatment know who is in the experimental or control group, are so powerful. Unfortunately, the double-blind approach is not feasible in most nursing research because nursing interventions are harder to disguise than medications.

In summary, experimental designs have some limitations that make them difficult to apply to real-world problems; nevertheless, experiments have a clear-cut superiority for testing causal hypotheses.

CONSUMER TIP

Researchers using an experimental design usually note this in their reports, but they may also refer to the designs as randomized designs or as clinical trials. After-only, before–after, and repeated-measures designs are the most commonly used experimental designs. The research report does not always identify which specific experimental design was used; this may have to be inferred from information about the data collection plan (in the case of after-only and before–after designs) or from such statements as: The participants were used as their own controls (in the case of a repeated-measures design). ■

Quasi-Experimental Research

Quasi-experimental research looks much like experiments because quasi-experiments also involve the manipulation of an independent variable (*i.e.,* the institution of a treatment). Quasi-experiments, however, lack either the randomization or control-group features that characterize true experiments, or both—features that strengthen the ability to make causal inferences.

Quasi-Experimental Designs

There are several quasi-experimental designs, but only the two most commonly used by nurse researchers are discussed here.

Nonequivalent Control-Group Design. The most frequently used quasi-experimental design is the **nonequivalent control-group before–after**

design, which involves a treatment and two or more groups of participants observed before and after its implementation. As an example, suppose we wanted to study the effect of primary nursing on nursing staff morale in a large metropolitan hospital. Because the new system of nursing care delivery is being implemented throughout the hospital, randomization is not possible. Therefore, we decide to collect comparison data from nurses in another similar hospital that is not instituting primary nursing. We decide to gather data on staff morale in both hospitals before implementing the primary nursing delivery system (the pretest) and again after its implementation in the first hospital (the posttest).

This quasi-experimental research design is identical to the before–after experimental design discussed in the previous section, *except* participants were not randomly assigned to the groups. The quasi-experimental design is weaker because, without randomization, *it cannot be assumed that the experimental and comparison groups are equivalent at the outset.* The design is, nevertheless, a strong one because the collection of pretest data allows us to determine whether the groups had similar morale initially. If the comparison and experimental groups responded similarly, on the average, at the pretest, we could be relatively confident that any posttest difference in self-reported morale was the result of the experimental treatment. (Note that in quasi-experiments, the term **comparison group** is usually used in lieu of *control group* to refer to the group against which outcomes in the treatment group are evaluated.)

Now suppose we had been unable to collect pretest data before primary nursing care was introduced (*i.e.,* only posttest data were collected). This design has a serious flaw because we have no basis for judging the initial equivalence of the two nursing staffs. If we found higher morale in the experimental group, could we conclude that primary nursing caused an improvement in staff morale? There could be several alternative explanations for posttest differences. Campbell and Stanley (1963), in fact, would call this **nonequivalent control-group after-only design** a **preexperimental design** rather than a quasi-experimental design because the researcher is severely constrained from making the desired inferences. Thus, even though quasi-experiments lack some of the controlling properties of experiments, the hallmark of quasi-experiments is the effort to introduce some controls.

Example of a nonequivalent control-group before–after design:

Wells et al. (2001) studied the effect of an abilities-focused educational program on the interactions of the institutionalized elderly and their caregivers. The educational program was implemented on one hospital unit and three other units were used for comparison. The researchers preferred this approach to randomization within units because information sharing among participants within the same unit would have contaminated the treatment condition. By collecting pretest data, the researchers learned that the two groups of patients were comparable with regard to demographic characteristics and diagnosis. However, the two groups of caregivers were different in terms of education and employment status.

Time-Series Design.   In the designs just described, a control group was used, but randomization was not. The next design has neither a control group nor randomization. Let us suppose that a hospital is adopting a requirement that all its nurses accrue a certain number of continuing education units before being eligible for a promotion or raise. The nurse administrators want to assess the consequences of this mandate on turnover rate, absentee rate, and number of raises and promotions awarded. For the purposes of this example, assume there is no other hospital that can serve as a reasonable comparison for this study. In such a case, the only kind of comparison that can be made is a before–after contrast. If the requirement were inaugurated in January, one could compare the turnover rate, for example, for the 3-month period before the new rule with the turnover rate for the subsequent 3-month period.

This **one-group before–after design** seems logical, but it has a number of problems. What if one of the 3-month periods is atypical, apart from the mandate? What about the effect of any other rules instituted during the same period? What about the effects of external factors, such as changes in the local economy? The design in question, which is also preexperimental, offers no way of controlling any of these factors.

The inability to obtain a meaningful control group, however, does not eliminate the possibility of conducting research with integrity. The previous design could be modified so that at least some of the alternative explanations for change in nurses' turnover rate could be ruled out. One such design is the **time-series design,** which involves the collection of data over an extended time period and the introduction of the treatment during that period. The present study could be designed with four observations before the new continuing education rule and four observations after it. For example, the first observation might be the number of resignations between January and March in the year before the new rule, the second observation might be the number of resignations between April and June, and so forth. After the rule is implemented, data on turnover similarly would be collected for four consecutive 3-month periods, giving us observations five through eight.

Although the time-series design does not eliminate all the problems of interpreting changes in turnover rate, the extended time perspective strengthens a researcher's ability to attribute change to the intervention. This is because the time-series design rules out the possibility that changes in resignations represent a random fluctuation of turnover measured at only two points.

Example of a time-series design:

Reynolds and Neidig (2002) used a time-series design to assess the effect of a combination of antiretroviral medications on the frequency, severity, and distress related to nausea among HIV-infected patients. Measurements were taken before the intervention and then once a week for 12 consecutive weeks once the treatment was initiated.

Advantages and Disadvantages of Quasi-Experiments

One strength of quasi-experiments is that they are practical. It is sometimes not feasible to conduct true experiments. Nursing research often occurs in natural settings, where it is difficult to deliver an innovative treatment randomly to some people but not to others. Quasi-experimental designs introduce some research control when full experimental rigour is not possible.

The major disadvantage of quasi-experiments is that cause-and-effect inferences that researchers often seek cannot be made as easily as with experiments. With quasi-experiments, there are alternative explanations for observed results. Suppose we wanted to evaluate the effect of a nursing intervention for infants of heroin-addicted mothers on infants' weight gain. If we use no comparison group or if we use a nonequivalent control group and then observe a weight gain, we must ask the following questions: Is it plausible that some external factor influenced the gain? Is it plausible that pretreatment group differences resulted in differential weight gains? Is it plausible that the changes would have occurred without an intervention? If the answer to any of these **rival hypotheses** is yes, inferences about treatment effectiveness are weakened. With quasi-experiments, there is almost always at least one plausible rival explanation.

CONSUMER TIP

Researchers often do not identify their studies as quasi-experimental or preexperimental. If a study involves a treatment or intervention (*i.e.,* if the researcher has control over the independent variable) and if the report does not explicitly mention random assignment or the use of an experimental design, it is probably safe to conclude that the design is quasi-experimental or preexperimental. ■

Nonexperimental Research

Many research problems cannot be addressed with an experimental or quasi-experimental design. For example, suppose we are interested in studying the effect of widowhood on physical and psychological functioning. Our independent variable here is widowhood versus nonwidowhood. Clearly, we cannot manipulate widowhood; people lose their spouses by a process that is neither random nor subject to research control. Thus, we would have to proceed by taking the two groups (widows and nonwidows) as they naturally occur and comparing their psychological and physical well-being. There are various reasons for doing **nonexperimental research,** including situations in which the independent variable is inherently nonmanipulable or in which it would be unethical to manipulate the independent variable. There are also research questions for which an experimental design is not appropriate, such as studies whose purpose is description.

Types of Nonexperimental Research

One class of nonexperimental research is known as ***ex post facto*** (or **correlational**) **research.** The literal translation of the Latin term *ex post facto* is "from after the fact," indicating that the research has been conducted after variation in the independent variable has occurred.

The basic purpose of *ex post facto* or correlational research is essentially the same as that of experimental research: to study relationships among variables. However, it is difficult to infer causal relationships in *ex post facto* studies. In experiments, the investigator makes a prediction that a deliberate variation in *X*, the independent variable, will result in changes to *Y*, the dependent variable. In *ex post facto* research, on the other hand, the investigator does not control the independent variable—the presumed causative factor—because it has already occurred. It is risky to draw cause-and-effect conclusions in such a situation. A famous research dictum is relevant: *correlation does not prove causation.* That is, the mere existence of a relationship between variables is not enough to warrant the conclusion that one variable caused the other, even if the relationship is strong.

Ex post facto research that is designed to shed light on causal relationships is sometimes described as either retrospective or prospective. **Retrospective studies** are *ex post facto* investigations in which a phenomenon observed in the present is linked to phenomena occurring in the past. In a retrospective study, the investigator focuses on a presently occurring outcome and then tries to ascertain the antecedent factors that have caused it. For example, in retrospective lung cancer research, the investigator begins with a sample of those who have lung cancer and a sample of those who do not. The researcher then looks for differences between the groups in antecedent behaviours or conditions, such as smoking habits.

Prospective studies, by contrast, start with an examination of a presumed cause and then go forward to the presumed effect. For example, in prospective lung cancer studies, researchers start with samples of smokers and nonsmokers and later compare the two groups in terms of lung cancer incidence. Prospective studies are more costly than retrospective studies but are considerably stronger. For one thing, any ambiguity concerning the temporal sequence of phenomena is resolved in prospective research (*i.e.,* the smoking is known to precede the lung cancer). In addition, samples are more likely to be representative of smokers and nonsmokers, and investigators may be in a position to impose controls to rule out competing explanations for observed effects.

> ### Example of a prospective study:
> Gardner and Sibthorpe (2002) conducted a prospective study to predict the level of recovery of patients admitted to an intensive care unit. Illness severity on admission was found to predict survival, functional status, and psychosocial recovery 6 months later. Researchers can sometimes strengthen a retrospective study, using a **case-control design.**

This design involves comparing "cases" with a certain condition (*e.g.,* women with breast cancer) with controls (women without breast cancer) who are selected to be similar to the cases with regard to key background factors (*e.g.,* age, family history of breast cancer). If the researcher can demonstrate

> **Example of a retrospective case-control study:**
>
> Heitkemper et al. (2001) used a retrospective design in their study of factors contributing to the onset of irritable bowel syndrome (IBS). Women with and without IBS (who were similar in background characteristics) were compared in terms of their history of sexual and physical abuse. They found that abusive experiences were more prevalent among women with IBS.

similarity between cases and controls with regard to extraneous traits, the inferences regarding the presumed cause of the disease are enhanced.

A second broad class of nonexperimental research is **descriptive research.** The purpose of descriptive studies is to observe, describe, and document aspects of a situation. For example, an investigator may wish to determine the percentage of teenaged mothers who receive inadequate prenatal care. Sometimes, a report refers to the study design as a **descriptive correlational study,** meaning that the researcher was interested primarily in describing relationships among variables, without necessarily seeking to establish a causal connection. For example, a researcher might be interested in documenting the relationship between fatigue and psychological distress. Because the intent in these situations is not to explain or to understand the underlying causes of the variables of interest, a nonexperimental design is appropriate.

> **Example of a descriptive study:**
>
> Harrisson et al. (2002) conducted a study to describe psychological and work factors related to well-being among two distinct groups of health care providers. The researchers described levels of hardiness, psychological distress, and perceived work support among nursing assistants and registered nurses in Quebec.

Advantages and Disadvantages of Nonexperimental Research

The major disadvantage of nonexperimental research is its inability to reveal causal relationships conclusively. *Ex post facto* studies are susceptible to faulty interpretation because the researcher works with preexisting groups that have formed through self-selection. Kerlinger and Lee (2000), noted research methodologists, indicates that "**self-selection** occurs when the members of the groups being studied are in the groups, in part, because they differentially possess traits or characteristics extraneous to the research problem, characteristics that possibly influence or are otherwise related to the variables of the research problem" (p. 349). In other words, preexisting differences may be a plausible alternative explanation for any observed group differences on the dependent variable.

As an example of the interpretive problems in *ex post facto* studies, suppose we were interested in studying differences in the level of depression of cancer patients who do or do not have adequate social support (*i.e.,* assistance and emotional sustenance through a social network). The independent variable is social support and the dependent variable is depression. Suppose we found that patients without social support are more depressed than the pa-

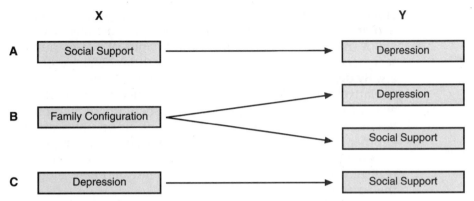

FIGURE 8-2 Alternative explanations for relationship between depression and social support in cancer patients.

tients with adequate social support. We could interpret this finding to mean that people's emotional state is influenced by the adequacy of their social supports. This relationship is diagrammed in Figure 8–2A. There are, however, alternative explanations for the findings. Perhaps there is a third variable that influences *both* social support and depression, such as the patients' family structure (*e.g.,* whether they are married). It may be that the availability of a significant other is a powerful influence on how depressed cancer patients feel *and* on the quality of their social support. These relationships are diagrammed in Figure 8–2B. A third possibility may be reversed causality, as shown in Figure 8–2C. Depressed cancer patients may find it more difficult to elicit needed social support from others than patients who are more cheerful. In this interpretation, it is the person's emotional state that causes the amount of received social support, and not the other way around. The point here is that *ex post facto* results should be interpreted cautiously, especially if the research has no theoretical basis.

CONSUMER TIP

Be prepared to think critically when a researcher claims to be studying the "effects" or "impacts" of an independent variable on a dependent variable in a nonexperimental study. For example, if the title of a report were "The Effects of Dieting on Depression," the study would likely be nonexperimental (*i.e.,* participants were not randomly assigned to dieting or not dieting). In such a situation, you might ask: "Did dieting have an effect on depression?" or "Did depression have an effect on dieting?" or "Did a third variable (*e.g.,* being overweight) have an effect on both?" ■

Despite the interpretive problems associated with *ex post facto* studies, they continue to play a crucial role in nursing because many interesting problems are not amenable to experimentation. Correlational research is often an efficient and effective means of collecting a large amount of data about a problem area. For example, it would be possible to collect extensive information about the health histories and eating habits of a large number of people. Researchers could then examine which health problems correlate with which diets. By doing this, a large number of interrelationships could be discovered in a relatively short time. By contrast, an experimenter looks at only a few variables at a time. For example, one experiment might manipulate foods with different cholesterol levels to observe the effects on physical symptoms, whereas another experiment might manipulate protein consumption, and so forth.

One final advantage is that nonexperimental research tends to be high in realism. Correlational and descriptive research can seldom be criticized for their artificiality.

CONSUMER TIP

Retrospective *ex post facto* studies are more common in nursing than prospective studies. Research reports, however, rarely point out that the design is retrospective. You will have to determine whether the researcher measured the dependent variable in the present and then attempted to identify its antecedent causes or determinants. By contrast, researchers almost always make explicit reference to the use of a prospective design. ■

RESEARCH DESIGN AND THE TIME DIMENSION

The research design incorporates decisions about when and how often data will be collected in a study. In many nursing studies, data are collected at a single point in time; other studies involve data collection on more than one occasion. Indeed, several designs involving multiple measurements have already been discussed, such as the pretest–posttest experimental design, the time-series design, and the prospective design.

There are four situations in which it is appropriate to design a study with multiple points of data collection:

1. *Time-related processes.* Certain research problems involve phenomena that evolve over time. Examples include healing, learning, growth, recidivism, and physical development.
2. *Time-sequenced phenomena.* It is sometimes important to ascertain the sequencing of phenomena. For example, if it is hypothesized that infertility contributes to depression, it would be important to determine that depression did not precede the fertility problem.
3. *Comparative purposes.* Sometimes, multiple data points are used to compare phenomena over time. For example, a study might document trends in the incidence of child abuse over a 10-year period. Another example is a time-series study, in which the intent is to determine whether changes over time can be attributed to an intervention.

4. *Enhancement of research control.* Some research designs involve collecting data at multiple points to enhance the interpretability of the results. For example, in nonequivalent control-group designs, the collection of preintervention data allows the researcher to detect and control for initial group differences.

Because of the importance of the time dimension in designing research, studies are often categorized in terms of how they deal with time. The major distinction is between cross-sectional and longitudinal designs.

Cross-Sectional Designs

Cross-sectional studies involve the collection of data at one point in time. The phenomena under study are captured during one data collection period. Cross-sectional designs are especially appropriate for describing the status of phenomena or relationships among phenomena at a fixed point. For example, a researcher might study whether psychological symptoms in menopausal women are correlated contemporaneously with physiologic symptoms. Retrospective studies are almost always cross-sectional. Data with regard to the independent and dependent variables are collected concurrently (*e.g.*, the lung cancer status of respondents and their smoking habits), but the independent variable usually captures events or behaviours occurring in the past.

When cross-sectional designs are used to study time-related phenomena, the designs are weaker than longitudinal ones. Suppose, for example, we were studying changes in attitudes of nursing students toward nursing research as they progress through a 4-year baccalaureate program. One way to investigate this would be to survey students when they are freshmen and survey them again as seniors. On the other hand, we could use a cross-sectional design by surveying members of these two classes at one point in time and then comparing their responses. If seniors had more positive attitudes toward research than freshmen, it might be inferred that nursing students become socialized professionally by their educational experiences. To make this kind of inference, the researcher must assume that the seniors would have responded as the freshmen responded had they been questioned 3 years earlier, or, conversely, that freshmen would be more favourable toward research if they were surveyed again 3 years later.

The main advantage of cross-sectional designs is that they are economical and easy to manage. There are, however, problems in inferring changes and trends over time using a cross-sectional design. The amount of social and technologic change that characterizes our society makes it questionable to assume that differences in the behaviours, attitudes, or characteristics of different age groups are the result of the passage through time rather than cohort or generational differences. In the previous example, seniors and freshmen may have different attitudes toward nursing research independent of any experiences they had during their 4 years of education. In cross-sectional studies, there are frequently alternative explanations for any observed differences.

Example of a cross-sectional study:

Mindell and Jacobson (2000) used a cross-sectional design to study sleep patterns and the presence of sleep disorders among pregnant women. Their sample included women at four points in pregnancy: at 8 to 12 weeks, 18 to 22 weeks, 25 to 28 weeks, and 35 to 38 weeks. They concluded that sleep disturbances were particularly common in late pregnancy.

Longitudinal Designs

Research projects designed to collect data over an extended time period are referred to as **longitudinal studies.** The main value of longitudinal designs is their ability to demonstrate changes over time and the temporal sequencing of phenomena, which is an essential criterion for establishing causality.

Three types of longitudinal studies deserve special mention: trend, panel, and follow-up studies. **Trend studies** are investigations in which samples from a general population are studied over time with respect to some phenomenon. Different samples are selected at repeated intervals, but the samples are always drawn from the same population. Trend studies permit researchers to examine patterns and rates of change and to make predictions about future directions. For example, trend studies have been conducted to analyze the number of students entering nursing programs and to forecast future supplies of nursing personnel.

In **panel studies,** the same participants supply the data at two or more points in time. The term *panel* refers to the sample of people involved in the study. Panel studies typically yield more information than trend studies because the investigator can examine patterns of change and reasons for the changes. The same people are contacted at two or more points in time; therefore, the researcher can identify those who did and did not change and then isolate the characteristics of the subgroups in which change occurred. Panel studies are appealing as an approach to studying change but are difficult and expensive to manage. The most serious problem is the loss of participants at different points in the study. Subject **attrition** causes problems for the researcher because those who drop out of the study may differ in important respects from those who continue to participate; hence, the generalizability of the findings may be impaired.

Example of a panel study:

Wilson et al. (2000) explored relationships among family dynamics, paternal–fetal and maternal–fetal attachment, and infant temperament. They first gathered data from pregnant women and their partners during the third trimester of pregnancy. Parental data from the first round of data collection were then linked to the infant's temperament about 1 year later when the child was 8 to 9 months old.

Follow-up studies are undertaken to determine the subsequent status of participants with a specified condition or those who have received a specified intervention. For example, patients who have received a particular nursing intervention or clinical treatment may be followed up to ascertain the long-term effects of the treatment. To take a nonexperimental example, samples of premature infants may be followed up to assess their later perceptual and motor development. Prospective studies usually fall in this category.

> **Example of a follow-up study:**
>
> Rennick et al. (2002) conducted a follow-up study of 120 children after discharge from a pediatric intensive care unit and ward. Data on the children's sense of control over their health, medical fears, posttraumatic stress, and changes in behaviours were collected before discharge and at 6 weeks and 6 months after discharge.

In longitudinal studies, the number of data collection periods and the time intervals between data collection points depend on the nature of the study. When change or development is rapid, numerous time points at relatively short intervals may be required to document the pattern and to make accurate forecasts. By convention, however, the term *longitudinal* implies multiple data collection points over an extended period. Our earlier example of a time-series study, which involved the collection of data on nurse turnover rates over a 2-year period, would be considered longitudinal. However, a time-series design involving the collection of patient data on vital signs preoperatively and postoperatively at hourly intervals over a 2-day period would not be described as longitudinal.

SPECIFIC TYPES OF QUANTITATIVE RESEARCH

This section describes some specific types of quantitative nursing research that vary according to the study's purpose rather than the dimensions outlined in Table 8-1.

Surveys

A **survey** obtains information regarding the prevalence, distribution, and interrelationships of variables within a population. Political opinion polls, such as those conducted by Gallup, are examples of surveys. Surveys collect information on people's actions, knowledge, intentions, opinions, and attitudes. Survey data are based on **self-reports;** that is, the respondents answer questions posed by the researcher. The three most common methods of collecting survey data are personal, face-to-face interviews; interviews by telephone; and self-administered questionnaires distributed through the mail. Survey research is highly flexible because it can be applied to many populations, it can focus on a wide range of topics, and its information can be used for many purposes. Survey information tends, however, to be relatively superficial. Survey research is better suited to extensive rather than intensive analysis. Although surveys can be performed within the context of large-scale experiments, surveys are usually done as part of a nonexperimental study.

> ### Example of a survey:
> Roberts et al. (2001) were interested in learning more about new mothers' use of maternal–infant health services and its associated costs following hospital postpartum discharge. Using self-administered questionnaires before discharge and a telephone interview at 4 weeks after discharge, the researchers surveyed 1250 mothers in the province of Ontario.

Evaluations

Evaluations are used to find out how well a program, treatment, practice, or policy works. Clinical nurses, nurse administrators, and nursing educators often need to pose such questions as the following: How are current practices working? Is there a more effective way to do things? Should a new practice be adopted? Which approach is most effective? In this era of accountability, evaluations of the effectiveness of nursing actions are common. Evaluations can employ experimental, quasi-experimental, or nonexperimental designs and can be either cross-sectional or longitudinal.

There are various types of evaluations. A **process analysis** (or an **implementation analysis**) is undertaken to obtain descriptive information about the process of implementing a new program or procedure and about its functioning in actual operation. An **outcome analysis** documents the extent to which the goals of a program are attained (*i.e.,* the extent to which positive outcomes occur). An **impact analysis** attempts to identify (usually using an experimental design) the impacts or **net effects** of an intervention (*i.e.,* the effects over and above what would have occurred in the absence of the intervention). Finally, evaluations sometimes include a **cost–benefit analysis** to determine whether the monetary benefits of the program outweigh the costs.

> ### Example of an evaluation:
> Edgar et al. (2001) evaluated the effect of a short-term psychoeducational coping skills training intervention, called Nucare, on oncology patients' psychosocial distress, well-being, and optimism. Eligible patients were randomly assigned to one of four groups: Nucare presented on an individual basis, Nucare presented in a group format, a nondirective supportive group, and a no-intervention control group. Measures of distress, well-being, and optimism were evaluated every 4 months during 1 year. Women with breast cancer who received Nucare presented in an individual format showed more significant improvements in measures of psychosocial distress and well-being over time compared with those in the control group.

Outcomes Reseach

Outcomes research, designed to document the effectiveness of health care services, is gaining momentum in nursing and health care fields. Outcomes research overlaps with evaluation research, but evaluations typically appraise a specific new intervention, whereas outcomes research is a more global assessment of health care services. The impetus for outcomes research comes from the quality assessment and quality assurance functions that grew out of the professional standards review organizations (PSROs) in the 1970s. Outcomes research represents a response to the increasing demand from policymakers, insurers, and the public to justify care practices and systems in terms of both improved patient outcomes and costs. Specific efforts to appraise and document the quality of nursing care—as distinct from the care provided by the overall health care system—are not numerous. A major obstacle is attribution, that is, linking the outcomes of interest to specific nursing actions or interventions, distinct from the actions or interventions of other members of the health care team.

Example of outcomes research:

Hagan et al. (2000) conducted an outcomes study to evaluate a hotline telephone service (telenursing) in the province of Quebec. Callers' ratings of perceived accessibility, satisfaction with care, and the development and use of self-care abilities subsequent to the use of telenursing were assessed. Researchers found, among other things, that of the 4696 callers, most were highly satisfied with the telephone service, most followed nurses' advice, and most carried out self-care measures as recommended. In addition, half the respondents stated that, without this service, they would have used emergency departments and a third of respondents reported that they would have consulted a doctor in private practice.

TECHNIQUES OF RESEARCH CONTROL

A major purpose of research design in quantitative studies is to maximize the researcher's control over the research situation. This section describes what is meant by research control and then discusses methods of achieving it.

Research Control

Research control is concerned with eliminating possible extraneous influences on the dependent variable so that the true relationship between the independent and dependent variables can be understood. Research control attempts to exclude contaminating factors that might obscure the relationship between the variables that are of central interest. A detailed example should clarify this point.

Suppose we wanted to study whether teenaged women are at higher risk than older mothers of having low-birth-weight infants because of their age. In other words, we want to test whether something about the maturational development of women causes differences in the birth weights of their infants.

Existing studies have shown that, in fact, teenagers have a higher rate of low-birth-weight infants than women in their twenties. The question, however, is whether age itself causes this difference or whether there are other **mediating variables** that intervene in the relationship between maternal age and infant birth weight.

We would want a study design that controls other influences on the dependent variable. But which variables should be controlled? To answer this, we must ask the following crucial question: What variables affect the dependent variable and at the same time are related to the independent variable?

In the present study, the dependent variable is infant birth weight and the independent variable is maternal age. Two variables that are candidates for concern (there are other possibilities) are the nutritional habits of the mother and the amount of prenatal care received. Teenagers have been found to have less-adequate diets during pregnancy and are also less likely to obtain adequate prenatal care than older women. Both nutrition and the amount of care could, in turn, affect the baby's birth weight. Thus, if these two mediating factors are not controlled, any observed relationship between the mother's age and her baby's weight at birth could be caused by the mother's age, by her diet, or by her prenatal care.

These three possible explanations are shown schematically.

1. Mother's age → infant birth weight
2. Mother's age → adequacy of prenatal care → infant birth weight
3. Mother's age → nutritional adequacy → infant birth weight

The arrows symbolize a causal mechanism or an influence. The researcher's task is to design a study in which the true explanation is made clear. If the researcher is testing the first explanation, then both nutrition and prenatal care must be controlled.

How can the researcher impose this control? The general principle underlying various control methods is this: the competing influences—the extraneous variables—must be held constant. The extraneous variables must somehow be handled in such a way that, *in the context of the study,* they are not related to the independent variable or dependent variable.

Research control is a fundamental feature of quantitative studies. The world is complex, and variables are interrelated in complicated ways. In quantitative studies, it is difficult to examine this complexity directly. Researchers analyze a few relationships at one time and put the pieces together like a jigsaw puzzle. That is why even modest quantitative studies can make contributions to knowledge. The extent of the contribution, however, is often related to how well a researcher controls contaminating influences. In reading reports, you will need to consider whether the researcher has, in fact, appropriately controlled extraneous variables.

Controlling External Factors

Various external factors, such as the research environment, can affect study variables. In carefully controlled quantitative research, steps are taken to minimize situational contaminants (*i.e.,* to achieve **constancy of conditions** for the collection of data) so that the researcher can be confident that the conditions are not influencing the data.

The environment has been found to influence people's emotions and behaviour, and therefore investigators strive to control the environmental context of the study. Control over the environment is most easily achieved in laboratory experiments, in which all participants are brought into an environment structured by the researcher. Researchers have less freedom to control studies that occur in natural settings, but some opportunities exist. For example, in interview studies, researchers can restrict data collection to one type of setting (*e.g.,* the respondents' homes).

A second external factor that may need to be controlled is time. Depending on the research topic, the dependent variable may be influenced by the time of day or the time of year in which the data are collected. In these cases, the researcher should ensure that constancy of time is maintained. If an investigator were studying fatigue or perceptions of well-being, it would matter whether the data were gathered in the morning, afternoon, or evening or in the summer as opposed to the winter.

Another aspect of maintaining constancy of conditions concerns the communications to the participants. To ensure constancy of communication, formal scripts are often prepared. In research involving the implementation of a treatment, formal **research protocols,** or specifications for the interventions, are developed. For example, in an experiment to test the effectiveness of a new medication, care would be needed to ensure that the participants in the experimental group received the same chemical substance and the same dosage, that the substance was administered in the same way, and so forth.

Controlling Intrinsic Factors

Control of study participants' characteristics is especially important. For example, suppose we were investigating the effects of an innovative physical training program on the cardiovascular functioning of residents in nursing homes. In this study, variables such as the participants' age, gender, and smoking history would be extraneous variables; each is likely to be related to the outcome variable (cardiovascular functioning), independent of the physical training program. In other words, the effects that these variables have on the dependent variable are extraneous to the research topic. In this section, we review methods of controlling extraneous participant characteristics.

Methods of Controlling Participant Characteristics
Randomization.   We have already discussed the most effective method of controlling participant characteristics: randomization. The primary function of randomization is to secure comparable groups, that is, to equalize the groups with respect to the extraneous variables. A distinct advantage of random

assignment, compared with other methods of controlling extraneous variables, is that randomization controls all possible sources of extraneous variation, without any conscious decision on the researcher's part about which variables need to be controlled. In our example of the physical training intervention, random assignment of participants to an experimental (intervention) group and control (no intervention) group would be the ideal control mechanism. Presumably, these two groups would be comparable in terms of age, gender, smoking history, and thousands of other preintervention characteristics. Randomization within a repeated-measures context is especially powerful. In a repeated-measures design, participants serve as their own controls, thereby totally controlling all extraneous variables.

Example of randomization:

Using an experimental before and after design, Hartford et al. (2002) tested the effectiveness of an information and support telephone intervention for reducing anxiety in patients who have undergone coronary artery bypass grafting and their partners. Patient–partner dyads were randomly assigned through computer-generated numbers to either the treatment or the control group (usual care). The researchers found that the treatment group was similar to the control group in terms of age, gender, marital status, education, employment, occupation, diagnosis, and procedures undergone.

Homogeneity.   When randomization is not feasible, other methods of controlling extraneous participant characteristics can be used. The first alternative is **homogeneity,** in which only participants who are homogeneous with respect to the extraneous variables are included in the study. The extraneous variables, in this case, are not allowed to vary. In the example of the physical training program, if gender were considered a confounding variable, the researcher could recruit only men (or only women) as participants. If the researcher were concerned about the confounding effect of the participants' ages on physical fitness, participation could be limited to those within a specified age range. This strategy of using a homogeneous subject pool is easy, but its limitation is that the findings can be generalized only to the type of participants who took part. If the physical training program was found to have beneficial effects on the cardiovascular functioning of men aged 65 to 75 years, its usefulness for improving the cardiovascular status of women in their eighties would need to be tested in a separate study.

Example of homogeneity:

Zauszniewski and Chung (2001) studied the effects of depressive symptoms and learned resourcefulness on the health practices of persons with diabetes. They restricted their sample to adult women with type 2 diabetes who had no history of a mental disorder.

Matching.   A third method of dealing with extraneous variables is matching. **Matching** involves using information about participant characteristics to form comparison groups. For example, suppose the researcher began with a sample of nursing home residents already participating in the physical training program. A comparison group of nonparticipating residents could be created by matching participants, one by one, on the basis of important extraneous variables (*e.g.,* age and gender). This procedure results in groups known to be comparable in terms of the extraneous variables of concern. Matching is the technique used to form comparable groups in case-control designs.

Matching has some drawbacks as a control technique. To match effectively, the researcher must know in advance what the relevant extraneous variables are. Second, after two or three variables, it becomes difficult to match. Suppose we wanted to control the age, gender, race, and length of nursing home stays of the participants. Thus, if participant 1 in the physical training program is an African-American woman, aged 80 years, whose length of stay is 5 years, the researcher must seek another woman with these same or similar characteristics as a comparison group counterpart. With more than three variables, the matching procedure becomes extremely cumbersome. Thus, matching as a control technique is usually used only when more powerful procedures are not feasible.

Example of matching:

Benzies et al. (in press) followed parents of preterm and full-term infants for a 7-year period to study the relationship between children's characteristics and family environmental factors during the child's first year of life and subsequent behavioural problems at age 7. At recruitment, the sample consisted of 56 families with a preterm infant and 58 families with a full-term infant. To ensure that the groups were similar, participants were matched in terms of hospital of birth and infant gender.

Statistical Control.   Yet another method of controlling extraneous variables is through statistical analysis. Many readers are unfamiliar with basic statistical procedures, let alone sophisticated techniques such as those referred to here. Therefore, a detailed description of powerful statistical control mechanisms, such as **analysis of covariance,** will not be attempted. You should recognize, however, that nurse researchers are increasingly using powerful statistical techniques to control extraneous variables. A brief description of analysis of covariance is presented in Chapter 13.

Example of statistical control:

Wishart et al. (2000) evaluated a community-based visiting/walking program provided by volunteers to reduce caregiver burden among those caring for a cognitively impaired relative. The researchers knew in advance that the caregiver's level of education could influence their report of caregiver burden. Through statistical control, the two groups of caregivers (the intervention and control groups) were made comparable so that observed differences in caregiver burden could not be attributed to group differences in level of education.

Evaluation of Control Methods

Overall, random assignment is the most effective approach to controlling extraneous variables because randomization tends to cancel out individual variation on all possible extraneous variables. Repeated-measures designs are especially powerful, but they cannot be applied to all nursing research problems because of the possibility of carryover effects. The three remaining alternatives described here have two disadvantages in common. First, the researcher must know the relevant extraneous variables in advance. To select homogeneous samples, match, or perform an analysis of covariance, researchers must decide which variables to control. Second, these three methods control only for preidentified characteristics, possibly leaving others uncontrolled.

Although randomization is the best mechanism for controlling extraneous participant characteristics, randomization is not always possible. If the independent variable cannot be manipulated, other techniques must be used. It is far better to use matching or analysis of covariance than simply to ignore the problem of extraneous variables.

✓ CONSUMER TIP

In nursing studies that are not experimental, statistical procedures such as analysis of covariance are the most frequently used methods of controlling extraneous variables. Matching, which was a commonly used control technique a few decades ago, has become much less prevalent since computers have become widely available for statistical analysis. ■

INTERNAL AND EXTERNAL VALIDITY

In evaluating the merits of a quantitative study, you will need to pay careful attention to its research design. One useful framework for evaluating the adequacy of a research design in a quantitative study is an assessment of its internal and external validity.

Internal Validity

Campbell and Stanley (1963), in a classic monograph, use the term **internal validity** to refer to the extent to which it is possible to make an inference that the independent variable is truly influencing the dependent variable. Experiments possess a high degree of internal validity because randomization to different groups enables the researcher to rule out competing explanations. With quasi-experiments and correlational studies, the investigator must always contend with rival hypotheses. Competing explanations, or **threats to internal validity,** have been grouped into several classes.

Threats to Internal Validity

History.   The **history threat** is the occurrence of events concurrent with the independent variable that can affect the dependent variable. For example, suppose we were studying the effectiveness of an outreach program to encourage flu shots among the community-dwelling elderly using a time-series design. Now let us further suppose that, at about the same time the outreach program was initiated, there was a national public media campaign focusing on the flu. Our dependent variable in this case, number of flu shots administered, is now subject to the influence of at least two forces, and it becomes impossible for us to disentangle the two effects. In an experiment, history is not typically an issue because external events are as likely to affect one group as another; however, history can be a threat in quasi-experimental and nonexperimental studies.

Selection. The **selection threat** encompasses biases resulting from preexisting differences between groups. When people are not assigned randomly to groups, the possibility always exists that groups being compared are not equivalent. In such a situation, the researcher contends with the possibility that any difference in the dependent variable is due to extraneous factors rather than to the independent variable. Selection biases are the most problematic threats to the internal validity of studies not using an experimental design but can be partially addressed using the control mechanisms described in the previous section.

Maturation. In a research context, the **maturation threat** arises from processes occurring within the participants as a result of time (*e.g.,* growth, fatigue) rather than the independent variable. For example, if we wanted to evaluate the effect of a special sensorimotor-development program for developmentally retarded children, we would have to contend with the fact that progress would occur even without the intervention. Maturation is a relevant consideration in many areas of nursing research. Remember that the term here does not refer to developmental changes exclusively but rather to any kind of change that occurs as a function of time. Thus, phenomena such as wound healing, postoperative recovery, and other bodily changes can occur with little nursing intervention, and thus maturation may be a rival explanation for posttreatment results. The one-group before–after design is particularly vulnerable to the maturation threat.

Mortality. The **mortality threat** arises from differential attrition from groups. The loss of participants during the study may differ among groups because of initial differences in interest, motivation, and the like. For example, suppose we used a nonequivalent control-group design to assess nurses' morale in two different hospitals, one of which initiated primary nursing. The dependent variable, nursing staff morale, is measured before and after the intervention. The comparison group, which may have no particular commitment to the study, may be reluctant to complete a posttest questionnaire. Those who do fill it out may be totally unrepresentative of the group as a whole; they may be highly critical of their work environment, for example. Thus, on the average, it may appear that the morale of nurses in the comparison hospital declined, but this might only be an artifact of the mortality of a select segment of this group.

Internal Validity and Research Design

Quasi-experimental, preexperimental, and correlational studies are especially susceptible to threats to internal validity. The four threats described previously represent alternative explanations that compete with the independent variable as an influence on the dependent variable. *The aim of a good quantitative research design is to rule out these competing explanations.* The control mechanisms previously reviewed are strategies for improving the internal validity of studies.

Experimental designs normally eliminate competing explanations, but this is not always the case. For example, if constancy of conditions is not maintained for experimental and control groups, history might be a rival explanation for obtained results. Experimental mortality is, in particular, a salient threat in experiments. Because the experimenter does different things with the experimental and control groups, participants may drop out of the study differentially among these groups. This is particularly likely to happen if the experimental treatment is stressful, inconvenient, or time-consuming or if the control condition is boring or aggravating. When this happens, the participants remaining in the study may differ from those who left, thereby nullifying the initial equivalence of the groups.

You should pay careful attention to the possibility of competing explanations for reported results, especially in studies that do not use an experimental design. When the investigator does not have control over critical extraneous variables, caution in interpreting the results and drawing conclusions from them is appropriate.

External Validity

The term **external validity** refers to the generalizability of the research findings to other settings or samples. Quantitative studies are rarely conducted with the intention of discovering relationships among variables for a single group of people. If a nursing intervention is found to be successful, others would want to adopt the procedure. Therefore, an important question is whether the intervention would work in another setting or with different patients.

One aspect of a study's external validity concerns the adequacy of the sampling design. If the characteristics of the sample are representative of those of the population, the generalizability of the results is enhanced. Sampling designs are described in Chapter 10.

Various characteristics of the environment or research situation also affect the study's external validity. For example, when a treatment is new (*e.g.,* a new curriculum for nursing students), participants and researchers alike might alter their behaviour. People may be either enthusiastic or skeptical about new methods of doing things. Thus, the results may reflect reactions to the novelty rather than to the intrinsic qualities of the treatment.

Occasionally, the demands for internal and external validity conflict. If a researcher exercises tight control over a study to maximize internal validity, the setting may become too artificial to generalize to a more naturalistic environment. Therefore, a compromise must sometimes be reached. The importance of replicating studies in different settings with new participants cannot be overemphasized.

CRITIQUING QUANTITATIVE RESEARCH DESIGNS

The overriding consideration in evaluating a research design is whether the design enables the researcher to answer the research question. This must be determined in terms of both substantive and methodologic issues.

Substantively, the issue is whether the researcher selected a design that matches the aims of the research. If the research purpose is descriptive or exploratory, an experimental design is inappropriate. If the researcher is searching to understand the full nature of a phenomenon about which little is known, a highly structured design that allows little flexibility might block insights (flexible designs are discussed in Chap.9). We have discussed research control as a mechanism for reducing bias, but in certain situations, too much control can introduce bias, for example, when the researcher tightly controls the ways in which the phenomena under study can be manifested and thereby obscures their true nature.

Methodologically, the main design issues in quantitative studies are whether the research design provides the most accurate, unbiased, interpretable answers possible to the research question and whether it yields replicable results. Box 8-1 provides questions to assist you in evaluating the methodologic aspects of quantitative research designs.

RESEARCH EXAMPLES

Following are descriptions of the research designs used in three actual nursing studies. Use the guidelines in Box 8-1 to evaluate the research designs, referring to the full reports (cited at the end of the chapter), if necessary.

Research Example of an Experimental Evaluation

Arthur and her colleagues (2000) conducted a clinical trial to evaluate the effect of a preoperative intervention on preoperative and postoperative outcomes among patients awaiting coronary artery bypass graft (CABG) surgery. The evaluation included an impact analysis related to patient outcomes and a cost–benefit analysis.

Research Summary
In their study, Arthur and colleagues compared individuals waiting to undergo a CABG who received a multidimensional preoperative intervention with those who only received usual care. Patients who met the study criteria

BOX 8-1

GUIDELINES FOR CRITIQUING RESEARCH DESIGNS IN QUANTITATIVE STUDIES

1. Given the nature of the research question, what type of design is most appropriate? How does this correspond to the type of design used?

2. Does the design used in the study involve an intervention? If yes, was an experimental, quasi-experimental, or preexperimental design used—and was this the most appropriate design?

3. If the design is nonexperimental, why didn't the researcher manipulate the independent variable? Was the decision regarding manipulation appropriate?

4. Was the study longitudinal or cross-sectional? Was the number of points of data collection appropriate, given the research question?

5. What type of comparisons were called for in the research design (*e.g.,* was the study design within-subjects or between-subjects)? Are these comparisons the most appropriate for illuminating the relationship between the independent and dependent variables?

6. Can the study be described as a survey, an evaluation, or outcomes research?

7. What procedures, if any, did the researcher use to control external (situational) factors and intrinsic (subject characteristic) factors? Were these procedures appropriate and adequate?

8. To what extent is the study internally valid? What types of alternative explanations must be considered (*i.e.,* what are the threats to the study's internal validity)? Does the research design enable the researcher to draw causal inferences about the relationship among study variables?

9. To what extent is the study externally valid?

10. What are the major limitations of the design used? Are these limitations acknowledged by the researcher and taken into account in interpreting the results?

and agreed to participate were randomly assigned to either group. The sample consisted of 123 patients in each group. Participants in the intervention group received an 8-week individualized preoperative intervention that included exercise training twice per week in a supervised environment, education and reinforcement, and monthly nurse-initiated telephone calls to answer questions and provide reassurance. Participants in the control group were followed by their primary care physicians, cardiologists, or surgeons.

The research team was interested in evaluating the effect of the intervention on two main areas: (1) postoperative hospital length of stay and related costs of care and (2) health-related outcomes such as physical performance, quality of life, anxiety, and use of health services by patients.

Findings indicated that overall the intervention group spent 1 less day in hospital than the control group with a net cost saving of approximately $133 per patient per day, when considering the intervention and related physical performance tests costs. In addition, the intervention group reported better health-related quality of life during the waiting period, which continued up to 6 months after surgery. Mortality rates did not differ between the two groups.

Clinical Relevance

In several Canadian provinces, there is high demand for CABG but increasing budgetary constraints means that patients in need of CABG are often placed on waiting lists. Recent publications suggest that this waiting period may be used productively to manage distress and improve health outcomes. The researchers systematically studied whether an innovative intervention during the wait period would make a difference. Because waiting time related to health services is now a common phenomenon, Arthur and her colleagues addressed an issue of considerable significance to both patients and the health care system.

Their findings are persuasive because they used a rigourous research design. By randomly assigning the participants to either the standard care control group or the special intervention group, the researchers could be reasonably confident that the intervention, rather than any preexisting group differences, resulted in shorter hospital stays and better quality of life. In fact, the researchers documented that the experimental and control groups were comparable in terms of such factors as medical background (*e.g.*, number of aortocoronary bypasses, resting heart rate, blood pressure, and use of beta-blockers), and gender—attesting to the success of the randomization. As such, the clinical implications of this study are many. As health care costs continue to spiral upward, it may be financially beneficial for hospitals to consider programs similar to that of Arthur and her colleagues, in which a multidimensional preoperative intervention is used during the waiting period.

Research Example of a Quasi-Experimental Study

Bull, Hansen, and Gross (2000) used a quasi-experimental design to assess the effect of a professional–patient partnership model of discharge planning with elders hospitalized with heart failure on various health-related outcomes (*e.g.*, quality of life, psychological distress, health locus of control, patient's satisfaction with health services, readmission to hospital and emergency use, and family reaction to caregiving).

The sample consisted of 180 elder–caregiver dyads. The discharge planning model was implemented in one hospital and a nonequivalent control group was secured through a different hospital that did not adopt the new model. The two hospitals were matched in terms of size, type, and the discharge planning practices used in the hospitals' cardiac units. Data on a range of measures (including health status, patient satisfaction, and health locus of control) were collected from patients and caregivers predischarge, and then again at 2 weeks and 2 months after discharge. Data were gathered in both hospitals before and then again after the intervention was implemented, thus combining features of a nonequivalent control-group design with that of a mini-time series. Because postintervention data from the comparison group in the second hospital were contaminated (the hospital introduced an innovation that weakened comparisons), postintervention data from the experimental group were compared with two rather than three comparison groups, as originally planned (*i.e.*, patients from both hospitals before the new model was implemented). The three groups of elders were found to be comparable in terms of demographics and predischarge measures of health. The two comparison groups were combined for the analysis, due to the absence of any significant differences between them.

Findings indicated that elders in the treatment group felt better prepared to manage care, reported more continuity of information about care management, and felt they were in better health than elders in the comparison group. Moreover, elders in the treatment group who were readmitted to the hospital spent fewer days in the hospital than their counterparts in the comparison group. The strength of the design makes it possible to draw inferences about the effectiveness of the innovative discharge planning model, even in the absence of randomization.

Clinical Relevance

Nurses can play an important role in promoting involvement of patients and caregivers in discharge planning. The results from this study suggest that the professional–patient partnership model can facilitate elder and caregiver participation in planning. Nurses in practice might incorporate elements of this model in assisting patients and caregivers to plan for discharge. For example, they can explore patient and caregiver postdischarge needs and preferences, encourage them to ask questions regarding their care, and refer them to appropriate resources.

Results from this study also indicate that more than half the elders and caregivers in both the control and intervention groups reported difficulty evaluating and managing symptoms after discharge. Patients who had been ingesting food that had a high salt content, for instance, did not realize that salt contributes to fluid retention nor that fluid retention is related to heart failure. This suggests that patients and caregivers need to learn not only about how to relieve symptoms, but also how to recognize readily potential contributors to these symptoms.

Findings also suggest that the provision of information to caregivers pertaining to the elder's condition, medication, and diet may reduce frustration and distress related to caregiving and contribute to more positive health outcomes.

Nurse administrators might wish to evaluate the feasibility of similar discharge planning models that take into consideration patients and family preferences and the key role of caregivers in planning for discharge.

Research Example of a Nonexperimental Survey

Loiselle and colleagues (2001) conducted a survey of first-time mothers regarding the breastfeeding information and support that was provided to them by health professionals.

Research Summary

Loiselle and her colleagues sought to document women's perceptions of the breastfeeding support received from hospital- and community-based health professionals within a multiethnic community. The researchers examined differences in the perceptions of Canadian-born and immigrant women. A telephone survey was used to gather data for this descriptive, nonexperimental study.

The sample for this study consisted of 108 first-time mothers, who were surveyed at 3 weeks postpartum. The survey instrument was administered by telephone by a trained interviewer. The interview included questions about the women's impressions of professional support for breastfeeding, whether recommended breastfeeding practices had been delivered, and the nature and sources of breastfeeding informational support received. Questions about support included ones relating to health care professionals' emotional support (*e.g.,* "helped you to feel confident about breastfeeding"), instrumental support (*e.g.,* "gave good 'hands-on' help with breastfeeding"), and informational support (*e.g.,* "got enough information about breastfeeding").

Loiselle and her colleagues found that, overall, women's evaluations of professional support for breastfeeding were positive, even though they reported breastfeeding practices that fell short of recommended standards. Immigrant women were more likely than Canadian-born women to experience hospital practices detrimental to breastfeeding success, but were more likely to receive professional breastfeeding support in the community. Significant differences were also found between Canadian-born and immigrant women's sources of breastfeeding informational support.

Clinical Relevance

Health professionals are in a key position to enhance breastfeeding success through the provision and mobilization of timely, consistent, and culturally sensitive forms of support, particularly for first-time mothers. A lack of accurate knowledge about and negative attitudes toward breastfeeding are acknowledged as significant barriers to the promotion and support of breastfeeding by health professionals. In addition, inconsistent or conflicting breastfeeding information from professionals is identified frequently as detrimental to the initiation of breastfeeding. Given the context of an increasingly culturally diverse population, an enhanced understanding of similarities and discrepancies in the breastfeeding needs and resources of both Canadian-born and immigrant women is needed for health professionals to best support optimal breastfeeding practices among all Canadians. This study took place in

Quebec; therefore, the study should be replicated to determine its applicability in other provinces and countries.

● ● ● ● ● *SUMMARY POINTS*

* The **research design** is the researcher's overall plan for answering the research question. In quantitative studies, the design indicates whether there is an intervention, the type of intervention, the nature of any comparisons, the methods used to control extraneous variables, and the timing and location of data collection.
* **Experimental research** involves **manipulation** (the researcher manipulates the independent variable by introducing a **treatment**), control (including the use of a **control group** that is compared with the experimental group), and **randomization** (wherein participants are allocated to experimental and control groups at random to make the groups comparable at the outset).
* The **after-only design** involves collecting data only once—after random assignment and the introduction of the treatment.
* In the **before–after** (or **pretest–posttest**) design, data are collected both before and after the experimental manipulation.
* **Factorial designs,** in which two or more variables are manipulated simultaneously, allow researchers to test both **main effects** (effects from the experimentally manipulated variables) and **interaction effects** (effects resulting from combining the treatments).
* **Between-subjects designs,** in which different groups of people are compared, contrast with **within-subjects designs,** which involve comparisons of the same participants.
* In a **repeated-measures design** (or **crossover design**), research participants are exposed to more than one experimental condition and serve as their own controls.
* When an experiment is used to test the efficacy of a clinical treatment in a large, heterogeneous population, the study is referred to as a **clinical trial.**
* **Quasi-experimental research** involves manipulation but lacks a comparison group or randomization. Quasi-experiments are designs in which controls are introduced to compensate for these missing components. By contrast, **preexperimental designs** have no such safeguards.
* **The nonequivalent control-group before–after design** involves the use of a **comparison group** that was not created through random assignment and the collection of pretreatment data that permits an assessment of initial group equivalence.
* In a **time-series design,** there is no comparison group; information on the dependent variable is collected over a period of time before and after the treatment.

- **Nonexperimental research** includes **descriptive research**—studies that summarize the status of phenomena—and *ex post facto* (or **correlational**) studies that examine relationships among variables but involve no manipulation of the independent variable.
- Researchers use **retrospective** and **prospective** *ex post facto* designs to infer causality, but the findings from such studies are usually open to several interpretations.
- **Cross-sectional designs** involve the collection of data at one point in time, whereas longitudinal designs involve data collection at two or more points over an extended time period. Three types of **longitudinal studies,** which are used to study changes or development over time, are **trend studies, panel studies,** and **follow-up studies.**
- **Survey research** examines the characteristics, attitudes, behaviours, and intentions of a group of people by asking individuals to answer questions either through interviews or self-administered questionnaires.
- **Evaluations** involve the collection and analysis of information relating to the effects and functioning of a program or procedure.
- **Outcomes research** is undertaken to document the effectiveness and quality of health care services and the end results of patient care.
- **Research control** is used to control external factors that could affect the study outcomes (*e.g.,* the environment) and to control intrinsic participant characteristics that are extraneous to the research question.
- Techniques for controlling participant characteristics include **homogeneity** (restricting the selection of participants to eliminate variability on the extraneous variable); **matching** (matching participants on a one-to-one basis to make groups comparable on the extraneous variables); statistical procedures, such as **analysis of covariance;** and randomization—the most effective control procedure because it controls all possible extraneous variables without the researcher having to identify or measure them.
- **Internal validity** concerns the degree to which the results of a study can be attributed to the independent variable. **Threats to internal validity** include **history, selection, maturation,** and **mortality** (caused by participant **attrition**).
- **External validity** refers to the ability to generalize study findings to other samples and settings.

➤➤➤➤ *CRITICAL THINKING ACTIVITIES*

Chapter 8 of the accompanying *Study Guide to Accompany Essentials of Nursing Research,* 5th edition, offers various exercises and study suggestions for reinforcing the concepts presented in this chapter. In addition, you can address the following:

1. Read the first of the actual research studies in the Appendix of this book and then answer the questions in Box 8-1.

2. Read the full study by Arthur and colleagues (2000) that was described as a research example of an experimental study. What were the independent and dependent variables in this study? What, in your opinion, were the key extraneous variables? To what extent did the research design control these variables?

For additional review, see questions 81–105 on the study CD provided with Polit: Study Guide to Accompany Essentials of Nursing Research.

SUGGESTED READINGS

Methodologic References

Campbell, D.T., & Stanley, J.C. (1963). *Experimental and quasi-experimental designs for research.* Chicago: Rand McNally.

Kerlinger, F.N., & Lee, H.B. (2000). *Foundations of behavioral research.* (4th ed.). Orlando, FL: Harcourt College Publishers.

Lazarsfeld, P. (1955). Foreword. In H. Hyman (Ed.), *Survey design and analysis.* New York: The Free Press.

Polit, D.F., & Beck, C.T. (2003). *Nursing research: Principles and methods.* (7th Ed.). Philadelphia: Lippincott Williams & Wilkins.

Substantive References

Arthur, H. M., Daniels, C., McKelvie, R. S., Hirsh, J., & Rush, B. (2000). The effects of a pre-operative intervention on pre and post-operative outcomes in patients awaiting elective CABG surgery in Ontario: A randomized controlled trial. *Annals of Internal Medicine, 133,* 253–262.

Benzies, K. M., Harrison, M. J., & Magill-Evans, J. (in press). Parenting stress, marital quality, and child behavior problems at age 7 years. *Public Health Nursing.*

Bull, M. J., Hansen, H. E., & Gross, C.R. (2000). A professional -patient partnership model of discharge planning with elders hospitalized with heart failure. *Applied Nursing Research, 13,* 19–28.

Edgar, L., Rosberger, Z., & Collet, J.-P. (2001). Lessons learned: Outcomes and methodology of a coping skills intervention trial comparing individual and group formats for patients with cancer. *International Journal of Psychiatry in Medicine, 31,* 289–304.

Gardner, A., & Sibthorpe, B. (2002). Will he get back to normal? Survival and functional status after intensive care therapy. *Intensive Critical Care Nursing, 18,* 138–145.

Goulet, C., Gevry, H., Gauthier, R. J., Lepage, L., Fraser, W., & Aita, M. (2001). A controlled clinical trial of home care management versus hospital care management for preterm labour. *International Journal of Nursing Studies, 38,* 259–69.

Hagan, L., Morin, D., & Lépine, R. (2000). Evaluation of telenursing outcomes: Satisfaction, self-care practices, and cost savings. *Public Health Nursing, 17,* 305–313.

Harrisson, M., Loiselle, C. G., Duquette, A., & Semenic, S. E. (2002). Hardiness, work support and psychological distress among nursing assistants and registered nurses in Quebec. *Journal of Advanced Nursing, 38,* 584–591.

Hartford, K., Wong, C., & Zakaria, D. (2002). Randomized controlled trial of a telephone intervention by nurses to provide information and support to patients and their partners after elective coronary artery bypass graft surgery: Effects of anxiety. *Heart & Lung, 31,* 199–206.

Heitkemper, M., Jarrett, M., Taylor, P., Walker, E., Landenburger, K., & Bond, E. F. (2001). Effect of sexual and physical abuse on symptom experiences in women with irritable bowel syndrome. *Nursing Research, 50,* 15–23.

Loiselle, C. G., Semenic, S. E., Côté, B., Lapointe, M., & Gendron, R. (2001). Impressions of breastfeeding information and support among first-time mothers within a multiethnic community. *Canadian Journal of Nursing Research, 33,* 31–46.

Milne, J. (2000). The impact of information on health behaviors of older adults with urinary incontinence. *Clinical Nursing Research, 9,* 161–176.

Mindell, J. A., & Jacobson, B. J. (2000). Sleep disturbances in pregnancy. *Journal of Obstetric, Gynecologic, and Neonatal Nursing, 29,* 590–597.

Pridham, K., Kosorok, M. R., Greer, F., Carey, P., Kayata, S., & Sondel, S. (1999). The effects of ad libitum feelings and formula caloric density on premature infant dietary intake and weight gain. *Nursing Research, 48,* 86–93.

Rennick, J. E., Johnston, C. C., Dougherty, G., Platt, R., & Ritchie, J. (2002). Children's psychological responses after critical illness and exposure to invasive technology. *Developmental and Behavioral Pediatrics, 23,* 133–144.

Reynolds, N. R., & Neidig, J. L. (2002). Characteristics of nausea reported by HIV-infected patients initiating combination antiretroviral regimens. *Clinical Nursing Research, 11,* 71–88.

Roberts, J., Sword, W., Watt, S., Gafni, A., Krueger, P., Sheehan, D., & Soon-Lee, K. (2001). Costs of postpartum care: Examining associations from the Ontario Mother and Infant Survey. *Canadian Journal of Nursing Research, 33,* 19–34.

Wells, D. L., Dawson, P. L., Sidani, S., Craig, D., & Pringle, D. (2001). Effects of an abilities focused program of morning care on the behaviors of residents and on caregivers' perceptions of caregiving. In S.G. Funk, E. M. Tornquist, J. Leeman, M. S. Miles, & J. S. Harrell (Eds.), *Key aspects of preventing and managing chronic illness* (pp. 316–329). New York: Springer Publishing.

Wilson, M. E., White, M. A., Cobb, B., Curry, R., Greene, D., & Popovitch, D. (2000). Family dynamics, parental-fetal attachment, and infant temperament. *Journal of Advanced Nursing, 31,* 204–210.

Winkelman, C. (2000). Effect of backrest position on intracranial and cerebral perfusion pressures in traumatically brain-injured adults. *American Journal of Critical Care, 9,* 373–382.

Wishart, L., Macerollo, J., Loney, P., King, A., Beaumont, L., Browne, G., & Roberts, J. (2000). "Special Steps": An effective visiting/walking program for persons with cognitive impairment. *Canadian Journal of Nursing Research, 31,* 57–71.

Zauszniewski, J. A., & Chung, C. W. (2001). Resourcefulness and health practices of diabetic women. *Research in Nursing & Health, 24,* 113–121.

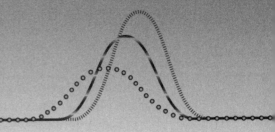

Understanding Qualitative Research Design

THE DESIGN OF QUALITATIVE STUDIES
Characteristics of Qualitative Research
Design
Qualitative Design and Planning
Phases in a Qualitative Study
Qualitative Design Features
QUALITATIVE RESEARCH TRADITIONS
Overview of Qualitative Research Traditions
Ethnography
Phenomenology
Grounded Theory
**INTEGRATION OF QUALITATIVE AND QUANTITATIVE
APPROACHES**
Rationale for Integrated Designs

Applications of Integrated Designs
Integration Strategies
CRITIQUING QUALITATIVE AND INTEGRATED DESIGNS
RESEARCH EXAMPLES
Research Example of a Grounded Theory
Study
Research Example of an Ethnographic Study
Research Example of an Integrated Study
SUMMARY POINTS
CRITICAL THINKING ACTIVITIES
SUGGESTED READINGS
Methodologic References
Substantive References

Student Objectives

On completion of this chapter, the student will be able to:

○ describe the characteristics of and rationale for an emergent design in qualitative research
○ describe the three major phases typical in the design of a qualitative study
○ identify the major research traditions for qualitative research and describe the domain of inquiry of each
○ describe the characteristics of ethnographic, phenomenological, and grounded theory studies
○ identify several advantages of an integrated qualitative and quantitative design and describe specific applications
○ define new terms in the chapter

New Terms

Being-in-the-world	Ethology
Black box	Etic perspective
Bracketing	Grounded theory
Bricolage	Hermeneutics
Cognitive anthropology	Historical research
Constant comparison	Integrated design
Corporeality	Intuiting
Discourse analysis	Macroethnography
Ecological psychology	Microethnography
Embodiment	Multimethod research
Emergent design	Phenomenology
Emic perspective	Relationality
Essence	Researcher as instrument
Ethnography	Spatiality
Ethnomethodology	Symbolic interaction
Ethnonursing research	Tacit knowledge
Ethnoscience	Temporality

THE DESIGN OF QUALITATIVE STUDIES

As we have seen, quantitative researchers specify a research design before collecting any data and adhere to that design after the study is underway. In qualitative research, by contrast, study design elements typically evolve over the course of the project. Decisions about how best to obtain data, from whom to obtain data, how to schedule data collection, and how long each data collection session should last are made in the field, as the study unfolds. The design for a qualitative study is an **emergent design**—a design that emerges as the researcher makes ongoing decisions reflecting what has already been learned. As noted by Lincoln and Guba (1985), an emergent design in qualitative studies is not the result of researchers' sloppiness or laziness, but rather of their desire to base the inquiry on the realities and viewpoints of those under study—realities and viewpoints that are not known or understood at the outset.

CONSUMER TIP

Design decisions for a qualitative study are usually summarized in the method section of a report (*e.g.,* a decision to interview a subset of study participants a second time), but the decision-making process for design decisions is rarely described. ■

Characteristics of Qualitative Research Design

Qualitative inquiry has been guided by a number of different disciplines, and each has developed methods best suited to address questions of particular interest. However, some general characteristics of qualitative research design tend to apply across disciplines. Qualitative design has the following characteristics:

- It is flexible and elastic, capable of adjusting to what is being learned during the course of data collection
- It typically involves a merging together of various data collection strategies
- It tends to be holistic, striving for an understanding of the whole
- It requires the researcher to become intensely involved, usually remaining in the field for lengthy periods of time
- It requires the researcher to become the research instrument
- It requires ongoing analysis of the data to formulate subsequent strategies and to determine when field work is done

With regard to the second characteristic, qualitative researchers tend to put together a complex array of data, derived from various sources. This tendency has been described as **bricolage,** and the qualitative researcher has been referred to as a *bricoleur,* a person who "is adept at performing a large number of diverse tasks, ranging from interviewing to observing, to interpreting personal and historical documents, to intensive reflection and introspection" (Denzin & Lincoln, 1994, p. 2).

Qualitative Design and Planning

Although design decisions are not specified in advance, the qualitative researcher typically does advance planning that can support an emergent design. In the absence of planning, flexibility in the design might actually be constrained. For example, a researcher might project a 6-month period for data collection but might also plan (financially and emotionally) for the possibility of spending longer in the field to pursue emerging data collection opportunities.

In other words, the qualitative researcher plans for broad contingencies that may be expected to pose decision opportunities after the study has begun. Advance planning is especially important with regard to the following:

- Selection of a broad research tradition (described in the next section) that will guide certain design and analytic decisions
- Selection of the study site and identification of settings within the site that are likely to be especially fruitful for data collection
- Identification of the key "gatekeepers" who can provide (or deny) access to important sources of data and can make arrangements for gaining entrée
- Determination of the maximal time available for the study, given costs and other constraints
- Identification of all needed equipment for the collection and analysis of data in the field (*e.g.,* audio and video recording equipment, laptop computers, etc.)

Thus, qualitative researchers plan for various circumstances, but decisions about how they will deal with them must be resolved when the social context of time, place, and human interactions is better understood.

Phases in a Qualitative Study

Although the exact form of a qualitative study is not specified in advance, Lincoln and Guba (1985) noted that a naturalistic inquiry typically progresses through three broad phases while the researcher is in the field:

1. *Orientation and overview.* Quantitative researchers generally believe they know what they do not know (*i.e.,* they know the type of knowledge they expect to obtain by doing a study and then strive to obtain it). A qualitative researcher, by contrast, enters the study "not knowing what is not known" (*i.e.,* not knowing what it is about the phenomenon that will drive the inquiry forward). Therefore, the first phase of many qualitative studies is to get a handle on what is salient about the phenomenon of interest.
2. *Focused exploration.* The second phase is a more focused scrutiny and in-depth exploration of aspects of the phenomenon judged to be salient. The questions asked and the types of people invited to participate in the study are shaped by the understandings developed in the first phase.
3. *Confirmation and closure.* In the final phase, qualitative researchers undertake efforts to establish that their findings are trustworthy, often by going back and discussing their understanding with study participants. Phase 3 activities are described in Chapter 12.

The three phases are not discrete but rather overlap to a greater or lesser degree in different projects. For example, even the first few interviews or observations are typically used as a basis for selecting subsequent informants, even though the researcher is still striving to understand the scope of the phenomenon and to identify its major dimensions. The various phases might take only a few weeks to complete—or they may take many months.

Qualitative Design Features

Some of the design features of quantitative studies (see Chap. 8) also apply to qualitative studies. However, qualitative design features are often *post hoc* characterizations of what happened in the field rather than features specifically planned in advance. To further contrast qualitative and quantitative research design, we refer to the design elements identified in Table 8-1 in Chapter 8.

Control Over the Independent Variable

Qualitative researchers do not conceptualize their studies as having independent and dependent variables, and they rarely control or manipulate any aspect of the setting under study. Qualitative research is almost always nonexperimental—although, as we discuss later in this chapter, a qualitative study sometimes can be embedded within an experimental project.

Type of Group Comparisons

Qualitative researchers typically do not plan in advance to make group comparisons because the intent of most qualitative studies is to describe thoroughly and explain a phenomenon. Nevertheless, patterns emerging in the data sometimes suggest that certain comparisons are relevant and illuminating.

Example of qualitative comparisons:

Katz (2001) described the experience of screening for HIV in pregnancy from the perspective of pregnant women. Katz discovered that, although there were commonalities in the experiences of the women who consented to the screening and those who declined, those who chose to be screened experienced unique thoughts and feelings.

Number of Data Collection Points

Qualitative research, like quantitative research, can be either cross-sectional, with one data collection point, or longitudinal, with multiple data collection points over an extended time, to observe the evolution of some phenomenon. Sometimes, a qualitative researcher plans in advance for multiple sessions, but in other cases, the decision to study a phenomenon longitudinally may be made in the field after preliminary data have been collected and analyzed.

Examples of the time dimension in qualitative studies:

Cross-sectional: Dewar and Lee (2000) examined how people with a catastrophic illness or injury managed their circumstances. In a single interview, the researchers asked participants (who had endured their condition for between 3 and 25 years) to describe their coping processes over time.

Longitudinal: Fergus, Gray, Fitch, Labrecque, and Phillips (2002) studied patient-provided support for spouse caregivers. Thirty-four men with prostate cancer and their female caregivers were interviewed three times over a 1-year period to examine how caregiving and caregiving support evolved.

Occurrence of the Independent and Dependent Variables

Qualitative researchers typically would not apply the terms *retrospective* or *prospective* to their studies. Nevertheless, in trying to elucidate the full nature of some phenomenon, they may look back retrospectively (with the assistance of study participants) for antecedent events leading to the occurrence of some phenomenon. Qualitative researchers may also study the evolution of some phenomenon prospectively.

Examples of exploring influences and causes in qualitative designs:

Retrospective exploration: Manns and Chad (2001) investigated the components of quality of life for persons with quadriplegic and paraplegic spinal cord injury. Fifteen people were asked to recollect how their spinal cord injury may or many not have affected what was important to them and how they defined quality of life.

Prospective exploration: Olson et al. (2002) conducted a prospective study over a 6-month period to explore why some cancer patients develop fatigue and others do not.

Research Setting

Qualitative researchers collect their data in real-world, naturalistic settings. And, whereas a quantitative researcher usually strives to collect data in one type of setting to maintain constancy of conditions (*e.g.,* conducting all interviews in study participants' homes), qualitative researchers may deliberately strive to study their phenomena in a variety of natural contexts.

Examples of variation in settings:

Long et al. (2002) conducted a 2-year qualitative study to examine nurses' role within multiprofessional rehabilitation teams in the United Kingdom. Forty-nine individuals were recruited. Their pathways through rehabilitation services were observed for 6 months in a variety of settings, including homes, outpatient clinics, hospital wards, and nursing homes.

QUALITATIVE RESEARCH TRADITIONS

There are many different types of qualitative studies, but there unfortunately is no readily agreed-on taxonomy for the various approaches. Some authors have categorized qualitative studies in terms of analysis styles; others have classified studies according to their focus. One useful system is to describe qualitative research according to disciplinary traditions. These traditions vary in their conceptualization of what questions are important to ask to understand human experiences. This section provides an overview of qualitative research traditions, and subsequent sections describe three traditions that have been especially useful for nurse researchers.

Overview of Qualitative Research Traditions

The research traditions that have provided an underpinning for qualitative studies come primarily from anthropology, psychology, and sociology. As shown in Table 9-1, each discipline has tended to focus on one or two broad domains of inquiry.

The discipline of anthropology is concerned with human cultures. **Ethnography** is the primary research tradition within anthropology and provides a framework for studying the meanings, patterns, and experiences of a defined cultural group in a holistic fashion. **Ethnoscience** (or **cognitive anthropology**) focuses on the cognitive world of a culture, with particular emphasis on the semantic rules and the shared meanings that shape behaviour. Ethnoscience often relies on quantitative as well as qualitative data.

Phenomenology, which has its disciplinary roots in both philosophy and psychology, is concerned with the lived experiences of humans. A closely related research tradition is **hermeneutics,** which uses the lived experiences of people as a tool for better understanding the social, cultural, political, and historical context in which those experiences occur. Hermeneutic inquiry often focuses on meaning—how socially and historically conditioned individuals interpret the world within their given context.

The discipline of psychology has several qualitative research traditions that focus on human behaviour. Human **ethology,** which is sometimes

TABLE 9-1. Overview of Qualitative Research Traditions

DISCIPLINE	DOMAIN	RESEARCH TRADITION	AREA OF INQUIRY
Anthropology	Culture	Ethnography	Holistic view of a culture
		Ethnoscience (cognitive anthropology)	Mapping of the cognitive world of a culture; a culture's shared meanings, semantic rules
Psychology or philosophy	Lived experience	Phenomenology	Experiences of individuals within their lifeworld
		Hermeneutics	Interpretations and meanings of individuals' experiences
Psychology	Behaviour and events	Ethology	Behaviour observed over time in natural context
		Ecological psychology	Behaviour as influenced by the environment
Sociology	Social settings	Grounded theory	Social structural processes within a social setting
		Ethnomethodology	Manner by which shared agreement is achieved in social settings
Sociolinguistics	Human communication	Discourse analysis	Forms and rules of conversation

described as the biology of human behaviour, studies human behaviour as it evolves in its natural context. Human ethologists use observational methods to discover universal behavioural structures. **Ecological psychology** focuses more specifically on the environment's influence on human behaviour and attempts to identify principles that explain the interdependence of humans and their environmental context.

Sociologists study the social world and have developed several research traditions of importance to qualitative researchers. The **grounded theory** tradition (described briefly in Chap. 7 and discussed more fully in a later section of this chapter) seeks to understand the key social psychological and structural processes that occur in a social setting. **Ethnomethodology** seeks to discover how people make sense of everyday activities and interpret their social world to behave in socially acceptable ways. Within this tradition, researchers attempt to understand a social group's norms and assumptions that are so deeply ingrained that members no longer think about the underlying reasons for their behaviours.

The domain of inquiry for sociolinguists is human communication. The tradition often referred to as **discourse analysis** seeks to understand the rules, mechanisms, and structure of conversations. The data for discourse analysis typically are transcripts from naturally occurring conversations, such as those between nurses and their patients.

Finally, **historical research**—the systematic collection and critical evaluation of data relating to past occurrences—is also a tradition that relies primarily on qualitative data. Usually, historical research is undertaken to answer questions concerning causes, effects, or trends relating to past events that may shed light on present behaviours or practices. It is important not to confuse historical research with a review of the literature about historical events. Like other types of research, historical inquiry has as its goal the discovery of new knowledge, not the summary of existing knowledge. Nurses have used historical research methods to examine a wide range of phenomena in both the recent and more distant past.

 CONSUMER TIP

Some qualitative research reports do not identify a research tradition (*e.g.*, ethnography or phenomenology) but simply describe the study as qualitative. A research tradition may need to be inferred from information about the types of questions that were asked and the methods used to collect and analyze data. ■

Researchers in each of the qualitative research traditions have developed methodologic guidelines for the design and conduct of relevant studies. Thus, after a researcher has identified what aspect of the human experience is of greatest interest, typically a wealth of advice is available with regard to methods likely to be productive.

CONSUMER TIP

A research report will sometimes identify more than one tradition as having provided the framework for a qualitative inquiry. For example, Gibson and Kenrick (1998) studied the experience of living with peripheral vascular disease in a sample of 9 patients who had had vascular bypass surgery. They described their investigation as a phenomenological study that used a grounded theory method. However, such "method slurring" (Baker, Wuest, & Stern, 1992) has been criticized because each research tradition has different intellectual assumptions and methodologic prescriptions. ■

Ethnography

Ethnography, as noted previously, focuses on the culture of a group of people. Ethnographic researchers can study both broadly defined cultures (*e.g.,* a Samoan village culture), in what is sometimes referred to as a **macroethnography,** and more narrowly defined ones (*e.g.,* the culture of homeless shelters) in a **microethnography.** An underlying assumption of the ethnographer is that every human group evolves a culture that guides the members' view of the world and the way they structure their experiences.

The aim of the ethnographer is to learn from (rather than to study) members of a cultural group. Ethnographic researchers sometimes refer to emic and etic perspectives. An **emic perspective** is the way the members of the culture envision their world—it is the insiders' view. The **etic perspective,** by contrast, is the outsiders' interpretation of the experiences of that culture. Ethnographers strive to acquire an emic perspective of cultures. Moreover, they strive to reveal **tacit knowledge,** information about the culture that is so deeply embedded in cultural experiences that members do not talk about it or may not even be consciously aware of it.

Ethnographers undertake extensive field work to learn about the cultural group in which they are interested. Ethnographic research typically is a labour-intensive and time-consuming endeavour; months and even years of field work may be required. The study of a culture requires a certain level of intimacy with members of the cultural group, and such intimacy can only be developed over time and by working directly with those members as an active participant. The concept of **researcher as instrument** is frequently used by anthropologists to describe the significant role the ethnographer plays in analyzing and interpreting a culture.

Three types of information are usually sought by ethnographers: cultural behaviour (what members of the culture do), cultural artifacts (what members of the culture make and use), and cultural speech (what people say). This implies that the ethnographer relies on various data sources, including observations, in-depth interviews, records, charts, and other types of physical evidence (photographs, diaries, letters, etc.). Ethnographers typically conduct in-depth interviews with about 25 to 50 informants.

The products of ethnographic research are rich and holistic descriptions of the culture under study. Ethnographers also make interpretations of the culture, describing normative behavioural and social patterns. Among health care researchers, ethnography provides information about the health beliefs and health practices of a culture or subculture. Ethnographic inquiry can thus facilitate understanding of behaviours affecting health and illness. Many nurse researchers have undertaken ethnographic studies. Indeed, Madeleine Leininger has coined the phrase **ethnonursing research,** which she defines as "the study and analysis of the local or indigenous people's viewpoints, beliefs, and practices about nursing care behavior and processes of designated cultures" (1985, p. 38).

> **Example of an ethnographic study:**
>
> Li and Browne (2000) conducted an ethnographic study that focused on the perspectives of Asian Canadian immigrants of mental illness and access to mental health services. Personal interviews were conducted with 60 Asian immigrants living in Northern British Columbia. Through these interviews, the researchers learned six themes that defined a mental health problem. In addition, they found that poor English language ability and lack of understanding of mainstream culture were major barriers to gaining access to mental health facilities.

Phenomenology

Phenomenology, rooted in a philosophical tradition developed by Husserl and Heidegger, is an approach to thinking about people's life experiences.

The phenomenological researcher asks the question: "What is the essence of this phenomenon as experienced by these people and what does it *mean?*"

The phenomenologist assumes there is an **essence**—an essential invariant structure—that can be understood, in much the same way that the ethnographer assumes that cultures exist. The phenomenologist investigates subjective phenomena in the belief that critical truths about reality are grounded in people's lived experiences.

There are two "schools" of phenomenology: descriptive phenomenology and interpretive phenomenology (hermeneutics). Descriptive phenomenology was developed first by Husserl (1962), who was primarily interested in the question: "What do we know as persons?" His philosophy emphasized descriptions of the meaning of human experience. Heidegger, a student of Husserl, moved away from his professor's philosophy into interpretive phenomenology. To Heidegger (1962), the critical question is: "What is being?" He stressed interpreting and understanding—not just describing—human experience. The focus of phenomenological inquiry, then, is what people experience in regard to a phenomenon (descriptive phenomenology) and how they interpret those experiences (hermeneutics). The phenomenologist believes that lived experience gives meaning to each person's perception of a particular phenomenon. The goal of phenomenological inquiry is to describe fully lived experience and the perceptions to which it gives rise. Four aspects of lived experience that are of interest to phenomenologists are lived space, or **spatiality;** lived body, or **corporeality;** lived time, or **temporality;** and lived human relation, or **relationality.**

Phenomenologists believe that human existence is meaningful and interesting because of people's consciousness of that existence. The phrase **being-in-the-world** (or **embodiment**) is a concept that acknowledges people's physical ties to their world; they think, see, hear, feel, and are conscious through their bodies' interaction with the world.

In a phenomenological study, the main data source is in-depth conversations, with the researcher and informant as full co-participants. The researcher helps the informant to describe lived experiences without leading the discussion. Through in-depth conversations, the researcher strives to gain entrance into the informants' world, to have full access to their experiences as lived. Sometimes, two separate interviews or conversations may be needed. Typically, phenomenological studies involve a small number of study participants, often 10 or fewer. For some phenomenological researchers, the inquiry includes not only gathering information from informants but also efforts to experience the phenomenon in the same way, typically through participation, observation, and introspective reflection.

Although there are a number of methodologic interpretations of phenomenology, a descriptive phenomenological study often involves the following four steps: bracketing, intuiting, analyzing, and describing. **Bracketing** refers to the process of identifying and holding in abeyance preconceived beliefs and opinions about the phenomenon under study. The researcher brackets out the world and any presuppositions in an effort to confront the data in pure form. **Intuiting** occurs when the researcher remains open to the meanings attributed to the phenomenon by those who have experienced it. Phenomenological researchers then proceed to the analysis phase (*i.e.*, extracting significant statements, categorizing, and making sense of the essential meanings of the phenomenon). (Chap. 14 provides further information regarding the analysis of data collected in phenomenological studies.) Finally, the descriptive phase occurs when the researcher comes to understand and define the phenomenon. An important distinction between descriptive and interpretive phenomenology is that in an interpretive phenomenological study, bracketing does not occur. For Heidegger, it was not possible to bracket one's being-in-the-world. Hermeneutics presupposes prior understanding on the part of the researcher.

The phenomenological approach is especially useful when a phenomenon of interest has been poorly defined or conceptualized. The topics appropriate to phenomenology are ones that are fundamental to the life experiences of humans; for health researchers, these include such topics as the meaning of stress, the experience of bereavement, and the quality of life with a chronic illness.

> **🔲** | **Example of a phenomenological study:**
>
> Racher (2002) conducted a phenomenological study of the lived experience of rural elderly couples and their ability to continue to live independently in the community. The study involved interviews with a sample of 19 frail elderly couples who lived independently in rural communities.

Grounded Theory

Grounded theory has become a strong research tradition that began more as a systematic method of qualitative research than as a philosophy. Grounded theory was developed in the 1960s by two sociologists, Glaser and Strauss (1967), whose theoretical roots were in **symbolic interaction,** which focuses on the manner in which people make sense of social interactions and the interpretations they attach to social symbols, such as language.

Grounded theory is an approach to the study of social processes and social structures. The focus of most grounded theory studies is the evolution of a social experience—the social and psychological stages and phases that characterize a particular event or process. As noted in Chapter 7, the primary purpose of the grounded theory approach is to generate comprehensive explanations of phenomena that are grounded in reality.

Grounded theory methods constitute an entire approach to the conduct of field research. For example, a study that truly follows the precepts of Glaser and Strauss does not begin with a focused research question; the question emerges from the data. A fundamental feature of grounded theory research is that data collection, data analysis, and sampling of participants occur simultaneously. A procedure referred to as **constant comparison** is used to develop and refine theoretically relevant categories and to identify the basic problem. The categories elicited from the data are constantly compared with data obtained earlier so that commonalities and variations can be determined, and categories can be condensed and collapsed. As data collection proceeds, the inquiry becomes increasingly focused on emerging theoretical concerns and on core processes. Data analysis within a grounded theory framework is described more fully in Chapter 14.

In-depth interviews are the most common data source in a grounded theory study, but observational methods and existing documents may also be used. Typically, a grounded theory study involves interviews with a sample of about 25 to 50 informants.

Grounded theory has become an important research method for the study of nursing phenomena and has contributed to the development of many middle-range theories of phenomena relevant to nurses. Most qualitative nursing studies that identify a research tradition claim grounded theory as the tradition to which they are linked.

⊞ ***Example of a grounded theory study:***

Kushner and Harrison (2002) conducted a grounded theory study during a 2-year period to examine the process used by mothers to cope with the stress of managing multiple responsibilities in family, health, and paid work. The women experienced stress from continous demands in paid and family health-related work. This stress was compounded by conflicting demands, inadequate support, time constraints, inflexible expectations, and compromised personal resources. Twenty mothers took part in face-to-face and telephone interviews.

INTEGRATION OF QUALITATIVE AND QUANTITATIVE APPROACHES

An emerging trend, and one that we believe will gain momentum, is the integration of qualitative and quantitative data within single studies or coordinated clusters of studies. This section discusses the rationale for such **integrated designs** and presents a few applications.

Rationale for Integrated Designs

The dichotomy between quantitative and qualitative data represents the key epistemologic and methodologic distinction within the social and behavioural sciences. Some argue that the paradigms that underpin qualitative and quantitative research are fundamentally incompatible. Others, however, believe that many areas of inquiry can be enriched through the judicious blending of qualitative and quantitative data, that is, by undertaking **multimethod research.** The advantages of an integrated design include:

- *Complementarity.* Qualitative and quantitative data are complementary, representing words and numbers, the two fundamental languages of human communication. Researchers address their problems with methods that are fallible, but the strengths and weaknesses of quantitative and qualitative data are complementary. By using multiple methods, the researcher can allow each method to do what it does best, possibly avoiding the limitations of a single approach.
- *Incrementality.* It is sometimes argued that qualitative methods are well suited to hypothesis-generating research early in the development of a research problem area and that quantitative methods are needed as the problem area matures for verification. However, the evolution of knowledge is rarely linear and unidirectional. The need for in-depth insights is rarely confined to the beginning of an inquiry in an area, and subjective experiences may need to be tested continuously. Thus, progress on a topic tends to be incremental, relying on multiple feedback loops. It can be productive to build a loop into the design of a single study, thereby potentially speeding progress toward understanding.

- *Enhanced validity.* When a researcher's hypothesis or model is supported by multiple and complementary types of data, the researcher can be more confident about the validity of the results. The integration of qualitative and quantitative data can provide opportunities for testing alternative interpretations of the data and for examining the extent to which context helped to shape the results.
- *Creating new frontiers.* Researchers sometimes find that qualitative and quantitative data are inconsistent with each other. This lack of congruity—when it happens in the context of a single investigation—can lead to insights that can push a line of inquiry further. Inconsistencies in separate studies may reflect differences in study participants and circumstances rather than theoretically meaningful distinctions that merit further study. In a single study, discrepancies can be used as a springboard for further exploration.

CONSUMER TIP

Integrated studies rarely combine qualitative and quantitative findings in a single report. Typically, the quantitative findings are reported in one journal article, and the qualitative findings appear in a separate article in a different journal. However, the authors often summarize the results of the other component of the study in the introduction or discussion section of the report. ■

Applications of Integrated Designs

Researchers make decisions about study design and procedures based on the specific objectives of their investigations. The integration of qualitative and quantitative data can be used to address various research goals.

1. *Instrumentation.* Qualitative data are sometimes collected for the development and validation of formal, quantitative instruments for research or clinical purposes. The questions for a formal instrument are sometimes derived from clinical experience, theory, or prior research. When a construct is new, however, these mechanisms may be inadequate to capture its full complexity and dimensionality. A researcher's knowledge base, no matter how rich, is personal and limited, and thus nurse researchers sometimes gather qualitative data as the basis for generating questions for quantitative instruments that are subsequently subjected to rigorous testing.

Example of instrumentation:

Beck and Gable (2000) developed the Postpartum Depression Screening Scale, an instrument that screens new mothers for the mood disorder that can develop after delivering a baby. The items in the scale were based on in-depth interviews of three different samples of mothers suffering from postpartum depression.

2. *Explicating and validating constructs.* Multimethod research is often used to develop a comprehensive understanding of a construct or to validate the construct's dimensions. Such research may be undertaken when a little-researched phenomenon has been identified as worthy of further scrutiny or when there is a body of existing research in which some serious gaps have been identified or doubts have been raised about the prevailing conceptualization.

Example of explication and validation:

Reece and Harkless (1996) conducted a multimethod study to examine the maternal experiences of women older than 35 years. The researchers administered an existing quantitative measure of maternal experience and also asked their respondents probing questions about their motherhood experience, which they analyzed qualitatively for emerging themes. They found that several new dimensions arose in the qualitative portion of the research not captured by the quantitative scale.

3. *Illustration.* Qualitative data are sometimes used to illustrate the meaning of quantitative descriptions or relationships. Such illustrations help to clarify important concepts and further serve to corroborate the findings from the statistical analysis. The illustrations help to illuminate the analysis and give guidance to the interpretation of results. Qualitative materials can be used to illustrate specific statistical findings and to provide more global and dynamic views of the phenomena under study, often in the form of illustrative case studies.

Example of illustrating with qualitative data:

Polit et al. (2000) used data from the ethnographic component of a study of poor urban families to illustrate how food insecurity and hunger—reported by more than half of the sample from the survey component of the study—were experienced and managed.

4. *Understanding relationships and causal processes.* Quantitative methods can demonstrate that variables are systematically related but may fail to provide insights about why they are related. Interpretations are often speculative, representing new hypotheses that could be tested in another study. When a study integrates qualitative and quantitative data, however, the researcher may be in a stronger position to derive meaning immediately from the statistical findings.

Example of illuminating with qualitative data:

In the previously mentioned multicomponent study of poor urban families, Polit et al. (2000) found from the survey data that differences in the food insecurity of poor women were related to differences in their sources of income, and yet the differences in the hunger of their children were more modest. The ethnographic data revealed that differences were small largely because of the lengths to which mothers, regardless of income source, went to protect their children from hunger.

5. *Theory building, testing, and refinement.* The most ambitious application of an integrated approach is in the area of theory development. A theory gains acceptance as it escapes disconfirmation, and the use of multiple methods provides great opportunity for potential disconfirmation of a theory. If the theory can survive these assaults, it can provide a stronger context for the organization of clinical and intellectual work.

Example of theory building:

Salazar and Carter (1993) conducted a study that promoted the development of theory in the area of decision making. These researchers sought to identify the factors that influence the decision of working women to practice breast self-examination (BSE). The first phase of the study involved in-depth interviews with 19 women, selected on the basis of how frequently they practiced BSE. The qualitative analysis led to the development of a hierarchical scheme of factors influencing the BSE decision. The researchers then used the hierarchy as the basis for developing a questionnaire that was administered to 52 women. A complex statistical analysis was used to identify factors in the decision hierarchy that best distinguished BSE performers and nonperformers.

Integration Strategies

The ways in which a researcher can design a study to integrate qualitative and quantitative methods are almost limitless. The three following scenarios are especially common:

1. *Embedding qualitative approaches within a survey.* After the researcher has gained the cooperation of a survey sample, he or she may be in a good position to collect more in-depth data with a subset of the initial respondents. If the collection of in-depth data can be postponed until after the analysis of quantitative data, the researcher can probe into the reasons for any obtained results. The second-stage respondents, in other words, can be used as informants to help the researcher interpret outcomes.

Example of embedding qualitative approaches into a survey:

Boydell et al. (2000) directed a large-scale multimethod study of homeless people in Toronto. Some 330 homeless adults were surveyed, using a formal interview that yielded quantitative data. Subsequently, some 29 participants were purposively selected from the larger sample for in-depth questioning about their inner view of their lives and experiences.

2. *Embedding quantitative measures into field work.* Although qualitative data prevail in field studies, field researchers can sometimes profit from the collection of more structured information, either from the study participants or from a larger or more representative sample. Having already gained entrée into the community and the trust and cooperation of its members, the field researcher may be in an ideal position to pursue a survey or a record-extraction activity. For example, if the researcher's in-depth field work focused on family violence, community-wide police and hospital records could be used to gather systematic data amenable to statistical analysis.

Example of quantitative measures in field work:

Moore (1999) conducted an in-depth study of social interaction in a special care unit for cognitively impaired older people. The rich qualitative data were gathered through observations and in-depth interviews with staff and family members. The researcher contextualized the study and developed a better understanding of the participants by administering several structured, quantitative instruments, such as the Mini-Mental State Examination and the Katz Index of Activities of Daily Living.

3. *Qualitative data in experimental and quasi-experimental research.* Qualitative data can often enrich experimental or quasi-experimental studies. Through in-depth, unstructured approaches, the researcher can better understand qualitative differences between groups, including differences in the experiences and processes underlying experimental effects. Qualitative data may be especially useful when the researcher is evaluating complex interventions. When an experimental treatment is straightforward (*e.g.,* a new drug), it might be easy to interpret the results. However, many nursing interventions are more complicated; they may involve new ways of interacting with patients or new approaches to organizing the delivery of care. At the end of the experiment, even when hypothesized results are obtained, people may ask, "What was it that really caused the group differences?" In-depth qualitative data may help researchers to address the **black box** question—understanding what it is about the intervention that is driving any observed effects. Finally, the use of qualitative methods in nursing intervention studies can play a role in making nursing work more visible and accessible to other nurses, policymakers, and the public (Sandelowski, 1996).

Example of qualitative data in an experimental clinical trial:

Whittemore and a team of researchers (2000) were involved in a clinical trial of alternative social support interventions, admnistered by nurse versus peer advisors, for patients who had had a myocardial infarction. Patients, who were randomly assigned to 3 groups (nurse advisors, peer advisors, or control group), were compared in terms of health outcomes. The qualitative part of the study, which was designed to better understand the *experiences* of the peer advisors, was based on written logs and individual and group interviews.

CRITIQUING QUALITATIVE AND INTEGRATED DESIGNS

Evaluating a qualitative design is often difficult. Qualitative researchers do not always document design decisions and are even less likely to describe the process by which such decisions were made. Researchers often do, however, indicate whether the study was conducted within a specific qualitative tradition. This information can be used to come to some conclusions about the study design. For example, if a report indicated that the researcher conducted 1 month of field work for an ethnographic study, there would be reason to suspect that insufficient time had been spent in the field to obtain a true emic perspective of the culture under study.

Most qualitative studies, quite appropriately, do not collect any quantitative data. However, it might be useful to consider how and in what way the addition of quantitative data might have improved the study design. Conversely, not all integrated studies are well suited to a multimethod approach; hence, integrated studies should be carefully evaluated in terms of the incremental value of having both types of data in a single study.

The guidelines in Box 9-1 are designed to assist you in critiquing the designs of qualitative and integrated studies.

RESEARCH EXAMPLES

Nurse researchers have conducted studies within all of the qualitative research traditions described in this chapter. Table 9-2 provides several examples of research questions addressed within various traditions. In this section, we present more detailed descriptions of three nursing studies, including two multimethod investigations.

Research Example of a Grounded Theory Study

Small, Brennan-Hunter, Best, and Solberg (2002) conducted a grounded theory study to understand what parents experienced as a result of their adolescent children's smoking behaviour. Their research report appeared in *Qualitative Health Research*.

Research Summary
Small and her colleagues chose a grounded theory approach "because of the scarcity of knowledge in the area of parenting adolescents who smoke and

<table>
<tr><td>BOX 9-1 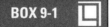</td><td>GUIDELINES FOR CRITIQUING QUALITATIVE AND INTEGRATED DESIGNS</td></tr>
</table>

1. Is the research tradition within which the qualitative study was undertaken identified? What was that tradition? If no research tradition is identified, can one be inferred?

2. Does the research question appear to be congruent with the research tradition (*i.e.,* is the domain of inquiry for the study congruent with the domain encompassed by the tradition)? Do the data sources and general methods of the study appear consistent with the tradition?

3. How well is the research design described? Are design decisions explained and justified?

4. Does the design appear thoughtful and appropriate? Does the design lend itself to a thorough, in-depth, intensive examination of the phenomenon of interest? What design elements might have strengthened the study (*e.g.,* would a longitudinal perspective have been preferable, although a cross-sectional design was used)?

5. Is the study exclusively qualitative, or were both qualitative and quantitative data collected? Could the study have been strengthened by the inclusion of some quantitative data?

6. If both qualitative and quantitative data were collected, were they used in a complementary fashion? How (if at all) did the inclusion of both types of data contribute to enhanced theoretical insights, enhanced validity, or movement toward new frontiers?

TABLE 9-2. Examples of Qualitative Studies Within Various Traditions

RESEARCH TRADITION	RESEARCH QUESTION
Ethnography	What are First Nations parents' beliefs about childhood immunization and vaccine-preventable diseases? (Tarrant & Gregory, 2003)
Phenomenology	What is the experience of men living with pain of fibromyalgia type? (Paulson, Danielson, & Söderberg, 2002)
Ethology	What are the social acts through which nurses and patients negotiate in interactions? (Spiers, 2002)
Grounded theory	How do women make sense of depression as they live with and manage it in their daily lives? (Schreiber & Hartrick, 2002)
Ethnomethodology	How is the work of surgical nurses organized in the U.K. health service? (Wakefield, 2000)
Discourse analysis and history	What historically situated discourse was used at the Hadamar trial in defense of the actions and inactions of nurses in Nazi Germany? (Lagerwey, 1999)

the need to develop an explanatory model of the process nonsmoking parents experience in their interactions with adolescents who smoke" (p. 1203). They recruited a sample of 25 nonsmoking parents with children who smoked through junior high and high schools in a Canadian city. Participants were asked to talk abaout their experience during in-depth interviews. The early interviews asked broad and exploratory questions, but in later interviews the researchers asked more focused and direct questions when they "required information that was more specific to expand on certain aspects of the parents' experiences" (p. 1204).

In this study, consistent with grounded theory methods, data collection and analysis occurred simultaneously in an interactive process. Data analysis began when the first interview transcript was completed, and increasingly guided subsequent data collection. Data were analyzed using the constant comparative method.

Based on their analysis, the researchers developed an explanatory model that they represented with a diagram depicting relationships among the themes they discovered. The model, which they called "Struggling to Understand," was validated by presenting and discussing it with eight additional parents. In the model, the parents' attempt to understand was reflected by their passage through four stages: discovering the smoking, facing the problem, reflecting, and waiting it out. Each of these stages consisted of several activities on the part of the parents. For example, with Stage 1 (discovering the smoking), the process entailed seeing the evidence, putting the pieces together, and confirming the behaviour.

Clinical Relevance

Ample evidence suggests that rearing adoloscents is challenging to many parents. Studies have consistently found that during adolescence children like to experiment, take risks, and be autonomous from their parents. Smoking is one risky behaviour that adolescents may experiment with and subsequently adopt. Small and colleagues point out that, as in other studies, parents in their study were not expecting their children to be smoking and, as a result, missed or dismissed early signs that indicated their children were starting to smoke.

The findings of this study suggest that nonsmoking parents struggled to understand their adolescents' smoking and that this behaviour caused parents emotional distress. Faced with this stressor parents attempted to deal with the adolescents' behaviour in a number of ways. One coping strategy used by the parents was to hope that their children would quit smoking; however, smoking remained an ongoing source of stress. An important recommendation made by the researchers is the need for the development of programs designed to assist parents with prevention and intervention strategies related to adolescent smoking in addition to the current antismoking campaigns aimed directly at the adolescents.

Research Example of an Ethnographic Study

Varcoe (2001) conducted a study to describe the relationship between the social context in which health care is provided and nurses' care for women who have been abused. She used an ethnographic approach to collect data in the emergency units of two urban hospitals and the communities they served. This study was also informed by a feminist understanding of violence and oppression.

Research Summary

To conduct her study Varcoe chose to use an ethnographic approach because the ethnographic method is well suited to study the culture of a group of people in a particular setting. This method offered the researcher opportunities to build a comprehensive picture of a specific culture in an environment through 200 hours of observations and interviews. Varcoe spent 2 years in the field to collect data in the emergency units of two urban hospitals and the communities they served to describe nursing practice in relation to violence against women. Varcoe spent this length of time in the setting because as an ethnographer her intent was to learn from rather than study the nurses and the women served by these nurses in the emergency departments. She combined observations, while paired with 1 of the 8 nurses who volunteered, with interviews of 25 health care providers and 5 abused patients on the two units. These were complemented with interviews of 5 nurses who worked in other emergency departments and 9 other health care providers (admitting clerks, social workers, physicians, and hospital adminstrators).

Varcoe reported several themes regarding abuse from her analysis: abuse unrecognized, abuse obscured through efficient patient processing, and abuse obscured through stereotypical thinking. When the abuse was recognized by health care workers their behaviour could be categorized according to three overlapping patterns: doing nothing, influencing choices, and offering choices. In this study, findings suggest that decisions about what patients deserved for types and levels of care incorporated subjective judgments about patient acuity and social judgments about patients. The researcher found that, similar to previous research, the nurses who participated in this study felt considerable moral distress over the judgmental attitudes they noticed in others and in themselves.

Clinical Relevance

According to several studies, including this one by Varcoe, violence against women is a significant issue nationally and globally. This research was important because is provides a rich understanding of emergency nursing and practices in relation to abuse. The study findings point to the fact that nurses who participanted in this study seldom recognized abuse; therefore, for them this study was critical in increasing their alertness and attentiveness about the extent of abuse and how they dealt with it; they believed that they overlooked it or, when they did recognize it, did nothing to deal with it and thus provided care that they considered inadequate.

This study points out that improved practice in relation to violence against women goes beyond the care and concern of nurses. Congruent with Varcoe's beliefs, care must be approached on the basis of effective health care outcomes, rather than based simply on efficiency in processing of patients. This change requires determination and adequate resources. The findings of this study also point to the importance of continuing education of practicing nurses who work in practice settings where they are likely to see individuals seeking care as a result of abuse. Aspects to be included in these continuing education opportunities should include the nature of abuse, how to recognize it, and how to intervene appropiately.

Research Example of an Integrated Study

Connelly, Bott, Hoffart, and Taunton (1997) conducted a multimethod research project that focused on the retention of staff nurses. Their research is an example of construct explication and theory building through the integration of qualitative and quantitative methods.

Research Summary

The study by Connelly and her colleagues was primarily quantitative and involved the development of a sophisticated statistical model designed to predict nurse retention. The researchers measured four types of factors that they believed could predict retention: characteristics of the managers (*e.g.,* leadership style), characteristics of the organization (*e.g.,* promotional opportunity), work characteristics (*e.g.,* group cohesion), and characteristics of the nurses themselves (*e.g.,* education, marital status). The variables in the model had all been verified in the research literature; nevertheless, their cumulative predictive power was relatively low.

In the final year of the project, the researchers did a qualitative study to examine whether a different research approach might produce an additional construct that belonged in the retention model. A total of 21 staff nurses who had low scores on an Intent to Stay Scale that had been administered to them in the first year of the project—but who had nevertheless remained working in the same hospital—were interviewed in depth about their reasons for staying, their possible reasons for leaving, and the positive and negative aspects of their employment.

The researchers found that there was some correspondence between the information obtained through the in-depth interviews and the variables included in their model, thereby validating aspects of the model. However, new themes also emerged during the qualitative interviews, for example, variables such as location close to home, fringe benefits, ability to provide high-quality care, and ability to transfer among units within the hospital. The advantages of having used a multimethod design were described as follows:

Triangulation helped us attain three benefits. First, the careful comparison of quantitative and qualitative data added support for the variables in the retention model. Second, the comparison also showed new dimensions about nurse retention, thereby contributing to a more complete understanding of nurse retention. (. . .) Third, the researchers were able to make suggestions for revision of the quantitative instrument. (Connelly et al., 1997, p. 301)

Clinical Relevance

The study by Connelly and co-researchers has implications for nursing administrators, who are routinely confronted with the disruptive effects of staff turnover. The findings suggest that certain factors should be of particular concern to administrators attempting to achieve nurse retention. These include personal job stress, situational job stress, routinization, instrumental communication, and distributive justice—all of which are amenable to modification through carefully conceived institutional policies. It is noteworthy that these factors, which were significant predictors of nurse retention in the quantitative portion of the study, were validated through the in-depth qualitative interviews, adding credibility to these findings.

Administrators also need to consider the new dimensions discovered in the qualitative data as critical pieces in the puzzle of retaining nurses in their workforce. For example, the issue of nurses' ability to give quality time can be addressed through nurse-to-patient ratios; nurses need time to be caring and to sit with their patients and give their full attention.

● ● ● ● ● *SUMMARY POINTS*

- Qualitative research typically involves an **emergent design**—a design that emerges in the field as the study unfolds.
- As **bricoleurs,** qualitative researchers tend to be creative and intuitive, putting together an array of data drawn from many sources in an effort to arrive at a holistic understanding of a phenomenon.
- Although qualitative design is elastic and flexible, qualitative researchers nevertheless can plan for broad contingencies that can be expected to pose decision opportunities for the design of the study in the field.
- A naturalistic inquiry typically progresses through three broad phases in the field: an orientation and overview phase to determine what it is about the phenomenon under investigation that is salient, a focused exploration phase that closely examines important aspects of the phenomenon, and a confirmation and closure phase to confirm findings.
- Qualitative research traditions have their roots in anthropology (*e.g.,* **ethnography** and **ethnoscience**), philosophy (**phenomenology and hermeneutics**), psychology (**ethology, ecological psychology**), sociology (**grounded theory, ethnomethodology, symbolic interaction**), and sociolinguistics (**discourse analysis**).
- Ethnography focuses on the culture of a group of people and relies on extensive field work. The ethnographer strives to acquire an **emic,** or in-

sider's, perspective of the culture under study; the outsider's perspective is known as **etic.**

- Phenomenology seeks to discover the essence and meaning of a phenomenon as it is experienced by people. In descriptive phenomenology, the researcher strives to **bracket** out any preconceived views and to **intuit** the essence of the phenomenon by remaining open to the meanings attributed to it by those who have experienced it. Bracketing is not a feature of interpretive (hermeneutic) phenomenology.

- **Grounded theory,** an approach to studying social psychological processes and social structures, aims to discover theoretical precepts grounded in the data. This approach uses **constant comparison:** categories elicited from the data are constantly compared with data obtained earlier so that shared themes and variations can be determined.

- In some studies, an **integrated design** that combines qualitative and quantitative data in a single investigation (multimethod research) can be advantageous because qualitative and quantitative approaches have complementary strengths and weaknesses.

- In nursing, one of the most frequent uses of **multimethod research** has been in the area of instrument development. Integrated designs are also used in efforts to illustrate, to interpret relationships and causal processes, and to develop theory.

▶ ▶ ▶ ▶ *CRITICAL THINKING ACTIVITIES*

Chapter 9 of the accompanying *Study Guide to Accompany Essentials of Nursing Research,* 5th edition, offers various exercises and study suggestions for reinforcing the concepts presented in this chapter. In addition, you can address the following:

1. Read the introduction and method section from the qualitative study in the Appendix of this book, and then answer relevant questions in Box 9-1.

2. In Chapter 8, one of the research examples was a quantitative study by Arthur and her colleagues (2000), who evaluated an intervention for patients awaiting CABG surgery. How might qualitative data have enriched this study? (*Annals of Internal Medicine, 133,* 253–262)

3. In Li and Browne's study, used as an example of an ethnographic study in this chapter, what might the focal research question have been in a phenomenological study? In a hermeneutic study? In a grounded theory study?

*For additional review, see questions 106–124 on the study CD provided with Polit: *Study Guide to Accompany Essentials of Nursing Research.*

SUGGESTED READINGS

Methodologic References

Baker, C., Wuest, J., & Stern, P. N. (1992). Method slurring: The grounded theory/phenomenology example. *Journal of Advanced Nursing, 17,* 1355–1360.

Carey, J. W. (1993). Linking qualitative and quantitative methods: Integrating cultural factors into public health. *Qualitative Health Research, 3,* 298–318.

Chesla, C. A. (1992). When qualitative and quantitative findings do not converge. *Western Journal of Nursing Research, 14,* 681–685.

Creswell, J. W. (1998). *Qualitative inquiry and research design: Choosing among five traditions.* Thousand Oaks, CA: Sage.

Denzin, N. K., & Lincoln, Y. S. (Eds.). (1994). *Handbook of qualitative research.* Thousand Oaks, CA: Sage.

Glaser, B. G., & Strauss, A. L. (1967). *The discovery of grounded theory: Strategies for qualitative research.* Chicago: Aldine.

Heidegger, M. (1962) *Being and time.* New York: Harper & Row.

Husserl, E. (1962). *Ideas: General introduction to pure phenomenology.* New York: MacMillan.

Leininger, M. M. (Ed.). (1985). *Qualitative research methods in nursing.* New York: Grune & Stratton.

Lincoln, Y. S., & Guba, E. G. (1985). *Naturalistic inquiry.* Newbury Park, CA: Sage.

Morse, J. M. (1991). *Qualitative nursing research: A contemporary dialogue.* Newbury Park, CA: Sage.

Morse, J. M. (1999). Qualitative methods: The state of the art. *Qualitative Health Research, 9,* 393–406.

Morse, J. M., & Field, P. A. (1995). *Qualitative research methods for health professionals* (2nd ed.). Thousand Oaks, CA: Sage.

Sandelowski, M. (1996). Using qualitative methods in intervention studies. *Research in Nursing & Health, 19,* 359–364.

Streubert, H. J., & Carpenter, D. R. (1995). *Qualitative research in nursing: Advancing the humanistic imperative.* Philadelphia: J. B. Lippincott.

Substantive References

Beck, C. T., & Gable, R. (2000). Postpartum Depression Screening Scale: Development and psychometric testing. *Nursing Research, 49,* 272–282.

Boydell, K. M., Goering, P., & Morrell-Bellai, T. L. (2000). Narratives of identity: Re-presentation of self in people who are homeless. *Qualitative Health Research, 10,* 26–38.

Connelly, L. M., Bott, M., Hoffart, N., & Taunton, R. L. (1997). Methodological triangulation in a study of nurse retention. *Nursing Research, 46,* 299–302.

Dewar, A.L., & Lee, E.A. (2000). Bearing illness and injury. *Western Journal of Nursing Research, 22,* 912–926.

Fergus, K. D., Gray, R. E., Fitch, M. I., Labrecque, M., & Phillips, C. (2002). Active consideration: Conceptualizing patient-provided support for spouse caregivers in the context of prostate cancer. *Qualitative Health Research, 12,* 492–514.

Gibson, J. M. E., & Kenrick, M. (1998). Pain and powerlessness: The experience of living with peripheral vascular disease. *Journal of Advanced Nursing, 27,* 737–745.

Grant Kalischuk, R., & Davies, B. (2001). A theory of healing in the aftermath of youth suicide. *Journal of Holistic Nursing, 19,* 163–186.

Katz, A. (2001). HIV screening in pregnancy: What women think. *Journal of Obstetric, Gynecologic, and Neonatal Nursing, 30,* 184–191.

Kushner, K. E., & Harrison, M. J. (2002). Employed mothers: Stress and balance-focused coping. *Canadian Journal of Nursing Research 34,* 47–65.

Lagerwey, M. D. (1999). Nursing ethics at Hadamar. *Qualitative Health Research, 9,* 759–772.

Li, H. Z.., & Browne, A. J. (2000). Defining mental illness and accessing mental health services: Perspectives of Asian Canadians. *Canadian Journal of Community Mental Health, 19,* 143–159.

Long, A. F., Kneafsey, R., Ryan, J., & Berry, J. (2002). The role of the nurse within the multi-professional rehabilitation team. *Journal of Advanced Nursing, 37,* 70–78.

Manns, P. J., & Chad, K. E. (2001). Components of quality of life for persons with a quadriplegic spinal cord injury. *Qualitative Health Research, 11,* 795–811.

Moore, K. D. (1999). Dissonance in the dining room: A study of social interaction in a special care unit. *Qualitative Health Research, 9,* 133–155.

Morgan, D. G., & Stewart, N. J. (1999). The physical environment of special care units: Needs of residents with dementia from the perspective of staff and family caregivers. *Qualitative Health Research, 9,* 105–118.

Olson, K., Tom, B., Hewitt, J., Whittingham, J., Buchanan, L., & Ganton, G. (2002). Evolving routines: Preventing fatigue associated with lung and colerectal cancer. *Qualitative Health Research, 12,* 655–670.

Paulson, M., Danielson, E., & Söderberg, S. (2002). Struggling for a tolerable existence: The meaning of men's lived experiences fo living with pain of fibromyalgia type. *Qualitative Health Research, 12,* 238–249.

Polit, D. F., London, A. S., & Martinez, J. M. (2000). *Food security and hunger in poor, mother-headed families in four U.S. cities.* New York: MDRC.

Racher, F. E. (2002). Synergism of frail rural elderly couples: Influencing interdependent independence. *Journal of Gerontological Nursing, 28,* 32–39.

Reece, S. M., & Harkless, G. (1996). Divergent themes in maternal experience in women older than 35 years of age. *Applied Nursing Research, 9,* 148–153.

Salazar, M. K., & Carter, W. B. (1993). Evaluation of breast self-examination beliefs using a decision model. *Western Journal of Nursing Research, 15,* 403–418.

Schreiber, & Hartrick (2002). Keeping it together: How women use the biomedical explanatory model to manage the stigma of depression. *Issues in Mental Health Nursing, 23,* 91–105.

Small, S. P., Brennan-Hunter, A. L., Best, D. G., & Solberg, S. M. (2002). Struggling to understand: The experience of nonsmoking parents with adolescents who smoke. *Qualitative Health Research, 12,* 1202–1219.

Spiers, J. (2002). The interpersonal context of negotiating care in home care nurse–patient interactions. *Qualitative Health Research, 12,* 1033–1057.

Tarrant, M., & Gregory, D. (2003). Exploring childhood immunization uptake with First Nations mothers in north-western Ontario, Canada. *Journal of Advanced Nursing, 41,* 63–72.

Varcoe, C. (2001). Abuse obscured: An ethnographic account of emergency nursing in relation to violence against women. *Canadian Journal of Nursing Research, 32,* 95–115.

Wakefield, A. (2000). Ethnomethodology: The problems of unique adequacy. *NT Research, 5,* 46–53.

Whittemore, R., Rankin, S. H., Callahan, C. D., Leder, M. C., & Carroll, D. L. (2000). The peer advisor experience providing social support. *Qualitative Health Research, 10,* 260–276.

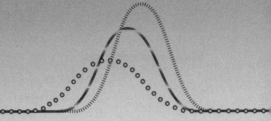

Examining Sampling Plans

BASIC SAMPLING CONCEPTS IN QUANTITATIVE RESEARCH
Populations
Samples and Sampling
Strata
Sampling Rationale
NONPROBABILITY SAMPLING
Convenience Sampling
Quota Sampling
Purposive Sampling
Evaluation of Nonprobability Sampling
PROBABILITY SAMPLING
Simple Random Sampling
Stratified Random Sampling
Cluster Sampling
Systematic Sampling
Evaluation of Probability Sampling

SAMPLE SIZE IN QUANTITATIVE STUDIES
SAMPLING IN QUALITATIVE RESEARCH
The Logic of Qualitative Sampling
Types of Qualitative Sampling
Sample Size
CRITIQUING THE SAMPLING PLAN
Evaluating Quantitative Sampling Plans
Evaluating Qualitative Sampling Plans
RESEARCH EXAMPLES
Research Example of a Quantitative Study
Research Example of a Qualitative Study
SUMMARY POINTS
CRITICAL THINKING ACTIVITIES
SUGGESTED READINGS
Methodologic References
Substantive References

Student Objectives

On completion of this chapter, the student will be able to:

○ describe the rationale for sampling in research studies
○ distinguish between nonprobability and probability samples and compare their advantages and disadvantages
○ identify several types of nonprobability and probability samples and describe their main characteristics
○ identify differences in the logic and evaluation criteria used in sampling approaches for quantitative versus qualitative studies
○ identify several approaches to theoretical/purposive sampling in qualitative studies
○ evaluate the sampling method and sample size in a research study
○ define new terms in the chapter

New Terms

Accessible population	Quota sampling
Accidental sampling	Random selection
Cluster sampling	Response rate
Convenience sampling	Sample size
Data saturation	Sampling
Disproportionate sample	Sampling bias
Elements	Sampling error
Eligibility criteria	Sampling frame
Extreme/deviant case sampling	Sampling interval
Judgmental sampling	Simple random sampling
Maximum variation sampling	Snowball sampling
Multistage sampling	Strata
Network sampling	Stratified random sampling
Nonprobability sampling	Systematic sampling
Nonresponse bias	Target population
Population	Theoretical sampling
Power analysis	Typical case sampling
Probability sampling	Volunteer sample
Proportionate sample	Weighting
Purposive (purposeful) sampling	

Sampling is a process familiar to all of us—we gather information, make decisions, and formulate predictions about phenomena based on contact with a limited portion of them. Researchers, too, derive knowledge and draw conclusions from samples. In testing the efficacy of a nursing intervention for cancer patients, a nurse researcher reaches conclusions without testing the intervention with every victim of the disease. However, researchers cannot afford to draw conclusions about the effectiveness of nursing interventions based on faulty samples. The consequences of erroneous inferences are more momentous in nursing research than in private decision making.

Quantitative and qualitative researchers have different approaches to sampling. Quantitative researchers select samples that allow them to generalize their results by developing an appropriate plan before data collection begins. Qualitative researchers are not as concerned with issues of generalizability but rather want to achieve an in-depth, holistic understanding of the phenomenon of interest. They allow sampling decisions to emerge during the course of data collection based on informational and theoretical needs. Because formal sampling designs are more relevant to quantitative than to qualitative research, most of this chapter is devoted to sampling plans for quantitative studies.

BASIC SAMPLING CONCEPTS IN QUANTITATIVE RESEARCH

Sampling is an important step in the research process for quantitative studies. Let us first consider some terms associated with sampling—terms that are used primarily (but not exclusively) in connection with quantitative studies.

Populations

A **population** is the entire aggregation of cases that meets a specified set of criteria. For instance, if a nurse researcher were studying Canadian nurses with doctoral degrees, the population could be defined as all Canadian citizens who are registered nurses and who have acquired a PhD or other doctoral-level degree. Other possible populations might be all the cardiac patients hospitalized in University Hospital in 2002, all Canadian women older than 60 years of age who have Alzheimer disease, or all the children in Edmonton with cystic fibrosis. Thus, a population may be broadly defined, involving millions of people, or narrowly specified to include only several hundred people.

Populations are not restricted to human participants. A population might consist of all the hospital records on file in the Belleview Hospital, or all the Canadian high schools with a school-based clinic that dispenses contraceptives. Whatever the basic unit, the population comprises the aggregate of entities in which the researcher is interested.

Quantitative researchers specify the characteristics that delimit the population through the **eligibility criteria** for inclusion in their studies. For example, consider the population of Canadian nursing students. Would this population include part-time students? Would registered nurses returning to school for a baccalaureate degree be included? The researcher establishes these criteria to determine whether a person qualifies as a member of the population. A reader of a research report needs to know the eligibility criteria to understand the population to which the findings can be generalized.

> **BB** *Example of eligibility criteria:*
>
> Davis et al. (2002) undertook a study to evaluate a strategy to promote early detection of anxiety disorders in asthmatics. The eligibility criteria for the study included the following: (1) 18 years of age or older; (2) able to read, write, and speak English; (3) objective evidence of asthma, based on the Canadian Consensus Guidelines; and (4) no other major medical problems (*e.g.,* cardiovascular disease, cancer, insulin-dependent diabetes).

Researchers sample from an **accessible population** in the hope of generalizing to a target population. The **target population** is the entire population in which the researcher is interested. The accessible population comprises cases from the target population that are accessible to the researcher as a pool of participants. For example, the researcher's target population might consist of all diabetic patients in Canada, but, in reality, the population that is accessible to a researcher might consist of diabetic patients who are members of a particular health region.

> **⬚ CONSUMER TIP:**
>
> In some quantitative research reports, the researchers do not clearly identify the population under study. In others, the population is not clarified until the discussion section, when an effort is made to discuss the group to which the study findings can be generalized. ■

Samples and Sampling

Sampling is the process of selecting a portion of the population to represent the entire population. A sample, then, is a subset of the population. The entities that make up the samples and populations are **elements.** In nursing research, the elements are usually humans.

Samples and sampling plans vary in their adequacy. *The overriding consideration in assessing a sample in a quantitative study is its representativeness*—the extent to which the sample is similar to the population. Unfortunately, there is no method for ensuring that a sample is representative. Certain sampling plans are less likely to result in biased samples than others, but there is never a guarantee of a representative sample. Researchers operate under conditions in which error is possible, but an important role of the researcher is to minimize or control those errors. Consumers must assess the researcher's success in having done so.

There are two broad categories of sampling plans: probability sampling and nonprobability sampling. With a **probability sample,** researchers are able to specify the probability that each element of the population will be included in the sample. Probability samples use random selection in choosing the sample units, and therefore some confidence can be placed in their representativeness. In **nonprobability samples,** elements are selected by nonrandom methods. There is no way to estimate the probability of including each element in a nonprobability sample, and every element usually does not have a chance for inclusion.

Strata

Populations consist of subpopulations, or strata. **Strata** are mutually exclusive segments of a population based on a specified characteristic. For instance, a population consisting of all registered nurses in Canada could be divided into two strata based on gender. Alternatively, we could specify three strata consisting of nurses younger than 30 years, nurses aged 30 to 45 years, and nurses aged 46 years or older. Strata are used in the sample selection process to enhance the sample's representativeness.

Sampling Rationale

Researchers work with samples rather than with populations because it is more economical and efficient to do so. Researchers have neither the time nor the resources to study all members of a population. Furthermore, it is unnecessary to do so because it is usually possible to obtain reasonably accurate information from a sample. Samples, thus, are practical means of collecting data.

Still, data from samples can lead to erroneous conclusions. Finding 50 participants to take part in a study is easy, but it is difficult to select 50 subjects who are not a biased subset of the population. **Sampling bias** is the systematic over-representation or under-representation of some segment of the population in terms of a characteristic relevant to the research question.

Sampling bias is affected by the homogeneity of the population. If the elements in a population were all identical on the critical attribute, any sample would be as good as any other. Indeed, if the population were completely homogeneous (*i.e.,* exhibited no variability at all), a single element would be a sufficient sample for drawing conclusions about the population. For many physical or physiologic attributes, it may be safe to assume a reasonable degree of homogeneity. For example, the blood in a person's veins is relatively homogeneous; hence, a single blood sample chosen haphazardly from a patient is adequate for clinical purposes. Most human attributes, however, are not homogeneous. Variables, after all, derive their name from the fact that traits vary from one person to the next. Age, blood pressure, stress level, and health habits are all attributes that reflect the heterogeneity of humans.

CONSUMER TIP:

The sampling plan is usually discussed in the method section of a research report, sometimes in a separate subsection with the heading "Sample," "Subjects," or "Study Participants." A description of sample characteristics, however, may be reported in the results section. If the researcher has undertaken analyses to detect sample biases in a quantitative study, these may be described in either the method or results section (*e.g.,* the researcher might compare the characteristics of patients who were invited to participate in the study but who declined to do so with those of patients who actually became subjects). ■

NONPROBABILITY SAMPLING

Three primary methods of nonprobability sampling are used in quantitative studies: convenience, quota, and purposive sampling.

Convenience Sampling

Convenience sampling (or **accidental sampling**) entails the use of the most conveniently available people as study participants. A nurse who distributes questionnaires about breastfeeding intentions to the first 100 available pregnant women is using a convenience sample. The problem with convenience sampling is that available participants might be atypical of the population; therefore, the price of convenience is the risk of bias and erroneous findings. Convenience samples do not necessarily comprise people known to the researchers. Stopping people at a street corner to ask them questions is sampling by convenience. People select themselves as pedestrians on certain streets, and self-selection generally leads to bias.

Another type of convenience sampling is **snowball sampling** (or **network sampling**). With this approach, early sample members are asked to refer others who meet the study's eligibility criteria. This method of sampling is most often used when the population consists of people with specific traits who might be difficult to identify by ordinary means (*e.g.*, women who stopped breastfeeding their infants within 1 month after birth).

Convenience sampling is the weakest form of sampling for quantitative studies. When the phenomena of interest are heterogeneous, there is no other sampling method in which the risk of bias is greater—and there is no way to evaluate the biases. You should exercise caution in interpreting findings and generalizing results from quantitative studies that used convenience samples.

Example of convenience sampling:

Hamel et al. (2002) conducted an experimental study to determine whether an individualized intervention for older community-dwelling adults increased their discussion and completion of advanced directives (ADs). The study participants were a convenience sample of 74 older adults who belonged to a senior centre in Manitoba and who had attended an educational session on ADs.

Quota Sampling

With quota sampling, the researcher uses knowledge about the population to build some representativeness into the sampling plan. A **quota sample** is one in which the researcher identifies strata of the population and specifies the number (the quota) of elements needed from those strata in the sample. By using information about the composition of the population, the investigator can ensure that diverse segments are represented.

Let us use as an example a researcher interested in studying the attitudes of undergraduate nursing students toward working on an AIDS unit. The accessible population for this study is a nursing school with an enrollment of 1000 undergraduates, and a sample size of 200 students is desired. With a convenience sample, the researcher could simply distribute questionnaires to students in classrooms. Suppose, however, that the researcher suspects that male and female students, as well as members of the four classes, have different attitudes toward working with AIDS patients. A convenience sample could easily sample too many or too few students from these subgroups. Table 10-1 presents some fictitious data showing the numbers of students in each strata, both for the population and for a hypothetical convenience sample. As Table 10-1 shows, the convenience sample seriously overrepresents first year students and women and underrepresents men and fourth year students. In a quota sample, the researcher can guide the selection of subjects so that the sample includes an appropriate number of cases from each stratum. The bottom panel of Table 10-1 shows the number of cases that would be required from each stratum in a quota sample.

If we continue with this example, you may better appreciate the problem of inadequate representation of the strata. Suppose a key question in this study was: "Would you be willing to work on a unit that cared exclusively for AIDS patients?" The percentage of students in the population who would respond "yes" to this question is shown in the first column of Table 10-2. Of course, these values would not be known by the researcher; they are displayed

TABLE 10-1. Numbers and Percentages of Students in Strata of a Population, Convenience Sample, and Quota Sample

	YEAR 1	YEAR 2	YEAR 3	YEAR 4	TOTAL
POPULATION					
Males	25 (2.5%)	25 (2.5%)	25 (2.5%)	25 (2.5%)	100 (10%)
Females	225 (22.5%)	225 (22.5%)	225 (22.5%)	225 (22.5%)	900 (90%)
TOTAL	250 (25%)	250 (25%)	250 (25%)	250 (25%)	1000 (100%)
CONVENIENCE SAMPLE					
Males	2 (1%)	4 (2%)	3 (1.5%)	1 (0.5%)	10 (5%)
Females	98 (49%)	36 (18%)	37 (18.5%)	19 (9.5%)	190 (95%)
TOTAL	100 (50%)	40 (20%)	40 (20%)	20 (10%)	200 (100%)
QUOTA SAMPLE					
Males	5 (2.5%)	5 (2.5%)	5 (2.5%)	5 (2.5%)	20 (10%)
Females	45 (22.5%)	45 (22.5%)	45 (22.5%)	45 (22.5%)	180 (90%)
TOTAL	50 (25%)	50 (25%)	50 (25%)	50 (25%)	200 (100%)

TABLE 10-2. Students Willing to Consider Working with AIDS Patients

	NUMBER IN POPULATION	NUMBER IN CONVENIENCE SAMPLE	NUMBER IN QUOTA SAMPLE
Year 1 males	2	0	0
Year 2 males	6	1	1
Year 3 males	8	1	2
Year 4 males	12	0	3
Year 1 females	6	2	1
Year 2 females	16	2	3
Year 3 females	30	4	7
Year 4 females	45	3	9
Number of willing students	125	13	26
Total number of students	1000	200	200
Percentage	12.5%	6.5%	13.0%

to illustrate a point. Within the population, males and older students are more likely than females and younger students to express willingness to work on a unit with AIDS patients, yet these are the groups under-represented in the convenience sample. Thus, there is a sizable discrepancy between the population and sample values: nearly twice as many students in the population are favorable toward working with AIDS patients (12.5%) than in the convenience sample (6.5%). The quota sample, on the other hand, does a reasonably good job of reflecting the population's views.

Quota sampling is a relatively easy way to enhance the representativeness of a nonprobability sample. Researchers stratify on the basis of extraneous variables that, in their estimation, would reflect important differences in the dependent variable under investigation. Such variables as age, gender, ethnicity, socioeconomic status, and medical diagnosis are most likely to be used.

Except for the identification of the key strata, quota sampling is procedurally similar to convenience sampling. The subjects are a convenience sample from each stratum of the population. Because of this fact, quota sampling shares many of the same weaknesses as convenience sampling. For instance, if the researcher were required by the quota sampling plan to interview 20 male nursing students, a trip to the dormitories might be a convenient method of recruiting those subjects. Yet this approach would fail to give any representation to male students living off campus, who may have distinctive views about working with AIDS patients. Despite its problems, however, quota sampling is an important improvement over convenience sampling for quantitative studies.

Example of quota sampling:

Jahraus et al. (2002) evaluated the effect of an education program on the perceived adequacy of knowledge of patients with breast cancer receiving radiation therapy. Quota sampling was used to ensure that a minumum of 20 participants were recruited from three age categories assumed to represent women in premenopausal, perimenopausal, and postmenopausal stages.

Purposive Sampling

Purposive sampling (or **judgmental sampling**) is based on the assumption that a researcher's knowledge about the population can be used to "hand pick" the cases to be included in the sample. The researcher might decide purposely to select the widest possible variety of respondents or might choose subjects who are judged to be typical of the population in question or particularly knowledgeable about the issues under study. Sampling in this subjective manner, however, provides no external, objective method for assessing the typicalness of the selected participants. Nevertheless, this method can be advantageous in certain instances. For example, newly developed instruments can be effectively pretested and evaluated with a purposive sample of divergent types of people. Also, as discussed in the next section, purposive sampling is frequently used by qualitative researchers.

Example of purposive sampling:

Alexander et al. (2002) conducted a retrospective chart review study to evaluate a sedation protocol for intubated critically ill children who had been admitted to the PICU over a 5-month period. The sampling plan involved purposive sampling designed to obtain a group of critically ill children who were considered typical of the children admitted to the unit (based on types of illness) and who were intubated during their stay.

Evaluation of Nonprobability Sampling

Nonprobability samples are rarely representative of the target population—some segment of the population is likely to be systematically under-represented. Only a small fraction of the characteristics in which quantitative nurse researchers are interested are sufficiently homogeneous to render sampling bias an irrelevant consideration.

Why, then, are nonprobability samples used at all in quantitative research? Clearly, the advantage of these sampling designs lies in their convenience and economy. Probability sampling requires resources and time. There may be no option but to use a nonprobability sampling plan. Researchers using a nonprobability sample out of necessity must be cautious about their conclusions, and you as reader should be alert to the possibility of sampling bias.

> **CONSUMER TIP:**
>
> Research reports are not always explicit about the type of sampling approach used. This is particularly apt to be true with nonprobability sampling plans. If the sampling design is not specified, it is probably safe to assume that a sample of convenience was used. ■

PROBABILITY SAMPLING

Probability sampling involves the random selection of elements from the population. Random selection should not be confused with random assignment, which was described in Chapter 8. Random assignment is the process of allocating subjects to different treatments on a random basis in experimental designs. Random assignment has no bearing on how subjects in the experiment were selected in the first place. A **random selection** process is one in which each element in the population has an equal, independent chance of being selected. The four most commonly used probability sampling designs are simple random, stratified random, cluster, and systematic sampling.

Simple Random Sampling

Simple random sampling is the most basic probability sampling design. Because more complex probability sampling designs incorporate features of simple random sampling, the procedures are briefly described so that you can appreciate what is involved.

After the population has been defined, the researcher establishes a **sampling frame,** the technical name for the actual list of the population elements. If nursing students attending the University of Alberta constituted the population, then a student roster would be the sampling frame. If the population were 400-bed or larger general hospitals in Canada, then a list of all those hospitals would be the sampling frame. In actual practice, a population is sometimes defined in terms of an existing sampling frame. For example, a researcher might use a telephone directory as a sampling frame. In such a case, the population would be defined as the residents of a certain community who have telephones and who have a listed number. After a listing of the population elements has been developed or located, the elements are numbered consecutively. A table of random numbers or a computer is then used to draw, at random, a sample of the desired size.

Samples selected randomly in such a fashion are not subject to researcher biases. There is no *guarantee* that the sample will be representative of the population, but random selection does guarantee that differences between the sample and the population are purely a function of chance. The probability of selecting a markedly deviant sample through random sampling is low, and this probability decreases as the sample size increases.

Simple random sampling is a labourious process. The development of the sampling frame, enumeration of all the elements, and selection of the sample elements are time-consuming chores, particularly with a large population. Moreover, it is rarely possible to get a complete listing of population elements; hence, other methods are often used.

> **Example of random sampling:**
> Cowin (2001) developed and rigourously tested a new self-concept instrument for nurses with samples of nursing students and working nurses. The sampling frame for working nurses included all nurses registered in the New South Wales Nurses Registration Board confidential database. The instrument was mailed to 2000 randomly selected working nurses.

Stratified Random Sampling

In **stratified random sampling,** the population is divided into homogeneous subsets from which elements are selected at random. As in quota sampling, the aim of stratified sampling is to enhance the sample's representativeness. The most common procedure for drawing a stratified random sample is to group together those elements that belong to a stratum and to randomly select the desired number of elements.

The researcher may sample either proportionately (in relation to the size of the stratum) or disproportionately. If an undergraduate population in a school of nursing consisted of 10% Chinese, 5% Aboriginals, and 85% whites, a **proportionate sample** of 100 students, with racial background as the stratifying variable, would consist of 10, 5, and 85 students from the respective subpopulations. Researchers often use a **disproportionate sample** whenever comparisons between strata of unequal membership size are desired. In the example at hand, the researcher might select 20 Chinese, 20 Aboriginals, and 60 whites to ensure a more adequate representation of the viewpoints of the two racial minorities. (When disproportionate sampling is used, however, it is necessary to make a mathematical adjustment—known as **weighting**—to the data to arrive at the best estimate of overall population values.)

By using stratified random sampling, researchers can sharpen the precision and representativeness of the final sample. Stratified sampling may, however, be impossible if information on the stratifying variables is unavailable (*e.g.,* a student roster might not include information on race and ethnicity). Furthermore, a stratified sample requires even more labour than simple random sampling because the sample must be drawn from multiple enumerated listings.

> **Example of stratified random sampling:**
> Hagan et al. (2000) conducted a survey to assess patient satisfaction and adherence to nurses' advice about self-care measures among patients of the Quebec telenursing

service. The province-wide survey was conducted with a stratified random sample of 4696 callers. The sample was stratified by type of services received (central and local, local only, and based on health region they covered) and the callers' age (18 years old or less, 19–44 years old, and 65 years old or older).

Cluster Sampling

For many populations, it is impossible to obtain a listing of the elements. For example, there is no listing of all full-time nursing students in Canada. Large-scale quantitative studies rarely use simple or stratified random sampling. The most common procedure for large-scale surveys is cluster sampling.

In **cluster sampling,** there is a successive random sampling of units. The first unit to be sampled is large groupings, or clusters. For example, in drawing a sample of nursing students, the researcher might first draw a random sample of nursing schools. The usual procedure for selecting a general sample of citizens is to sample such administrative units as provinces, cities, census tracts, and then households, successively. Because of the successive stages of sampling, this approach is often referred to as **multistage sampling.**

For a specified number of cases, cluster sampling tends to contain more sampling error than simple or stratified random sampling. Nevertheless, cluster sampling is more economical and practical when the population is large and widely dispersed.

Example of cluster sampling:

Trinkoff et al. (2000) studied nurses' substance abuse, using data from a two-stage cluster sample. In the first stage, 10 states in the United States were selected using a complex stratification procedure. In the second stage, registered nurses were selected from each state (a total sample of 3600) by simple random sampling.

Systematic Sampling

Systematic sampling involves the selection of every *k*th case from some list or group, such as every 10th person on a patient list. Systematic sampling designs can be applied in such a way that an essentially random sample is drawn. First, the size of the population is divided by the size of the desired sample to obtain the sampling interval width. The **sampling interval** is the standard distance between the selected elements. For instance, if we wanted a sample of 50 from a population of 5000, our sampling interval would be 100 (5000/50 = 100). In other words, every 100th case on the sampling frame would be sampled. Next, the first case would be selected randomly, using a table of random numbers. If the random number chosen is 73, the people corresponding to numbers 73, 173, 273, 373, and so forth would be included in the sample. Systematic sampling conducted in this manner is essentially identical to simple random sampling and in most cases is preferable because the same results are obtained in a more convenient and efficient manner.

🔲 ***Example of systematic random sampling:***

Then et al. (2001) conducted a study to compare the clinical manifestations of first-time acute myocardial infarction in three age groups of men and women who presented to the emergency departments of three acute tertiary care hospitals. Phase 1 of the study involved a retrospective chart review of a systematic random sample of patient charts.

Evaluation of Probability Sampling

Probability sampling is the only reliable method of obtaining representative samples in quantitative studies. Probability sampling avoids the risk of conscious or unconscious biases. If all the elements in the population have an equal probability of being selected, there is a high likelihood that the sample will represent the population adequately. A further advantage is that probability sampling allows researchers to estimate the magnitude of sampling error. **Sampling error** is the difference between population values (*e.g.,* the average heart rate of the population) and sample values (*e.g.,* the average heart rate of the sample). It is rare that a sample is perfectly representative of a population and contains no sampling error; however, probability sampling permits estimates of the degree of expected error. On the other hand, probability sampling is expensive and demanding. Unless the population is narrowly defined, it is beyond the scope of most researchers to draw a probability sample.

SAMPLE SIZE IN QUANTITATIVE STUDIES

Sample size—the number of subjects in a sample—is a major issue in conducting and evaluating quantitative research. There is no simple equation to determine how large a sample is needed, but quantitative researchers are generally advised to use the largest sample possible. The larger the sample, the more representative it is likely to be. Every time a researcher calculates a percentage or an average based on sample data, the purpose is to estimate a population value. The larger the sample, the smaller the sampling error.

Let us illustrate this notion with an example of estimating monthly aspirin consumption in a nursing home facility (Table 10-3). The population is 15 nursing home residents whose aspirin consumption averages 16 per month. Two simple random samples with sample sizes of 2, 3, 5, and 10 were drawn from the population of 15 residents. Each sample average on the right represents an estimate of the population average, which we know is 16. (Under ordinary circumstances, the population value would be unknown to us, and we would draw only one sample.) With a sample size of 2, our estimate

TABLE 10-3. Comparison of Population and Sample Values and Averages in Nursing Home Aspirin Consumption Example

NUMBER IN GROUP	GROUP	VALUES (MONTHLY NUMBER OF ASPIRINS CONSUMED)	AVERAGE
15	Population	2, 4, 6, 8, 10, 12, 14, 16, 18, 20, 22, 24, 26, 28, 30	16.0
2	Sample 1A	6, 14	10.0
2	Sample 1B	20, 28	24.0
3	Sample 2A	16, 18, 8	14.0
3	Sample 2B	20, 14, 26	20.0
5	Sample 3A	26, 14, 18, 2, 28	17.6
5	Sample 3B	30, 2, 26, 10, 4	14.4
10	Sample 4A	18, 16, 24, 22, 8, 14, 28, 20, 2, 6	15.8
10	Sample 4B	14, 18, 12, 20, 6, 14, 28, 12, 24, 16	16.4

might have been wrong by as many as 8 aspirins (sample 1B). As the sample size increases, the average gets closer to the population value, and differences in the estimates between samples A and B get smaller. As the sample size increases, the probability of getting a deviant sample diminishes because large samples provide the opportunity to counterbalance atypical values.

Researchers can estimate how large the sample should be for an adequate test of the research hypotheses through **power analysis** (Cohen, 1988). A simple example can illustrate the basic principle of power analysis. Suppose a researcher were testing a new intervention to help people quit smoking; smokers would be randomly assigned to either an experimental or a control group. How many smokers should be used in the study? When using power analysis, the researcher must estimate how large the group difference will be (*e.g.,* the difference in the average number of cigarettes smoked in the week after the intervention). This estimate might be based on previous research, on the researcher's personal experience, or on other factors. When expected differences are large, it does not take a large sample to ensure that the differences will be revealed in a statistical analysis; but when small differences are predicted, large samples are needed. Cohen (1988) claims that, for new areas of research, group differences are likely to be small. In our example, if a small group difference in postintervention smoking were expected, the sample size needed to test the effectiveness of the new program, assuming standard statistical criteria, would be about 800 smokers (400 per group). If a medium-sized difference were expected, the total sample size would still be several hundred smokers.

When samples are too small, quantitative researchers run the risk of gathering data that will not confirm the study hypotheses—even when those hypotheses are correct. Large samples are no assurance of accuracy, however.

With nonprobability sampling, even a large sample can harbour extensive bias. A large sample cannot correct for a faulty sampling design; nevertheless, a large nonprobability sample is preferable to a small one. When critiquing quantitative studies, you must assess both the sample size and the sample selection method to judge how representative the sample likely was.

CONSUMER TIP:

The sampling plan is often one of the weakest aspects of quantitative nursing studies (this is also true of quantitative research in other disciplines). Most nursing studies use samples of convenience, and many are based on samples that are too small to provide an adequate test of the research hypotheses. Most quantitative studies are based on samples of fewer than 200 subjects, and a great many studies have fewer than 100 subjects. Power analysis is not used by many nurse researchers, and research reports typically offer no justification for the size of the study sample. (When a power analysis is performed, the minimum power that is generally considered acceptable is .80). Small samples run a high risk of leading researchers to erroneously reject their research hypotheses. Therefore, you should be especially prepared to critique the sampling plan of studies that fail to support research hypotheses. ■

SAMPLING IN QUALITATIVE RESEARCH

Qualitative studies use small, nonrandom samples. This does not mean that qualitative researchers are unconcerned with the quality of their samples, but rather that they use different criteria for selecting study participants. This section examines considerations that apply to sampling in qualitative studies.

The Logic of Qualitative Sampling

Quantitative research is concerned with measuring attributes and relationships in a population, and therefore a representative sample is needed to ensure that the measurements accurately reflect and can be generalized to the population. The aim of most qualitative studies is to discover meaning and to uncover multiple realities; therefore, generalizability, as quantitative researchers use this term, is not a guiding criterion.

The qualitative researcher asks such questions as: "Who would be an information-rich data source for my study?" "Whom should I talk to first, or what should I observe, to maximize my understanding of the phenomenon?" Clearly, with these types of questions, a critical first step in qualitative sampling is the selection of a setting with high potential for "information richness."

As the study progresses, new sampling questions emerge, such as the following: "Whom can I talk to or observe to confirm my understandings? Challenge or modify my understandings? Enrich my understandings? Broaden the utility of the constructs to explain different situations?" Thus, as with the overall design in qualitative studies, sampling design is an emergent one that capitalizes on early learnings to guide subsequent direction.

Types of Qualitative Sampling

Qualitative researchers usually eschew probability samples. A random sample is not the best method of selecting people who will make good informants (*i.e.*, people who are knowledgeable, articulate, reflective, and willing to talk at length with the researcher).

Qualitative researchers may begin with a convenience sample (sometimes referred to in qualitative studies as a **volunteer sample**), especially if the researcher needs potential informants to come forward to identify themselves (*e.g.*, by placing notices in newspapers for people with certain experiences). Qualitative researchers also use snowball sampling, asking early informants to make referrals for other study participants.

Example of snowball sampling:

Browne and Fiske (2001) did an ethnographic study of First Nations women's encounters with mainstream health care services. The researchers used snowball sampling as one approach to make contact with the 10 women who were invited to participate in the study.

Although qualitative sampling may begin with volunteer informants and may be supplemented with new participants through snowballing, most qualitative studies eventually evolve to a purposive sampling strategy. In qualitative research, purposive sampling is often referred to as **theoretical sampling** (especially in grounded theory studies) or **purposeful sampling.** That is, regardless of how initial participants are selected, the researcher usually strives to select sample members purposefully based on the information needs emerging from the early findings. Whom to sample next depends on who has been sampled already.

Example of theoretical sampling:

Perry (2002) conducted a grounded theory study to explore the evolving caring process among women giving care to husbands with Alzheimer disease. The researchers initially recruited sample members from a support group, a day care center, and diagnostic and outreach clinics. As the study progressed, emerging themes provided direction for theoretical sampling. For example, to better understand the evolution of what Perry caled "interpretive caring" as the disease progressed, participants whose husbands were in both the middle and advanced stages of Alzheimer disease were sought.

Within purposive sampling, several alternative strategies have been identified (Patton, 1990), only a few of which are mentioned here:

- **Maximum variation sampling** involves purposefully selecting cases with a wide range of variation on dimensions of interest
- **Extreme/deviant case sampling** provides opportunities for learning from the most unusual and extreme informants (*e.g.,* outstanding successes and notable failures)
- **Typical case sampling** involves selection of participants who will illustrate or highlight what is typical or average

---

Example of maximum variation sampling:

McIntyre et al. (2001) studied the experiences of women living with the decision to seek and have an abortion. They selected 14 women varying in age, social background, economic situation, political perspectives, marital status, range of geographical locations in Western Canada, whether they already had children or not, and whether they had had a previous abortion.

Maximum variation sampling is often the sampling mode of choice in qualitative research because it is useful in documenting the scope of a phenomenon and in identifying important patterns that cut across variations. Other strategies can also be used advantageously, however, depending on the nature of the research question.

 CONSUMER TIP:

A qualitative research report will not necessary use such terms as "maximum variation sampling," but may describe the researcher's intent in selecting study participants. ■

Sample Size

There are no firmly established criteria or rules for sample size in qualitative research. Sample size is largely a function of the purpose of the inquiry, the quality of the informants, and the type of sampling strategy used. For example, a larger sample is likely to be needed with maximum variation sampling than with typical case sampling. Patton argues that purposive samples "be judged on the basis of the purpose and rationale of each study and the sampling strategy used to achieve the study's purpose. The sample, like all other aspects of qualitative inquiry, must be judged in context. . . ." (1990, p. 185).

In qualitative research, sample size should be determined on the basis of informational needs. Hence, a guiding principle in sampling is **data saturation** (*i.e.,* sampling to the point at which no new information is obtained and redundancy is achieved). Redundancy can typically be achieved with a fairly small number of cases, if the information from each is of sufficient depth. Phenomenologic studies are typically based on samples of 10 or fewer study participants. Grounded theory or ethnographic studies are more likely to involve samples of 20 to 50 people.

> ☑ **CONSUMER TIP:**
>
> The sample size adequacy of quantitative studies can be estimated by consumers after the fact through power analysis. However, sample size adequacy in a qualitative study is more difficult to judge on the basis of reading a research report because the main criterion is redundancy of information, which is difficult for consumers to judge. Some qualitative reports explicitly state that data saturation was achieved. ■

CRITIQUING THE SAMPLING PLAN

The sampling plan of a research study—particularly a quantitative study—merits particular scrutiny because, if the sample is seriously biased or too small, the findings may be misleading or just plain wrong. In critiquing a description of a sampling plan, you should consider two issues. The first is whether the researcher has adequately described the sampling plan. Ideally, a research report includes a description of the following aspects of the sample:

- The type of sampling approach used (*e.g.,* convenience, snowball, purposive, simple random)
- The population under study and the eligibility criteria for sample selection in quantitative studies; the nature of the setting and study group in a qualitative one
- The number of participants in the study and a rationale for the sample size
- A description of the main characteristics of the participants (*e.g.,* age, gender, medical condition, race, ethnicity, and so forth) and, in a quantitative study, of the population
- In quantitative studies, the number and characteristics of potential subjects who declined to participate in the study and of subjects who agreed to participate but who subsequently withdrew

If the description of the sample is inadequate, you may not be in a position to deal with the second and principal issue, which is whether the researcher made good sampling decisions.

Evaluating Quantitative Sampling Plans

We have stressed that the main criterion for assessing the adequacy of a sampling plan in quantitative research is whether the sample is representative of the population. You will never be able to know for sure, of course, but if the sampling strategy is weak or if the sample size is small, there is reason to suspect some bias. The extent of this bias depends on several factors, including the population's homogeneity. When the researcher has adopted a sampling plan in which the risk for bias is high, he or she should have taken steps to estimate the direction and degree of this bias so that readers can draw some informed conclusions.

Even with a rigorous sampling plan, the sample may contain some bias if not all people invited to participate in a research study agree to do so. If certain segments of the population refuse to cooperate, then a biased sample can result, even when probability sampling is used. The research report ideally should provide information about **response rates** (*i.e.,* the number of people participating in a study relative to the number of people sampled), and about possible **nonresponse bias**—differences between participants and those who declined to participate.

In developing the sampling plan, the researcher makes decisions regarding the specification of the population as well as the selection of the sample. If the target population is defined broadly, the researcher may have missed opportunities to control extraneous variables, and the gap between the accessible and the target population may be too great. Your job as reviewer is to come to conclusions about the reasonableness of generalizing the findings from the researcher's sample to the accessible population and from the accessible population to a broader target population. If the sampling plan is seriously flawed, it may be risky to generalize the findings at all without further replication of the results with another sample.

Box 10-1 presents some guiding questions for critiquing the sampling plan of a quantitative research report.

Evaluating Qualitative Sampling Plans

In a qualitative study, the sampling plan can be evaluated in terms of its adequacy and appropriateness (Morse, 1991). *Adequacy* refers to the sufficiency and quality of the data the sample yielded. An adequate sample provides data

---

BOX 10-1 **GUIDELINES FOR CRITIQUING QUANTITATIVE SAMPLING DESIGNS**

1. Is the target or accessible population identified and described? Are eligibility criteria specified? To whom can the study results be generalized?

2. Are the sample selection procedures clearly described? What type of sampling plan was used?

3. How adequate is the sampling plan in terms of yielding a representative sample?

4. Did some factor other than the sampling plan affect the representativeness of the sample (*e.g.,* a low response rate)?

5. Are possible sample biases identified?

6. Is the sample size sufficiently large? Was the sample size justified on the basis of a power analysis or other rationale?

without any "thin" spots. When the researcher has truly obtained saturation with a sample, informational adequacy has been achieved, and the resulting description or theory is richly textured and complete.

Appropriateness concerns the methods used to select a sample. An appropriate sample is one resulting from the identification and use of study participants who can best supply information according to the conceptual requirements of the study. The researcher must use a strategy that will yield the fullest possible understanding of the phenomenon of interest. A sampling approach that excludes negative cases or that fails to include participants with unusual experiences may not meet the information needs of the study.

Further guidance to critiquing sampling in a qualitative study is presented in Box 10-2.

RESEARCH EXAMPLES

Below, we describe at some length the sampling plans of two nursing studies, one quantitative and the other qualitative. The guidelines in Boxes 10-1 and 10-2 can be used to evaluate the research samples.

Research Example of a Quantitative Study

Zboril-Benson (2002) conducted a study to profile the reasons for absenteeism among registered nurses in Saskatchewan, Canada.

Research Summary

The population in Zboril-Benson's study was registered nurses working in acute care and long-term care settings in the province of Saskatchewan. The researcher had an excellent sampling frame, a listing of all registered nurses in the Saskatchewan Registered Nurses Association database. The sampling frame identified whether the nurses were working in the two settings of interest. Zboril-Benson randomly selected a sample of 2000 registered nurses from the total population of 4936 nurses. Although Zboril-Benson did not provide a rationale for her sample size, she presumably sought to include a large and diverse representation of nurses. She undoubtedly also realized that, with a mailed questionnaire, her eventual sample size would be reduced by nonreponse.

The 2000 potential participants were mailed a questionnaire and a cover letter explaining the study. To increase response rates, Zboril-Benson sent out a reminder letter with another copy of the survey to the total sample 1 month after the initial mailing. A total of 1079 usable surveys were returned, for a response rate of 54%. Although the response rate is relatively low, the resulting sample was sufficiently large for the researcher's statistical analysis. Unfortunately, the research report did not provide information about the extent to which survey respondents were representative of the population (*i.e.,* there was no discussion of how respondents and nonrespondents may have differed). Of course, the absence of such information does not mean that a response bias analysis was not done.

Zboril-Benson found that 44% of the sample had not been absent in the previous 3 months. Participants who reported absenteeism had been absent an average of 2.9 days. The most frequent absence-producing event was fatigue associated with work overload. Nurses working in acute care had higher absenteeism than nurses working in long-term care. Adequate staffing was the most frequently suggested strategy to decrease absenteeism among participants who offered recommendations.

Clinical Relevance

Given the current shortage of nurses and the projected rise in this shortage over the next decade, absenteeism is a major problem for employers because it affects cost and standards of care. Thus, Zboril-Benson's efforts to identify the reasons for absenteeism among registered nurses has considerable relevance.

Zboril-Benson used a strong sampling strategy that enhanced the likelihood that a diverse sample of nurses from Saskatchewan would be included in the sample. Indeed, every nurse working in acute care and long-term care settings had an equal probability of being invited to participate in the survey. The response rate of 54%, typical for a mailed survey, is rather low, and so caution must be taken in interpreting the results in the absence of information about how representative respondents were of the population. Nevertheless, the findings suggest some strategies to decrease absenteeism. Collaborative efforts between employers and registered nurses may be needed to develop methods of enhancing job satisfaction, improving retention, and reducing job strain. As the health care environment continues to experience stressors such as nursing shortages and difficulties with recruitment and retention, the day-to-day work of nurses and the care of patients may be greatly affected.

Research Example of a Qualitative Study

Wuest (2001) undertook a grounded theory study to develop a middle-range theory that captures the common processes of women's caring in a wide array of circumstances.

Research Summary

Wuest noted that there are social and political trends that place increasing demands on women to provide care. She argued that a conceptualization of caring that captures the full range of women's caring experiences could have consequences for health and social policy. She undertook an in-depth grounded theory study within a feminist framework that combined new data with data she had previously gathered in earlier studies.

Theoretical sampling was particularly important in Wuest's study because she sought to develop an explanatory theory that was reflective of the complex reality and diversity of women's caring experiences. Wuest used theoretical sampling not only to guide her selection of new participants as the study progressed, but also to "sample" from other data sources: "Theoretical sampling took many forms: choosing new participants on the basis of what they could contribute, looking for comparisons in data already collected, returning to participants to ask new questions, observing participants, and looking at literature and other written data" (p. 172). As an example of her approach to sampling participants, Wuest began by interviewing women who were raising children and discovered such issues as the competing demands of caring for spouse versus caring for children, and caring for parents versus caring for their own family. This led her to ask, "Are there other problematic properties of *demands*?" and subsequently to seek as study participants women who had greater demands (*e.g.*, mothers of physically disabled children) and fewer demands (*e.g.*, widows with adult children). Wuest sampled women until she achieved saturation and had a sufficiently large number of participants to conduct a detailed analysis. She conducted 32 new interviews with 21 women who had diverse characteristics and caring responsibilities, and also drew on 43 previously collected interviews.

Wuest's grounded theory provided insight into the process she called *precarious ordering,* which accounts for the complex strategies that women use to manage the dissonance created by the competing and changing caring demands in their lives. The theory demonstrates the power and resilience in women's management through the interrelated processes of *setting boundaries, negotiating,* and *repatterning care.*

Clinical Relevance

Wuest's grounded theory of precarious ordering makes visible the many facets and strategies of women's caring that often are invisible. This visibility is necessary for alerting clinicians to the complexities and habitually changing caring demands placed on women. In discovering the process of precarious ordering where women set limits on caring demands, the linkages between caring and the negative consequences of women's health emerged. Implications for nursing practice with women of all ages can be derived from the different phases of this grounded theory to help promote women's health and well-being. For example, in setting boundaries, two strategies used by women were discovered, those being, "attending to one's own voice" and "determining legitimacy." Nurses can design specific interventions for women based on these identified strategies to help them set limits on the number, nature, and intensity of their caring demands. As patient advocates, nurses can also use the findings of Wuest's grounded theory to help change public policy that can result in modified caring demands and more accessible and suitable resources for women.

● ● ● ● ● *SUMMARY POINTS*

- **Sampling** is the process of selecting a portion of the population, which is an entire aggregate of cases.
- An **element** (the basic unit about which information is collected) can be included in a sample if it meets the researcher's **eligibility criteria.**
- Researchers usually sample from an **accessible population** rather than an entire **target population.**
- The main consideration in assessing a sample in a quantitative study is its representativeness—the extent to which the sample is similar to the population and avoids bias. **Sampling bias** refers to the systematic over-representation or under-representation of some segment of the population.
- The principal types of **nonprobability sampling** (wherein elements are selected by nonrandom methods) are **convenience, quota,** and **purposive sampling.** Nonprobability sampling designs are convenient and economical; a major disadvantage is their potential for bias.
- **Convenience sampling** (or **accidental sampling**) uses the most readily available or most convenient group of people for the sample. **Snowball sampling** is a type of convenience sampling in which referrals for potential participants are made by those already in the sample.
- **Quota sampling** divides the population into homogeneous **strata** (subgroups) to ensure representation of those subgroups in the sample; within each stratum, the researcher selects participants by convenience sampling.
- In **purposive** (or **judgmental**) **sampling,** participants are "hand picked" to be included in the sample based on the researcher's knowledge about the population.
- **Probability sampling** designs, which involve the **random selection** of **elements** from the population, yield more representative samples than nonprobability designs and permit estimates of the magnitude of

sampling error. Probability samples, however, are expensive and demanding.

- **Simple random sampling** involves the selection on a random basis of elements from a **sampling frame** that enumerates all the elements.
- **Stratified random sampling** divides the population into homogeneous subgroups from which elements are selected at random.
- **Cluster sampling** (or **multistage sampling**) involves the successive selection of random samples from larger to smaller units by either simple random or stratified random methods.
- **Systematic sampling** is the selection of every *k*th case from a list. By dividing the population size by the desired sample size, the researcher establishes the **sampling interval,** which is the standard distance between the selected elements.
- Researchers can use a procedure known as **power analysis** to estimate sample size needs. Large samples are preferable to small ones because larger samples tend to be more representative. However, even a large sample does not guarantee representativeness.
- Qualitative researchers use the theoretical demands of the study to select articulate and reflective informants with certain types of experience in an emergent way, capitalizing on early learnings to guide subsequent sampling decisions.
- Qualitative researchers thus most often use **purposive** or **theoretical sampling** to guide them in selecting data sources that maximize information richness. Various strategies can be used to sample purposively, including sampling to maximize variation, to select typical cases, and to learn from extreme cases.
- The criteria for evaluating qualitative sampling are informational adequacy and appropriateness.

➤➤➤➤ *CRITICAL THINKING ACTIVITIES*

Chapter 10 of the accompanying *Study Guide to Accompany Essentials of Nursing Research,* 5th edition, offers various exercises and study suggestions for reinforcing the concepts presented in this chapter. In addition, you can address the following:

1. Read the introduction and method section from the two studies in the Appendix of this book and then answer relevant questions in Box 10-1 or Box 10-2 or both.

2. Read the full research report of Zboril-Benson's (2000) study, which was used as research example in this chapter. What could the researcher have done to increase the representativeness of her research sample? What information could the researcher have provided to indicate whether the response rates of Saskatchewan nurses resulted in any biases in the findings?

*For additional review, see questions 122–135 on the study CD provided with Polit: Study Guide to Accompany Essentials of Nursing Research

SUGGESTED READINGS

Methodologic References

Cohen, J. (1988). *Statistical power analysis for the behavioral sciences* (2nd. ed.). Mahwah, NJ: Erlbaum.

Morse, J. M. (1991). Strategies for sampling. In J. M. Morse (Ed.), *Qualitative nursing research: A contemporary dialogue*. Newbury Park, CA: Sage.

Patton, M. Q. (1990). *Qualitative evaluation and research methods* (2nd ed.). Newbury Park, CA: Sage.

Substantive References

Alexander, E., Carnevale, F. A., & Razack, S. (2002). Evaluation of a sedation protocol for intubated critically ill children. *Intensive and Critical Care Nursing, 18,* 292–301.

Baker, C., Varma, M., & Tanaka, C. (2001). Sticks and stones: racism as experienced by adolescents in New Brunswick. *Canadian Journal of Nursing Research, 33,* 87–105.

Browne, A. J., & Fiske, J. (2001). First Nations women's encounters with mainstream health care services. *Western Journal of Nursing Research, 23,* 126–147.

Cowin, L. (2001). Measuring nurses' self-concept. *Western Journal of Nursing Research, 23,* 313–325.

Davis, T. M. A., Ross, C. J. M., & MacDonald, G. F. (2002). Screening and assessing adult asthmatics for anxiety disorders. *Clinical Journal of Nursing Research, 11,* 173–189.

Hagan, L., Morin, D., & Lepine, R. (2000). Evaluation of telenursing outcomes: Satisfaction, self-care practices, and cost savings. *Public Health Nursing, 17,* 305–313.

Hamel, C. F., Guse, L. W., Hawranik, P. G., & Bond J. B., Jr. (2002). Advance directives and community-dwelling older adults. *Western Journal of Nursing Research, 24,* 143–158.

Jahraus, D., Soklosky, S., Thurston, N., & Guo, D. (2002). Evaluation of an education program for patients with breast cancer receiving radiation therapy. *Cancer Nursing, 25,* 266–275.

McIntyre, M., Anderson, B., & McDonald, C. (2001). The intersection of relational and cultural narratives: women's abortion experiences. *Canadian Journal of Nursing Research, 33,* 47–62.

Perry, J. (2002). Wives giving care to husbands with Alzheimer's disease: A process of interpretive caring. *Research in Nursing & Health, 25,* 307–316.

Then, K. L., Rankin, J. A., & Fotonoff, D. A. (2001). Atypical presentation of acute myocaridal infarction in 3 age groups. *Heart & Lung, 30,* 285–293.

Trinkoff, A. M., Zhou, Q., Storr, C. L., & Soeken, K. L. (2000). Workplace access, negative perscription, job strain, and substance use in registered nurses. *Nursing Research, 49,* 83–90.

Wuest, J. (2001). Precarious ordering: toward a formal theory of women's caring. *Health Care Women International, 22,* 167–193.

Zboril-Benson LR. (2002). Why nurses are calling in sick: The impact of health-care restructuring. *Canadian Journal of Nursing Research, 33*(4), 89–107.

PART IV

COLLECTION OF RESEARCH DATA

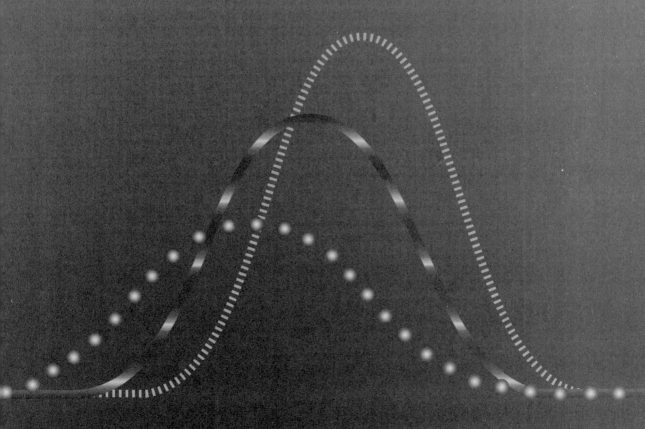

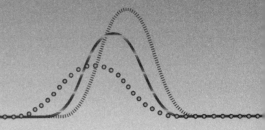

Scrutinizing Data Collection Methods

OVERVIEW OF DATA COLLECTION AND DATA SOURCES
    Existing Data Versus New Data
    Key Dimensions of Data Collection Methods
SELF-REPORT METHODS
    Unstructured and Semistructured Self-Report Techniques
    Structured Self-Report Techniques
    Scales and Other Special Forms of Structured Self-Reports
    Evaluation of Self-Report Methods
    Critiquing Self-Reports
OBSERVATIONAL METHODS
    Unstructured Observational Methods
    Structured Observational Methods
    Evaluation of Observational Methods
    Critiquing Observational Methods

BIOPHYSIOLOGIC MEASURES
    Uses of Biophysiologic Measures in Nursing Research
    Types of Biophysiologic Measures
    Evaluation of Biophysiologic Measures
    Critiquing Biophysiologic Measures
IMPLEMENTING THE DATA COLLECTION PLAN
RESEARCH EXAMPLES
    Research Example of Structured Self-Report and Biophysiologic Measures
    Research Example of Unstructured Self-Report and Observation
SUMMARY POINTS
CRITICAL THINKING ACTIVITIES
SUGGESTED READINGS
    Methodologic References
    Substantive References

Student Objectives

On completion of this chapter, the student will be able to:

○ evaluate a researcher's decision to use existing data versus collecting new data

○ discuss the four dimensions along which data collection approaches vary

○ critique a researcher's decisions regarding the data collection plan and its implementation

○ define new terms in the chapter

Self-Reports

○ distinguish between and evaluate structured and unstructured self-reports; open-ended and closed-ended questions; and interviews and questionnaires

○ identify several types of structured and unstructured self-report techniques

○ evaluate a researcher's decision to use a self-report approach

Observation

○ identify several types of phenomena that lend themselves to observation

○ distinguish between and evaluate structured and unstructured observations and describe various methods of collecting such observational data

○ identify methods of sampling observations

○ evaluate a researcher's decision to use an observational data collection approach versus an alternative approach (*e.g.*, self-report)

Biophysiologic Measures

○ describe the major features, advantages, and disadvantages of biophysiologic measures

○ evaluate a researcher's decision to use a biophysiologic measure as well as the choice of the specific measure

New Terms

Acquiescence response set bias	Grand tour question
Biophysiologic measure	Historical research
Bipolar adjectives	*In vitro* measures
Category system	*In vivo* measures
Checklist	Instrument
Closed-ended question	Interview schedule
Completely unstructured interviews	Item
Counterbalancing	Life history
Diary	Likert scale
Event sampling	Log
Extreme response set bias	Methodologic notes
Field notes	Mobile positioning
Fixed-alternative question	Moderator
Focus group interview	Multiple positioning
Focused interview	Nay-sayer

Observation
Observational methods
Observational notes
Open-ended question
Participant observation
Personal notes
Pretest
Projective technique
Q sort
Questionnaire
Rating scale
Reactivity
Records
Response alternatives
Response set biases
Scale
Secondary analysis

Self-report
Semantic differential
Semistructured interview
Single positioning
Social desirability response set bias
Structured observation
Structured self-report
Summated rating scale
Theoretical notes
Time sampling
Topic guide
Unstructured observation
Unstructured self-report
Vignette
Visual analog scale
Yea-sayer

The phenomena in which a researcher is interested must be translated into concepts that can be measured, observed, or recorded. The task of selecting or developing methods for gathering data is among the most challenging in the research process. Without appropriate data collection methods, the validity of research conclusions is easily challenged.

OVERVIEW OF DATA COLLECTION AND DATA SOURCES

There are many alternative approaches to data collection, and these approaches vary along several dimensions. This introductory section provides an overview of some of the important dimensions.

Existing Data Versus New Data

One of the first data decisions an investigator makes concerns the use of existing data versus new data gathered specifically for the study. Most of this chapter is devoted to methods researchers use to generate new data, but they sometimes can take advantage of existing information. A meta-analysis (see Chap. 6) is one type of study that relies on available data, that is, from research reports.

Historical research typically relies on available data. Data for historical research are usually in the form of written, narrative records of the past: diaries, letters, newspapers, minutes of meetings, reports, and so forth. Nurses have used historical research methods to examine a wide range of phenomena.

> **Example of the use of historical data:**
>
> Wilson et al. (2002), a team of researchers from six disciplines, studied the 20th century influences on location of death in Canada. Data were obtained from diverse sources such as Canadian government documents, various databases, and books. Findings of the study indicate that the two key influences on location of death are developments in health care and health systems and reduced availability of home-based caregivers.

Sometimes researchers perform a **secondary analysis,** which is the use of data gathered in a previous study, often by other researchers, to test new hypotheses or address new research questions. A secondary analysis can be performed with both quantitative and qualitative data.

> **Examples of secondary analysis:**
>
> *Quantitative example:* Wong and Wong (2002) used data from the National Population Health Survey to examine the prevalent trends of self-reported lifestyle cardiovascular disease risk factors in adult women.
>
> *Qualitative example:* Skillen et al. (2001) did a secondary analysis of data from 56 transcribed in-depth interviews. The original descriptive study explored organizational factors and work hazards. The secondary analysis resulted in a framework describing ideologies of female public health nurses related to their workplace environmental risks.

An important existing data source for nurse researchers is **records.** Hospital records, nursing charts, physicians' order sheets, and care plan statements all constitute rich data sources. Records are an economical and convenient source of information. Because the researcher was not responsible for collecting and recording information, however, he or she may be unaware of the records' limitations, biases, or incompleteness. If the records available for use are not the entire set of all possible records, the investigator must deal with the issue of the records' representativeness. Existing records have been used in both qualitative and quantitative nursing studies.

> **Example of a study using records:**
>
> Wilson (2002) studied end-of-life dependency among dying patients, using healthcare records of all deceased persons who received care over a 6-month period in one Canadian hospital and one home care department.

Key Dimensions of Data Collection Methods

If existing data are not available or are unsuitable for the research question, new data must be collected. In developing a data collection plan, the investigator makes many important decisions. A primary decision concerns the basic form of data collection to use. Three types of approach have been used most frequently by nurse researchers: self-reports, observations, and biophysiologic measures. **Self-reports** are participants' responses to questions posed by the researcher, such as in an interview. Direct **observation** of people's behaviours, characteristics, and circumstances is an alternative to self-reports for certain types of research questions. Nurses are increasingly using **biophysiologic measures** to assess important clinical variables. Sections of this chapter are devoted to these three major types of data collection.

Regardless of the approach used, data collection methods vary along several important dimensions:

- *Structure.* Research data are often collected in a highly structured manner; the same information is gathered from all participants in a comparable, prespecified way. Sometimes, however, it is more appropriate to be flexible and to allow participants to reveal relevant information in a naturalistic way.
- *Quantifiability.* Data that will be analyzed statistically must be gathered in such a way that they can be quantified. On the other hand, data that are to be analyzed qualitatively are collected in narrative form. Structured data collection approaches tend to yield data that are more easily quantified.
- *Obtrusiveness.* Data collection methods differ in terms of the degree to which people are aware of their status as study participants. If participants are fully aware of their role in a study, their behaviour and responses might not be normal. When data are collected unobtrusively, however, ethical problems may emerge.
- *Objectivity.* Some data collection approaches require more subjective judgment than others. Quantitative researchers generally strive for methods that are as objective as possible. In qualitative research, however, the subjective judgment of the investigator is considered a valuable tool.

Sometimes, the research question dictates where on these four dimensions the data collection method will lie. For example, questions that are best suited for a qualitative study normally use methods that are low on structure, quantifiability, obtrusiveness, and objectivity, whereas research questions appropriate for a survey tend to require methods that are high on all four dimensions. However, researchers often have latitude in selecting or designing appropriate data collection plans.

CONSUMER TIP

Researchers describe their data collection plan in the method section of a research report. In a report for a quantitative study, the specific data collection methods are often described in a subsection with the heading "Measures" or "Instruments." The actual steps taken to collect the data are sometimes described in a separate subsection with the heading "Procedures." ■

SELF-REPORT METHODS

In the human sciences, a good deal of information can be gathered by direct questioning of people. If, for example, we were interested in learning about patients' perceptions of hospital care, nursing home residents' fear of death, or women's knowledge about menopause, we would likely try to obtain information by posing questions to a sample of relevant people. For some research variables, alternatives to direct questioning exist, but the unique ability of humans to communicate verbally on a sophisticated level ensures that self-reports will never be eliminated from nurse researchers' repertoire of data collection techniques.

The self-report approach consists of a range of techniques that vary in the degree of structure imposed. At one extreme are loosely structured methods that do not involve a formal written set of questions. At the other extreme are tightly structured methods involving the use of formal documents such as questionnaires. Some characteristics of different self-report approaches are discussed next.

Unstructured and Semistructured Self-Report Techniques

Unstructured or loosely structured **self-report** methods offer flexibility. When these methods are used, the researcher does not have a set of questions that must be asked in a specific order and worded in a given way. Instead, the researcher starts with some general questions or topics and allows the respondents to tell their stories in a naturalistic, narrative fashion. In other words, unstructured or semistructured self-reports, usually obtained in interviews, tend to be conversational in nature.

Unstructured interviews, which are used by researchers in all qualitative research traditions, encourage respondents to define the important dimensions of a phenomenon and to elaborate on what is relevant to them, rather than being guided by the investigator's *a priori* notions of relevance. Unstructured interviews are the mode of choice when researchers do not have a clear idea of what it is they do not know.

Types of Unstructured Self-Reports

There are several approaches to collecting unstructured self-report data. **Completely unstructured interviews** are used when the researcher has no preconceived view of the content or flow of information to be gathered. Their aim is to elucidate the respondents' perceptions of the world without imposing the researcher's views. Typically, the researcher begins by posing a broad **grand tour question** such as, "What happened when you first learned that you had AIDS?" Subsequent questions are more focused and are guided by initial responses. Ethnographic and phenomenological studies often use unstructured interviews.

Example of a study using unstructured interviews:

McIntyre et al. (2001) explored women's choices concerning abortions. The interviews, which were audiotaped, began by generating conversation between each of the 14 women and one of the researchers. There was no attempt to standardize the conversations. The researchers encouraged each of the women to explore by prompting, eliciting examples, and posing questions.

Focused (or **semistructured**) **interviews** are used when a researcher has a list of topics that must be covered in an interview. The interviewer uses a written **topic guide** to ensure that all question areas are covered. The interviewer's function is to encourage participants to talk freely about all the topics on the guide.

Example of a study using a semistructured interview:

Werezak and Stewart (2002) conducted a study to explore the process of learning to live with early-stage dementia. Data were obtained from the participants using semistructured interviews. Coding and analysis of these interviews led the researchers to develop a preliminary theory encompassing six categories. A second, unstructured interview was conducted to verify and clarify the emerging theory.

Focus group interviews are interviews with groups of about 5 to 15 people whose opinions and experiences are solicited simultaneously. The interviewer (or **moderator**) guides the discussion according to a topic guide or set of questions. The advantages of a group format are that it is efficient and can generate a great deal of dialogue, but some people are uncomfortable expressing their views or describing their experiences in front of a group.

Example of a study using focus group interviews:

Rodney et al. (2002) studied nurses' ethical decision making. Data were collected from focus groups held with advanced-practice nurses, other practicing nurses, and third and fourth year nursing students from a variety of settings, agencies, and units.

Life histories are narrative self-disclosures about life experiences. With this approach, the researcher asks the respondents to describe, in chronological sequence, their experiences regarding a specified theme, either orally or in writing. Some researchers have used this approach to obtain a total life health history.

Example of a study using life histories:

Abrums (2000) explored the meaning of death and the experience of grieving among deeply religious members of a store-front church. Life history interviews were used to analyze these concepts.

Diaries have been used by some researchers, who ask participants to maintain a daily log about some aspect of their lives for a specified time period. Nurse researchers have used health diaries to collect information about how people prevent illness, maintain health, experience morbidity, or treat health problems.

Example of a study using diaries:

Arthur et al. (2001) conducted research to develop and implement a community-based support group for women with heart disease. Two groups of women (n=16) met monthly for 5 months to develop the program. Between the sessions participants kept diaries of their experiences. The diaries, combined with videotapes, session transcriptions, field notes, and final evaluation constituted the data for this study.

Gathering Unstructured Self-Report Data

Researchers gather unstructured self-report data to develop a construction of a phenomenon that is consistent with that of the participants. This goal requires researchers to take steps to overcome communication barriers and to enhance the flow of meaning. For example, a researcher who is studying a subgroup that uses distinctive terms should strive before going into the field to understand those terms and their nuances.

Although unstructured interviews are conversational in nature, this does not mean that researchers enter into them casually. The conversations are purposeful ones that require advance thought and preparation. For example, the wording of questions should make sense to respondents and reflect their world view. In addition to being good questioners, the researchers must be good listeners. Only by attending carefully to what the respondent is saying can the in-depth interviewer develop appropriate follow-up questions.

Unstructured interviews are typically long—sometimes lasting several hours. The issue of how best to record such abundant information is a difficult one. Some researchers take sketchy notes as the interview progresses, filling in the details after the interview is completed. Many prefer tape recording the interviews for later transcription. Although some respondents are self-conscious when their conversation is recorded, they typically forget about the presence of recording equipment after a few minutes.

Structured Self-Report Techniques

A structured approach to collecting self-report data is appropriate when researchers know in advance exactly what they need to know and can, therefore, frame appropriate questions to obtain the needed information. **Structured self-report** data are usually collected by means of a formal, written document referred to as an **instrument.** The instrument is known as the **interview schedule** when the questions are asked orally in either a face-to-face or telephone format and as the **questionnaire** when respondents complete the instrument themselves in a paper-and-pencil or computerized format. Some features of structured self-report instruments are discussed next.

Question Form

In a totally structured instrument, respondents are asked to respond to the same questions in the same order, and they are given the same set of options for their responses. **Closed-ended questions** (also referred to as **fixed-alternative questions**) are ones in which the **response alternatives** are specified by the researcher. The alternatives may range from a simple yes or no to complex expressions of opinion. The purpose of using questions with fixed alternatives is to ensure comparability of responses and to facilitate analysis.

Many structured instruments, however, also include some **open-ended questions,** which allow participants to respond to questions in their own words. When open-ended questions are included in questionnaires, respondents must write out their responses. In interviews, the interviewer writes down responses verbatim or uses a tape recorder for later transcription. Some examples of open-ended and closed-ended questions are presented in Box 11-1.

Both open-ended and closed-ended questions have strengths and weaknesses. Closed-ended questions are more difficult to construct than open-ended ones but easier to administer and, especially, to analyze. Furthermore, closed-ended questions are more efficient because people can complete more closed-ended questions than open-ended ones in a given amount of time. Also, in questionnaires, respondents may be unwilling to compose lengthy written responses to open-ended questions.

The major drawback of closed-ended questions is that researchers might overlook some potentially important responses. Another concern is that closed-ended questions can be superficial; open-ended questions allow for richer and fuller information if the respondents are verbally expressive and cooperative. Finally, some respondents object to choosing from alternatives that do not reflect their opinions precisely.

Instrument Construction

Researchers generally begin by developing an outline of the instrument's content. Questions for the content areas are then drafted or, if possible, borrowed or adapted from other instruments. Researchers must carefully monitor the wording of each question for clarity, sensitivity to the respondent's psychological state, freedom from bias, and (in questionnaires) reading level. Questions must then be sequenced in a psychologically meaningful order that encourages cooperation and candor.

Draft instruments are usually critically reviewed by peers or colleagues and then pretested with a small sample of respondents. A **pretest** is a trial run to determine whether the instrument is clearly worded, free from major biases, and useful in generating desired information. In large studies, the development and pretesting of self-report instruments may take many months to complete.

| BOX 11-1 | **EXAMPLES OF QUESTION TYPES** |

Open-Ended

- What led to your decision to stop smoking?
- What did you do when you discovered you had AIDS?

Closed-Ended

1. Dichotomous Question

Have you ever been hospitalized?

  ❑ 1. Yes
  ❑ 2. No

2. Multiple-Choice Question

How important is it to you to avoid a pregnancy at this time?

  ❑ 1. Extremely important
  ❑ 2. Very important
  ❑ 3. Somewhat important
  ❑ 4. Not at all important

3. "Cafeteria" Question

People have different opinions about the use of estrogen-replacement therapy for women in menopause. Which of the following statements best represents your point of view?

  ❑ 1. Estrogen replacement is dangerous and should be totally banned.
  ❑ 2. Estrogen replacement may have some undesirable side effects that suggests the need for caution in its use.
  ❑ 3. I am undecided about my views on estrogen-replacement therapy.
  ❑ 4. Estrogen replacement has many beneficial effects that merit its promotion.
  ❑ 5. Estrogen replacement is a wonder cure that should be administered routinely to menopausal women.

4. Rank-Order Question

People value different things about life. Below is a list of principles or ideals that are often cited when people are asked to name things they value most. Please indicate the order of importance of these values to you by placing a 1 beside the most important, 2 beside the next most important, and so forth.

  ❑ Achievement and success
  ❑ Family relationships
  ❑ Friendships and social interaction
  ❑ Health
  ❑ Money
  ❑ Religion

5. Forced-Choice Question

Which statement most closely represents your point of view?

  ❑ 1. What happens to me is my own doing.
  ❑ 2. Sometimes I feel I don't have enough control over my life.

(continued)

BOX 11-1 *(Continued)*

6. Rating Question

On a scale from 0 to 10, where 0 means extremely dissatisfied and 10 means extremely satisfied, how satisfied are you with the nursing care you received during your hospitalization?

Extremely dissatisfied   Extremely satisfied

0   1   2   3   4   5   6   7   8   9   10

Interviews Versus Questionnaires

Researchers using a structured self-report approach must decide whether to use an interview or a questionnaire. You should be aware of the limitations and strengths of these alternatives because the decision may affect the findings. Questionnaires, relative to interviews, have the following advantages:

- Questionnaires are less costly and require less time and effort to administer; this is a particular advantage if the sample is geographically dispersed.
- Questionnaires offer the possibility of complete anonymity, which may be crucial in obtaining information about illegal or deviant behaviours or about embarrassing characteristics.
- The absence of an interviewer ensures that there will be no biases reflecting the respondent's reaction to the interviewer rather than to the questions themselves.

Example of a study using questionnaires:

Laschinger et al. (2001) studied the impact of structural and psychological empowerment on job strain in nursing work settings based on Kanter's structural empowerment model. Questionnaires were mailed to a random sample of 404 Canadian staff nurses.

The strengths of interviews far outweigh those of questionnaires. These strengths include the following:

- The response rate tends to be high in face-to-face interviews. Respondents are less likely to refuse to talk to an interviewer than to ignore a questionnaire, especially a mailed questionnaire. Low response rates can lead to bias because respondents are rarely a random subset of those whom the researcher intended for inclusion in the study.
- Many people simply cannot fill out a questionnaire; examples include young children, the blind, and the very elderly. Interviews are feasible with most people.

- Questions are less likely to be misinterpreted by respondents because the interviewer can determine whether questions have been understood.
- Interviewers can produce additional information through observation of respondents' living situation, level of understanding, degree of cooperativeness, and so on, all of which can be useful in interpreting responses.

Most advantages of face-to-face interviews also apply to telephone interviews. Complicated or detailed instruments are not well suited to telephone interviewing, but for relatively brief instruments, the telephone interview combines relatively low costs with high response rates.

Example of a study using structured interviews:

Roberts et al. (2002) conducted structured telephone interviews with cancer patients who were recently discharged from an Australian hospital and who had been offered a hospital-based cancer support nurse service. The interview asked about the patient's use, perceptions, and satisfaction with the service.

Scales and Other Special Forms of Structured Self-Reports

Several special types of structured self-report are used by nurse researchers. These include composite social–psychological scales, vignettes, projective techniques, and Q sorts.

Composite Scales

Social–psychological scales are often incorporated into a questionnaire or interview schedule. A **scale** is a device designed to assign a numeric score to people to place them on a continuum with respect to attributes being measured, like a scale for measuring weight. Social-psychological scales quantitatively discriminate among people with different attitudes, fears, motives, perceptions, personality traits, and needs.

The most common scaling technique is the Likert scale, named after social psychologist Rensis Likert. A **Likert scale** consists of several declarative statements (or **items**) that express a viewpoint on a topic. Respondents are asked to indicate the degree to which they agree or disagree with the opinion expressed by the statement. Table 11-1 presents an illustrative, 6-item Likert scale for measuring attitudes toward the mentally ill. In this example, agreement with positively worded statements and disagreement with negatively worded statements are assigned higher scores. The first statement is positively phrased; agreement indicates a favourable attitude toward the mentally ill. Because the item has five response alternatives, a score of 5 would be given to someone strongly agreeing, 4 to someone agreeing, and so forth. The responses of two hypothetical respondents are shown by a check or an X, and their item scores are shown in the right-hand columns. Person 1, who agreed with the first statement, has a score of 4, whereas person 2, who strongly disagreed, has a score of 1. The second statement is negatively worded, and so the scoring is re-

TABLE 11-1. Example of a Likert Scale to Measure Attitudes Toward the Mentally Ill

DIRECTION OF SCORING*		RESPONSES†					SCORE	
		SA	A	?	D	SD	Person 1 (✓)	Person 2 (X)
+	1. People who have had a mental illness can become normal, productive citizens after treatment.	✓				X	4	1
−	2. People who have been patients in mental hospitals should not be allowed to have children.		X		✓		5	3
−	3. The best way to handle patients in mental hospitals is to restrict their activity as much as possible.		X	✓			4	2
+	4. Many patients in mental hospitals develop normal, healthy relationships with staff members and other patients.			✓	X		3	2
+	5. There should be an expanded effort to get the mentally ill out of institutional settings and back into their communities.	✓				X	5	1
−	6. Because the mentally ill cannot be trusted, they should be kept under constant guard.		X			✓	5	2
						TOTAL SCORE	26	11

*Researchers would not indicate the direction of scoring on a Likert scale administered to subjects. The scoring direction is indicated in this table for illustrative purposes only.
†SA, strongly agree; A, agree; ?, uncertain; D, disagree; SD, strongly disagree.

versed—a 1 is assigned to those who strongly agree, and so forth. This reversal is necessary so that a high score will consistently reflect positive attitudes toward the mentally ill. A person's total score is determined by summing item scores; hence, these scales are sometimes called **summated rating scales.** The total scores of the two hypothetical respondents, shown at the bottom of Table 11-1, reflect a considerably more positive attitude toward the mentally ill on the part of person 1 (score = 26) than person 2 (score = 11). The summation feature of Likert scales makes it possible to make fine discriminations among people with different viewpoints. A single Likert question allows people to be put into only five categories. A 6-item scale, such as the one in Table 11-1, permits much finer gradation—from a minimum possible score of 6 (6 × 1) to a maximum possible score of 30 (6 × 5).

> **Example of a study using a Likert scale:**
>
> Profetto-McGrath et al. (2003) studied the relationship between nurses' research utilization (RU) and critical thinking dispositions (CTDs). Nurses' CTDs were measured using a 6-item Likert scale. An example of an item from the California Critical Thinking Disposition Inventory used to measure the CTD is: "The truth always depends on your point of view."

Another technique for measuring attitudes is the **semantic differential** (SD). With the SD, respondents are asked to rate a concept (*e.g.,* primary nursing, team nursing) on a series of **bipolar adjectives,** such as good/bad, strong/weak, effective/ineffective, important/unimportant. Respondents are asked to place a check at the appropriate point on a 7-point scale that extends from one extreme of the dimension to the other. An example of an SD format is shown in Figure 11-1. The SD has the advantage of being flexible and easy to construct. The concept being rated can be virtually anything—a person, concept, controversial issue, and so on. The scoring procedure for SD responses is similar to that for Likert scales. Scores from 1 to 7 are assigned to each bipolar scale response, with higher scores generally associated with the positively worded adjective. Responses are then summed across the bipolar scales to yield a total score.

> **Example of a study using a semantic differential:**
>
> Phillips et al. (2001) developed the Elder Image Scale, a semantic differential instrument that measures a caregiver's mental image of an elder derived from past associations and present observations. Example of adjective pairs include reasonable/unreasonable, even tempered/hot tempered, and considerate/abusive.

Another type of psychosocial measure is the **visual analog scale** (VAS), which can be used to measure subjective experiences, such as pain, fatigue, nausea, and dyspnea. The VAS is a straight line, the end anchors of which are labeled as the extreme limits of the sensation or feeling being measured. Participants are asked to mark a point on the line corresponding to the amount of sensation experienced. Traditionally, a VAS line is 100 mm in length, which facilitates the derivation of a score from 0 to 100 through simple measurement of the distance from one end of the scale to the participant's mark on the line. An example of a VAS is presented in Figure 11-2.

> **Example of a study using a visual analog scale:**
>
> Eller (2001) studied the quality of life in person living with HIV. A sample of 81 HIV-positive individuals completed a single-item Visual Analog Scale–Fatigue Scale. The scale is a 100-mm scale with the following anchors at each end: *not at all fatigued* and *most fatigued I ever felt.*

NURSE PRACTITIONERS

competent	7*	6	5	4	3	2	1	incompetent
worthless	1	2	3	4	5	6	7	valuable
important								unimportant
pleasant								unpleasant
bad								good
cold								warm
responsible								irresponsible
successful								unsuccessful

*The score values would not be printed on the form administered to actual subjects. The numbers are presented here solely for the purpose of illustrating how semantic differentials are scored.

FIGURE 11-1. Example of a semantic differential.

Scales permit researchers to efficiently quantify subtle gradations in the strength or intensity of individual characteristics. A good scale can be useful both for group-level comparisons (*e.g.,* comparing the stress levels of mastectomy patients before and after surgery) and for making individual comparisons (*e.g.,* predicting that patient X will not need as much emotional support as patient Y because of scores on a coping scale). Scales can be administered either verbally or in writing and are, therefore, suitable for use with most people.

Scales are susceptible to several common problems, however, the most troublesome of which are referred to as **response set biases.** The most important biases include the following:

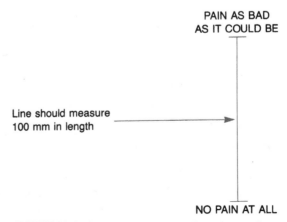

PAIN AS BAD
AS IT COULD BE

Line should measure
100 mm in length

NO PAIN AT ALL

FIGURE 11-2. Example of a visual analog scale.

- **Social desirability response set bias**—a tendency to misrepresent attitudes or traits by giving answers that are consistent with prevailing social views
- **Extreme response set bias**—a tendency to consistently express attitudes or feelings in extreme responses (*e.g.*, strongly agree), leading to distortions because extreme responses may not necessarily signify the greatest intensity
- **Acquiescence response set bias**—a tendency to agree with statements regardless of their content by people who are referred to as **yea-sayers.** The opposite tendency for other people (**nay-sayers**) to disagree with statements independently of the question content is less common.

These biases can be reduced through such strategies as **counterbalancing** positively and negatively worded statements, developing sensitively worded questions, creating a permissive, nonjudgmental atmosphere, and guaranteeing the confidentiality of responses.

Vignettes

Vignettes are brief descriptions of events or situations to which respondents are asked to react. The descriptions are structured to elicit information about respondents' perceptions, opinions, or knowledge about a phenomenon. The vignettes are usually written, narrative descriptions but can also be videotapes. The questions posed to respondents after the vignettes may be either open-ended (*e.g.*, "How would you recommend handling this situation?") or closed-ended (*e.g.*, "On the 9-point scale below, rate how well you believe the nurse handled the situation.").

Vignettes are an economical means of eliciting information about how people might behave in situations that would be difficult to observe in daily life. For example, we might want to assess how patients would react to or feel about nurses with different personal styles of interaction. In clinical settings, it would be difficult to expose patients to many nurses, all of whom have been evaluated as having different interaction styles.

The principal problem with vignettes concerns the validity of responses. If respondents describe how they would react in a situation portrayed in the vignette, how accurate is that description of their actual behaviour? Thus, although the use of vignettes can be profitable, the possibility of response biases should be recognized.

Example of a study using vignettes:

Arslanian-Engoren (2001) studied emergency department nurses' triage decisions in relation to patients' age and gender. She distributed vignettes for cases that contained identical cues for myocardial infarction but that differed in patient gender and age. Nurses perceived middle-aged men as needing more urgent triage than same-aged women with identical symptoms.

Projective Techniques

Most self-report methods depend on a respondent's capacity for self-insight and candor. **Projective techniques** are methods for obtaining psychological measurements through verbal self-report with a minimum of participants' conscious cooperation. Projective methods give free play to the participants' imagination by providing them with ambiguous stimuli that invite personal interpretations. The rationale underlying projective techniques is that the manner in which a person reacts to unstructured stimuli is a reflection of the person's needs, motives, attitudes, or personality traits.

Projective techniques are flexible: virtually any unstructured stimulus can be used to induce projective responses. The resulting data can often be analyzed either qualitatively or quantitatively. One class of projective methods uses pictorial materials, such as the Rorschach (inkblot) test. Verbal projective techniques present participants with ambiguous verbal stimuli rather than pictorial ones. For example, word-association methods present participants with a series of words to which participants respond with the first thing that comes to mind. A third class of projective measures is expressive methods, such as play techniques, drawing and painting, and role playing. The assumption is that people express their feelings and emotions by working with or manipulating various materials.

Projective measures have been controversial among researchers. Critics point out that a high degree of inference is required in gleaning information from projective tests, and data quality depends heavily on the researcher's interpretive skill. On the other hand, some people argue that projective methods probe the unconscious mind, encompass the whole personality, and provide data of breadth and depth unattainable by more traditional methods. One useful feature of projective instruments is that they are less susceptible to faking than self-report measures. Finally, some projective techniques are particularly useful with special groups, such as children or people with speech and hearing defects.

Example of a study using projective techniques:

Instone (2000) conducted a grounded theory study of children with HIV infection. The study included projective drawings, which were analyzed for themes of emotional distress, disturbed self-image, and social isolation.

Q Sorts

In a **Q sort,** the study participant is presented with a set of cards on which words, phrases, or statements are written. The participant is asked to sort the cards along a specified bipolar dimension, such as agree/disagree. Typically, there are between 60 and 100 cards to be sorted into 9 or 11 piles, with the number of cards to be placed in each pile predetermined by the researcher.

The sorting instructions and objects to be sorted in a Q sort can vary. For example, personality can be studied by writing descriptions of personality traits on the cards; participants can then be asked to sort items on a continuum from "exactly like me" to "not at all like me." Other applications include asking patients to rate nursing behaviours on a continuum from most helpful to least helpful or asking cancer patients to rate various aspects of their treatment on a most distressing to least distressing continuum.

Q sorts can be a powerful tool, but, like other data collection techniques, they also have drawbacks. On the positive side, Q sorts are versatile and can be applied to a wide variety of problems. Requiring people to place a predetermined number of cards in each pile eliminates many response biases that can occur in Likert scales. On the other hand, it is difficult and time-consuming to administer Q sorts to a large sample of people. Some critics argue that the forced distribution of cards according to the researcher's specifications is artificial and excludes information about how the participants would ordinarily distribute their responses.

> ### Example of a study using Q sorts:
> McCaughan et al. (2002) used Q sorts as an approach to studying nurses' perceptions of barriers that prevent them from using research in their decision making. The 60 statements used on the Q sort cards were derived from in-depth interviews and observations. An example of a Q sort statement is: "Statistics put me off research papers or other kinds of research information."

Evaluation of Self-Report Methods

Self-report techniques—the most common method of data collection in nursing studies—are strong with respect to their directness. If researchers want to know how people feel or what they believe, the most direct approach is to ask them. Moreover, self-reports frequently yield information that would be difficult, if not impossible, to gather by other means. Behaviours can be directly *observed,* but only if people are willing to manifest them publicly. It is usually impossible for a researcher to observe such behaviours as contraceptive practices or drug usage. Furthermore, observers can only observe behaviours occurring at the time of the study; self-report instruments can gather retrospective data about activities and events occurring in the past or about behaviours in which participants plan to engage in the future. Information about feelings, values, opinions, and motives can sometimes be inferred through observation, but behaviours and feelings do not always correspond exactly. People's actions do not always indicate their state of mind. Self-report instruments can be used to measure psychological characteristics through direct communication with the participants.

Despite these advantages, self-report methods share certain weaknesses. The most serious issue is the question of the validity and accuracy of self-reports: How can we be sure that respondents feel or act the way they say they do? How can we trust the information that respondents provide, particularly if the questions could potentially require them to admit to undesirable traits? Investigators often have no alternative but to assume that most respondents have been frank. Yet, we all have a tendency to present ourselves in the best light, and this may conflict with the truth. When reading research reports, you should be alert to potential biases in self-reported data, particularly with respect to behaviours or feelings that our society judges to be controversial or wrong.

You should also be familiar with the merits of unstructured and structured self-reports. In general, unstructured interviews are of greatest utility when a new area of research is being explored. An unstructured approach allows researchers to ascertain what the basic issues are, how sensitive or controversial the topic is, how individuals conceptualize and talk about a phenomenon, and what the range is of opinions or behaviours that are relevant to the topic. Unstructured methods may also help elucidate the underlying meaning of a pattern or relationship repeatedly observed in more structured research.

Unstructured methods, however, are extremely time-consuming and demanding. Also, unstructured self-reports are not appropriate for capturing the measurable aspects of a phenomenon, such as incidence (*e.g.,* the percentage of infertile couples who elect *in vitro* fertilization), duration (*e.g.,* average time period during which pregnancy was attempted before infertility treatment was sought), or magnitude (*e.g.,* the degree of stress experienced during infertility treatment). Structured self-reports are also especially appropriate when the researcher wants to test hypotheses concerning cause-and-effect relationships.

 CONSUMER TIP

Most nursing studies reported in nursing journals use a data collection plan that is structured and quantitative, but increasing numbers of nurses are undertaking qualitative studies. Most studies that collect self-report data incorporate one or more social–psychological scale. ■

Critiquing Self-Reports

One of the first questions you should ask is whether the researcher made the correct decision in obtaining the data by self-report rather than by an alternative method. Attention then should be paid to the adequacy of the actual methods used. Box 11-2 presents some guiding questions for critiquing self-reports.

It may be difficult to perform a thorough critique of self-report methods in studies that are reported in journals because detailed descriptions of the data collection methods are often not included. What you can expect is information about the following aspects of the self-report data collection:

- The degree of structure used in the questioning
- Whether interviews or questionnaires (or variants such as a projective method or Q sort) were used
- Whether a composite scale was administered
- How the instruments were administered (*e.g.,* by telephone, in person, by mail)
- The response rate

BOX 11-2 **GUIDELINES FOR CRITIQUING SELF-REPORTS**

1. Does the research question lend itself to a self-report method of data collection? Would an alternative method have been more appropriate?

2. Is the degree of structure consistent with the nature of the research question?

3. Given the research question and respondent characteristics, did the researcher use the best possible mode for collecting the data (*i.e.,* personal interviews, telephone interviews, or self-administered questionnaires)?

4. Do the questions included in the instrument or topic guide adequately cover the complexities of the problem under investigation?

5. If a composite scale was used, does its use seem appropriate? Does the scale adequately capture the target research variable?

6. If a vignette, projective technique, or Q sort was used, does its use seem appropriate?

Degree of structure is of special importance in assessing a data collection plan. The decision about an instrument's structure should be based on considerations that you can often evaluate. For example, respondents who are not very articulate are more receptive to instruments with closed-ended questions than to questioning that forces them to compose lengthy answers. Other considerations include the amount of time available (structured instruments are more efficient); the expected sample size (open-ended questions and unstructured interviews are difficult to analyze with large samples); the status of existing information on the topic (in a new area of inquiry, a structured approach may not be warranted); and, most important, the nature of the research question.

CONSUMER TIP

In research reports, descriptions of data collection instruments are often brief; therefore, it is not always possible to evaluate the data collection plan thoroughly. For example, if a study involved the administration of a measure of depression (*e.g.,* the Center for Epidemiological Studies Depression Scale, or CES-D), the research report most likely would not describe individual items on this scale—although the report should provide a reference to the appropriate source. Moreover, there is typically insufficient space in journals for the researcher to offer a rationale for the plan (*e.g.,* a rationale for why the CES-D was chosen instead of the Beck Depression Scale, or why depression was not measured through an approach other than structured self-report). Because of these facts, it may be difficult for you to undertake a detailed critique of the data collection plan. ∎

OBSERVATIONAL METHODS

For some research questions, direct observation of people's behaviour is an alternative to self-reports. Within nursing research, **observational methods** have broad applicability, particularly for clinical inquiries. Nurses are in an advantageous position to observe, relatively unobtrusively, the behaviours and activities of patients, their families, and health care staff. Observational methods can be used to gather such information as the characteristics and conditions of individuals (*e.g.,* the sleep–wake state of patients); verbal communication (*e.g.,* exchange of information at change-of-shift report); nonverbal communication (*e.g.,* facial expressions); activities (*e.g.,* geriatric patients' self-grooming activities); and environmental conditions (*e.g.,* architectural barriers in the homes of people with disabilities).

In observational studies, the researcher has flexibility with regard to several important dimensions:

- *The focus of the observation.* The focus can be broadly defined events (*e.g.,* patient mood swings), or it can be small, highly specific behaviours (*e.g.,* gestures, facial expressions).
- *Concealment.* As discussed in Chapter 4, researchers do not always tell people they are being observed because awareness of being observed may cause people to behave abnormally, thereby jeopardizing the validity of the observations. The problem of behavioural distortions due to the known presence of an observer is called **reactivity.**
- *Duration of observation.* Some observations can be made in a short period of time, but others, particularly those in ethnographic and other field studies, may require months or years in the field.
- *Method of recording observations.* Observations can be made through the human senses and then recorded by paper-and-pencil methods, but they can also be done with sophisticated technical equipment (*e.g.,* video equipment, specialized microphones and audio recording equipment, computers).

In summary, observational techniques can be used to measure a broad range of phenomena and are versatile along several key dimensions. Like self-report techniques, an important dimension for observational methods is degree of structure.

Unstructured Observational Methods

Qualitative researchers collect observational data with a minimum of structure and researcher-imposed constraints. Skilful **unstructured observation** permits researchers to see the world as the study participants see it, to develop a rich understanding and appreciation of the phenomena of interest, to extract meaning from events and situations, and to grasp the subtleties of cultural variation.

Naturalistic observations often are made in field settings through a technique called **participant observation.** A participant observer participates in the functioning of the group or institution under study and strives to observe and record information within the contexts, experiences, and symbols that are relevant to the participants. By assuming a participating role, the observer may have insights that would have eluded a more passive or concealed observer. Not all unstructured observational studies use participant observation, but most do, particularly in the case of ethnographic research.

Example of a nonparticipant unstructured observation:

Lotzark and Bottorff (2001) used ethological analysis to study the development of a nurse–patient relationship. Eight patients were observed via videotape (continous videotaping for 72 hours); their interactions with nurses were then analyzed qualitatively.

The Observer–Participant Role in Participant Observation

In participant observation, the role observers play in the social group under study is important because their social position determines what they are likely to see. That is, the behaviours that are likely to be available for observation depend on the observers' position in a network of relations.

The extent of the observers' actual participation in a group is best thought of as a continuum. At one extreme of the continuum is complete immersion in the setting, with the researcher assuming full participant status; at the other extreme is complete separation, with the researcher assuming an onlooker status. The researcher may in some cases assume a fixed position on this continuum throughout the study. For example, researchers studying the stress and coping of parents whose infant has died of sudden infant death syndrome might spend time observing the parents' interactions with each other and with other family members in their homes, but they would not likely participate in the life of the family as an actual family member.

On the other hand, the researcher's role as participant may evolve over the course of the fieldwork. The researcher may begin primarily as a bystander, with participation in group activities increasing over time. In other cases, it might be profitable to become immersed in a social setting quickly, with participation diminishing to allow more time for pure observation.

CONSUMER TIP

It is not unusual to find research reports that state that participant observation was used when in fact the description of the methods suggests that observation but not participation was involved. Some researchers appear to use the term "participant observation" to refer more generally to observations conducted in the field.

Leininger (1985) has offered the following 4-phase strategy as a possible model for participant observation: (1) primarily observation, (2) primarily observation with some participation, (3) primarily participation with some observation, and (4) reflective observation. In the initial phase, the researcher observes and listens to those under study, allowing observer and participants to become acquainted and to get more comfortable in interacting. In phase 2, observation is enhanced by a modest degree of participation. As the researcher participates more actively in the social group, the reactions of people to specific researcher behaviours can be more systematically studied. In phase 3, the researcher strives to become a more active participant, learning by the experience of doing rather than just watching and listening. In phase 4, the researcher reflects on the total process of what transpired.

The observer must overcome at least two major hurdles in assuming a satisfactory role vis-à-vis participants. The first is to gain entrée into the social group under investigation; the second is to establish rapport and develop trust within that group. Without gaining entrée, the study cannot proceed; but without the trust of the group, the researcher will typically be restricted to "front stage" knowledge—that is, information distorted by the group's protective facades (Leininger, 1985). The goal of the participant observer is to "get back stage"—to learn about the true realities of the group's experiences and behaviours. On the other hand, being a fully participating member does not *necessarily* offer the best perspective for studying a phenomenon—just as being an actor in a play does not offer the most advantageous view of the performance.

Example of a participant observation:

Valkenier et al. (2002) studied mothers' perspectives of an in-home nursing respite service. This study was carried out over a 2-year period. The participant observations occurred during home visits and included general observations to capture the family situation, the complexity of care, and the progress of nursing respite services.

Gathering Unstructured Observational Data

The participant observer typically places few restrictions on the nature of the data collected, in keeping with the goal of minimizing observer-imposed meanings and structure. Nevertheless, participant observers often do have a broad plan for the types of information to be gathered. Among the aspects of an observed activity likely to be considered relevant are the following:

1. *The physical setting—"where" questions.* Where is the activity happening? What are the main features of the physical setting? What is the context within which human behaviour unfolds?
2. *The participants—"who" questions.* Who is present? What are the characteristics of those present? How many people are there? What are their roles? Who is given free access to the setting—who "belongs"? What brings these people together?

3. *Activities—"what" questions.* What is going on? What are the participants doing? Is there a discernible progression of activities? How do the participants interact with one another? What methods do they use to communicate, and how frequently do they do so?

4. *Frequency and duration—"when" questions.* When did the activity begin and end? Is the activity a recurring one and, if so, how regularly does it recur? How typical of such activities is the one under observation?

5. *Process—"how" questions.* How is the activity organized? How are people interacting and communicating? How does the event unfold?

6. *Outcomes—"why" questions.* Why is the activity happening, or why is it happening in this manner? What kinds of things will ensue? What did not happen (especially if it ought to have happened) and why?

The next decision is to identify a way to sample observations and to select observational locations. Researchers generally use a combination of positioning approaches. **Single positioning** means staying in a single location for a period to observe transactions in that location. **Multiple positioning** involves moving around the site to observe behaviours from different locations. **Mobile positioning** involves following a person throughout a given activity or period.

Because participant observers cannot spend a lifetime in one site and cannot be in more than one place at a time, observation is usually supplemented with information from unstructured interviews or conversations. For example, informants may be asked to describe what went on in a meeting the observer was unable to attend, or to describe an event that occurred before the observer entered the field. In such cases, the informant functions as the observer's observer.

Recording Unstructured Observational Data
The most common forms of record keeping in participant observation studies are logs and field notes. A **log** is a daily record of events and conversations. **Field notes** may include the daily log but tend to be much broader, more analytic, and more interpretive. Field notes represent the observer's efforts to record information and also to synthesize and understand the data.

Field notes can be categorized according to their purpose. **Observational notes** are objective descriptions of events and conversations; information such as time, place, activity, and dialogue are recorded as completely as possible. **Theoretical notes** are interpretive attempts to attach meaning to observations. **Methodologic notes** are instructions or reminders about how subsequent observations will be made. **Personal notes** are comments about the researcher's own feelings during the research process.

The success of any participant observation study depends on the quality of the logs and field notes. It is clearly essential to record observations as quickly as possible, but participant observers cannot usually record information by openly carrying a clipboard or a tape recorder because this would undermine their role as ordinary participants of the group. Observers must develop the skill of making detailed mental notes that can later be written or tape-recorded. The use of laptop computers can greatly facilitate the recording and organization of notes in the field.

Structured Observational Methods

Structured observation differs from the unstructured techniques in the specificity of behaviours selected for observation, in the advance preparation of forms, and in the kinds of activity in which observers engage. The creativity of structured observation lies not in the observation itself but rather in the formulation of a system for accurately categorizing, recording, and encoding the observations and sampling the phenomena of interest.

Categories and Checklists

One approach to making structured observations is the construction of a category system. A **category system** represents an attempt to designate in a systematic, quantitative fashion the behaviours and events transpiring within a setting. A category scheme involves listing all those behaviours or characteristics that the observer is required to observe and record.

Some category systems are constructed so that all observed behaviours within a specified domain can be classified into one (and only one) category. A contrasting technique is to develop a system in which only particular types of behaviour are categorized. For example, if we were studying aggressive behaviour in autistic children, we might develop such categories as "strikes another child," "kicks or hits walls or floor," or "throws objects around the room." In this category system, many behaviours—all that are nonaggressive—would not be classified. Nonexhaustive systems are adequate for many purposes, but one risk is that resulting data might be difficult to interpret. When a large number of behaviours are not categorized, the investigator may have difficulty placing categorized behaviour into perspective.

> **Example of a nonexhaustive system:**
> Feldt (2000) created a checklist to capture the occurrence of nonverbal pain indicators. Observers indicate whether, during an observational session, subjects demonstrate such pain-related behaviours as nonverbal vocal complaints (*e.g.*, moans, grunts, sighs), facial grimaces (*e.g.*, furrowed brow, clenched teeth), and bracing (*e.g.*, clutching onto siderails). Behaviours unrelated to pain were not captured.

One of the most important requirements of a category system is the careful and explicit definition of the behaviours and characteristics to be observed. Each category must be carefully explained, giving observers clearcut criteria for assessing the occurrence of the phenomenon. Nevertheless, virtually all category systems require observer inference, to greater or lesser degree.

Examples of varying observer inference:

Low inference: Holditch-Davis et al. (2000) studied the interactions between mothers and their premature infants during periods of feeding and nonfeeding in relation to infant behaviours, such as sleep–wake states. Observers categorized sleep–wake states into four mutually exclusive categories: Sleep, Drowse/Transition, Alert, and Active Walking. The "Alert" category, for example, was defined as follows: "The infant's eyes are open and scanning. Motor activity is typically low, particularly during the first two weeks, but the infant may be active" (p. 325).

High inference: The Abnormal Involuntary Movement Scale (AIMS), which was developed by the National Institute for Mental Health, has been used by several nurse researchers for studying tardive dyskinetic movements. For example, Herman (1997) evaluated the clinical response of chronic schizophrenic patients to clozapine treatment using AIMS. This scale contains such broad categories as "incapacitation due to abnormal movements."

Even when such categories (incapacitation due to abnormal movements) are defined in detail, a heavy inferential burden is placed on the observer.

After a category system has been developed, the researcher constructs a **checklist,** which is the instrument used to record observed phenomena. The checklist is generally formatted with the list of behaviours from the category system on the left and space for tallying their frequency or duration on the right. The task of the observer using an exhaustive category system is to place *all* observed behaviours in one category for each integral unit of behaviour (*e.g.,* a sentence in a conversation, a time interval). Checklists based on exhaustive category systems are demanding because the recording task is continuous. With nonexhaustive category systems, categories of behaviours that may or may not be manifested by participants are listed. The observer's tasks are to watch for instances of these behaviours and to record their occurrence. With this type of checklist, the observer does not classify all behaviours of the people being observed, but rather identifies the occurrence and frequency of particular behaviours.

Rating Scales

Another approach to collecting structured observational data is through the use of rating scales. A **rating scale** is a tool that requires the observer to rate some phenomena in terms of points along a descriptive continuum. The observer may be required to make ratings of behaviour at intervals throughout the observation or to summarize an entire event or transaction after observation is completed.

Rating scales can be used as an extension of checklists, in which the observer records not only the occurrence of some behaviour but also some qualitative aspect of it, such as its magnitude or intensity. When rating scales are coupled with a category scheme in this fashion, considerably more information about the phenomena under investigation can be obtained. The disadvantage of this approach is that it places an immense burden on the observer, particularly if there is an extensive amount of activity.

⊞ ***Example of an observational rating scale:***

Drevenhorn et al. (2001) conducted an observational study of 21 Swedish public health nurses. They observed the nurses' interactions with hypertensive patients using an instrument called the Nurse Practitioner Rating Form. At the end of each observational session, nurses were rated on a scale from 1 to 7 in terms of communication activity. For example, a rating of 2 on the nurses' scale corresponds to the following: "Nurse does not attempt to identify client's feelings, has a disinterested manner, and does not individualize the approach."

Observational Sampling

Researchers must decide how and when structured observational systems will be applied. Observational sampling methods provide a mechanism for obtaining representative examples of the behaviours being observed. One system is **time sampling,** which involves the selection of time periods during which observations will occur. The time frames may be systematically selected (*e.g.,* every 30 seconds at 2-minute intervals) or selected at random.

Event sampling selects integral behaviours or events for observation. Event sampling requires researchers to either have knowledge about the occurrence of events or be in a position to wait for or precipitate their occurrence. Examples of integral events that may be suitable for event sampling include shift changes of nurses in a hospital, cast removals of pediatric patients, and cardiac arrests in the emergency room. This sampling approach is preferable to time sampling when the events of interest are infrequent and may be missed if time sampling is used. When behaviours and events are relatively frequent, however, time sampling enhances the representativeness of the observed behaviours.

Evaluation of Observational Methods

The field of nursing is particularly well suited to observational research. Nurses are often in a position to watch people's behaviours and may, by training, be especially sensitive observers. Moreover, some nursing problems are better suited to observation than to self-reports, such as when people cannot adequately describe their own behaviours. This may be the case when people are unaware of their own behaviour (*e.g.,* manifesting preoperative symptoms of anxiety), when people are embarrassed to report their activities (*e.g.,* displays of aggression or hostility), when behaviours are emotionally laden (*e.g.,* grieving behaviour among the bereaved), or when people are not capable of articulating their actions (*e.g.,* young children or the mentally ill). Observational methods have an intrinsic appeal for directly capturing behaviours and events. Furthermore, virtually no other data collection method can provide the depth and variety of information as observation. With this approach, humans—the observers—are used as measuring instruments and provide a uniquely sensitive and intelligent (if fallible) tool.

Several of the shortcomings of the observational approach have already been mentioned. These include possible ethical difficulties, reactivity of the observed when the observer is conspicuous, and lack of consent to being observed. However, one of the most pervasive problems is the vulnerability of observations to bias. A number of factors interfere with objective observations, including the following:

- Emotions, prejudices, and values of the observer may result in faulty inference.
- Personal interest and commitment may colour what is seen in the direction of what the observer wants to see.
- Anticipation of what is to be observed may affect what is observed.
- Hasty decisions before adequate information is collected may result in erroneous classifications or conclusions.

Observational biases probably cannot be eliminated, but they can be minimized through the careful training of observers.

As with self-reports, both unstructured and structured observational methods have advantages and disadvantages. Unstructured observational methods have the potential of yielding a richer understanding of human behaviours and social situations than is possible with structured procedures. With a skilful observer, participant observation can help the researcher "get inside" a situation and lead to a more complete understanding of its complexities. Furthermore, unstructured observational approaches are inherently flexible and, therefore, permit the observer freedom to reconceptualize the problem after becoming familiar with the situation. On the other hand, observer bias may pose a threat: once the researcher begins to participate in a group's activities, the possibility of emotional involvement becomes a salient issue. The researcher in a member role may develop a myopic view on issues of importance to the group. Another problem is that unstructured observational methods are more dependent on the observational and interpersonal skills of the observer.

Researchers generally choose an approach that matches the research problem—and their paradigmatic orientation. Unstructured observational methods are especially profitable for in-depth research in which the investigator wishes to establish an adequate conceptualization of the important issues in a social setting or to develop hypotheses. Structured observational methods are better suited to the formal testing of research hypotheses regarding measurable human behaviours.

Critiquing Observational Methods

As in the case of self-reports, the first question you should ask when critiquing an observational study is whether the data should have been collected by some other approach. The advantages and disadvantages of observational methods, discussed previously, should be helpful in considering the appropriateness of using observation.

BOX 11-3 **GUIDELINES FOR CRITIQUING OBSERVATIONAL METHODS**

1. Does the research question lend itself to an observational approach? Would an alternative method have been more appropriate?

2. Is the degree of structure consistent with the nature of the research question?

3. To what degree were observers concealed during data collection? If there was no concealment, what effect might the observers' presence have had on the behaviours being observed?

4. What was the focus of the observation? How much inference was required on the part of the observers, and to what extent did this affect the potential for bias?

5. Where did the observations take place? To what extent did the setting influence the naturalness of the behaviours observed?

6. How were data actually recorded (*e.g.,* on field notes, checklists)? Did the recording procedure appear appropriate?

7. What was the plan by which events or behaviours were sampled? Did this plan appear appropriate?

8. What steps were taken to minimize observer biases?

Some additional guidelines for critiquing observational studies are presented in Box 11-3.

A journal article should usually document the following aspects of the observational plan:

- The degree of structure in the observations
- The focus of the observations
- The degree to which the observer was concealed
- For unstructured methods, how entry into the observed group was gained, the relationship between the observer and those observed, the time period over which data were collected, and the method of recording data
- For structured methods, a description of the category system or rating scales and the settings in which observations took place
- The plan for sampling events and behaviours to observe

BIOPHYSIOLOGIC MEASURES

One result of the trend toward clinical, patient-centred studies is greater use of biophysiologic and physical variables. Clinical nursing studies involve biophysiologic instruments both for creating independent variables (*e.g.,* an intervention using biofeedback equipment) and for measuring dependent variables. For the most part, our discussion focuses on the use of biophysiologic measures as dependent variables.

Uses of Biophysiologic Measures in Nursing Research

Most nursing studies in which biophysiologic measures have been used fall into one of five classes:

1. Studies of basic biophysiologic processes that have relevance for nursing care. These studies involve normal, healthy participants or a subhuman animal species.

Example of a study of basic physiologic processes:

Bartfay and Bartfay (2002) used mice to study the dose-dependent effects of chronic iron overload on cardiovascular functioning. Iron-treated mice were compared with placebo-treated mice in terms of heart selenium concentrations and heart glutathione peroxidase activity.

2. Description of nursing actions and explorations of the ways in which nursing actions affect health outcomes. These studies do not focus on specific interventions, but rather are designed to document standard procedures or to learn how standard nursing procedures affect people.

Example of a study of physiologic outcomes of nursing actions:

Jellema et al. (2000) investigated the hemodynamic changes induced by manual lung hyperinflation (MLH) in patients with septic shock. Their intent was to assess if changes were sufficiently adverse to warrant prohibition of MLH as a routine procedure in caring for these patients.

3. Evaluations of a specific nursing procedure or intervention. These studies differ from the studies in the second category in that they involve the testing of a new intervention, usually in comparison with standard methods of care. Typically, these studies involve a hypothesis stating that the innovative nursing procedure will result in improved biophysiologic outcomes among patients.

Example of an evaluation:

Cheng and Boey (2002) evaluated the effectiveness of physical exercise on self-efficacy and exercise tolerance among a group of 43 cardiac patients who suffered from ischaemic heart disease or were recovering from myocardial infarction or percutaneous translumnial coronary angioplasty. The outcome measures included heart rate, walking distance, and walking time.

4. Studies to evaluate or improve the measurement and recording of bio-physiologic information gathered by nurses. Clinically, the accurate measurement of biophysiologic phenomena is crucial, and therefore some studies focus on improving clinical measurements.

Example of a study on clinical measurement:

Fallis and Christiani (1999) conducted a study to determine whether predictive mode axillary temperature measurement is accurate in full-term newborns. Electronic thermometer predictive and monitor mode axillary temperatures were compared.

5. Studies of the correlates of physiologic functioning in patients with health problems. Researchers study possible antecedents and consequences of biophysiologic indicators to gain insight into potential treatments or modes of care.

Example of a study of physiologic correlates:

Belza et al. (2001) examined relationships between functional performance (physical activity), functional capacity (*e.g.*, forced expiratory volume during spirometry), and symptom experiences in people with chronic obstructive pulmonary disease.

Types of Biophysiologic Measures

Biophysiologic measures include both *in vivo* and *in vitro* measures. **In vivo measures** are those performed directly within or on living organisms. Examples of *in vivo* measures include blood pressure, body temperature, and vital capacity measurement. *In vivo* instruments are available to measure all bodily functions, and technological advances continue to improve the ability to measure biophysiologic phenomena more accurately, conveniently, and rapidly.

Example of a study with in vivo measures:

Wipke-Tevis et al. (2001) conducted a study to compare the partial pressure of transcutaneous tissue oxygen ($TcPO_2$) in people with venous ulcers in four body positions, both with and without inspired oxygen. Tissue perfusion was measured with a Novametrix 840 PrO_2 and $PtcO_2$ monitor. Arterial oxygen saturation (SaO_2) was measured by an Oximax 100 pulse oximeter.

With **in vitro measures,** data are gathered from participants by extracting some biophysiologic material from them and subjecting it to laboratory analysis. The analysis is normally done by specialized laboratory technicians. *In vitro* measures include chemical measures (*e.g.*, the measurement of hormone, sugar, or potassium levels), microbiologic measures (*e.g.,* bacterial counts and identification), and cytologic or histologic measures (*e.g.,* tissue biopsies).

> **Example of a study with in vitro *measures*:**
>
> Bliss et al. (2001) compared the effects of a fibre supplement in community-living adults who were incontinent of loose or liquid stools. Stool specimens collected before and after the intervention were subjected to laboratory analysis.

Evaluation of Biophysiologic Measures

Biophysiologic measures offer a number of advantages to nurse researchers, including the following:

- Biophysiologic measures are relatively accurate and precise, especially when compared with psychological measures, such as self-report measures of anxiety, pain, and so forth.
- Biophysiologic measures are objective. Two nurses reading from the same spirometer output are likely to record the same tidal volume measurements, and two different spirometers are likely to produce identical readouts. Patients cannot easily distort measurements of biophysiologic functioning deliberately.
- Biophysiologic instrumentation provides valid measures of the targeted variables: thermometers can be depended on to measure temperature and not blood volume, and so forth. For nonbiophysiologic measures, the question of whether an instrument is really measuring the target concept is an ongoing concern.
- Because equipment for obtaining biophysiologic measurements is available in hospital settings, the cost to nurse researchers of collecting biophysiologic data may be low or nonexistent.

Biophysiologic measures also have a few disadvantages:

- The measuring tool may affect the variables it is attempting to measure. The presence of a sensing device, such as a transducer, located in a blood vessel partially blocks that vessel and, hence, alters the pressure-flow characteristics being measured.
- There are normally interferences that create artifacts in biophysiologic measures. For example, noise generated within a measuring instrument interferes with the signal being produced.
- Energy must often be applied to the organism when taking the biophysiologic measurements; extreme caution must continually be exercised to avoid damaging cells by high-energy concentrations.

In summary, biophysiologic measures are plentiful, tend to be accurate and valid, and are extremely useful in clinical nursing studies. However, care must be exercised in using them with regard to practical, ethical, medical, and technical considerations.

Critiquing Biophysiologic Measures

Biophysiologic measures offer the nurse researcher many advantages, as discussed previously, and their shortcomings are relatively minor. As always, however, the most important consideration in evaluating a data collection strategy is the appropriateness of the measures for the research question. The objectivity, accuracy, and availability of biophysiologic measures are of little significance if an alternative method would have resulted in a better measurement of the key concepts. Stress, for example, could be measured in various ways: through self-report (*e.g.,* through the use of a scale such as the State–Trait Anxiety Inventory); through direct observation of participants' behaviour during exposure to stressful stimuli; or by measuring heart rate, blood pressure, or levels of adrenocorticotropic hormone in urine samples. The choice of which measure to use must be linked to the way that stress is conceptualized in the research problem.

Additional criteria for assessing the use of biophysiologic measures are presented in Box 11-4. The general questions to consider are these: Did the researcher select the correct biophysiologic measure? Was care taken in the collection of the data? Did the researcher competently interpret the data?

 CONSUMER TIP

Many nursing studies integrate a variety of data collection approaches. In quantitative studies, structured self-reports combined with biophysiologic measures are especially common. Qualitative studies are especially likely to combine unstructured observations and self-reports. ■

IMPLEMENTING THE DATA COLLECTION PLAN

In addition to selecting methods for collecting data, researchers must develop and implement a plan for gathering the data. This involves decisions that could affect the quality of the data being collected.

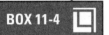 **GUIDELINES FOR CRITIQUING BIOPHYSIOLOGIC METHODS**

1. Does the research question lend itself to a biophysiologic approach? Would an alternative method have been theoretically more appropriate?

2. Was the proper instrumentation used to obtain the biophysiologic measurements? Would an alternative instrument or method have been more appropriate?

3. Does the researcher appear to have the skills necessary for proper interpretation of the biophysiologic measures?

BOX 11-5 **GUIDELINES FOR CRITIQUING DATA COLLECTION PROCEDURES**

1. Who collected the research data? Were the data collectors qualified for their role, or is there something about them (*e.g.,* their professional role, their relationship with study participants) that could undermine the collection of unbiased, high-quality data?

2. How were data collectors trained? Does the training appear adequate?

3. Where and under what circumstances were the data gathered? Were other people present during the data collection? Could the presence of others have created any distortions?

4. Did the collection of data place any undue burdens (in terms of time or stress) on participants? How might this have affected data quality?

One important decision concerns who will collect the data. In many studies, the researcher hires assistants to collect data rather than doing it personally. This is especially likely to be the case in large-scale quantitative studies. In other studies, nurses or other health care staff are asked to assist in the collection of data. From your perspective as a consumer, the critical issues are whether the people collecting data might have introduced any biases and whether they were able to produce valid and accurate data. In any research endeavour, adequate training of data collectors is essential.

Another issue concerns the circumstances under which data were gathered. For example, it may be critical to ensure total privacy to participants. In most cases, it is important for the researcher to create a nonjudgmental atmosphere in which participants are encouraged to be candid or behave naturally. Again, you as a consumer must ask whether there is anything about the way in which the data were collected that could have introduced bias or otherwise affected data quality.

In evaluating the data collection plan of a study, then, you should critically appraise not only the actual methods chosen but also the procedures used to collect the data. Box 11-5 provides some specific guidelines for critiquing the procedures used to collect research data.

RESEARCH EXAMPLES

In this section, we present summaries of actual nursing studies. Use the guidelines presented in this chapter to evaluate the researchers' data collection plans, referring to the original articles if necessary.

Research Example of Structured Self-Report and Biophysiologic Measures

Brooks-Brunn (2000) conducted a study to identify risk factors for the development of postoperative pulmonary complications (PPCs) after total abdominal hysterectomy. Her data sources included self-reports, chest examinations, and medical records.

Research Summary

In Brooks-Brunn's multisite study, 120 patients undergoing a total abdominal hysterectomy were included in the sample. The research design was prospective; the women were recruited into the sample preoperatively, and their PPC status was subsequently determined postoperatively.

Brooks-Brunn collected data on a wide range of risk factors that had previously been identified in the literature and that were accessible to the health care team. These included preoperative, intraoperative, and postoperative risk factors. Preoperative factors included information on the patients' health habits, demographic characteristics, and medical history. This information was obtained through a structured interview and review of medical charts. Information about intraoperative risk factors (*e.g.*, duration of anesthesia and location, direction, and length of the incision) was obtained from charts as well. Postoperative risk factors included the presence of a nasogastric tube and the initial method of pain management. After surgery, patients underwent a daily interview and chest examination. The dependent variable, presence or absence of PPCs, was based on a combination of biophysiologic measures, such as body temperature, abnormal breath sounds, and cough and sputum production.

In the research sample, 11% of subjects developed a PPC. Brooks-Brunn's results indicated that the patients most likely to develop a PPC were older, had a history of smoking, and had a history of cancer or congestive heart failure. Also, women at highest risk were those who had an upper (versus lower) abdominal surgical location and had a vertical incision. Factors that were not found to be reliably related to PPC risk included obesity, history of asthma, history of chronic obstructive pulmonary disease, duration of anesthesia during surgery, and type of analgesia used postoperatively.

Clinical Relevance

Postoperative pulmonary complications are relatively common and are associated with increased morbidity and mortality as well as longer hospital stay. Until Brooks-Brunn had undertaken her study, there had been little research on risk factors associated with PPCs among women undergoing gynecologic surgery.

The design for Brooks-Brunn's study was strong: prospective designs are always more reliable than retrospective designs. She also appeared to be thorough in assessing a wide variety of risk factors and drawing on several data sources. Another strength is that the sample was drawn from two sites. However, it was a relatively small sample for a correlational study; therefore, it would be unwise to generalize without further replications.

Nevertheless, the study does provide an important foundation for further identification of key risk factors. Furthermore, nurses can use the information from this study to be on the alert for patients who have the risk factors found to be correlated with PPC and, especially, for patients with multiple risk factors. When these high-risk patients are identified, nurses can then play a key role in preventing PPCs through patient education, assessment, and initiation of interventions both preoperatively and postoperatively. Nursing interventions can be designed to target risk factors that are modifiable and amenable to manipulation, such as smoking behaviour. The preoperative and postoperative periods provide nurses with a "window of opportunity" to promote smoking cessation in these high-risk patients.

Research Example of Unstructured Self-Report and Observation

Vivian and Wilcox (2000) conducted a study that focused on compliance communication (nurse–patient communication) in home health care. Their study combined observational and interview data.

Research Summary

In Vivian and Wilcox's (2000) study, *compliance communication* referred to communication about patient care for situations in which the patient or family had some degree of responsibility for carrying out the medical regime. Nurse–patient communication of 6 registered nurses and 25 adult patients from two home care agencies was the focus of this research.

Phase 1 of the study involved participant observation. Each of the 6 nurses was accompanied on a day of rounds. A total of 25 home visits were observed, with visits ranging from 15 to 75 minutes. In the car between home visits and at the close of each day, informal unstructured interviews with the nurses were conducted. During phase 2, a semistructured format was used to interview each of the nurses individually. This semistructured format focused on the topics of patient needs, nurse's role in home care, expectation for compliance, and strategies used to promote patient compliance. The in-depth interviews required between 1 and 1.5 hours to complete. In addition, the researcher and nurse spent between 15 and 30 minutes after the interview discussing patients who had been visited in phase 1. Finally, telephone interviews were held with 11 patients and 8 family members.

Data analysis revealed five categories of compliance communication: (1) education of patients and family members, (2) arrangement of additional support services, (3) removal of obstacles to compliance, (4) provision of positive reinforcement or rewards, and (5) use of threats or scare tactics. Educating patients and family members emerged as the strongest theme regarding the promotion of patient compliance.

Clinical Relevance

Patient noncompliance in carrying out treatment recommendations is a significant problem in contemporary health care. Noncompliance can result in wasting of health resources, frustration to clinicians, and potential threats to patients' health.

The researchers' use of multiple data collection methods on nurse–patient compliance communication was a strength of this study. By using participant observation in phase 1, the researchers were able to make observations that sharpened the saliency of their questions in the unstructured, semistructured, and telephone interviews they subsequently conducted. Moreover, by using both observation and interviews, the researchers were able to examine the degree of consistency between self-reports and actual behaviour. Finally, through their observations, they were able to study both verbal and nonverbal forms of communication.

Results of Vivian and Wilcox's study have clinical implications for nurses in achieving the goals of home care of moving patients toward self-care and independence. Based on their findings, Vivian and Wilcox suggested the following strategies for educating patients and their families: reinforcing compliance messages by repetition and reminders, inquiring why a patient is noncompliant, offering to help a patient in complying with a treatment regimen, having a patient practice compliance, and setting short-term goals related to compliance. Although some of these strategies may be unique to home care, these "sequential influence attempts" may also have relevance to non-home care situations.

● ● ● ● ● SUMMARY POINTS

- Some researchers use existing data in their studies—for example, those doing **historical research,** meta-analyses, **secondary analyses,** or an analysis of **records**.
- Data collection methods vary along four dimensions: structure, quantifiability, researcher obtrusiveness, and objectivity.
- The three principal data collection methods for nurse researchers are self-reports, observations, and biophysiologic measures.
- **Self-report** data are collected by means of an oral interview or written questionnaire. Self-report methods are an indispensable means of collecting data but are susceptible to errors of reporting.
- Unstructured self-reports, used in qualitative studies, include **completely unstructured interviews,** which are conversational discussions on the topic of interest; **focused** (or **semistructured) interviews,** using a broad **topic guide; focus group interviews,** which involve discussions with

small groups; **life histories,** which encourage respondents to narrate their life experiences regarding some theme; and **diaries,** in which respondents are asked to maintain daily records about some aspects of their lives.

- Structured self-reports usually use a formal **instrument**—a **question-naire** or **interview schedule**—that may contain a combination of **open-ended questions** (which permit respondents to respond in their own words) and **closed-ended questions** (which offer respondents fixed alternatives from which to choose).

- Questionnaires are less costly than interviews, offer the possibility of anonymity, and run no risk of interviewer bias; however, interviews yield a higher response rate, are suitable for a wider variety of people, and provide richer data than questionnaires.

- Social-psychological **scales** are self-report tools for quantitatively measuring the intensity of such characteristics as personality traits, attitudes, needs, and perceptions.

- **Likert scales** (or **summated rating scales**) present the respondent with a series of **items** worded favourably or unfavourably toward some phenomenon; responses indicating level of agreement or disagreement with each statement are scored and summed into a composite score.

- The **semantic differential (SD)** technique consists of a series of scales with **bipolar adjectives** (*e.g.,* good/bad) along which respondents rate their reactions toward phenomena.

- A **visual analog scale (VAS)** is used to measure, along a line designating a bipolar continuum, subjective experiences, such as pain, fatigue, and nausea.

- Scales are versatile and powerful but are susceptible to **response set biases**—the tendency of some people to respond to items in characteristic ways, independently of item content.

- **Vignettes** are brief descriptions of some event, person, or situation to which respondents are asked to react.

- **Projective techniques** encompass various data collection methods that rely on the participant's projection of psychological traits or states in response to vaguely structured stimuli.

- **Q sorts** involve the sorting of a set of statements into piles according to specified criteria.

- **Observational methods,** which include both structured and unstructured procedures, are techniques for acquiring data through the direct observation of phenomena.

- One type of **unstructured observation** is **participant observation,** in which the researcher gains entrée into the social group of interest and participates to varying degrees in its functioning while making in-depth observations of activities and events. **Logs** of daily events and **field notes** of the observer's experiences and interpretations constitute the major data collection instruments.

- **Structured observations,** which dictate what the observer should observe, often involve **checklists**—tools based on **category systems** for recording the appearance, frequency, or duration of prespecified behaviours or events. Alternatively, the observer may use a **rating scale** to rate some phenomenon along a dimension of interest (*e.g.,* fast/slow).

- Most structured observations use a sampling plan (such as **time sampling** or **event sampling**) for selecting the behaviours, events, and conditions to be observed.
- Observational techniques are a versatile and important alternative to self-reports; however, various observational biases can pose a threat to the validity and accuracy of observational data.
- Data may also be derived from **biophysiologic measures,** which can be classified as either ***in vivo* measurements** (those performed within or on living organisms) or ***in vitro* measurements** (those performed outside the organism's body, such as blood tests). Biophysiologic measures have the advantage of being objective, accurate, and precise.
- In developing a data collection plan, the researcher must decide who will collect the data, how the data collectors will be trained, and what the circumstances for data collection will be.

➤ ➤ ➤ ➤ **CRITICAL THINKING ACTIVITIES**

Chapter 11 of the accompanying *Study Guide to Accompany Essentials of Nursing Research,* 5th edition, offers various exercises and study suggestions for reinforcing the concepts presented in this chapter. In addition, you can address the following questions:

1. Read the Method section of one or both of the actual research studies in the Appendix of this book, paying particular attention to the data collection plan. Answer the relevant questions from Boxes 11-2 to 11-5 with regard to this study.

2. Read the Results section of the Vivian and Wilcox (2000) study that was used as a research example in this chapter. How might relevance and accuracy of the study findings have been jeopardized if only observation or only self-report had been used?

3. Read the study by Brooks-Brunn (2000), used as the quantitative research example in this chapter. Comment on the researcher's description of her data collection plan.

For additional review, see questions 136–155 on the study CD provided with Polit: Study Guide to Accompany Essentials of Nursing Research.

SUGGESTED READINGS

Methodologic References

Frank-Stromberg, M. (Ed.). (1988). *Instruments for clinical nursing research.* Norwalk, CT: Appleton & Lange.

Kerlinger, F. N., & Lee, H. B. (2000). *Foundations of behavioral research* (4th ed.). New York: Holt, Rinehart & Winston.

Leininger, M. M. (Ed.). (1985). *Qualitative research methods in nursing.* New York: Grune & Stratton.

Lofland, J., & Lofland, L. (1984). *Analyzing social settings: A guide to qualitative observation and analysis.* Belmont, CA: Wadsworth.

Polit, D. F., & Hungler, B. P. (2004). *Nursing research: Principles and methods* (7th ed.). Philadelphia: Lippincott Williams & Wilkins.

Rew, L., Bechtel, D., & Sapp, A. (1993). Self-as-instrument in qualitative research. *Nursing Research, 42,* 300–301.

Waltz, C. F., Strickland, O. L., & Lenz, E. R. (1991). *Measurement in nursing research* (2nd ed.). Philadelphia: F. A. Davis.

Substantive References

Abrums, M. (2000). Death and meaning in a storefront church. *Public Health Nursing, 17,* 132–142.

Arslanian-Engoren, C. (2001). Gender and age differences in nurses' triage decisions using vignette patients. *Nursing Research, 50,* 61–66.

Arthur, H. M., Wright, D. M., & Smith, K. M. (2001). Women and heart disease: The treatment may end but the suffering continues. *Canadian Journal of Nursing Research, 33*(3), 17–29.

Bartfay, W. J., & Bartfay, E. (2002). Decreasing effects of iron toxicosis on selenium and glutathione peroxidase activity. *Western Journal of Nursing Research, 24,* 119–131.

Belza, B., Steele, B. G., Hunziker, J., Lakshminaryan, S., Holt, L., & Buchner, D. (2001). Correlates of physical activity in chronic obstructive pulmonary disease. *Nursing Research, 50,* 195–202.

Bliss, D. Z., Jung, H., Savik, K., Lowry, A., MeMoine, M. Jensen, L. Werner, C., & Schaffer, K. (2001). Supplementation with dietary fiber improves fecal incontinence. *Nursing Research, 50,* 203–213.

Brandon, D. H., Holditch-Davis, D., & Beylan, M. (1999). Nursing care and the development of sleeping and waking behaviors in preterm infants. *Research in Nursing & Health, 22,* 217–229.

Brooks-Brunn, J. A. (2000). Risk factors associated with postoperative pulmonary complications following total abdominal hysterectomy. *Clinical Nursing Research, 9,* 27–46.

Cheng, T. Y. L., & Boey, K. M. (2002). The effectiveness of a cardiac rehabilitation program on self-efficacy and exercise tolerance. *Clinical Nursing Research, 11,* 10–21.

Drevenhorn, E., Hakansson, A., & Petersson, K. (2001). Counseling hypertensive patients: An observational study of 21 public health nurses. *Clinical Nursing Research, 10,* 369–386.

Eller, L. (2001). Quality of life in persons living with HIV. *Clinical Nursing Research, 10*(4), 401–423.

Fallis, W. M., & Christiani, P. (1999). Neonatal axillary temperature measurement: A comparison of electronic thermometer predictive and monitor modes. *Journal of Obstetric, Gynecologic, and Neonatal Nursing, 28,* 389–394.

Feldt, K. S. (2001). Checklist of nonverbal pain indicators. *Pain Management Nursing, 1,* 13–21.

Herman, M. (1997). Clinical response to clozapine treatment of 11 chronic patients in a state psychiatric ward. *Australian-New Zealand Journal of Mental Health Nursing, 6,* 129–133.

Holditch-Davis, D., Miles, M. S., & Belyea, M. (2000). Feeding and nonfeeding interactions of mothers and prematures. *Western Journal of Nursing Research, 22,* 320–334.

Instone, S. L. (2000). Perception of children with HIV infection when not told for so long. *Journal of Pediatric Health Care, 14,* 235–243.

Jellema, W. T., Groeneveld, J., van Goudoever, J., Wesseling, K. H., Westerhof, N., Lubbers, M. J., Kesecioglu, J., & van Lieshout, J. J. (2000). Hemodynamic effects of intermittent manual lung hyperinflation in patients with septic shock. *Heart & Lung, 29,* 356–366.

Laschinger, H. K., Finegan, J., Shamian, J., & Wilk, P. (2001). Impact of structural and psychological empowerment on job strain in nursing work settings: Expanding Kanter's model. *Journal of Nursing Administration, 31,* 260–272.

Lotzkar, M., & Bottorff, J. L. (2001). An observational study of the development of a nurse-patient relationship. *Clinical Nursing Research, 10,* 275–294.

Ludington-Hoe, S. M., Anderson, G. C., Simpson, S., Hollingsead, A., Argote, L. A., & Rey, H. (1999). Birth-related fatigue in 34–36-week preterm neonates: Rapid recovery with very early kangaroo (skin-to-skin) care. *Journal of Obstetric, Gynecologic, and Neonatal Nursing, 28,* 94–103.

McCaughan, D., Thompson, C., Cullum, N., Sheldon, T. A., & Thompson, D. R. (2002). Acute care nurses' perception of barriers to using research information in clinical decision-making. *Journal of Advanced Nursing, 39,* 46–60.

McIntyre, M., Anderson, B., & McDonald, C. (2001). The intersection of relational and cultural narratives: Women's abortion experiences. *Canadian Journal of Nursing Research 33,* 47–62.

Phillips, L. R., Brewer, B. B., & Torres de Ardon, E. (2001). The Elder Image Scale: a method for indexing history and emotion in family caregivers (*Journal of Nursing Measurement, 9,* 23–47.

Profetto-McGrath, J., Hesketh, K., Lang, S., & Estabrooks, C. A. (2003). A study of critical thinking and research utilization among nurses. *Western Journal of Nursing Research.*

Roberts, S., Schofield, P., Freeman, J., Hill, D., Akkerman, D., & Rodger, A. (2002). Bridging the information and support gap: Evaluation of a hospital-based cancer support nurse service. *Patient Education and Counseling, 47,* 47–55.

Rodney, P., Varcoe, C., Storch, J. L., McPherson, G., Mahoney, K., Brown, H., Pauly, B., Hartrick, G., & Starzomski, R. (2002). Navigating towards a moral horizon: A multitude qualitative study of ethical practice in nursing. *Canadian Journal of Nursing Research, 34,* 75–102.

Schneider, B. S., Correia, L. A., & Cannon, J. G. (1999). Sex differences in leukocyte invasion in injured murine skeletal muscle. *Research in Nursing & Health, 22,* 243–251.

Skillen, D. L., Olson, J. K., & Gilber, J. A. (2001). Framing personal risk in public health nursing. *Western Journal of Nursing Research, 23,* 664–678.

Valkenier, B. J., Hayes, V. E., & McElheran, P. (2002). Mothers' perspectives of an in-home nursing respite service: Coping and control. *Canadian Journal of Nursing Research 34*(1), 87–109.

Vivian, B. G., & Wilcox, J. R. (2000). Compliance communication in home health care: A mutually reciprocal process. *Qualitative Health Research, 10,* 103–116.

Werezak, L., & Stewart, N. (2002). Learning to live with early dementia. *Canadian Journal of Nursing Research, 34,* 67–85.

Wipke-Tevis, D. D., Scotts, N. A., Williams, D. A., Froelicher, E. S., & Hunt, T. K. (2001). Tissue oxygenation, perfusion, and position in patients with venous leg ulcers. *Nursing Research, 50,* 24–32.

Wong, J., & Wong, S. (2002). Trends in lifestyle cardiovascular risk factors in women: analysis from the Canadian National Population Health Survey. *International Journal of Nursing Studies, 39,* 229–242.

Wilson, D. M. (2002). The duration and degree of end-of-life dependency of home care clients and hospital inpatients. *Applied Nursing Research, 15,* 81–88.

Wilson, D. M., Smith, S., L., Anderson, M. C., Northcott, H. C., Fainsinger, R. L., Stingl, M. J., & Truman, C. D. (2002). Twentieth-century social and health-care influences on location of death in Canada. *Canadian Journal of Nursing Research 34,* 141–161.

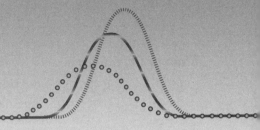

Evaluating Measurements and Data Quality

MEASUREMENT AND THE ASSESSMENT OF QUANTITATIVE DATA
 Measurement
 Reliability of Measuring Instruments
 Validity of Measuring Instruments
ASSESSMENT OF QUALITATIVE DATA
 Credibility
 Dependability
 Confirmability
 Transferability

CRITIQUING DATA QUALITY
RESEARCH EXAMPLES
 Research Example of a Quantitative Study
 Research Example of a Qualitative Study
SUMMARY POINTS
CRITICAL THINKING ACTIVITIES
SUGGESTED READINGS
 Methodologic References
 Substantive References

Student Objectives

On completion of this chapter, the student will be able to:

○ describe the major characteristics of measurement and identify major sources of measurement error

○ describe three aspects of reliability and specify how each aspect can be assessed

○ interpret the meaning of reliability coefficients

○ describe three different aspects of validity and specify how each aspect can be assessed

○ describe the four dimensions used in establishing the trustworthiness of qualitative data and identify methods of enhancing data quality in qualitative studies

○ evaluate the overall quality of a measuring tool or data collection approach used in a research study

○ define new terms in the chapter

New Terms

Audit trail
Coefficient alpha
Concurrent validity
Confirmability
Construct validity
Content validity
Credibility
Criterion-related validity
Cronbach's alpha
Data source triangulation
Dependability
Equivalence
Error of measurement
Face validity
Factor analysis
Inquiry audit
Internal consistency
Interobserver reliability
Interrater reliability
Investigator triangulation
Known-groups technique
Measurement
Member check
Method triangulation

Negative case analysis
Obtained score
Peer debriefing
Persistent observation
Predictive validity
Prolonged engagement
Psychometric evaluation
Quantification
Reliability
Reliability coefficient
Researcher credibility
Split-half technique
Stability
Stepwise replication
Subscales
Test–retest reliability
Theory triangulation
Thick description
Transferability
Triangulation
True score
Trustworthiness
Validity
Validity coefficient

Data collection methods vary in quality. An ideal data collection procedure is one that results in indicators of the constructs that are accurate, valid, and unbiased. For most concepts of interest to nurse researchers, few, if any, data collection procedures match this ideal. In this chapter, we discuss criteria for evaluating the quality of data obtained in both quantitative and qualitative research projects.

MEASUREMENT AND THE ASSESSMENT OF QUANTITATIVE DATA

In a quantitative study, data come from measures of an abstract construct. Before describing criteria for assessing quantitative measures, we briefly discuss the concept of measurement.

Measurement

Measurement involves rules for assigning numeric values to *qualities* of objects to designate the *quantity* of the attribute. No attribute inherently has a numeric value; human beings invent the rules to measure concepts. An often-quoted statement by an American psychologist, L. L. Thurstone, summarizes a position assumed by many quantitative researchers: "Whatever exists, exists in some amount and can be measured." The notion here is that attributes are not constant: they vary from day to day or from one person to another. This variability is capable of a numeric expression that signifies *how much* of an attribute is present. **Quantification** is used to communicate that amount. The purpose of assigning numbers is to differentiate among people who possess varying degrees of the critical attribute.

The definition of measurement also requires numbers to be assigned to objects according to rules rather than haphazardly. Quantification in the absence of rules would be meaningless. The rules for measuring temperature, weight, blood pressure, and other physical attributes are widely known and accepted. Rules for measuring many variables, however, have to be invented. What are the rules for measuring patient satisfaction? Pain? Depression? Whether the data are collected through observation, self-report, or some other method, the researcher must specify the criteria according to which numeric values are to be assigned.

Advantages of Measurement

A major strength of measurement is that it removes guesswork in gathering information. Consider how handicapped nurses and doctors would be in the absence of measures of body temperature, blood pressure, and so on. Because measurement is based on explicit rules, the information tends to be objective: two people measuring a person's weight using the same scale would likely get identical results. Two people scoring responses to a self-report stress scale would likely arrive at identical scores. Not all quantitative measures are completely objective, but most incorporate rules for minimizing subjectivity.

Quantitative measurement also makes it possible to obtain reasonably precise information. Instead of describing Nathan as "rather tall," for example, we can depict him as a man who is 1.9 meters tall. If we chose, or if the research required it, we could obtain even more precise height measurements. Because of the possibility for precision, the researcher can differentiate among people who possess different degrees of an attribute.

Finally, measurement is a language of communication. Numbers are less vague than words and are thus capable of communicating information to a broad audience. If a researcher reported that the average oral temperature of a sample of patients was "somewhat high," different readers might develop different conceptions about the physiologic state of the sample. If the researcher reported an average temperature of 37.5°C, however, there is no ambiguity.

Errors of Measurement

Researchers work with fallible measures. Values and scores from even the best measuring instruments have a certain amount of error. We can think of every piece of quantitative data as consisting of two parts: an error component and a true component. This can be written as an equation, as follows:

Obtained score = True score ± Error

The **obtained** (or observed) **score** could be, for example, a patient's heart rate or score on an anxiety scale. The **true score** is the true value that would be obtained if it were possible to have an infallible measure of the target attribute. The true score is hypothetical; it can never be known because measures are not infallible. The **error of measurement**—the difference between true and obtained scores—is the result of extraneous factors that affect the measurement and result in distortions.

Many factors contribute to errors of measurement. Among the most common are the following:

- *Situational contaminants.* Measurements can be affected by the conditions under which they are produced (*e.g.,* people's awareness of an observer can affect their behaviour; environmental factors, such as temperature, lighting, or time of day, can be sources of measurement error).
- *Response set biases.* A number of relatively enduring characteristics of respondents can interfere with accurate measures of an attribute (see Chap. 11).
- *Transitory personal factors.* Temporary personal factors (*e.g.,* fatigue, hunger, mood) can influence people's motivation to cooperate, act naturally, or do their best.
- *Administration variations.* Alterations in the methods of collecting data from one person to the next can affect obtained scores (*e.g.,* if some biophysiologic measures are taken before a feeding and others are taken postprandially, measurement errors might occur).
- *Item sampling.* Errors can be introduced as a result of the sampling of items used to measure an attribute. For example, a student's score on a

100-item research methods test will be influenced to a certain extent by which 100 questions are included.

This list is not exhaustive, but it illustrates that data are susceptible to measurement error from a variety of sources.

Reliability of Measuring Instruments

The **reliability** of a quantitative measure is a major criterion for assessing its quality. Reliability refers to the consistency with which an instrument measures the attribute. If a spring scale gave a reading of 50 kg for a person's weight one minute and a reading of 60 kg the next minute, we would naturally be wary of using such an unreliable scale. The less variation an instrument produces in repeated measurements of an attribute, the higher is its reliability.

Another way of defining reliability is in terms of accuracy. An instrument is reliable if its measures accurately reflect the true measures of the attribute. A reliable measure is one that maximizes the true score component and minimizes the error component of a score.

Three aspects of reliability are of interest to researchers collecting quantitative data: stability, internal consistency, and equivalence.

Stability

The **stability** of a measure is the extent to which the same scores are obtained when the instrument is used with the same people on separate occasions. Assessments of stability are derived through **test–retest reliability** procedures. The researcher administers the same measure to a sample of people on two occasions and then compares the scores.

Suppose, for example, we were interested in the stability of a self-report scale that measured self-esteem in adolescents. Because self-esteem is a fairly stable attribute that would not change markedly from one day to the next, we would expect a reliable measure of it to yield consistent scores on two separate tests. As a check on the instrument's stability, we arrange to administer the scale 3 weeks apart to a sample of teenagers. Fictitious data for this example are presented in Table 12-1. On the whole, differences on the two tests are not large. Researchers compute a **reliability coefficient,** a numeric index of a measure's reliability, to objectively determine exactly how small the differences are. Reliability coefficients (designated as *r*) range from .00 to 1.00.* The higher the value, the more reliable (stable) is the measuring instrument. In the example shown in Table 12-1, the reliability coefficient is .95, which is quite high.

---

* Computation procedures for reliability coefficients are not presented in this textbook, but formulas can be found in the references cited at the end of this chapter. Although reliability coefficients can, technically, be negative, (*i.e.,* less than .00), they are usually a positive number between .00 and 1.00.

TABLE 12-1. Fictitious Data for Test–Retest Reliability of Self-Esteem Scale

SUBJECT NUMBER	TIME 1 SCORE	TIME 2 SCORE
1	55	57
2	49	46
3	78	74
4	37	35
5	44	46
6	50	56
7	58	55
8	62	66
9	48	50
10	67	63

$r = .95$

CONSUMER TIP

For most purposes, reliability coefficients higher than .70 are satisfactory, but coefficients in the .85 to .95 range are far preferable. ■

The test–retest approach to estimating reliability has certain disadvantages. The major problem is that many traits of interest do change over time, independently of the instrument's stability. Attitudes, mood, knowledge, and so forth can be modified by intervening experiences between two measurements. Thus, stability indexes are most appropriate for relatively enduring characteristics, such as personality and abilities.

Example of test–retest reliability:

Tourigny (2000) tested a newly developed tool (*Échelle Descriptive des Comportements de l'Enfant Opéré, EDCO*) to assess anxiety, fear, and pain in children aged 3 to 10 who undergo day surgery. The test–retest reliability of the scale with a sample of hospitalized children (1 week between administration) was .88 (Tourigny, personal communication, January 16, 2003).

Internal Consistency

Ideally, psychosocial scales are composed of items that all measure the same critical attribute and nothing else. On a scale to measure empathy in nurses, it would be inappropriate to include an item that is a better measure of diagnostic competence than empathy. An instrument may be said to have **internal consistency** reliability to the extent that all its subparts measure the same characteristic. This approach to reliability assesses an important source of measurement error in multi-item measures: the sampling of items.

Many scales and tests contain multiple **subscales** or subtests, each of which tap distinct, but related, concepts (*e.g.*, a measure of independent functioning might include subscales for motor activities, communication, and socializing). The internal consistency of the subscales is typically assessed and, if subscale scores are summed for an overall score, the scale's internal consistency would also be assessed. ∎

One of the oldest methods for assessing internal consistency is the **split-half technique.** In this approach, the items comprising a test or scale are split into two groups (usually, odd versus even items) and scored, and then scores on the two half-tests are used to compute a reliability coefficient. If the two half-tests are really measuring the same attribute, the reliability coefficient will be high. More sophisticated and accurate methods of computing internal consistency estimates are now in use, most notably, **Cronbach's alpha** or **coefficient alpha.** This method gives an estimate of the split-half correlation for all possible ways of dividing the measure into two halves, not just odd versus even items. As with test–retest reliability coefficients, indexes of internal consistency range in value between .00 and 1.00. The higher the reliability coefficient, the more accurate (internally consistent) the measure.

Example of internal consistency reliability:

Lobchuk and Degner (2002) compared family caregivers' and patients' perceptions of symptom experiences in advanced-stage cancer. To assess perceptions pertaining to symptoms (*i.e.*, presence, frequency, severity, and distress), they used the Memorial Symptom Assessment Scale (MSAS), a 32-item instrument that had been found previously to have adequate reliability. In their study, the subscales' internal consistency coefficients ranged from .59 to .84.

Equivalence

The **equivalence** approach to estimating reliability—used primarily with structured observational instruments—determines the consistency or equivalence of the instrument by different observers or raters. As noted in Chapter 11, a potential weakness of direct observation is the risk for observer error. The degree of error can be assessed through **interrater** (or **interobserver**) **reliability,** which is estimated by having two or more trained observers make simultaneous, independent observations. The resulting data can then be used to calculate an index of equivalence or agreement. That is, a reliability coefficient can be computed to demonstrate the strength of the relationship between the observers' ratings. When two independent observers score some phenomenon congruently, the scores are likely to be accurate and reliable.

Example of interrater reliability:

Stewart et al. (1999) developed the Environment–Behaviour Interaction Code (EBIC), an observational coding system to classify the behaviour and environmental context of people with dementia. One version of the EBIC is a system for making ongoing observations in real time (event format); another is a global checklist developed for clinical outcome research (interval format). The mean percentages of agreement of raters were 78% for the event format and 96% for the interval format.

Interpretation of Reliability Coefficients

Reliability coefficients are an important indicator of an instrument's quality. A measure with low reliability prevents an adequate testing of a researcher's hypothesis. If data fail to confirm a research hypothesis, one possibility is that the measuring tool was unreliable—not necessarily that the expected relationships do not exist. Thus, knowledge of the reliability of an instrument is useful in interpretating research results.

Reliability estimates vary according to the procedure used to obtain them. Estimates of reliability computed by different procedures for the same instrument are not identical.

Example of different forms of reliability:

To better understand occupational stress among caregivers in rural nursing homes, Morgan et al. (2002) assessed the level of job strain among registered nurses, nursing aides, and activity workers. Job strain was assessed using three subscales of the Job Content Questionnaire (JCQ). Test–retest reliability was reported to be .90 for the JCQ, and the internal consistency coefficients of the three subscales ranged from .68 to .96.

In addition, reliability of an instrument is related to sample heterogeneity. The more homogeneous the sample (*i.e.,* the more similar the scores), the lower the reliability coefficient will be. This is because instruments are designed to measure differences, and if sample members are similar to one another, it is more difficult for the instrument to discriminate reliably among those who possess varying degrees of the attribute.

 CONSUMER TIP

If a research report provides information on the reliability of a quantitative scale without specifying the type of reliability measure used, it is probably safe to assume that internal consistency reliability was assessed by the Cronbach alpha method. ■

Validity of Measuring Instruments

The second important criterion for evaluating a quantitative instrument is its validity. **Validity** is the degree to which an instrument measures what it is supposed to be measuring. When researchers develop instruments to measure patients' perceived susceptibility to illness, they should take steps to ensure that the resulting scores validly reflect this variable and not something else.

The reliability and validity of an instrument are not totally independent. A measuring device that is not reliable cannot possibly be valid. An instrument cannot validly be measuring the attribute of interest if it is erratic or inaccurate. An instrument can be reliable, however, without being valid. Suppose we had the idea to measure patients' anxiety by measuring the circumference of their wrists. We could obtain highly accurate, consistent, and precise measurements of wrist circumferences, but they would not be valid indicators of anxiety. Thus, the high reliability of an instrument provides no evidence of its validity; the low reliability of a measure is evidence of low validity.

Like reliability, validity has a number of aspects and assessment approaches. One aspect is known as face validity. **Face validity** refers to whether the instrument looks as though it is measuring the appropriate construct. Although it is often useful for an instrument to have face validity, three other aspects of validity are of greater importance in assessments of an instrument: content validity, criterion-related validity, and construct validity.

CONSUMER TIP

In some studies, the focus is on data quality. That is, researchers undertake studies to examine the validity and reliability of instruments that could be used by clinicians or other nurse researchers. In these **psychometric evaluations,** information about data quality is carefully documented. ■

Content Validity

Content validity is concerned with adequacy of coverage of the content area being measured. Content validity is particularly relevant for tests of knowledge. In such a context, the validity question is: How representative are the questions on this test of the universe of all questions that might be asked on this topic?

Content validity is also relevant in measures of complex psychosocial traits. A person who wanted to develop a new instrument would begin by developing a thorough conceptualization of the construct of interest so that the measure would adequately capture the whole domain. Such a conceptualization might come from rich first-hand knowledge but is more likely to come from the results of a qualitative inquiry or from a literature review.

The content validity of an instrument is necessarily based on judgment. There are no totally objective methods for ensuring the adequate content coverage of an instrument. Experts in the content area are often called on to analyze the adequacy of items in representing the hypothetical content universe in the correct proportions. It is also possible to calculate a content validity index that indicates the extent of expert agreement, but ultimately the subjective judgments of the experts must be relied on.

EE | ***Example of content validity:***

Davies and Hodnett (2002) developed a scale to measure maternity care nurses' perceived self-efficacy for providing labour support, based on existing measures and a review of the literature. Content validity of the scale was judged by an expert panel of three obstetric nurses and one midwife, who were asked to rate the relevance of each scale item and to identify areas of omission.

Criterion-Related Validity

In a **criterion-related validity** assessment, the researcher seeks to establish the relationship between scores on an instrument and some external criterion. The instrument, whatever abstract attribute it is measuring, is said to be valid if its scores correspond strongly with scores on some criterion. One difficulty of criterion-related validation is finding a reliable and valid criterion. Researchers constructing an instrument to measure nursing effectiveness might use supervisory ratings as the criterion—but how could they be sure that the ratings were valid and reliable? Researchers must be content with less-than-perfect criteria.

After the criterion is established, the validity can be estimated easily. A **validity coefficient** is computed by using a mathematic formula that correlates scores on the instrument with scores on the criterion variable. The magnitude of the coefficient indicates how valid the instrument is. These coefficients (r) range between .00 and 1.00, with higher values indicating greater criterion-related validity. Coefficients of .70 or higher are desirable.

Sometimes, a distinction is made between two types of criterion-related validity. **Predictive validity** refers to an instrument's ability to differentiate between people's performances or behaviours on some future criterion. When a school of nursing correlates students' incoming SAT scores with their subsequent grade-point averages, the predictive validity of the SATs for nursing school performance is being evaluated. **Concurrent validity** refers to an instrument's ability to distinguish among people who differ in their present status on some criterion. For example, a test to differentiate between patients in a mental institution who could and could not be released could be correlated with current behavioural ratings of health care personnel. The difference between predictive and concurrent validity, then, is the difference in the timing of obtaining measurements on a criterion.

EE | ***Example of criterion-related validity:***

French et al. (2000) evaluated an expanded version of the Nursing Stress Scale (NSS), a tool used to asess work-related stress among nurses. Concurrent criterion-related validity of the expanded version of the scale (ENSS) was established by examining scale scores in relation to actual reports of how stressful nurses perceived their lives to be at the time of the study.

Construct Validity

Validating an instrument in terms of **construct validity** is difficult and challenging. Construct validity is concerned with the following question: What construct is the instrument actually measuring? The more abstract the concept, the more difficult it is to establish the construct validity of the measure; at the same time, the more abstract the concept, the less suitable it is to a criterion-related validation approach. What objective criterion is there for concepts such as empathy, grief, and separation anxiety?

Construct validation is addressed in several ways, but there is always an emphasis on testing relationships predicted on the basis of theoretical considerations. Constructs are explicated in terms of other concepts; the researcher makes predictions about the manner in which the construct will function in relation to other constructs.

One approach to construct validation is the **known-groups technique.** In this procedure, groups that are expected to differ on the critical attribute are administered the instrument, and group scores are compared. For instance, in validating a measure of fear of the labour experience, the scores of primiparas and multiparas could be contrasted. Women who had never given birth would likely experience more anxiety than women who had already had children; one might question the validity of the instrument if such differences did not emerge.

Another method of construct validation consists of an examination of relationships based on theoretical predictions. A researcher might reason as follows: According to theory, construct X is related to construct Y; instrument A is a measure of construct X, and instrument B is a measure of construct Y; scores on A and B are related to each other, as predicted by the theory; therefore, it is inferred that A and B are valid measures of X and Y. This logical analysis is fallible and does not constitute proof of construct validity, but it offers important evidence.

Another approach to construct validation uses a statistical procedure known as **factor analysis,** which is a method for identifying clusters of related items on a scale. The procedure is used to identify and group together different measures of some underlying attribute and to distinguish them from measures of different attributes.

In summary, construct validation uses both logical and empirical procedures. Like content validity, construct validity requires a judgment pertaining to what the instrument is measuring. Construct validity and criterion-related validity share an empirical component, but, in the latter case, there is a pragmatic, objective criterion with which to compare a measure rather than a second measure of an abstract theoretical construct.

Example of construct validity:

Dennis (in press) developed a short form of the Breastfeeding Self-Efficacy Scale (BSES), a tool to assess a mother's confidence in breastfeeding. She used the known-groups technique to validate the instrument; mean scores on the BSES validly differentiated between primiparas (*i.e.,* without previous breastfeeding experience) and multiparas with previous breastfeeding experience.

Interpretation of Validity

Like reliability, validity is not an all-or-nothing characteristic of an instrument. An instrument cannot really be said to possess or lack validity; it is a question of degree. The testing of an instrument's validity is not proved but rather is supported by an accumulation of evidence.

Strictly speaking, a researcher does not validate an instrument *per se* but rather some application of the instrument. A measure of anxiety may be valid for presurgical patients on the day before surgery but may not be valid for nursing students on the day of a final examination. Validation is a never-ending process: the more evidence that can be gathered that an instrument is measuring what it is supposed to be measuring, the greater the confidence researchers have in its validity.

 CONSUMER TIP

In many studies involving structured self-report or observational instruments, the research report provides validity and reliability information from an earlier study, usually conducted by the researcher who developed the measure. If the sample characteristics in the original study and the new study are similar, the citation provides valuable information about data quality in the new study. Researchers may also compute new reliability coefficients for the actual research sample—typically, internal consistency or interrater reliability. ■

ASSESSMENT OF QUALITATIVE DATA

The assessment procedures described thus far cannot be meaningfully applied to such qualitative materials as responses in unstructured interviews or participant observers' field notes. This does not imply, however, that qualitative researchers are unconcerned with data quality. The central question underlying the concepts of validity and reliability is: Do the measures used by the researcher yield data reflecting the truth? Certainly, qualitative researchers are as eager as quantitative researchers to have their findings reflect the true state of phenomena.

Many qualitative nurse researchers seek to evaluate the quality of their data and their findings through procedures that have been outlined by Lincoln and Guba (1985), two proponents of the naturalistic paradigm of inquiry. These researchers have suggested four criteria for establishing the **trustworthiness** of qualitative data and the ensuing analysis: credibility, dependability, confirmability, and transferability.

CONSUMER TIP

Qualitative research reports are uneven in the amount of information they provide about data quality. Some do not address data quality issues at all, whereas others elaborate in detail the steps the researcher took to confirm trustworthiness. The absence of information makes it difficult for consumers to come to conclusions about the believability of qualitative findings. ■

Credibility

Careful qualitative researchers take steps to improve and evaluate data **credibility,** which refers to confidence in the truth of the data. Lincoln and Guba note that the credibility of an inquiry involves two aspects: first, carrying out the investigation in a way that believability is enhanced and, second, taking steps to *demonstrate* credibility. Lincoln and Guba suggest various techniques for improving and documenting the credibility of qualitative data. A few that are especially relevant to the evaluation of qualitative studies are mentioned here.

Prolonged Engagement and Persistent Observation

Lincoln and Guba recommend activities that increase the likelihood of producing credible data and interpretations. A first and very important step is **prolonged engagement**—the investment of sufficient time in data collection activities to have an in-depth understanding of the culture, language, or views of the group under study and to test for misinformation. Prolonged engagement is also essential for building trust and rapport with informants.

Credible data collection also involves **persistent observation,** which refers to the researcher's focus on the aspects of a situation that are relevant to the phenomena being studied. As Lincoln and Guba note, "If prolonged engagement provides scope, persistent observation provides depth" (1985, p. 304).

Triangulation

Triangulation, another technique to enhance credibility, is the use of multiple referents to draw conclusions about what constitutes the truth. Denzin (1989) has identified four types of triangulation:

1. **Data source triangulation:** using multiple data sources in a study (*e.g.,* interviewing diverse key informants about the same topic)
2. **Investigator triangulation:** using more than one person to collect, analyze, or interpret a set of data
3. **Theory triangulation:** using multiple perspectives to interpret a set of data
4. **Method triangulation:** using multiple methods to address a research problem (*e.g.,* observations plus interviews)

Triangulation provides a basis for convergence on the truth. By using multiple methods and perspectives, researchers strive to distinguish true information from information with errors.

Example of triangulation:

Bottorff et al. (2001) identified critical elements of women-centred care within a multicultural context. More specifically, the researchers sought to document issues pertaining to cervical cancer screening practices among three ethnocultural groups in Canada: Asian, South Asian, and First Nations. Although the primary sources of data were from the women, the study also involved data triangulation wherein nurses and physicians working in the clinics and in the community were interviewed. Issues raised by women and providers were compared and contrasted.

External Checks: Peer Debriefing and Member Checks

Two other techniques for establishing credibility involve external checks on the inquiry. **Peer debriefing** is a session held with objective peers to review and explore various aspects of the inquiry. Peer debriefing exposes the investigator to the searching questions of others who are experienced in either qualitative research or in the phenomenon being studied, or both. These sessions can also be useful to researchers interested in testing some working hypotheses or in exploring new avenues in the emergent research design.

Member checks refers to providing feedback to study participants regarding preliminary findings and interpretations and securing the participants' reactions. Member checking can be carried out both informally in an ongoing way as data are being collected and more formally after data have been collected and analyzed. Lincoln and Guba consider member checking the most important technique for establishing the credibility of qualitative data.

Example of member checking:

Knoll and Johnson (2000) studied the experience of spouses who cared for their loved one after cardiac surgery. Data collection primarily involved unstructured, face-to-face, open-ended interviews conducted by the principal investigator. In these interviews, "the emerging themes were shared with the participants and they were asked to comment on whether the themes captured their experiences" (p. 66).

Searching for Disconfirming Evidence

Data credibility can be enhanced by the researcher's systematic search for data that challenge an emerging conceptualization or descriptive theory. The search for disconfirming evidence occurs through purposive sampling but is facilitated through other processes already described here, such as prolonged engagement and peer debriefings. The sampling of individuals who can offer conflicting viewpoints can greatly strengthen a comprehensive description of a phenomenon.

Lincoln and Guba refer to a similar activity of **negative case analysis**—a process by which researchers revise their hypotheses through the inclusion of cases that appear to disconfirm earlier hypotheses. The goal of this procedure is to refine a hypothesis or theory continuously until it accounts for all cases without exception.

Example of negative case analysis:

Varcoe (2001) explored the nature of nursing interventions with women who have been abused. Interviews were conducted with 30 health care providers and 5 women who had been abused. Interviews were transcribed and the author "continually sought competing and contradictory perspectives, using tensions between perspectives as points for analysis rather than as problems to be solved or choices to be made" (p. 100).

Researcher Credibility

Another aspect of credibility discussed by Patton (2002) is **researcher credibility,** the faith that can be put in the researcher. In qualitative studies, the researcher is the data collecting instrument—as well as the creator of the analytic process—and, therefore, the researcher's training, qualifications, and experience are important in establishing confidence in the data.

From your viewpoint as consumer, the research report should contain information about the researcher, including information about credentials and about any personal connections the researcher had to the people, topic, or community under study. For example, it is relevant for a reader of a report on AIDS patients' coping mechanisms to know that the researcher is HIV positive. Patton argues that the researcher should report "any personal and professional information that may have affected data collection, analysis and interpretation—negatively or positively. . . ." (1990, p. 566).

Dependability

The **dependability** of qualitative data refers to data stability over time and over conditions. It might be said that credibility (in qualitative studies) is to validity (in quantitative studies) what dependability is to reliability. Like the reliability–validity relationship in quantitative research, there can be no credibility in the absence of dependability.

One approach to assessing data dependability is to undertake a **stepwise replication.** This approach, which is conceptually similar to a split-half technique, involves having several researchers who can be divided into two teams. These teams deal with data sources separately and conduct, essentially, two independent inquiries through which data and conclusions can be compared.

Another technique relating to dependability is the **inquiry audit.** An inquiry audit involves a scrutiny of the data and relevant supporting documents by an external reviewer, an approach that also has a bearing on data confirmability, as we discuss next.

⊞ ***Example of dependability:***

Williams et al. (2000) used a stepwise replication and inquiry audit in their study of coping with normal results from predictive gene testing for neurodegenerative disorders. Ten participants were interviewed three times. Three researchers read through transcripts of the first set of interviews and made marginal notes for coding. The three researchers compared their codes and revised them until agreement was reached. All transcripts from the remaining interviews were coded independently, and the researchers met periodically to compare codes and reach a consensus. Once coding was completed, a qualitative nurse researcher reviewed the entire set of transcribed interviews and validated the findings with the three researchers.

Confirmability

Confirmability refers to the objectivity or neutrality of the data, such that two or more independent people would agree about the data's relevance or meaning. In qualitative studies, the issue of confirmability does not focus on the characteristics of the researcher (is he or she objective and unbiased?) but rather on the characteristics of the data (*i.e.*, are the data confirmable?).

Inquiry audits can be used to establish both the dependability and confirmability of the data. In an inquiry audit, the investigator develops an **audit trail,** which is a systematic collection of documentation that allows an independent auditor to come to conclusions about the data. Six classes of records are important in creating an adequate audit trail: (1) raw data (*e.g.*, field notes, interview transcripts), (2) data reduction and analysis products (*e.g.*, theoretical notes, documentation on working hypotheses), (3) process notes (*e.g.*, methodologic notes, notes from member check sessions), (4) materials relating to intentions and dispositions (*e.g.*, personal notes on intentions), (5) instrument development information (*e.g.*, pilot forms), and (6) data reconstruction products (*e.g.*, drafts of the final report).

After the audit trail materials are assembled, the inquiry auditor proceeds to audit, in a fashion analogous to a financial audit, the trustworthiness of the data and the meanings attached to them. Although the auditing task is complex, it is an invaluable tool for persuading others that qualitative data are worthy of confidence.

> *Example of confirmability:*
>
> In her research on mothering twins, Beck (2002) developed a 4-phased grounded theory entitled, "life on hold: releasing the pause button." In her report, Beck provided a partial audit trail for phase 3, which she called "striving to reset."

Transferability

In Lincoln and Guba's framework, **transferability** refers to the extent to which the findings from the data can be transferred to other settings or groups and is thus similar to the concept of generalizability. This is, to some extent, an issue relating to sampling and design rather than to the soundness of the data *per se.* As Lincoln and Guba note, however, a researcher's responsibility is to provide sufficient descriptive data in the research report for consumers to evaluate the applicability of the data to other contexts: "Thus the naturalist cannot specify the external validity of an inquiry; he or she can provide only the thick description necessary to enable someone interested in making a transfer to reach a conclusion about whether transfer can be contemplated as a possibility" (1985, p. 316). **Thick description** refers to a rich, thorough description of the research setting and the transactions and processes observed during the inquiry. Thus, if there is to be transferability, the burden of proof rests with researchers to provide sufficient information to permit judgments about contextual similarity.

CRITIQUING DATA QUALITY

If data are seriously flawed, the study findings cannot be meaningful. Therefore, it is important for you as a consumer to consider whether the researcher has taken appropriate steps to collect data that accurately reflect reality. In both qualitative and quantitative studies, you have the right—indeed, the obligation—to ask: "Can I trust the data?" "Do the data accurately reflect the true state of the phenomenon under study?"

In quantitative studies, you should expect some discussion of the reliability and validity of the measures—preferably, information collected directly with the sample under study (rather than evidence from other studies). You should be wary about the results of quantitative studies when the report provides no information about data quality or when it suggests unfavourable reliability or validity. Also, data quality deserves special scrutiny when the research hypotheses are not confirmed. There may be many reasons that hypotheses are not supported by data (*e.g.,* too small a sample or a faulty theory), but the quality of the measures is an important area of concern. When hypotheses are not supported, one possibility is that the instruments were not good measures of the research constructs. Box 12-1 provides some guidelines for critiquing data quality in quantitative studies.

Information about data quality is equally important in qualitative studies. You should be particularly alert to information on data quality when a single researcher has been responsible for collecting, analyzing, and interpreting all the data, as is frequently the case. Some guidelines for critiquing the trustworthiness of data in qualitative studies are presented in Box 12-2.

BOX 12-1 GUIDELINES FOR EVALUATING DATA QUALITY IN QUANTITATIVE STUDIES

1. Does there appear to be a strong congruence between the research variables as conceptualized (*i.e.,* as discussed in the introduction) and as operationalized (*i.e.,* as described in the method section)?

2. Do the rules for the measurement of the variables seem sensible? Were the data collected in such a way that measurement errors were minimized?

3. Does the report provide evidence of the reliability of the data? Does the evidence come from the research sample itself, or is it based on a prior study? If the latter, is it reasonable to believe that reliability would be similar for the research sample (*e.g.,* are the sample characteristics similar)?

4. If there is reliability information, what method of estimating reliability was used? Was this method appropriate? Is the reliability sufficiently high?

5. Does the report provide evidence of the validity of the measures? Does the evidence come from the research sample itself, or is it based on a prior study? If the latter, is it reasonable to believe that validity would be similar for the research sample (*e.g.,* are the sample characteristics similar)?

6. If there is validity information, what validity approach was used? Was this method appropriate? Does the validity of the instrument appear to be adequate?

BOX 12-2 GUIDELINES FOR EVALUATING DATA QUALITY IN QUALITATIVE STUDIES

1. Does the research report discuss efforts the researcher made to enhance or evaluate the trustworthiness of the data? If so, is the description sufficiently detailed and clear?

2. Which techniques (if any) did the researcher use to enhance and appraise the credibility of the data? Was the investigator in the field an adequate amount of time? Was triangulation used, and, if so, of what type? Did the researcher search for disconfirming evidence? Were there peer debriefings or member checks? Do the researcher's qualifications enhance the credibility of the data?

3. Which techniques (if any) did the researcher use to enhance and appraise the dependability, confirmability, and transferability of the data?

4. Were the procedures used to enhance and document data quality adequate? Given the procedures used (if any), what can you conclude about the trustworthiness of the data?

RESEARCH EXAMPLES

In this section, we present examples of the efforts researchers took to assess data in a quantitative and a qualitative study. Use the relevant guidelines in Boxes 12-1 and 12-2 to evaluate the researchers' activities.

Research Example of a Quantitative Study

Irvine and colleagues (2000) evaluated the psychometric properties of two health status measures: the Medical Outcome Study Short Form (SF-36) and the Quality of Life Profile, Senior Version (QOLPSV) within a home health care context. The study was designed to assess the patients' health status (*i.e.,* scores on the SF-36 and QOLPSV) at admission (T1) and discharge (T2) from the home care service, providing an indicator of patients' change in health status following receipt of home care services. The researchers' efforts to assess the reliability and validity of the SF-36 and QOLPSV are summarized below.

Research Summary

The main goal of their study was to evaluate the reliability and validity of the two different health outcome measures used to assess patients' health status. Data were collected from 50 individuals receiving home care nursing services. The SF-36 was administered first, followed by the QOLPSV. Internal consistency (Cronbach alpha) for the eight subscales of the SF-36 (*e.g.,* physical function, role function, mental function) ranged from .76 to .94 and from .47 to .82 for the nine subscales of the QOLPSV (*e.g,* physical being, social belonging, leisure becoming).

Construct validation for both scales was undertaken through testing a series of hypotheses. One hypothesis, for instance, was that nursing intensity (*i.e.,* the number of nursing diagnoses reflecting patients' needs for nursing resources) would be negatively related to patients' functional health status and quality of life baseline and outcome scores. Indeed, nursing intensity was found to be negatively associated with two SF-36 subscales (physical function and general health) at T1 and four of the subscales at T2 (physical function and role, vitality, and social function). Nursing intensity was also negatively related to one QOLPSV subscale (practical becoming) at T1 and five of its subscales at T2 (physical and spiritual being, physical and social belonging, and practical becoming). An additional hypothesis being tested was that health status scores would improve significantly from admission to the nursing agency to discharge or within 30 visits, whichever came first; statistical analysis indicated a significant improvement in health status scores for seven of the eight subscales of the SF-36 between T1 and T2 and four of the nine QOLPSV subscales.

In light of their findings, the authors concluded that the SF-36 "may be a better measure of health outcomes following nursing care than the brief version of the QOLPSV" (p. 53). They also suggested further testing of the SF-36 in community health settings.

Clinical Relevance

Financial constraints within the health care system and technologic breakthroughs mean that much of in-hospital care is now being shifted to home care. Because nurses form a large proportion of the home health care workforce, a better understanding of the contribution of nursing care to patient outcomes is needed. Questionnaires that assess changes in health outcomes could be used to assess the impact of nursing care on patient outcomes. One goal of this study was to evaluate the reliability and validity of the SF-36 and the QOLPSV as potential outcome measures related to nursing interventions in a community health setting. The acceptable levels of reliability and validity achieved for most of the subscales support their applicability to community health settings. Home care nurses could periodically assess any changes in health outcomes over time particularly by using the SF-36, because many of the SF-36 subscales were significantly associated with nursing intensity. In addition, should any deterioration in health outcomes be detected by the SF-36, nurses could then readily intervene to address the health issue. Further testing is needed, however, with different clinical populations and community health settings.

Research Example of a Qualitative Study

Banister (1999) conducted an ethnographic study to explore midlife women's perceptions of their changing bodies within the Western cultural context. The study involved in-depth interviews with 23 midlife women. Her efforts to enhance and document data quality are summarized below.

Research Summary

Data collection in this study was carried out in two phases. The first phase involved in-depth, unstructured interviews with study participants. The second phase involved gathering the participants into groups for verification of emerging domains and further theory development.

Methods used to strengthen the data's credibility included triangulation, peer debriefing, member checks, and the maintenance of a reflective journal by the researcher, who was herself a midlife woman. With respect to member checking, the author wrote, "To assure that the analysis accurately represented the social world of mid-life women, participants were invited to comment on the analyzed material throughout the research process and to suggest changes where they felt the materials did not reflect their experiences" (p. 525). Banister recognized that her position as a woman in midlife could both enhance and threaten the truth value of the study. She therefore maintained a reflective journal in which she reflected on reactions in the field and ways in which they might influence her interpretation and the representation of the women's experiences.

With respect to dependability and confirmability, Banister maintained an audit trail in a research journal that documented all of her methodologic decisions. Transferability was facilitated through rich description of the women and their contexts.

The results of this rigourous qualitative study indicated that women's midlife experience of their changing bodies is full of contradiction and change. Issues of loss, cultural influences that perpetuate ageism and sexism, lack of consistent information about menopause, questioning, redefining self, and self-care all played a central role in the women's lives during this time of transition.

Clinical Relevance

Growing proportions of women are entering midlife, and yet there appears to be little solid information about their perceptions, their situations, and their health care needs. Banister's study makes a contribution to our understanding of midlife women's experiences and the role that sociocultural and physiologic factors play in those experiences. Banister conducted a careful study that was strengthened by her steps to enhance and ensure data quality.

Banister found that a salient characteristic of the midlife experience of women was their questioning about their changing bodies and critically reflecting on the cultural construction of their realities—findings that have implications for clinical practice. Educating women regarding menopause and their changing bodies is a critical nursing intervention. Women need not only facts about what is happening to their changing bodies but also opportunities to discuss the ambiguity between cultural stereotypes of midlife women and their personal experiences. One such type of opportunity could be a support group facilitated by nurses in which cultural avoidance of issues facing midlife women could be openly discussed. By encouraging midlife women to reflect and question critically, health care providers can assist them to enhance the quality of their lives. The findings also suggest that nurses and other health care professionals could profitably engage in critically questioning their own assumptions and biases toward midlife women. These biases could influence the caring they provide these women. Nurses are in an excellent position given their many interactions with women to help demystify our society's attitudes and beliefs about the midlife transition in women's lives.

● ● ● ● ● SUMMARY POINTS

- **Measurement** involves a set of rules according to which numeric values are assigned to objects to represent varying degrees of some attribute.
- Few quantitative measuring instruments are infallible. Sources of measurement error include situational contaminants, response set biases, and transitory personal factors, such as fatigue.
- **Obtained scores** from an instrument consist of a **true score** component—the value that would be obtained if it were possible to have a perfect measure of the attribute—and an error component, or **error of measurement,** that represents measurement inaccuracies.

- **Reliability** is the degree of consistency or accuracy with which an instrument measures an attribute. The higher the reliability of an instrument, the lower the amount of error in the obtained scores.
- There are different methods for assessing an instrument's reliability and for computing a **reliability coefficient.** The **stability** aspect, which concerns the extent to which the instrument yields the same results on repeated administrations, is evaluated by **test–retest procedures.**
- The **internal consistency** aspect of reliability, which refers to the extent to which all the instrument's items are measuring the same attribute, is assessed using either the **split-half reliability technique** or, more likely, **Cronbach's alpha method.**
- When the focus of a reliability assessment is on establishing **equivalence** between observers in rating or coding behaviours, estimates of **interrater** (or **interobserver) reliability** are obtained.
- **Validity** is the degree to which an instrument measures what it is supposed to be measuring.
- **Content validity** is concerned with the sampling adequacy of the content being measured.
- **Criterion-related validity** focuses on the correlation between the instrument and an outside criterion.
- **Construct validity** refers to the adequacy of an instrument in measuring the construct of interest. One construct validation method is the **known-groups technique,** which contrasts the scores of groups that are presumed to differ on the attribute; another is **factor analysis,** a statistical procedure for identifying unitary clusters of items or measures.
- Qualitative researchers evaluate the **trustworthiness** of their data using the criteria of credibility, dependability, confirmability, and transferability.
- **Credibility,** roughly analogous to validity in a quantitative study, refers to the believability of the data. Techniques to improve the credibility of qualitative data include **prolonged engagement,** which strives for adequate scope of data coverage, and **persistent observation,** which is aimed at achieving adequate depth.
- **Triangulation** is the process of using multiple referents to draw conclusions about what constitutes the truth. The four major forms are **data source triangulation, investigator triangulation, theoretical triangulation,** and **method triangulation.**
- Two important tools for establishing credibility are **peer debriefings,** wherein the researcher obtains feedback about data quality and interpretation from peers, and **member checks,** wherein informants are asked to comment on the data and the researcher's interpretations.
- **Dependability** of qualitative data refers to the stability of data over time and over conditions and is somewhat analogous to the concept of reliability in quantitative studies.
- **Confirmability** refers to the objectivity or neutrality of the data. Independent inquiry audits by external auditors can be used to assess and document dependability and confirmability.

- **Transferability** is the extent to which findings from the data can be transferred to other settings or groups. Transferability can be enhanced through **thick descriptions** of the context of the data collection.

➤➤➤➤ *CRITICAL THINKING ACTIVITIES*

Chapter 12 of the accompanying *Study Guide to Accompany Essentials of Nursing Research,* 5th edition, offers various exercises and study suggestions for reinforcing the concepts presented in this chapter. In addition, you can address the following questions:

1. Read the method section from one or both of the actual research studies in the Appendix of this book, and then answer the questions in Boxes 12-1 and 12-2.

2. In the example in the text illustrating test–retest reliability, Tourigny (2000) calculated the reliability coefficient as .88. How do you explain such a high coefficient?

3. In the example in the text illustrating interrater reliability, Stewart and her colleagues (1999) found that the reliability was higher in the interval format than in the event format. Why do you think this occurred?

For additional review, see questions 156–171 on the study CD provided with Polit: Study Guide to Accompany Essentials of Nursing Research.

SUGGESTED READINGS

Methodologic References

Brink, P. J. (1991). Issues of reliability and validity. In J. M. Morse (Ed.). *Qualitative nursing research: A contemporary dialogue.* Newbury Park, CA: Sage.

Denzin, N. K. (1989). *The research act* (3rd ed.). New York: McGraw-Hill.

Lincoln, Y. S., & Guba, E. G. (1985). *Naturalistic inquiry.* Newbury Park, CA: Sage.

Meadows, L. M., & Morse, J. M. (2001). Constructing evidence within the qualitative project. In J. M. Morse, J. M. Swanson, & A. J. Kuzel (Eds.). *The nature of qualitative evidence* (pp.187–200). Thousand Oaks, CA: Sage.

Nunnally, J., & Bernstein, I. H. (1994). *Psychometric theory* (3rd ed.) New York: McGraw-Hill.

Patton, M. Q. (2002). *Qualitative evaluation and research methods* (3rd ed.). Thousand Oaks, CA: Sage.

Waltz, C. F., Strickland, O. L., & Lenz, E. R. (1991). *Measurement in nursing research* (2nd ed.). Philadelphia: F. A. Davis.

Substantive References

Banister, E. M. (1999). Women's mid-life experience of their changing bodies. *Qualitative Health Research, 9,* 520–537.

Beck, C.T. (2002). Releasing the pause button: Mothering twins during the first year of life. *Qualitative Health Research, 12,* 593–608.

Bottorff, J. L., Balneaves, L. G., Sent, L., Grewal, S., & Browne, A. J. (2001). Cervical cancer screening in ethnocultural groups: Case studies in women-centered care. *Women & Health, 33,* 29–46.

Davies, B. L., & Hodnett, E. (2002). Labor support: Nurses' self-efficacy and views about factors influencing implementation. *Journal of Obstetric, Gynecologic, and Neonatal Nursing, 31,* 48–56.

Dennis, C. L. (in press). The Breastfeeding Self-Efficacy Scale: Psychometric assessment of the short form. *Journal of Obstetric, Gynecologic, and Neonatal Nursing.*

French, S. E., Lenton, R., Walters, V., & Eyles, J. (2000). An empirical evaluation of an expanded nursing stress scale. *Journal of Nursing Measurement, 8,* 161–178.

Irvine, D., O'Brien-Pallas, L. L., Murray, M., Cockerill, R., Sidani, S., Laurie-Shaw, B. et al. (2000). The reliability and validity of two health status measures for evaluating outcomes of home care nursing. *Research in Nursing & Health, 23,* 43–54.

Knoll, S. & Johnson, J. (2000). Uncertainty and expectations: Taking care of cardiac surgery patients at home. *Journal of Cardiovascular Nursing, 14,* 64–75.

Lobchuk, M. M., & Degner, L. F. (2002). Symptom experiences: Perceptual accuracy between advanced-stage cancer patients and family caregivers in the home care setting. *Journal of Clinical Oncology, 20,* 3495–3507.

Morgan, D. G., Semchuk, K. M., Stewart, N. J., & D'Arcy, C. (2002). Job strain among staff of rural nursing homes: A comparison of nurses, aides and activity workers. *Journal of Nursing Administration, 32,* 152–161.

Stewart, N. J., Hiscock, M., Morgan, D. G., Murphy, P. B., & Yamamoto, M. (1999). Development and psychometric evaluation of the Environment–Behavior Interaction Code (EBIC). *Nursing Research, 48,* 261–268.

Tourigny, J. (2000). Un nouvel instrument pour mesurer la détresse d'un enfant opéré. [A new tool to assess distress among children undergoing surgery]. *L'infirmière du Québec, 8,* 18–29.

Varcoe, C. (2001). Abuse obscured: An ethnographic account of emergency nursing in relation to violence against women. *Canadian Journal of Nursing Research, 32,* 95–115.

Williams, J. K., Schutte, D.L., Evers, C., & Holkup, P. A. (2000). Redefinition: Coping with normal results from predictive gene testing for neurodegenerative disorders. *Research in Nursing & Health, 23,* 260–269.

PART V

ANALYSIS OF RESEARCH DATA

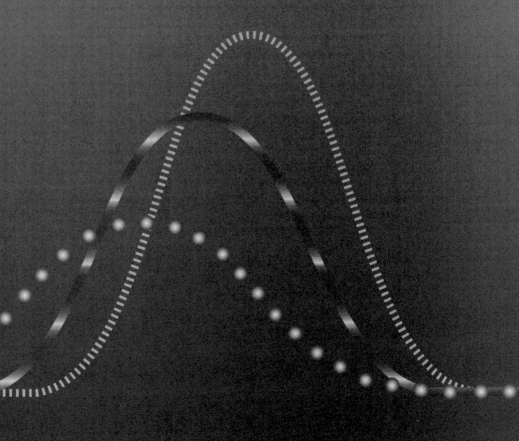

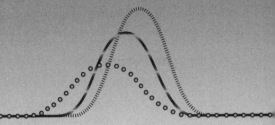

Analyzing Quantitative Data

LEVELS OF MEASUREMENT
DESCRIPTIVE STATISTICS
    Frequency Distributions
    Central Tendency
    Variability
    Bivariate Descriptive Statistics
INTRODUCTION TO INFERENTIAL STATISTICS
    Sampling Distributions
    Hypothesis Testing
BIVARIATE STATISTICAL TESTS
    t-Tests
    Analysis of Variance
    Chi-Squared Test
    Correlation Coefficients
    Guide to Bivariate Statistical Tests
MULTIVARIATE STATISTICAL ANALYSIS
    Multiple Regression
    Analysis of Covariance

    Other Multivariate Techniques
    Guide to Multivariate Statistical Analyses
READING AND INTERPRETING STATISTICAL INFORMATION
    Tips on Reading Text With Statistical Information
    Tips on Reading Statistical Tables
CRITIQUING QUANTITATIVE ANALYSES
RESEARCH EXAMPLES
    Research Example of Bivariate Inferential Statistics
    Research Example of Multivariate Statistical Analysis
SUMMARY POINTS
CRITICAL THINKING ACTIVITIES
SUGGESTED READINGS
    Methodologic References
    Substantive References

Student Objectives

On completion of this chapter, the student will be able to:

○ identify the four levels of measurement and describe and compare characteristics of each
○ distinguish descriptive and inferential statistics
○ describe the characteristics and shapes of frequency distributions
○ identify and compare measures of central tendency and variability and interpret these measures
○ interpret a correlation coefficient
○ describe the principle of sampling distributions
○ describe the logic and purpose of tests of statistical significance and describe hypothesis testing procedures
○ distinguish the characteristics and uses of parametric and nonparametric tests
○ specify the appropriate applications for *t*-tests, analysis of variance, chi-squared tests, and correlation coefficients and interpret the meaning of the calculated statistics
○ describe the applications and principles of multiple regression and analysis of covariance
○ understand the results of simple statistical procedures described in a research report
○ define new terms in the chapter

New Terms

Alpha
Analysis of covariance (ANCOVA)
Analysis of variance (ANOVA)
Bell-shaped curve
Bimodal distribution
Bivariate descriptive statistics
Causal modeling
Central tendency
Chi-squared test
Contingency table
Correlation
Correlation coefficient
Correlation matrix
Covariate
Cross-tabulation
Degrees of freedom
Dependent groups *t*-test
Descriptive statistics
Discriminant function analysis
Estimation procedures

F ratio
Factor analysis
Frequency distribution
Frequency polygon
Hypothesis testing
Independent groups *t*-test
Inferential statistics
Interaction effects
Interval measurement
Inverse relationship
Laws of probability
Level of measurement
Level of significance
Linear structural relations analysis
LISREL
Logistic regression
Logit analysis
Main effects
MANCOVA
MANOVA

Mean
Median
Mode
Multimodal distribution
Multiple comparison procedures
Multiple correlation analysis
Multiple correlation coefficient
Multiple regression analysis
Multivariate analysis of covariance
Multivariate analysis of variance
Multivariate statistics
N
Negative relationship
Negative skew
Nominal measurement
Nonparametric test
Nonsignificant result
Normal distribution
Null hypothesis
Odds
Odds ratio
Ordinal measurement
p value
Paired *t*-test
Parameter
Parametric test
Path analysis
Pearson's *r*
Perfect relationship
Positive relationship

Positive skew
Post hoc tests
Product–moment correlation coefficient
r
R
R²
Range
Ratio measurement
Repeated measures ANOVA
Sampling distribution of the mean
Sampling error
Skewed distribution
Spearman's rank-order correlation
Spearman's rho
Standard deviation
Standard error of the mean
Statistic
Statistical test
Statistically significant
Symmetric distribution
Test statistic
t-test
Two-way ANOVA
Type I error
Type II error
Unimodal distribution
Univariate descriptive statistics
Variability
Variance

The data collected in a study do not by themselves answer research questions or test research hypotheses. The data need to be systematically analyzed so that trends and patterns of relationships can be detected. This chapter describes statistical procedures for analyzing quantitative data, and Chapter 14 discusses the analysis of qualitative data.

LEVELS OF MEASUREMENT

A quantitative measure can be classified according to its **level of measurement.** This classification system is important because the types of statistical analysis that can be performed depend on the measurement level used. There are four major classes, or levels, of measurement:

1. **Nominal measurement,** the lowest level, involves using numbers simply to categorize characteristics. Examples of variables that are nominally measured include gender, blood type, and nursing specialty. The numbers assigned in nominal measurement do not convey quantitative information. If we establish a rule to code males as 1 and females as 2, the numbers have no numeric meaning. The number 2 here does not mean "more than" 1. Nominal measurement provides information only about categorical equivalence and nonequivalence; hence, the numbers cannot be treated mathematically. It is nonsensical, for example, to compute the average gender of the sample by adding the numeric values and dividing by the number of participants.

Example of nominal measurement:

Kodis et al. (2001) compared the change in patients' exercise capacity and lipid levels after coronary artery bypass graft surgery according to whether they had received clinic-based or home-based aerobic training. Type of exercise training received (clinic- versus home-based) was a nominal variable.

2. **Ordinal measurement** ranks objects based on their relative standing on a specified attribute. If a researcher rank-orders people from heaviest to lightest, this is ordinal measurement. As another example, consider this ordinal scheme for measuring ability to perform activities of daily living: 1 = is completely dependent; 2 = needs another person's assistance; 3 = needs mechanical assistance; and 4 = is completely independent. The numbers signify incremental ability to perform the activities of daily living independently. Ordinal measurement does not, however, tell us how much greater one level of an attribute is than another level. For example, we do not know if being completely independent is twice as good as needing mechanical assistance. As with nominal measures, the mathematic operations permissible with ordinal-level data are restricted.

Example of ordinal measurement:

Ross et al. (2001) studied family caregiving in long-term care facilities in the Ottawa-Carleton region. They asked their sample of 122 family members about frequency of visits, which was measured on the following ordinal scale: daily, several times a week, weekly, several times a month, or monthly.

3. **Interval measurement** occurs when the researcher can specify the ranking of objects on an attribute and the distance between those objects. Most educational and psychological tests (*e.g.,* the Scholastic Assessment Test, or SAT)* are based on interval scales. A score of 550 on

---

*The SAT is a standardized test used by some colleges and universities in the United States—and, less frequently, in Canada—for admission decisions.

the SAT is higher than a score of 500, which, in turn, is higher than 450. Moreover, the difference between 550 and 500 is presumed to be equivalent to the difference between 500 and 450. Interval scales expand analytic possibilities: interval-level data can be averaged meaningfully, for example. Many sophisticated statistical procedures require interval measurements.

> **Example of interval measurement:**
> King (2000), in a study designed to examine gender differences on early recovery from cardiac surgery, administered several psychosocial scales that were interval measures, including a social support scale and the Duke Activity Status Index.

4. **Ratio measurement** is the highest level of measurement. Ratio scales, unlike interval scales, have a rational, meaningful zero and therefore provide information about the absolute magnitude of the attribute. For example, the Centigrade scale for measuring temperature (interval measurement) has an arbitrary zero point. Zero on the thermometer does not signify the absence of heat; it would not be appropriate to say that 20°C is twice as hot as 10°C. Many physical measures, however, are ratio measures with a rational zero. A person's weight, for example, is a ratio measure. It is perfectly acceptable to say that someone who weighs 100 kg is twice as heavy as someone who weighs 50 kg. All the statistical procedures suitable for interval data are also appropriate for ratio-level data.

> **Example of ratio measurement:**
> Bell et al. (2001) conducted a study to examine the influence of personal, familial, and sociodemographic variables on breastfeeding duration. Many of the variables measured were on a ratio scale, including age of mother, income, gestational age, weight of infant, and number of days hospitalized.

Researchers generally strive to use the highest levels of measurement possible because higher levels yield more information and are amenable to more powerful analytic procedures than lower levels.

DESCRIPTIVE STATISTICS

Without statistics, quantitative data would be a chaotic mass of numbers. Statistical procedures enable the researcher to summarize, organize, interpret, and communicate numeric information. Statistics are classified as either descriptive or inferential. **Descriptive statistics** are used to describe and synthesize data. Averages and percentages are examples of descriptive statistics. When such indexes are calculated on data from a population, they are referred to as **parameters.** A descriptive index from a sample is a **statistic.**

Most scientific questions are about parameters; researchers calculate statistics to estimate them.

Frequency Distributions

Data that are not analyzed or organized are overwhelming. It is not even possible to discern general trends in the data without some structure. Consider the 60 numbers in Table 13-1. Let us assume that these numbers are the scores of 60 high school students on a 30-item test of knowledge about AIDS—scores that are on an interval scale. Visual inspection of the numbers in this table provides little insight on student performance.

Frequency distributions are a method of imposing order on numeric data. A **frequency distribution** is a systematic arrangement of numeric values from the lowest to the highest, together with a count (or percentage) of the number of times each value was obtained. The 60 test scores are presented as a frequency distribution in Table 13-2. This arrangement makes it convenient to see at a glance the highest and lowest scores, the most common score, where the scores clustered, and how many students were in the sample (total sample size is typically designated as **N** in research reports). None of this was easily discernible before the data were organized.

Some researchers display frequency data graphically in a **frequency polygon** (Fig. 13-1). In frequency polygons, scores are on the horizontal line (with the lowest value on the left), and the vertical line indicates frequency counts or percentages. Data distributions are sometimes described by their shapes. **Symmetric distribution** occurs if, when folded over, the two halves of a frequency polygon would be superimposed (Fig. 13-2). In an asymmetric or **skewed distribution,** the peak is off centre, and one tail is longer than the other. When the longer tail is pointed toward the right, the distribution has a **positive skew,** as in the first graph of Figure 13-3. Personal income is an example of a positively skewed attribute. Most people have moderate incomes, with only a few people with high incomes at the right end of the distribution. If the longer tail points to the left, the distribution has a **negative skew,** as in the second graph in Figure 13-3. Age at death is an ex-

TABLE 13-1. AIDS Knowledge Test Scores									
22	27	25	19	24	25	23	29	24	20
26	16	20	26	17	22	24	18	26	28
15	24	23	22	21	24	20	25	18	27
24	23	16	25	30	29	27	21	23	24
26	18	30	21	17	25	22	24	29	28
20	25	26	24	23	19	27	28	25	26

TABLE 13-2. Frequency Distribution of AIDS Knowledge Test Scores

SCORE	FREQUENCY	PERCENTAGE
15	1	1.7
16	2	3.3
17	2	3.3
18	3	5.0
19	2	3.3
20	4	6.7
21	3	5.0
22	4	6.7
23	5	8.3
24	9	15.0
25	7	11.7
26	6	10.0
27	4	6.7
28	3	5.0
29	3	5.0
30	2	3.3
	$N = 60$	100.0

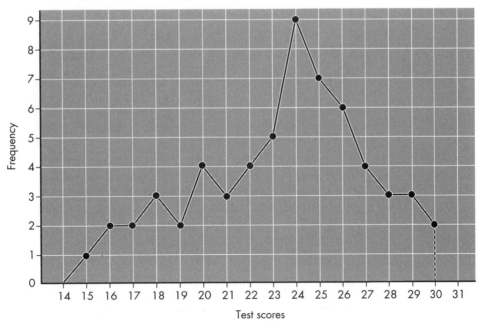

FIGURE 13-1. Frequency polygon of AIDS knowledge text scores.

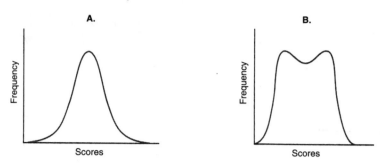

FIGURE 13-2. Examples of symmetric distributions.

ample of a negatively skewed attribute. Here, the bulk of people are at the far right end of the distribution, with relatively few people dying at an early age.

Another aspect of a distribution's shape concerns how many peaks or high points it has. A **unimodal distribution** has one peak (graph A, Fig. 13–2), whereas a **multimodal distribution** has two or more peaks—that is, two or more values of high frequency. A multimodal distribution with two peaks is a **bimodal distribution,** illustrated in graph B of Figure 13-2.

Some distributions have special names. Of particular interest is the **normal distribution** (sometimes referred to as a **bell-shaped curve**). A normal distribution is symmetric, unimodal, and not very peaked, as illustrated in graph A of Figure 13-2. Many attributes of humans (*e.g.*, height, intelligence, grip strength) have been found to approximate a normal distribution.

Example of frequency information:

Table 13-3 presents distribution information on sample characteristics from a study comparing family caregivers' and advanced-stage cancer patients' perceptions of patients' symptom experiences, frequency, severity, and distress (Lobchuk & Degner, 2002). This table shows, for some selected background characteristics, both the frequency (*N*) and percentage of sample members in various categories. For example, 60 participants (61.2%) were female and 38 (38.8%) were male.

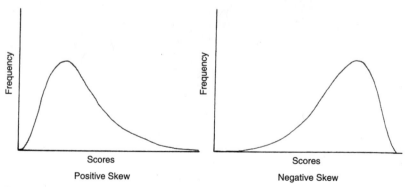

FIGURE 13-3. Examples of skewed distributions.

Central Tendency

For variables on an interval or ratio scale, a distribution of values is usually of less interest than an overall summary. The researcher asks such questions as: What was the average blood pressure of the patients after the intervention? How depressed was the typical mother after childbirth? These questions seek a single number that best represents the whole distribution. Such indexes of typicalness are measures of **central tendency.** To lay people, the term *average* is normally used to designate central tendency. There are three commonly used kinds of averages, or measures of central tendency: the mode, the median, and the mean.

- **Mode:** The mode is the number that occurs most frequently in a distribution. In the following distribution, the mode is 53:

  50 51 51 52 53 53 53 53 54 55 56

  The value of 53 was obtained four times, a higher frequency than for other numbers. The mode of the AIDS knowledge test scores was 24, as shown in Table 13-2. The mode, in other words, identifies the most popular value. The mode is used primarily for describing typical or

TABLE 13-3. Example of Table Showing Frequency Distribution Information: Patient Characteristics in Study of Perceptual Accuracy Between Advanced-Stage Cancer Patients and Family Caregivers in the Home Care Setting

CHARACTERISTICS	N = 98	PERCENTAGE
Marital status	Single: 2	2.0
	Married/common law: 74	75.5
	Divorced/separated: 5	5.1
	Widowed: 17	17.4
Gender	Female: 60	61.2
	Male: 38	38.8
Occupational status	Employed full-time: 7	7.1
	Employed part-time: 4	4.1
	Retired: 59	60.2
	Unemployed: 9	9.2
	On medical leave: 19	19.4
Current treatment*	None: 50	51.0
	Chemotherapy: 41	41.8
	Radiotherapy: 10	10.2
	Other: 2	2.0

Adapted from Lobchuk, M. M., & Degner, L. F. (2002). Symptom experiences: Perceptual accuracy between advanced-stage cancer patients and family caregivers in the home care setting. *Journal of Clinical Oncology, 20*(16), 3495–3507.
*Note: Numbers for current treatment add up to more than totals (i.e., > N = 98 and >100%) because some participants were undergoing more than one type of treatment for cancer.

high-frequency values for nominal measures. For example, in the study by Lobchuk & Degner (see Table 13-3), we could make the following statement: The typical (modal) patient was a married woman not currently undergoing cancer treatment.

- **Median:** The median is that point in a distribution above which and below which 50% of the cases fall. Consider the following set of values:

  2 2 3 3 4 5 6 7 8 9

  The value that divides the cases in half is midway between 4 and 5, and thus 4.5 is the median. For the AIDS knowledge test scores, the median is 24. An important characteristic of the median is that it does not take into account individual score values and is thus insensitive to extreme values. In the above set of values, if the value of 9 were changed to 99, the median would remain 4.5. Because of this property, the median is the preferred index of central tendency with highly skewed distributions and when a single typical value is of interest. In research reports, the median may be abbreviated as Md or Mdn.

- **Mean:** The mean is equal to the sum of all values divided by the number of participants—in other words, what people refer to as the average. The mean of the AIDS knowledge test scores is 23.42 (1405 ÷ 60). As another example, consider the following weights of eight people:

  50 55 61 66 72 78 86 92

  In this example, the mean is 70. Unlike the median, the mean is affected by the value of every score. If we were to exchange the 92-kg person for one weighing 132 kg, the mean weight would increase from 70 to 75 kg. A substitution of this kind would leave the median unchanged. In research reports, the mean is often symbolized as M or $\bar{X}$ (e.g., $\bar{X} = 70$).

For interval-level or ratio-level measurements, the mean, rather than the median or mode, is usually the statistic reported. Of the three indexes, the mean is the most stable: if repeated samples were drawn from a population, the means would fluctuate less than the modes or medians. Because of its stability, the mean generally is the best estimate of the central tendency of the population. When a distribution is highly skewed, however, the mean does not characterize the centre of the distribution; in such situations, the median is preferred. For example, the median is a better central tendency measure of family income than the mean because income is positively skewed.

Variability

Two sets of data with identical means could be quite different with respect to how spread out or dispersed the data are (*i.e.,* how different the people are from one another on the attribute of interest). The **variability** of two distributions could be different even when the means are identical.

Consider the distributions in Figure 13-4, which represent hypothetical scores of students from two high schools on the SAT. Both distributions have

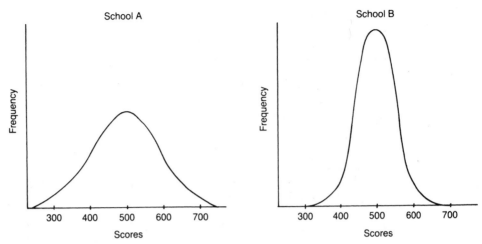

FIGURE 13-4. Two distributions of different variability.

an average score of 500, but the two groups of students are clearly different. In school A, there is a wide range of scores—from scores below 300 to some above 700. In school B, on the other hand, there are few low scorers but also few outstanding test achievers. School A is more heterogeneous (*i.e.,* more variable) than school B, whereas school B is more homogeneous than school A.

Researchers compute an index of variability to summarize the extent to which scores in a distribution differ from one another. Several such indexes have been developed, the most important of which are the range and the standard deviation.

- **Range:** The range is the highest score minus the lowest score in a distribution. In the example of the AIDS knowledge test scores, the range is 15 (30–15). In the distributions in Figure 13-4, the range for school A is 500 (750–250), whereas the range for school B is 300 (650–350). The chief virtue of the range is its ease of computation. Because it is based on only two scores, however, the range is unstable: from sample to sample drawn from the same population, the range tends to fluctuate considerably. Moreover, the range ignores score variations between the two extremes. In school B of Figure 13-4, if a single student obtained a score of 250 and another obtained a score of 750, the range of both schools would then be 500—despite large differences in their heterogeneity. For these reasons, the range is used largely as a gross descriptive index.
- **Standard deviation:** The most widely used variability index is the standard deviation. Like the mean, the standard deviation is calculated based on every value in a distribution. The standard deviation summarizes the average amount of deviation of values from the mean. In the AIDS knowledge test example, the standard deviation is 3.725.* In

---

* Formulas for computing the standard deviation, as well as other statistics discussed in this chapter, are not shown in this textbook. The emphasis here is on helping readers to understand the statistics and their applications. References at the end of the chapter can be consulted for computation formulas.

research reports, the standard deviation is often abbreviated as *s* or *SD*. Occasionally, the SD is simply shown in relation to the mean without a formal label, such as M = 4 (1.5) or M = 4 ± 1.5, where 4 is the mean and 1.5 is the standard deviation.†

An SD is more difficult to interpret than the range. With regard to the AIDS knowledge test, you might well ask, 3.725 what? What does the number mean? We will try to answer these questions from several angles. First, as discussed, the SD is an index of how variable scores in a distribution are. If two groups of students had means of 23 on the AIDS knowledge test, but one group had an SD of 7 and the other had an SD of 3, we would immediately know that the second group was more homogeneous (*i.e.,* their scores were more similar to one another).

The SD represents the average of deviations from the mean. The mean tells us the single best point for summarizing an entire distribution, and a SD tells us how much, on average, the scores deviate from that mean. In the AIDS test example, they deviated by an average of just under 4 points. An SD might thus be interpreted as an indication of our degree of error when we use a mean to describe an entire data set.

In normal and near-normal distributions, there are roughly three SDs above and below the mean. Suppose we had a normal distribution with a mean of 50 and an SD of 10 (Fig. 13-5). In such a distribution, a fixed percentage of cases fall within certain distances from the mean. Sixty-eight percent of all cases fall within 1 SD above and below the mean. Thus, in this example, nearly 7 of 10 scores are between 40 and 60. Ninety-five percent of the scores in a normal distribution fall within 2 SDs from the mean. Only a handful of cases—about 2% at each extreme—lie more than 2 SDs from the mean. Using this figure, we can see that a person who obtained a score of 70 achieved a higher score than about 98% of the sample.

Example of means and SDs:

Some measures of central tendency and variability from an actual nursing study are presented in Table 13-4. This study by Gibbins et al. (2002) compared the efficacy and safety of three interventions for relieving procedural pain associated with heel lances in preterm and term neonates. A total of 190 neonates were randomized to receive sucrose and nonnutritive sucking (*n* = 64), sucrose alone (*n* = 62), or, sterile water and nonnutritive sucking (*n* =64). Table 13-4 shows the means and SDs of infants' pain responses, 30 seconds and 60 seconds following a heel lance, as measured by the Premature Infant Pain Profile. The table indicates that pain scores were lowest for the sucrose and nonnutritive sucking group at both 30 and 60 seconds. There was more variability in pain scores at 60 seconds than at 30 seconds for all three groups, as can be seen by comparing SDs in parentheses.

†Occasionally, a research report will make a reference to an index of variability known as the **variance.** The variance is simply the value of the standard deviation squared. In the example of the AIDS knowledge test scores, the variance is 3.725^2, or 13.876.

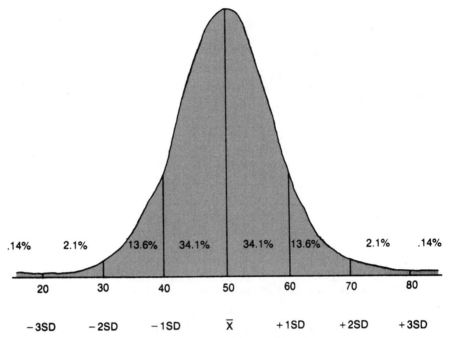

FIGURE 13-5. Standard deviations in a normal distribution.

Bivariate Descriptive Statistics

So far, our discussion has focused on descriptive indexes of single variables—**univariate** (one-variable) **descriptive statistics.** The mean, mode, SD, and so forth are used to describe one variable at a time. Research usually is concerned, however, with relationships. **Bivariate** (two-variable) **descriptive statistics** describe relationships between two variables.

TABLE 13-4. Example of Table Showing Central Tendency and Variability: Study of Efficacy and Safety of Sucrose for Procedural Pain Relief in Preterm and Term Neonates

| INTERVENTION GROUP | MEAN SCORES (SD) ON THE PREMATURE INFANT PAIN PROFILE | |
	30 Seconds	60 Seconds
Sucrose and nonnutritive sucking ($n = 64$)	8.16 (3.24)	8.78 (4.03)
Sucrose alone ($n = 62$)	9.77 (3.04)	11.20 (3.25)
Sterile water and nonnutritive sucking ($n = 64$)	10.19 (2.67)	11.20 (3.47)

Adapted from Gibbins et al. (2002). Efficacy and safety of sucrose for procedural pain relief in preterm and term neonates. *Nursing Research, 51,* 375–382.

Contingency Tables

A **contingency table** is a two-dimensional frequency distribution in which the frequencies of two variables are **cross-tabulated.** Suppose we have data on patients' gender and whether they are nonsmokers, light smokers (≤ 1 pack of cigarettes a day), or heavy smokers (>1 pack a day). Here, the question is whether there is a tendency for men to smoke more heavily than women or *vice versa.* Some fictitious data on these two variables are shown in a contingency table in Table 13-5. Six cells are created by placing one variable (gender) along the vertical dimension and the other variable (smoking status) along the horizontal dimension. After all subjects are allocated to the appropriate cells, percentages can be computed. This simple procedure allows us to see at a glance that, in this sample, women were more likely than men to be nonsmokers (45.4% versus 27.3%) and less likely to be heavy smokers (18.2% versus 36.4%). Contingency tables usually are used with nominal data or ordinal data that have few levels or ranks. In the present example, gender is a nominal measure, and smoking status is an ordinal measure.

Example of a contingency table:

Table 13-6 presents a cross-tabulation table from an actual study that examined the extent of communication between nursing research and nursing practice in the literature. Documents relating to nursing published in Canada and the United States in 1989 were analyzed to see if authors of research articles cited research articles more often than practice articles, and if authors of practice articles were more likely to cite other practice articles than research articles. In the sample of 1446 citations, research articles were more likely to have research citations (56.3%) than to have practice citations (43.7%), whereas practice articles were more likely to have practice citations (57.5%) than research citations (42.5%).

TABLE 13-5. Contingency Table for Gender and Smoking Status Relationship

	GENDER					
	Female		**Male**		**Total**	
SMOKING STATUS	*n*	%	*n*	%	*N*	%
Nonsmoker	卌卌 10	45.4	卌 I 6	27.3	16	36.4
Light smoker	卌 III 8	36.4	卌 III 8	36.4	16	36.4
Heavy smoker	IIII 4	18.2	卌 III 8	36.4	12	27.3
TOTAL	22	50.0	22	50.0	44	100.0

TABLE 13-6. Example of a Contingency Table: Associations Between Citing and Cited Article Types, for Sample of Citations in 1989 Nursing Documents			
	ARTICLE CITED		
Citing Article	**Research Citation**	**Practice Citation**	**Total**
Research article	241 (56.3%)	187 (43.7%)	428
Practice article	433 (42.5%)	585 (57.5%)	1018
Total	674 (46.6%)	772 (53.4%)	1446

Adapted from O'Neill, A. L., & Duffey, M. A. (2000). Communication of research and practice knowledge in nursing literature. *Nursing Research, 49,* 224–230.

A comparison of Tables 13-5 and 13-6 illustrates that cross-tabulated data can be presented in one of two ways: cell percentages can be computed on the basis of either row totals or column totals. In Table 13-5, the number 10 in the first cell (female nonsmokers) was divided by the column totals (*i.e.,* by the total number of women—22) to arrive at the percentage (45%) of women who were nonsmokers. (The table might well have shown 63% in this cell—the percentage of nonsmokers who were women). In Table 13-6, the number 241 in the first cell (number of research articles with research citations) was divided by the row total of 428 (total number of all research articles) to yield the percentage of 56.3%. Computed the other way, the researchers would have gotten 35.8% (241 ÷ 674), the percentage of research citations from a research article. Either approach is acceptable, although the former is usually preferred because then the percentages in a column add up to 100%.

 CONSUMER TIP

You may need to spend an extra minute when examining cross-tabulation tables to determine which total—row or column—was used as the basis for calculating percentages. ■

Correlation

The most common method of describing the relationship between two variables is through **correlation** procedures. The correlation question is: To what extent are two variables related to each other? For example, to what degree are anxiety test scores and blood pressure measures related? This question can be answered quantitatively by calculating a **correlation coefficient,** which describes the *intensity* and *direction* of a relationship.

Two variables that are related are height and weight: tall people tend to weigh more than short people. The relationship between height and weight would be a **perfect relationship** if the tallest person in a population was the heaviest, the second tallest person was the second heaviest, and so on. The correlation coefficient summarizes how "perfect" a relationship is. The possible values for a correlation coefficient range from -1.00 through .00 to $+1.00$. If height and weight were perfectly correlated, the correlation coefficient expressing this would be 1.00 (the actual correlation coefficient is in the vicinity of .50 to .60 for a general population). Height and weight have a **positive relationship** because greater height tends to be associated with greater weight.

When two variables are unrelated, the correlation coefficient is zero. One might anticipate that a woman's dress size is unrelated to her intelligence. Large women are as likely to perform well on tests of mental ability as small women. The correlation coefficient summarizing such a relationship would presumably be in the vicinity of .00.

Correlation coefficients running between .00 and -1.00 express a **negative** or **inverse relationship.** When two variables are inversely related, increments in one variable are associated with decrements in the second. For example, there is a negative correlation between depression and self-esteem. This means that, on average, people with *high* self-esteem tend to be *low* on depression. If the relationship were perfect (*i.e.,* if the person with the highest self-esteem score had the lowest depression score and so on), then the correlation coefficient would be -1.00. In actuality, the relationship between depression and self-esteem is usually moderate—in the vicinity of $-.40$ or $-.50$. Note that the higher the *absolute value* of the coefficient (*i.e.,* the value disregarding the sign), the stronger the relationship. A correlation of $-.80$, for instance, is much stronger than a correlation of $+.20$.

The most commonly used correlation index is the **product–moment correlation coefficient** (also referred to as **Pearson's r**), which is computed with interval or ratio measures. The correlation index generally used for ordinal measures is **Spearman's rank-order correlation** (r_s), sometimes referred to as **Spearman's rho.**

It is difficult to offer guidelines on what should be interpreted as strong or weak relationships. This determination depends on the nature of the variables. If we were to measure patients' body temperature both orally and rectally, a correlation (**r**) of .70 between the two measurements would be low. For most psychosocial variables (*e.g.,* stress and severity of illness), however, an *r* of .70 would be rather high. Perfect correlations ($+1.00$ and -1.00) are extremely rare.

In research reports, correlation coefficients are often reported in tables displaying a two-dimensional **correlation matrix,** in which every variable is displayed in both a row and a column. To read a correlation matrix, one finds the row for one variable and reads across until the row intersects with the column for the second variable.

Example of a correlation matrix:

Table 13-7 presents a correlation matrix from a study that examined relationships among eight nursing-related hospital variables and 30-day postadmission mortality rates for hospitalized patients (Tourangeau et al. 2002). The table lists, on the left, the eight nursing-related hospital variables in the matrix: nursing staffing dose, nursing skill mix, availability of professional role support, years of RN experience on the clinical unit, nurse capacity to work, condition of nursing practice environment, continuity of care, and physician expertise; 30-day mortality rates is the ninth variable. The numbers in the top row, from 1 to 9, correspond to the nine variables: 1 is nursing staffing dose, 2 is nursing skill mix and so on. At the intersection of row 1 and column 1, we find the value 1.00, which simply indicates that the variable "nursing staffing dose" is perfectly correlated with itself. The next entry represents the correlation between nursing skill mix and nursing staffing dose. The value of $-.47$ indicates a moderate negative relationship between these two variables: As nursing skill mix increases, nursing staffing dose decreases. On the other hand, an increase in availability of professional role support is positively correlated with an increase in nursing skill mix (.53). The strongest correlation is between physician expertise and availability of professional role support ($-.59$) and the weakest correlation is between nurse capacity to work and nursing skill mix ($-.04$).

INTRODUCTION TO INFERENTIAL STATISTICS

Descriptive statistics are useful for summarizing data, but usually researchers do more than simply describe. **Inferential statistics,** which are based on the **laws of probability,** provide a means for drawing conclusions about a population, given data from a sample.

TABLE 13-7. Example of a Correlation Matrix: Study of Nurse Staffing and Patient Outcomes								
	1	**2**	**3**	**4**	**5**	**6**	**7**	**8**	**9**
1. Nursing staffing dose	1.00								
2. Nursing skill mix	−.47	1.00							
3. Availability of professional role support	−.41	.53	1.00						
4. Years of RN experience on the clinical unit	−.08	−.12	−.11	1.00					
5. Nurse capacity to work	−.05	−.04	.08	−.25	1.00				
6. Condition of nursing practice environment	−.12	.20	.41	.06	−.16	1.00			
7. Continuity of care	−.06	.39	.33	−.14	.21	−.10	1.00		
8. Physician expertise	.24	−.51	−.59	.28	−.35	−.09	−.45	1.00	
9. 30-day mortality rate	.21	−.21	−.18	−.20	−.30	−.08	−.17	.19	1.00

Adapted from Tourangeau, A. E., Giovannetti, P., Tu, J. V., & Wood, M. (2002). Nursing-related determinants of 30-day mortality for hospitalized patients. *Canadian Journal of Nursing Research, 33,* 71–88.

Sampling Distributions

When estimating population characteristics, it is important to obtain representative samples, and probability (random) sampling is best suited to securing such samples. Inferential statistical procedures are based on the assumption of random sampling from populations, although this assumption is widely violated.

Even with random sampling, however, sample characteristics are seldom identical to those of the population. Suppose we had a population of 30,000 nursing school applicants. The mean SAT score for the population is 500 and the SD is 100. Now suppose that we do not know these parameters but that we must estimate them based on scores from a random sample of 25 students. Should we expect a mean of exactly 500 and an SD of 100 for this sample? It would be improbable to obtain identical values. Let us say that, instead, we calculated a mean of 505. If a completely new random sample of 25 students were drawn and another mean computed, we might obtain a value such as 497. Sample statistics fluctuate and are unequal to the corresponding population parameter because of **sampling error.** The challenge for a researcher is to determine whether sample values are good estimates of population parameters.

A researcher works with only one sample, but to understand the logic of inferential statistics, we must perform a mental exercise. Consider drawing a sample of 25 students from the population of applicants, calculating a mean, replacing the 25 students, and drawing a new sample. Each mean is considered a separate datum. If we drew 5000 samples, we would have 5000 means (data points) that could be used to construct a frequency polygon, as shown in Figure 13-6. This kind of distribution is called a **sampling distribution of the mean.** A sampling distribution is a theoretical rather than an actual distribution because in practice no one draws consecutive samples from a population and plots their means. Statisticians have demonstrated that (1) sampling distributions of means follow a normal distribution and (2) the mean of a sampling distribution composed of an infinite number of sample means is equal to the population mean. In the present example, the mean of the sampling distribution is 500, the same value as the mean of the population.

Remember that when scores are normally distributed, 68% of the cases fall between +1 SD and −1 SD from the mean. Because a sampling distribution of means is normally distributed, the probability is 68 of 100 that any randomly drawn sample mean lies within the range of values between +1 SD and −1 SD of the mean. The problem, then, is to determine the value of the SD of the sampling distribution—which is called the **standard error of the mean** (or SEM). The word *error* signifies that the sample means comprising the distribution contain some error in their estimates of the population mean. The smaller the standard error (*i.e.,* the less variable the sample means), the more accurate are the means as estimates of the population value.

Because no one actually constructs a sampling distribution, how can its SD be computed? Fortunately, there is a formula for estimating the SEM from

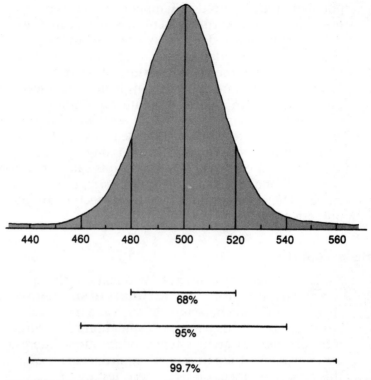

FIGURE 13-6. Sampling distribution of a mean.

data from a single sample, using two pieces of information: the sample's SD and sample size. In the present example, the SEM has been calculated as 20, as shown in Figure 13-6. This statistic is an estimate of how much sampling error there would be from one sample mean to another in an infinite number of samples of 25 students.

We can now estimate the probability of drawing a sample with a certain mean. With a sample size of 25 and a population mean of 500, the chances are about 95 of 100 that a sample mean would fall between the values of 460 and 540—2 SDs above and below the mean. Only 5 times of 100 would the mean of a randomly selected sample exceed 540 or be less than 460. In other words, only 5 times of 100 would we be likely to draw a sample whose mean deviates from the population mean by more than 40 points.

Because the SEM is partly a function of sample size, we need only increase sample size to increase the accuracy of our estimate. Suppose that instead of using a sample of 25 applicants to estimate the population's average SAT score, we use a sample of 100. With this many students, the SEM would be 10 rather than 20. In this situation, the probability of obtaining a sample whose mean is greater than 520 or less than 480 would be about 5 in 100. The chances of drawing a sample with a mean very different from that of the population are reduced as sample size increases because large numbers promote the likelihood that extreme cases will cancel each other out.

You may be wondering why you need to learn about these abstract statistical notions. Consider, though, that what we are talking about concerns how likely it is that a researcher's results are accurate. As an intelligent consumer, you need to evaluate critically how believable research results are so that you can decide whether to incorporate the findings into nursing practice. The concepts underlying the standard error are important in such an evaluation and are related to issues we stressed in Chapter 10 on sampling. First, the more homogeneous the population is on the critical attribute (*i.e.,* the smaller the SD), the more likely it is that results calculated from a sample will be accurate. Second, the larger the sample size, the greater is the likelihood of accuracy. The concepts discussed in this section are the basis for statistical hypothesis testing.

Hypothesis Testing

Statistical inference consists of two major techniques: estimation of parameters and hypothesis testing. **Estimation procedures** are used to estimate a single population characteristic, such as a mean value (*e.g.,* the mean temperature of appendicitis patients). Estimation procedures, however, are not common because researchers typically are more interested in relationships between variables than in estimating the accuracy of a single sample value. For this reason, we focus on hypothesis testing.

Statistical **hypothesis testing** provides objective criteria for deciding whether hypotheses should be accepted as true or rejected as false. Suppose a nurse researcher hypothesizes that maternity patients exposed to a teaching film on breastfeeding will breastfeed longer than mothers who do not see the film. The researcher subsequently learns that the mean number of days of breastfeeding is 131.5 for 25 experimental subjects and 125.1 for 25 control subjects. Should the researcher conclude that the hypothesis has been supported? True, the group differences are in the predicted direction, but the results might simply be due to sampling fluctuations. The two groups might *happen* to be different by chance, regardless of exposure to the film; perhaps in another sample, the group means would be nearly identical. Hypothesis testing helps researchers to make objective decisions about study results. Researchers need such a mechanism to help them decide which results are likely to reflect chance differences and which are likely to reflect true hypothesized effects.

The procedures used in testing hypotheses are based on rules of negative inference. In the above example, the researcher found that those who had seen the teaching film breastfed longer, on average, than those who had not. There are two possible explanations for this outcome: (1) the experimental treatment was successful in encouraging breastfeeding or (2) the difference was due to chance factors (*e.g.,* differences in the characteristics of the two groups even before the film was shown).

The first explanation is the researcher's scientific hypothesis, and the second is the **null hypothesis.** The null hypothesis, it may be recalled, states that there is no relationship between the independent and dependent variables. Statistical hypothesis testing is basically a process of disproof or rejection. It cannot be demonstrated directly that the scientific hypothesis is correct. But it is possible to show, using theoretical sampling distributions, that the null hypothesis has a high probability of being incorrect, and such evidence lends support to the scientific hypothesis.

The rejection of the null hypothesis, then, is what the researcher seeks to accomplish through **statistical tests.** Although null hypotheses are accepted or rejected on the basis of sample data, the hypothesis is made about population values. The real interest in testing hypotheses, as in all statistical inference, is to use a sample to draw conclusions about a population.

Type I and Type II Errors

Researchers decide whether to accept or reject the null hypothesis by determining how probable it is that observed group differences are due to chance. Because information about the population is not available, it cannot be asserted flatly that the null hypothesis is or is not true. The researcher must be content to say that the hypothesis is either probably true or probably false. Statistical inferences are based on incomplete information; hence, there is always a risk of making an error.

A researcher can make two types of error: (1) rejection of a true null hypothesis or (2) acceptance of a false null hypothesis. Figure 13-7 summarizes the possible outcomes of a researcher's decision. An investigator makes a **Type I error** by rejecting the null hypothesis when it is, in fact, true. For instance, if we concluded that the experimental treatment was effective in promoting breastfeeding when, in fact, group differences were due to sampling error, we would have made a Type I error. In the reverse situation, we might conclude that observed differences in breastfeeding were due to random sampling fluctuations when, in fact, the experimental treatment did have an effect. Acceptance of a false null hypothesis is called a **Type II error.**

	The actual situation is that the null hypothesis is:	
	True	False
True (Null accepted)	Correct decision	Type II error
False (Null rejected)	Type I error	Correct decision

The researcher calculates a test statistic and decides that the null hypothesis is:

FIGURE 13-7. Outcomes of statistical decision making.

CONSUMER TIP

Type II errors are especially likely to occur when small samples are used to estimate population values. If a research report indicates that a research hypothesis was not supported by the data, consider whether a Type II error might have occurred as a result of inadequate sample size. ■

Level of Significance

The researcher does not know when an error in statistical decision making has been committed. The validity of a null hypothesis could only be ascertained by collecting data from the population, in which case there would be no need for statistical inference.

The degree of risk in making a Type I error is controlled by the researcher, who selects a **level of significance.** Level of significance is the phrase used to signify the probability of making a Type I error. The two most frequently used levels of significance (referred to as **alpha** or α) are .05 and .01. With a .05 significance level, we accept the risk that of 100 samples, a true null hypothesis would be rejected 5 times. In 95 of 100 cases, however, a true null hypothesis would be correctly accepted. With a .01 significance level, the risk of making a Type I error is lower; in only 1 sample of 100 would we erroneously reject the null hypothesis. By convention, the minimal acceptable alpha level for scientific research is .05.

Naturally, researchers would like to reduce the risk of committing both types of error. Unfortunately, lowering the risk of a Type I error increases the risk of a Type II error. The stricter the criterion for rejecting a null hypothesis, the greater the probability of accepting a false null hypothesis. However, researchers can reduce the risk of a Type II error simply by increasing their sample size.*

Tests of Statistical Significance

Within a hypothesis testing framework, the researcher uses study data to compute a **test statistic.** For every test statistic, there is a related theoretical sampling distribution, analogous to the sampling distribution of means. Hypothesis testing uses theoretical distributions to establish probable and improbable values for the test statistics, which are, in turn, used as a basis for accepting or rejecting the null hypothesis.

A simple example will illustrate the process. Suppose we wanted to test the hypothesis that the average SAT score for students applying to nursing schools is higher than that for all other students taking the SAT, whose mean score is 500. The null hypothesis is that there is no difference in the mean population scores of students who do or do not apply to nursing school. Let us say that the mean score for a sample of 100 nursing school applicants is

---

* The risk of committing a Type II error can be estimated through power analysis. In many nursing studies, the risk of a Type II error is high because of small sample size, suggesting a need for greater use of power analysis among nurse researchers.

525, with an SD of 100. Using statistical procedures, we can test the null hypothesis that the mean of 525 is a chance fluctuation from the population mean of 500.

In hypothesis testing, researchers assume that the null hypothesis is true and then gather evidence to disprove it. Assuming a mean of 500 for the nursing school applicant population, a sampling distribution can be constructed with a mean of 500 and an SD equal to 10. In this example, 10 is the SEM, calculated from a formula that used the sample SD of 100 for a sample of 100 students. This is shown in Figure 13-8. Based on normal distribution characteristics, we can determine probable and improbable values of sample means from the nursing school applicant population. If, as is assumed, the population mean is actually 500, 95% of all sample means would fall between 480 and 520 because 95% of the cases are within 2 SDs of the mean. The obtained sample mean of 525 lies in the region considered improbable if the null hypothesis is correct, assuming that our criterion of improbability is an alpha level of .05. The improbable range beyond 2 SDs corresponds to only 5% (100%–95%) of the sampling distribution. We would thus reject the null hypothesis that the mean of the nursing school applicant population equals 500. We would not be justified in saying that we have proved the research hypothesis because the possibility of having made a Type I error remains.

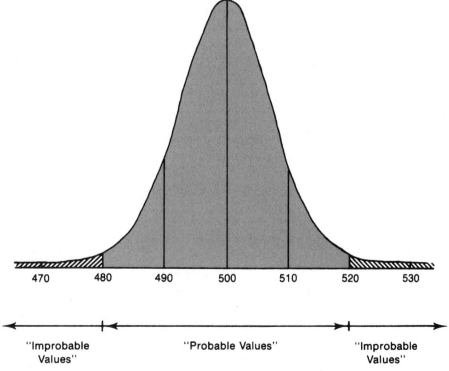

FIGURE 13-8. Sampling distribution for hypothesis testing example of SAT scores.

Researchers reporting the results of hypothesis tests state that their findings are **statistically significant.** The word *significant* should not be read as important or meaningful. In statistics, the term *significant* means that obtained results are not likely to have been due to chance, at some specified level of probability. A **nonsignificant result** means that any observed difference or relationship could have been the result of a chance fluctuation.

CONSUMER TIP

Inferential statistics are usually more difficult to understand than descriptive statistics. It may help to keep in mind that inferential statistics are just a tool to help us evaluate whether the results are likely to be real and replicable, or simply spurious. As recommended in Chapter 3, you can overcome much of the abstruseness of the results section by translating the basic thrust of the research findings into everyday language. ■

Parametric and Nonparametric Tests

The bulk of the tests that we discuss in this chapter—and also most tests used by researchers—are **parametric tests.** Parametric tests are characterized by three attributes: (1) they focus on population parameters; (2) they require measurements on at least an interval scale; and (3) they involve other assumptions about the variables under consideration, such as the assumption that the variables are normally distributed in the population.

Nonparametric tests, by contrast, are not based on the estimation of parameters and involve less restrictive assumptions about the shape of the distribution of the critical variables. Nonparametric tests are usually applied when the data have been measured on a nominal or ordinal scale.

Parametric tests are more powerful than nonparametric tests and are generally preferred when variables are measured on at least the interval scale. Nonparametric tests are most useful when the data under consideration cannot in any manner be construed as interval measures or when the data distribution is markedly nonnormal.

Overview of Hypothesis Testing Procedures

In the next section, various statistical procedures for testing research hypotheses are discussed. The emphasis is on explaining applications of statistical tests and on interpreting their meaning rather than on computations.

Each statistical test described in this chapter has a particular application and can be used only with particular kinds of data; however, the overall process of testing hypotheses is basically the same for all tests. The steps that a researcher takes are the following:

1. *Determining which test statistic to use.* The researcher must consider such factors as whether a parametric test is justified, which levels of measurement were used for the measures, and, if relevant, how many groups are being compared.

2. *Selecting the level of significance.* A level of .05 is usually acceptable, but, in some cases, the level is set more stringently at .01 or .001.
3. *Computing a test statistic.* The researcher then calculates a test statistic based on the collected data, using appropriate computation formulas.
4. *Calculating degrees of freedom.* The term **degrees of freedom** (***df***) is used throughout hypothesis testing to refer to the number of observations free to vary about a parameter. The concept is too complex for full elaboration here, but the computation of degrees of freedom is easy.
5. *Comparing the test statistic to a tabled value.* Theoretical distributions have been developed for all test statistics, and values for these distributions are available in tables. The tabled values enable the researcher to determine whether the computed test statistic value is beyond what is probable if the null hypothesis is true. The researcher examines a table for the test used, obtains a tabled value corresponding to the relevant degrees of freedom and significance level, and compares the tabled value to the computed test statistic. If the tabled value is smaller than the absolute value of the test statistic, the results are statistically significant; if the tabled value is larger, the results are nonsignificant.

When a computer is used for the analysis, the researcher follows only the first step and then gives the necessary commands to the computer. The computer calculates the test statistic, degrees of freedom, and the *actual* probability that the relationship being tested is due to chance. For example, the computer may print that the probability (*p*) of an experimental group doing better on a measure of postoperative recovery than the control group on the basis of chance alone is .025. This means that fewer than 3 times of 100 (or only 25 times of 1000) would a group difference of the size observed occur by chance. This computed probability can then be compared with the desired level of significance. In the present example, if the significance level were .05, the results would be significant because .025 is more stringent than .05. If .01 was the significance level, the results would be nonsignificant (sometimes abbreviated *NS*). Any computed probability level greater than .05 (*e.g.,* .20) indicates a nonsignificant relationship (*i.e.,* one that could have occurred on the basis of chance in more than 5 of 100 samples). In the section that follows, several specific statistical tests and their applications are described.

BIVARIATE STATISTICAL TESTS

You will find that researchers use a wide variety of statistical tests to make inferences about the validity of their hypotheses. Some of the most frequently used bivariate tests are briefly described and illustrated below.

t-Tests

A common research situation is the comparison of two groups of people on a dependent variable. The appropriate procedure for testing the statistical significance of a difference between the means of two groups is the parametric test known as the **t-test.**

Suppose a researcher wanted to test the effect of early discharge of maternity patients on their perceived maternal competence. The researcher administers a scale of perceived maternal competence 1 week after delivery to 10 primiparas who were discharged early (*i.e.,* within 24 hours of delivery) and to 10 others who remained in the hospital for longer periods. Some hypothetical data for this example are presented in Table 13-8. The mean scores for the two groups are 19.0 and 25.0, respectively. Is this difference a true population difference—is it likely to be replicated in other samples of early-discharge and later-discharge mothers? Or is the group difference just the result of chance fluctuations? The 20 scores, 10 for each group, vary from one person to another. Some variability reflects individual differences in perceived maternal competence. Some of the variability could also be due to measurement error (unreliability of the researcher's scale), some could be the result of the participants' moods on that particular day, and so forth. The research question is: Can a significant portion of the variability be attributed to the independent variable—time of discharge from the hospital? The *t*-test allows the researcher to answer this question objectively.

The formula for the *t* statistic uses group means, sample size, and variability to calculate a value for *t*. In the present example, the computed value of *t* is 2.86. Next, degrees of freedom are calculated. Here, the degrees of freedom are equal to the total sample size minus 2 ($df = 20 - 2 = 18$). Then, the tabled value for *t* with 18 degrees of freedom is determined. For a level of .05, the tabled value of *t* is 2.10. *This value establishes an upper limit to what is probable if the null hypothesis is true.* Thus, the calculated *t* of 2.86, which is larger than the tabled value of the statistic, is improbable (*i.e.,* statistically signifi-

---

TABLE 13-8. Fictitious Data for *t*-Test Example: Scores on a Perceived Maternal Competence Scale for Two Groups of Mothers

REGULAR-DISCHARGE MOTHERS	EARLY-DISCHARGE MOTHERS
30	23
27	17
25	22
20	18
24	20
32	26
17	16
18	13
28	21
29	14
Mean = 25.0	Mean = 19.0

$t = 2.86; df = 18; p < .05$

cant). We are now in a position to say that the primiparas discharged early had significantly lower perceptions of maternal competence than those who were not discharged early. The group difference in perceived maternal competence is sufficiently large that it is unlikely to reflect merely chance fluctuations. In fewer than 5 of 100 samples would a difference this great be found by chance alone.

The situation we just described calls for an **independent groups *t*-test:** The study participants in the two groups were different people, independent of each other. There are certain situations for which this type of test is not appropriate. For example, if means for a single group of people measured before and after an intervention were being compared, the researcher would compute a **paired *t*-test** (also known as a **dependent groups *t*-test**), using a different formula.

⊞ *Example of a t-test:*

Table 13-9 presents the results of four independent t-tests from a study that compared the psychosocial adjustment of children diagnosed with inflammatory bowel disease (IBD) with that of children with functional gastrointestinal complaints (FGI) (Gold et al., 2000). Three standardized tests were administered to capture children's psychosocial adjustment: (1) the Children Behaviour Checklist to measure social competence and behaviour problems, (2) the Children's Depression Inventory to measure depression, and (3) the Piers-Harris Children's Self-Concept Scale to measure self-concept. Children with FGI complaints were significantly more depressed ($p = .03$), had a less defined self-concept ($p = .01$), and had more behaviour problems than those with IBD ($p = .02$).

TABLE 13-9. Example of a Table with *t*-Tests: Inflamatory Bowel Disease and Functional Gastrointestinal Complaints Study

	INFLAMMATORY BOWEL DISEASE		FUNCTIONAL GASTROINTESTINAL COMPLAINTS			STATISTIC	
	Mean	SD	Mean	SD	N	t	p
Children's Depression Inventory	4.81	3.98	7.50	5.78	62	2.2	.034
Piers-Harris Children's Self-Concept Scale	64.61	8.44	60.35	11.86	62	2.7	.01
Children Behaviour Checklist-social competence	46.35	7.92	49.17	8.79	54	1.2	.22
Children Behaviour Checklist-behaviour problems	51.57	10.29	58.73	12.37	61	2.5	.02

Adapted from Gold, N., Issenman, R., Roberts, J., & Watt, S. (2000). Well-adjusted children: An alternate view of children with inflammatory bowel disease and functional gastrointestinal complaints. *Inflammatory Bowel Diseases, 6*(1), 1–7.

Analysis of Variance

Analysis of variance (ANOVA) is a parametric procedure used to test mean group differences of three or more groups. The statistic computed in an ANOVA is the **F ratio.** ANOVA decomposes the total variability of a dependent variable into two components: variability attributable to the independent variable and variability due to all other sources (*e.g.,* individual differences, measurement error). Variation between groups is contrasted with variation within groups to yield an F ratio.

Suppose we wanted to compare the effectiveness of different instructional techniques to teach high school students about AIDS. One group of students is exposed to a film on AIDS, a second group is given a special lecture, and a third control group receives no special instruction. The dependent variable is the student's score on the AIDS knowledge test the day after the intervention. The null hypothesis is that the group population means for AIDS knowledge test scores are the same, whereas the research hypothesis predicts that they are different.

The 60 test scores shown in Table 13-1 are reproduced in Table 13-10, according to treatment group. As Table 13-10 shows, there is variation from one student to the next within a group, and there are also group differences. The mean test scores are 25.35, 24.75, and 20.35 for groups A, B, and C, respectively. These means are different, but are they significantly different? Or do the differences reflect random fluctuations?

An ANOVA applied to these data yields an F ratio of 18.64. In ANOVA, two types of degrees of freedom are calculated: between groups (the number of groups minus 1) and within groups (the total number of subjects minus the

TABLE 13-10. Fictitious Data for One-Way ANOVA: Instructional Mode Effects on AIDS Knowledge Test Scores

FILM GROUP (A)		LECTURE GROUP (B)		CONTROL GROUP (C)	
26	25	22	24	15	33
20	29	24	25	26	19
16	30	27	21	24	20
25	27	23	27	18	22
25	29	23	25	20	18
23	28	26	21	20	24
26	26	22	24	19	18
25	25	24	29	21	23
24	27	24	28	17	20
23	28	30	26	17	24
Mean 25.35		24.75		20.35	

$F = 18.64$; $df = 2.57$; $p < .001$.

number of groups). In this example, then, $df = 2$ and 57. In a table of values for a theoretical F distribution, we would find that the value of F for 2 and 57 df, for an alpha of .05, is 3.16. Because our obtained F value of 18.64 exceeds 3.16, we reject the null hypothesis that the population means are equal. The observed group differences in mean test scores would be obtained by chance in fewer than 5 samples of 100. (Actually, the probability of achieving an F of 18.64 by chance is less than 1 in 1000.) In research reports, tables displaying ANOVA results are usually organized in a format similar to that used in Table 13-9 for t-tests, with descriptive statistics on the dependent variables for the groups being compared, followed by the value of the test statistic (F) and the probability level.

The data in our example support the hypothesis that the instructional interventions affect students' knowledge about AIDS, but we cannot tell from these results whether treatment A was significantly more effective than treatment B. Statistical analyses known as **multiple comparison procedures** (also called *post hoc* **tests**) are needed. The function of these procedures is to isolate the comparisons between group means that are responsible for rejecting the overall ANOVA null hypothesis. Note that it is *not* appropriate to use a series of t-tests (group A versus B, A versus C, and B versus C) in this situation because this would increase the risk of a Type I error.

Example of an ANOVA:

Wilson (2002) studied dependency in dying persons in relation to the setting of the person's care. Three groups of patients who died were compared using ANOVA: (a) hospital inpatients, (b) home care patients who died at home, and (c) home care patients who died in the hospital. Wilson found that the mean number of days of total dependency was highest among the transferred (group c) patients (mean = 81.3), and was especially high compared with the hospital inpatients (mean = 13.8). The ANOVA F test was significant beyond the .01 level.

ANOVA also can be used to test the effect of two (or more) independent variables on a dependent variable (*e.g.*, when a factorial experimental design has been used). Suppose we wanted to determine whether the two instructional techniques discussed previously were equally effective in helping first year and second year high school students acquire knowledge about AIDS. We could set up a design in which first year and second year would be randomly assigned, separately, to the two modes of instruction. Some hypothetical data, shown in Table 13-11, reveal the following about two **main effects:** On average, people in the film group scored higher than those in the lecture group (25.35 versus 24.75), and second year students scored higher than first year students (26.20 versus 23.90). In addition, there is an **interaction effect:** First year students scored higher when exposed to the lecture, whereas second year students scored higher when exposed to the film. By performing a **two-way ANOVA** on these data, it would be possible to ascertain the statistical significance of these differences.

TABLE 13-11. Fictitious Data for Two-Way (2 × 2) ANOVA Example: Instructional Mode and Year in School in Relation to Test Scores

YEAR IN SCHOOL	INSTRUCTIONAL MODE						
	Film			Lecture			
First year	26	20	$\bar{X} = 23.3$	22	24	$\bar{X} = 24.5$	First year mean = 23.90
	16	25		27	33		
	25	23		23	26		
	26	25		22	24		
	24	23		24	30		
Second year	25	29	$\bar{X} = 27.4$	24	25	$\bar{X} = 25.0$	Second year mean = 26.20
	30	27		21	27		
	29	28		27	25		
	26	25		21	24		
	27	28		28	26		
Film group mean	25.35		Lecture group mean	24.75			Grand mean = 25.05

A type of ANOVA known as **repeated measures ANOVA** is often used when the means being compared are means at different points in time (*e.g.,* mean blood pressure at 2, 4, and 6 hours after surgery). This is analogous to a dependent groups *t*-test, extended to three or more points of data collection, because it is the same people being measured multiple times. When two or more groups are measured several times, a repeated measures ANOVA provides information about a main effect for time (do the measures differ significantly over time?); a main effect for groups (do the group means differ significantly?); and an interaction effect (do the groups differ more at certain times?).

> **CONSUMER TIP**
>
> Experimental repeated measures designs (see Chap. 8) call for either a dependent groups *t*-test or a repeated measures ANOVA because the same people are measured more than once after being randomly assigned to a different ordering of treatments. However, repeated measures ANOVA can also be used in studies that do not involve an experimental repeated measures design if outcomes are measured more than once. ■

Chi-Squared Test

The **chi-squared** (χ^2) **test** is a nonparametric procedure used to test hypotheses about the proportion of cases that fall into various categories, as when a contingency table has been created. Consider the following example. A researcher is interested in studying the effect of planned nursing instruction on patients' compliance with a self-medication regimen. The experimental group is instructed by nurses who are implementing a new instructional approach based on Orem's Self-Care Model. A second (control) group of patients is cared for by nurses who continue their usual mode of instruction. The research hypothesis is that a higher proportion of people in the experimental than in the control group will comply with the regimen. Some hypothetical data for this example are presented in Table 13-12.

The chi-squared statistic is computed by summing differences between the observed frequencies in each cell and frequencies that would be expected if there were no relationship between the independent and dependent variable. In this example, the value of the computed chi-squared statistic is 18.18, which we can compare with the value from a theoretical chi-squared distribution. For the chi-squared statistic, the degrees of freedom are equal to the number of rows minus 1 times the number of columns minus 1. In the present case, $df = 1 \times 1$, or 1. With one degree of freedom, the value that must be exceeded to establish significance at the .05 level is 3.84. The obtained value of 18.18 is substantially larger than would be expected by chance. Thus, we can conclude that a significantly larger proportion of patients in the experimental group (60%) than in the control group (30%) were compliant.

Example of a chi-squared test:

King (2000) compared males and females in their recovery following cardiac surgery over a 3-month period. Throughout the study, the two groups differed on several characteristics. For example, at 1 month postoperatively women were significantly more likely than men to experience angina ($\chi^2 = 5.24$, $p = .02$) and shortness of breath ($\chi^2 = 4.62$, $p = .03$).

Correlation Coefficients

Pearson's r is both descriptive and inferential. As a descriptive statistic, r summarizes the magnitude and direction of a relationship between two variables. As an inferential statistic, r is used to test hypotheses about population correlations. The null hypothesis is that there is no relationship between two variables of interest.

TABLE 13-12. Observed Frequencies for a Chi-Squared Example On Patient Compliance

	EXPERIMENTAL	CONTROL	TOTAL
Compliant	60	30	90
Noncompliant	40	70	110
TOTAL	100	100	200

$\chi^2 = 18.18$; $df = 1$; $p < .001$.

Suppose we were studying the relationship between patients' self-reported level of stress (higher scores imply more stress) and the pH level of their saliva. With a sample of 50 patients, we find that $r = -.29$. This value indicates a tendency for people with high stress scores to have lower pH levels than those with low stress scores. But we need to ask whether this finding can be generalized to the population. Does the coefficient of $-.29$ reflect a random fluctuation, observed only in this particular sample, or is the relationship significant? Degrees of freedom for correlation coefficients are equal to the number of participants minus 2, or 48 in this example. In a statistical table for correlation coefficients, the tabled value for r with $df = 48$ and a .05 significance level is .282. Because the absolute value of the calculated r is .29 and thus larger than .282, the null hypothesis can be rejected. There is a significant, modest relationship between patients' self-reported level of stress and the acidity of their saliva.

Example of correlation coefficients:

Forchuk et al. (2002) described the relationships between smoking behaviour and severity of psychiatric symptoms among individuals with schizophrenia. The researchers reported, among other things, that both addiction ($r = .30$, $p < .01$) and automatic (habit) behaviour ($r = .33$, $p < .01$) scores were positively related to severity of psychiatric symptoms.

Guide to Bivariate Statistical Tests

The selection and use of a statistical test depends on several factors, such as the number of groups and the levels of measurement of the research variables. To aid you in evaluating the appropriateness of statistical procedures used in studies, a chart summarizing the major features of several tests is presented in Table 13-13. This table does not include every test you may encounter in research reports, but it does include the bivariate statistical tests most often used by nurse researchers.

MULTIVARIATE STATISTICAL ANALYSIS

Nurse researchers have become increasingly sophisticated, and many now use complex **multivariate statistics** to analyze their data. We use the term *multivariate* to refer to analyses dealing with at least three—but usually many more—variables simultaneously. This evolution has resulted in increased rigour in nursing studies, but one unfortunate side effect is that it is becoming more challenging for novice consumers to understand research reports.

Given the introductory nature of this text and the fact that many of you are not proficient with even basic statistical procedures, it is not possible to describe in detail the complex analytic procedures that now appear in nursing journals. However, we present some basic information that might assist you in reading reports in which two commonly used multivariate statistics are used: multiple regression and analysis of covariance (ANCOVA).

TABLE 13-13. Guide to Widely Used Bivariate Statistical Tests

NAME	TEST STATISTIC	PURPOSE	MEASUREMENT LEVEL* IV	DV
PARAMETRIC TESTS				
t-Test for independent groups	*t*	To test the difference between two independent group means	Nominal	Interval, ratio
t-Test for dependent groups	*t*	To test the difference between two dependent groups means	Nominal	Interval, ratio
Analysis of variance (ANOVA)	*F*	To test the difference among the means of three or more independent groups, or of more than one independent variable	Nominal	Interval, ratio
Repeated measures ANOVA	*F*	To test the difference among means of three or more related groups or sets of scores	Nominal	Interval, ratio
Pearson's *r*	*r*	To test the existence of a relationship between two variables	Interval, ratio	Interval, ratio
NONPARAMETRIC TESTS				
Chi-squared test	χ^2	To test the difference in proportions in two or more independent groups	Nominal	Nominal
Mann-Whitney *U*-test	*U*	To test the difference in ranks of scores on two independent groups	Nominal	Ordinal
Kruskal-Wallis test	*H*	To test the difference in ranks of scores of three or more independent groups	Nominal	Ordinal
Wilcoxon signed ranks test	*T(Z)*	To test the difference in ranks of scores of two related groups	Nominal	Ordinal
Friedman test	χ^2	To test the difference in ranks of scores of three or more related groups	Nominal	Ordinal
Phi coefficient	ϕ	To test the magnitude of a relationship between two dichotomous variables	Nominal	Nominal
Spearman's rank-order correlation	r_s	To test the existence of a relationship between two variables	Ordinal	Ordinal

*Measurement level of the independent variable (IV) and dependent variables (DV).

Multiple Regression

Correlations enable researchers to make predictions. For example, if the correlation between SAT scores and grades in a nursing program were .60, nursing school administrators could make predictions—albeit imperfect predictions—about applicants' future academic performance. Because two variables are rarely perfectly correlated, researchers often strive to improve their ability to predict a dependent variable by including more than one independent variable in the analysis. For example, a researcher might predict that an infant's birth weight is related to the amount of prenatal care the mother received. The researcher could collect data on birth weight and number of prenatal visits and then compute a correlation coefficient to determine whether a significant relationship between the two variables exists (*i.e.,* whether prenatal care could help predict infant birth weight). Birth weight is affected by many other factors, however, such as gestational period and mothers' nutritional practices during the pregnancy and their smoking behaviour. Many researchers, therefore, perform an analysis called **multiple regression analysis** (or **multiple correlation analysis**) that allows them to use more than one independent variable to explain or predict a dependent variable. (In multiple regression, the dependent variables are interval- or ratio-level variables. Independent variables are either interval- or ratio-level variables or dichotomous nominal-level variables, such as male/female.)

When several independent variables are used to predict a dependent variable, the resulting statistic is the **multiple correlation coefficient,** symbolized as **R.** Unlike the bivariate correlation coefficient *r*, R does not have negative values. R varies from .00 to 1.00, showing the *strength* of the relationship between several independent variables and a dependent variable, but not *direction.*

There are several ways of evaluating R. One is to determine whether R is statistically significant, that is, whether the overall relationship between the independent variables and the dependent variable is likely to be real or the result of chance sampling fluctuations. This is done through the computation of an F statistic that can be compared with tabled F values.

A second way of evaluating R is to determine whether the addition of new independent variables adds further predictive power. For example, a researcher might find that the R between infant birth weight on the one hand and maternal weight and prenatal care on the other is .30. By adding a third independent variable—let's say maternal smoking behaviour—R might increase to .36. Is the increase from .30 to .36 statistically significant? In other words, does knowing whether the mother smoked during her pregnancy improve our understanding of the birth-weight outcome, or does the increased R value simply reflect a relationship peculiar to this sample of women? Multiple regression procedures provide a way of answering this question.

The magnitude of the R statistic is also informative. Researchers would like to predict a dependent variable perfectly. In the birth-weight example, if it were possible to identify all the factors that lead to differences in infants' weight, the researcher could collect the relevant data to obtain an R of 1.00. Usually, the value of R in a nursing research study is much smaller, seldom higher than .60. An interesting feature of the R statistic is that, when squared, it can be interpreted as the proportion of the variability in the dependent variable accounted for by the independent variables. If a researcher predicting infant birth weight achieved an R of .80 ($R^2 = .64$), we could say that the independent variables accounted for nearly two thirds (64%) of the variability in infants' birth weights. One third of the variability, however, is caused by factors not identified or measured. Researchers usually report multiple correlation results in terms of R^2 rather than R.

Multiple regressions yield information about how each independent variable is related to the dependent variable. Although it is beyond our scope to explain how to read multiple regression tables, you should recognize that multiple regression analysis indicates whether an independent variable is significantly related to the dependent variable *even when* the other independent variables are controlled. Let us assume that our birth-weight researcher used 10 independent variables to predict or explain infant birth weight. If the amount of prenatal care received during pregnancy continued to be significantly related to the birth-weight outcome, this would mean that prenatal care was truly correlated with birth weight even with the other nine variables (which might be the extraneous variables) controlled. The example in the next section explains this concept in greater detail.

Example of multiple regression:

Duncan et al. (2001) examined predictors of emotional abuse experienced by nurses practicing in Alberta and British Columbia. Multiple regression was used to predict emotional abuse from personal, interpersonal, and organizational variables. The value of R was .36. Thus, the identified variables accounted for 13.2% of the variability in emotional abuse (*i.e.*, $R^2 = .132$).

Analysis of Covariance

Analysis of covariance (ANCOVA), which is essentially a combination of ANOVA and multiple regression, is used to control extraneous variables statistically. This approach can be especially valuable in certain types of research situations, such as when a nonequivalent control group design is used. The initial equivalence of the experimental and comparison groups in these studies is always questionable; thus, the researcher must consider whether the results were influenced by preexisting group differences. When experimental control through randomization is lacking, ANCOVA offers the possibility of *post hoc* statistical control.

Because the concept of statistical control may mystify you, we will explain the underlying principle with a simple illustration. Suppose we were interested in testing the effectiveness of a special training program on physical fitness, using as subjects the employees of two companies. Employees of one company receive the experimental physical fitness intervention, and those of the second company do not. The employees' score on a physical fitness test is the dependent variable. The research question is: Can some of the individual differences in performance on the physical fitness test be attributed to participation in the special program? Physical fitness is also related to other, extraneous characteristics of the study participants (*e.g.*, their age)—characteristics that might differ between the two intact groups.

Figure 13-9 illustrates how ANCOVA works. The large circles represent total variability (*i.e.*, the total extent of individual differences) in physical fitness scores for both groups. A certain amount of variability can be explained by age differences: Younger people tend to perform better on the test than older ones. This relationship is represented by the overlapping small circle on the left in part A of Figure 13-9. Another part of the variability can be explained by participation in the physical fitness program, represented here by the overlapping small circle on the right. In part A, the fact that the two small circles (age and program participation) themselves overlap indicates that there is a relationship between these two variables. In other words, people in the experimental group are, on average, either older or younger than those in the comparison group. Because of this relationship, which could distort the results of the study, age should be controlled.

ANCOVA can accomplish this by statistically removing the effect of the extraneous variable (age) on physical fitness. This is designated in part A of Figure 13-9 by the darkened area of the large circle. Part B illustrates that the analysis would examine the effect of program participation on fitness scores *after* removing the effect of age (called a **covariate** in ANCOVA). With the variability associated with age removed, we get a more precise estimate of the training program's effect on physical fitness. Note that even after removing variability resulting from age, there is still individual variability not associated with program participation (the bottom half of the large circle) that is not explained. This means that analytic precision could be further enhanced

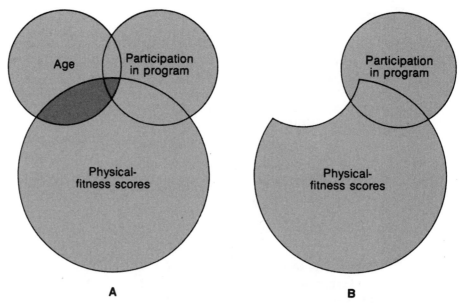

FIGURE 13-9. Schematic diagram illustrating the principle of analysis of covariance.

by controlling additional extraneous variables (*e.g.,* nutritional habits, smoking status). ANCOVA can accommodate multiple extraneous variables.

ANCOVA tests the significance of differences between group means after adjusting scores on the dependent variable to eliminate the effect of the covariates. This adjustment uses multiple regression procedures. The ANCOVA procedure produces *F* statistics—one for evaluating the significance of the covariates and another for evaluating the significance of group differences—that can be compared with tabled values of *F* to determine whether to accept or reject the null hypothesis. ANCOVA, like multiple regression analysis, is an extremely powerful and useful analytic technique for controlling extraneous or confounding influences on dependent measures.

Example of ANCOVA:

Johnston et al. (in press) studied the efficacy of maternal skin-to-skin contact—called kangaroo care (KC)—for lowering preterm infants' pain responses to heel lance. In the experimental group, infants were held in KC for 30 minutes prior to heelstick and remained in KC for the duration of the procedure. In the control group, infants were in a prone position in the isolette. ANCOVA was used to control for group differences with respect to extraneous characteristics such as severity of illness, order of exposure to the intervention, and study sites. The analyses revealed that, after adjusting for extraneous factors, infants in the KC group had significantly lower pain scores than infants in the control group.

Other Multivariate Techniques

Several other related multivariate techniques increasingly are being used in nursing studies. We mention these techniques briefly to acquaint you with terms you might encounter in the research literature.

Discriminant Function Analysis

In multiple regression analysis, the dependent variable is a measure on either the interval or ratio scale. **Discriminant function analysis** is used to make predictions about membership in groups, that is, about a dependent variable measured on the nominal scale. For example, a researcher might wish to use several independent variables to predict membership in such groups as complying versus noncomplying cancer patients, overweight versus normal-weight people, or normal pregnancies versus those terminating in a miscarriage. In discriminant function analysis, as in multiple regression, the independent variables are either interval- or ratio-level measures or dichotomous nominal variables (*e.g.,* smoker versus nonsmoker).

Logistic Regression

Logistic regression (or **logit analysis**) analyzes the relationships between multiple independent variables and a nominal-level dependent variable. It is thus used in situations similar to discriminant function analysis, but it uses a different statistical estimation procedure that many prefer for nominal-level dependent variables. Logistic regression transforms the probability of an event occurring (*e.g.*, that a woman will practise breast self-examination or not) into its **odds** (*i.e.*, into the ratio of one event's probability relative to the probability of a second event). After further transformations, the analysis examines the relationship of the independent variables to the transformed dependent variable. For each predictor, the logistic regression yields an **odds ratio,** which is the factor by which the odds change for a unit change in the predictors.

Example of logistic regression:

Bottorff et al. (2002) used logistic regression to explore whether sociodemographic and other factors predict women's interest in genetic testing for breast cancer risk. Their analysis revealed that the one variable that significantly differentiated women with and without an interest in genetic testing was a family history of breast cancer. The odds ratio for having at least one first- or second-degree relative with breast cancer was 2.34, indicating that women with a close relative with breast cancer were nearly 2½ times more likely to express interest in genetic testing than those with no reported family history.

Factor Analysis

Factor analysis is widely used by researchers seeking to develop, refine, or validate complex instruments. The major purpose of factor analysis is to reduce a large set of variables into a smaller, more manageable set. Factor analysis disentangles complex interrelationships among variables and identifies which variables go together as unified concepts or factors. For example, suppose a researcher has prepared 50 Likert statements aimed at measuring women's attitudes toward menopause. It would not be appropriate to combine all 50 items to form a scale score because there are various dimensions, or themes, to women's attitudes toward menopause. One dimension may relate to the issue of aging, another may concern the loss of ability to reproduce, and so on. These various dimensions should serve as the basis for subscale construction, and factor analysis offers an objective, empirical method for doing so.

Example of factor analysis:

Rosberger et al. (2002) carried out a factor analysis to identify the main dimensions of coping, using the Ways of Coping Questionnaire, in a sample of 235 oncology patients 6 months after diagnosis. Three factors were identified: positive problem solving, escape/avoidance, and seeking social support.

Multivariate Analysis of Variance

Multivariance analysis of variance (MANOVA) is the extension of ANOVA to more than one dependent variable. This procedure is used to test the significance of differences between the means of two or more groups on two or more dependent variables, considered simultaneously. For instance, if a researcher wanted to examine the effect of two methods of exercise treatment on both diastolic and systolic blood pressure, then a MANOVA would be appropriate. Covariates can also be included, in which case the analysis would be called a **multivariate analysis of covariance (MANCOVA).**

Causal Modeling

Causal modeling involves the development and statistical testing of a hypothesized explanation of the causes of a phenomenon. **Path analysis,** which is based on multiple regression, is a widely used approach to causal modeling. Alternative methods of testing causal models are also being used by nurse researchers, the most important of which is **linear structural relations analysis,** more widely known as **LISREL.** Both LISREL and path analysis are highly complex statistical techniques whose utility relies on a sound underlying causal theory.

Guide to Multivariate Statistical Analyses

In selecting a multivariate analysis, the researcher must attend to such issues as the number of independent variables, the number of dependent variables, the measurement level of all variables, and the desirability of controlling extraneous variables. Table 13-14 is an aid to help you evaluate the appropriateness of multivariate statistics used in research reports. This chart includes the major multivariate analyses used by nurse researchers.

READING AND INTERPRETING STATISTICAL INFORMATION

Statistical findings are communicated in the results section of a research report and are reported in the text as well as in tables (or, less frequently, figures). This section provides some assistance in reading and interpreting statistical information.

Tips on Reading Text With Statistical Information

There are usually three types of information reported in the results section. First, there are descriptive statistics (such as those shown in Table 13-4), which typically provide readers with a basic overview of the participants' characteristics and their performance on the dependent variables. Information about the subjects' background characteristics enables readers to draw conclusions about the groups to which the findings might be generalized. Second, some researchers provide statistical information that enables readers to evaluate the extent of any biases. For example, researchers sometimes compare the characteristics of people who did and did not agree to participate in the study (*e.g.,* using *t*-tests). Or, in a quasi-experimental design, evidence of the preintervention comparability of the experimental and comparison groups might be presented so that readers can evaluate the study's internal

TABLE 13-14. Guide to Widely Used Multivariate Statistical Analyses

| NAME | PURPOSE | MEASUREMENT LEVEL* | | | NUMBER OF: | | |
		IV	DV	COV	IVs	DVs	COVs
Multiple correlation, regression	To test the relationship between two or more IVs and 1 DV; to predict a DV from two or more IVs	N, I, R	I, R		2+	1	
Analysis of covariance (ANCOVA)	To test the difference between the means of two or more groups, while controlling for one or more covariate	N	I, R	N, I, R	1+	1	1+
Multivariate analysis of variance (MANOVA)	To test the difference between the means of two or more groups for two or more DVs simultaneously	N	I, R		1+	2+	
Multivariate analysis of covariance (MANCOVA)	To test the difference between the means of two or more groups for two or more DVs simultaneously, while controlling for one or more covariate	N	I, R	N, I, R	1+	2+	1+
Factor analysis	To determine the dimensionality or structure of a set of variables						
Discriminant analysis	To test the relationship between two or more IVs and one DV; to predict group membership; to classify cases into groups	N, I, R	N		2+	1	
Logistic regression	To test the relationship between two or more IVs and one DV; to predict the probability of an event; to estimate relative risk (odds ratios)	N, I, R	N		2+	1	

*Measurement level of the independent variable (IV), dependent variable (DV), and covariates (Cov): N = nominal, I = interval, R = ratio.

validity. Finally, inferential statistics relating to the research questions or hypotheses are presented. If the findings do not support the researcher's hypotheses, further analyses might be undertaken to help unravel the meaning of the results.

The text of research reports normally tells the readers certain facts about the statistical tests that were performed, including (1) what test was used, (2) the actual value of the calculated statistic, (3) the degrees of freedom, and (4) the level of statistical significance. Examples of how the results of various statistical tests would likely be reported in the text are shown below.

1. *t*-test: $t = 1.68$; $df = 160$; $p = .09$
2. Chi-squared: $\chi^2 = 6.65$; $df = 2$; $p < .05$
3. Pearson's *r*: $r = .26$; $df = 100$; $p < .01$
4. ANOVA: $F = 0.18$; $df = 1, 69$, NS

Note that the significance level is sometimes reported as the actual computed probability that the null hypothesis is correct, as in example 1. In this case, the observed group differences could be found by chance in 9 of 100 samples; thus, this result is not statistically significant because the differences have an unacceptably high chance of being spurious. The probability level is sometimes reported simply as falling below or above the researchers' significance criterion, as in examples 2 and 3. In both cases, the results are statistically significant because the probability of obtaining such results by chance alone is less than 5 (or 1) in 100. Note that you need to be careful to read the symbol that follows the **p value** (the probability value) correctly: The symbol < means less than, that is, the results are statistically significant; the symbol > means greater than, that is, the results are not statistically significant. When results do not achieve statistical significance at the desired level, researchers simply may indicate that the results were not significant (NS), as in example 4.

Statistical information is normally noted parenthetically following a sentence describing the findings, as in the following example: The patients in the experimental group had a significantly lower rate of infection than those in the control group ($\chi^2 = 7.99$, $df = 1$, $p < .01$). In reading a research report, it is not important to absorb numeric information regarding the actual statistical test. For example, the actual value of χ^2 has no inherent interest. What is important is to grasp whether the statistical tests indicate that the research hypotheses are supported (as demonstrated by significant results) or not supported (as demonstrated by nonsignificant results).

Tips on Reading Statistical Tables

The use of tables in the results section allows the researcher to condense a considerable amount of statistical information into a compact space and also prevents redundancy. Consider, for example, putting information from a correlation matrix (see Table 13-7) into the text: "The correlation between nursing staff dose and nursing skill mix was $-.47$; the correlation between nursing staff dose and availability of professional role support was $-.41$. . . ."

Unfortunately, although tables are efficient, they may be daunting and difficult to decipher. Part of the problem is the lack of standardization in table preparation. There is no universally accepted method of presenting *t*-test information, for example, and so each table may present a new challenge. Another problem is that some researchers try to include an enormous amount of information in their tables; we deliberately used tables of relative simplicity and clarity as examples in this chapter.

We know of no magic solution for helping you to comprehend tables in research reports, but we have a few suggestions. First, read the text and the tables simultaneously because the text may help to unravel what the table is trying to communicate. Second, before trying to understand the numbers in a table, try to glean as much information as possible from the accompanying words. Table titles and footnotes often communicate critical pieces of information. The table headings should be carefully reviewed because these indicate what the variables in the analyses were (often listed in the far left-hand column of the table as row labels) and what statistical information is included (usually specified in the top row as the column headings). Third, you may find it helpful to consult the glossary of symbols in Box 13-1 to determine the meaning of a statistical symbol included in a report table. Note that not all symbols in Box 13-1 were described in this chapter; therefore, it may be necessary to refer to a statistics textbook, such as that of Polit (1996), for further information. We recommend that you devote some extra time to making sure you have grasped what the tables are conveying and that, for each table, you write out a sentence or two that summarizes some of the tabular information in "plain English."

CONSUMER TIP

In tables, probability levels associated with the significance tests are sometimes presented directly, as in Table 13-9. Here, the actual significance of each *t*-test is indicated in the last column, headed "*p*." However, researchers often indicate significance levels in tables through asterisks placed next to the value of the test statistic. By convention, one asterisk signifies $p < .05$, two asterisks signify $p < .01$, and three asterisks signify $p < .001$ (there is usually a key at the bottom of the table that indicates what the asterisks mean). Thus, if this system had been used in Table 13-9, the first *t* would have been presented as 2.2* (significant at or below the .05 level), the second *t* would have been shown as 2.7** (the .01 level), and the third *t* would have been shown as 1.2 with no asterisks (nonsignificant). ■

CRITIQUING QUANTITATIVE ANALYSES

For novice research consumers, it is often difficult to critique statistical analyses. We hope this chapter has helped to demystify what statistics are all about, but we also recognize the limited scope of this presentation. Although it would be unreasonable to expect you to now be adept at evaluating statistical analyses, there are certain things you should routinely look for in reviewing research reports. Some specific guidelines are presented in Box 13-2.

BOX 13-1 **GLOSSARY OF SELECTED STATISTICAL SYMBOLS**

This list contains some commonly used symbols in statistics. The list is in approximate alphabetical order, with English and Greek letters intermixed. Nonletter symbols have been placed at the end.

a Regression constant, the intercept

α Greek alpha; significance level in hypothesis testing, probability of Type I error

b Regression coefficient, slope of the line

β Greek beta, probability of a Type II error; also, a standardized regression coefficient (beta weight)

χ^2 Greek chi squared, a test statistic for several nonparametric tests

CI Confidence interval around estimate of a population parameter

df Degrees of freedom

η^2 Greek eta squared, index of variance accounted for in ANOVA context

f Frequency (count) for a score value

F Test statistic used in ANOVA, ANCOVA and other tests

H_0 Null hypothesis

H_1 Alternative hypothesis; research hypothesis

λ Greek lambda, a test statistic used in several multivariate analyses (Wilks' lambda)

μ Greek mu, the population mean

M Sample mean (alternative symbol For $\overline{X}$)

MS Mean square, variance estimate in ANOVA

n Number of cases in a subgroup of the sample

N Total number of cases or sample members

p Probability that observed data are consistent with null hypothesis

r Sample Pearson's product–moment correlation coefficient

r_s Spearman's rank-order correlation coefficient

R Multiple correlation coefficient

R^2 Coefficient of determination, proportion of variance in *dependent variable* attributable to *independent variables*

R_c Canonical correlation coefficient

ρ Greek rho, population correlation coefficient

SD Sample standard deviation

(continued)

BOX 13-1   *(Continued)*

SEM	Standard error of the mean
σ	Greek sigma (lowercase), population standard deviation
Σ	Greek sigma (uppercase), sum of
SS	Sum of squares
t	Test statistics used in *t*-tests (sometimes called Student's *t*)
U	Test statistic for the Mann-Whitney *U*-test
$\overline{X}$	Sample mean
x	Deviation score
Y'	Predicted value of Y, dependent variable in regression analysis
z	Standard score in a normal distribution
$\|\|$	Absolute value
$\leq$	Less than or equal to
$\geq$	Greater than or equal to
$\neq$	Not equal to

The first issue is whether the data and the research problem lend themselves to quantitative analysis. Not all information collected in research projects is quantitative, nor should it necessarily be converted to numbers. In Chapter 14, we discuss how researchers go about analyzing qualitative information.

Another aspect of the critique should focus on the decisions about what analyses to include in the report. Researchers generally perform many more analyses than can be reported in a short journal article. You should determine whether the reported statistical information adequately describes the sample and important research variables and reports the results of statistical tests for all hypotheses. You might also wish to consider whether the author included statistical information that was not really needed, given the stated aims of the study. Another presentational issue concerns the researcher's judicious use of tables to summarize statistical information.

A thorough critique also addresses whether the researcher used the appropriate statistical procedures. Tables 13-13 and 13-14 provide summaries of the most frequently used statistical tests—although we do not expect that you will readily be able to determine the appropriateness of the tests used in a study without further statistical instruction. The major issues to consider are

BOX 13-2   **GUIDELINES FOR CRITIQUING QUANTITATIVE ANALYSES**

1. Does the report include any descriptive statistics? Do these statistics sufficiently describe the major characteristics of the researcher's data set?

2. Were the correct descriptive statistics used (*e.g.,* were percentages reported when a mean would have been more informative)?

3. Does the report include any inferential statistical tests? If not, should it have (*e.g.,* were groups compared without information on the statistical significance of group differences)?

4. Was a statistical test performed for each of the hypotheses or research questions?

5. Do the selected statistical tests appear to be appropriate (*e.g.,* are the tests appropriate for the level of measurement of key variables)?

6. Were any multivariate procedures used? If not, should multivariate analyses have been conducted—would the use of a multivariate procedure strengthen the internal validity of the study?

7. Were the results of any statistical tests significant? Nonsignificant? What do the tests tell you about the plausibility of the research hypotheses?

8. Was an appropriate amount of statistical information reported? Were important analyses omitted, or were unimportant analyses included?

9. Were tables used judiciously to summarize statistical information? Is information in the text and tables totally redundant? Are the tables clear, with a good title and carefully labeled headings?

10. Is the researcher sufficiently objective in reporting the results?

the number of independent and dependent variables, the levels of measurement of the research variables, the number of groups (if any) being compared, and the appropriateness of using a parametric test. When the researcher has not used a multivariate technique, you might consider whether the bivariate analysis adequately tests the relationship between the independent and dependent variables. For example, if a *t*-test or ANOVA was used, could the internal validity of the study have been enhanced through the statistical control of extraneous variables, using ANCOVA?

Finally, you can be alert to possible exaggerations or subjectivity in the reported results. The researcher should never claim that the data proved, verified, confirmed, or demonstrated that the hypotheses were correct or incorrect. Hypotheses should be described as being *supported* or *not supported, accepted* or *rejected.*

The main task for beginning consumers in reading a results section of a research report is to understand the meaning of the statistical tests. What do the quantitative results indicate about the researcher's hypothesis? How believable are the findings? The answer to such questions form the basis for interpreting the research results, a topic discussed in Chapter 15.

RESEARCH EXAMPLES

The statistical techniques described in this chapter are widely used methods of statistical analysis. Two research examples are described below. Use the guidelines in Box 13-2 to appraise the analytic decisions made by the researchers, referring to the original studies as needed.

Research Example of Bivariate Inferential Statistics

Research Summary

Goulet and colleagues (2001) conducted a clinical trial to test the effects of home care management for women in preterm labour. A sample of 250 women experiencing preterm labour were randomly assigned to an experimental group receiving home care or to a control group receiving hospital care management. The two groups of women were compared in terms of antenatal stress, social support satisfaction, family functioning, and neonate's gestational age and birth weight. The researchers used t-tests to compare the two groups on neonatal outcomes. These analyses revealed that there were no significant differences between the two groups in terms of infants' gestational age ($t = .06$, $p = .956$) or birth weight ($t = .53$, $p = .599$).

With respect to maternal outcomes, the data were analysed using a repeated measures analysis of variance (ANOVA) in which differences between the two groups over three time periods were examined. Time 1 (T1) was at the point of randomization, time 2 (T2) was 1 week later, and time 3 (T3) was 2 weeks after randomization. The researchers found no significant group differences in antenatal stress at T1 ($p = .797$), T2 ($p = .420$), or T3 ($p = .533$). Similarly, the two groups of mothers had comparable scores on measures of global stress and family functioning at all three time periods. However, there was a significant difference between the experimental and control groups with respect to the women's satisfaction with support from male partners, at T3 only ($p = .024$). There were no significant differences between groups with respect to women's satisfaction with support from others at any of the three time periods.

Clinical Relevance

Goulet and colleagues (2001) used a strong design to compare women in preterm labour who received either home care or hospital care in terms of several neonatal and maternal outcomes. The researchers assigned mothers to either home care with nurse visitation or hospital care randomly, thereby enhancing the internal validity of the study. The statistical analyses (t-tests and repeated measures ANOVA and ANCOVA) were appropriate, as researchers increased precision and internal validity by using analysis of covariance when indicated.

Although several results were not statistically significant, they have some clinical significance (although replication of the study is strongly indicated). The findings suggest that home care management is as safe and effective as hospital managed care for women experiencing preterm labour. Women therefore could be provided with the option to receive care in either setting. Moreover, the home setting may enhance closeness between women and their families. This type of care also could provide opportunities for health care professionals to observe families in their home environment and to identify special needs that may require reliance on childcare services. However, the potential effects of transfering the burden of care from the hospital to the family may require more collaborative efforts among hospital, community health care agencies, and families.

Research Example of Multivariate Statistical Analysis

Research Summary

Johnson and her colleagues (1999) conducted an evaluation of a nurse-delivered smoking cessation intervention for hospitalized patients with cardiac disease. The research design was a nonequivalent control group before–after design, using smokers admitted to two inpatient cardiac units in a large Canadian hospital. Patients in one unit received the intervention, which involved two in-hospital contacts followed by 3 months of telephone support. Patients in the other unit received no special intervention.

The main outcome measures in the study were (1) self-reported smoking status 6 months after enrollment and (2) self-reported smoking cessation self-efficacy, measured using the Smoking Abstinence Self-Efficacy Scale. When factor analyzed, this 20-item Likert scale revealed three factors that were used to form three subscales: a positive/social subscale, a negative/affective subscale, and a habit/addictive subscale.

Using t-tests and χ^2 tests, the researchers compared the baseline characteristics of the experimental and comparison group in terms of age, gender, marital status, education, and other demographic characteristics. Although the two groups were found to be similar in most respects, the experimental group was found to be significantly more affluent and significantly less likely to have been admitted for cardiac surgery. The groups were similar in terms of smoking histories.

Six months after enrollment in the study, 30.8% of control subjects and 46.0% of experimental subjects reported they were not smoking. A χ^2 test indicated that, although sizeable, this difference was not statistically significant. The researchers then conducted a logistic regression to predict smoking abstinence based on group assignment, while controlling for important covariates (*e.g.,* income, surgical status, prior smoking history). They found that those in the control group were about three times as likely as those in the experimental group to resume smoking, net of background factors (odds ratio = 3.18), which was significant at the .05 level.

Multiple regression was used to predict scores on the three subscales of the self-efficacy scale. These analyses revealed that, with background variables controlled, being in the treatment group was a significant predictor of scores on the positive/social and habit/addictive subscales. The total amounts of variance accounted for in these regression analyses were 33% and 39%, respectively. The researchers concluded that the results of the study were encouraging.

Clinical Relevance

Scientific evidence supports a strong association between smoking and morbidity and mortality rates from respiratory and cardiovascular diseases. Smoking cessation, however, can decrease these morbidity and mortality rates. A brief smoking cessation intervention designed to be implemented by nurses working on a hospital unit has considerable appeal.

Caution should be used, however, in applying the results of this study to clinical practice for a number of reasons. First, the researchers used a quasi-experimental design. Their analytic strategy, which controlled for a number of background characteristics, did, however, strengthen the internal validity of the study. Second, only 50 subjects were enrolled in the experimental group and 52 in the control group. No power analysis had been done to determine whether this sample size yielded an acceptable level of power to detect significant differences. Third, smoking status was measured solely by self-report. The subject's report of smoking status was not biochemically validated.

The findings of this study have more implications for future research than for immediate clinical practice. Because of the encouraging effectiveness of the nurse-delivered smoking cessation intervention, further research is indicated using a more rigorous design.

● ● ● ● ● *SUMMARY POINTS*

- There are four major **levels of measurement:** (1) **nominal measurement**—the classification of characteristics into mutually exclusive categories; (2) **ordinal measurement**—the ranking of objects based on their relative standing to each other on an attribute; (3) **interval measurement**—indicating not only the ranking of objects but also the amount of distance between them; and (4) **ratio measurement**—distinguished from interval measurement by having a rational zero point.
- **Descriptive statistics** enable the researcher to synthesize and summarize quantitative data.
- In a **frequency distribution,** a method of imposing order on raw data, numeric values are ordered from lowest to highest, accompanied by a count of the number (or percentage) of times each value was obtained; **frequency polygons** display frequency information graphically.

- A set of data may be completely described in terms of the shape of the distribution, central tendency, and variability.
- The shape may be **symmetric** or **skewed,** with one tail longer than the other; it may also be **unimodal** with one peak (*i.e.,* one value of high frequency), or **multimodal** with more than one peak.
- A **normal distribution** (bell-shaped curve) is symmetric, unimodal, and not too peaked.
- Measures of **central tendency** represent the average or typical value of a measure. The **mode** is the value that occurs most frequently in the distribution; the **median** is the point on a scale above which and below which 50% of the cases fall; and the **mean** is the arithmetic average of all the scores. The mean is usually the preferred measure of central tendency because of its stability.
- Measures of **variability**—how spread out the data are—include the range and standard deviation. The range is the distance between the highest and lowest scores, and the **standard deviation** indicates how much, on average, the scores deviate from the mean.
- **Bivariate descriptive statistics** describe the degree and magnitude of relationships between two variables.
- A **contingency table** is a two-dimensional frequency distribution in which the frequencies of two nominal- or ordinal-level variables are **cross-tabulated.**
- **Correlation coefficients** describe the direction and magnitude of a relationship between two variables. The values range from -1.00 for a perfect negative correlation, to .00 for no relationship, to $+1.00$ for a perfect positive correlation. The most frequently used correlation coefficient is the **product–moment correlation coefficient (Pearson's r),** used with interval- or ratio-level variables.
- **Inferential statistics,** which are based on the **laws of probability,** allow researchers to make inferences about a population based on data from a sample; they offer a framework for deciding whether the **sampling error** that results from sampling fluctuation is too high to provide reliable population estimates.
- The **sampling distribution of the mean** is a theoretical distribution of the means of many different samples drawn from the same population. Sampling distributions are the basis for inferential statistics.
- The **standard error of the mean**—the standard deviation of this theoretical distribution—indicates the degree of average error of a sample mean; the smaller the standard error, the more accurate are the estimates of the population value based on the mean of a sample.
- **Hypothesis testing** through statistical procedures enables researchers to make objective decisions about the results of their studies.
- The **null hypothesis** states that no relationship exists between the variables and that any observed relationship is due to chance or sampling fluctuations; rejection of the null hypothesis lends support to the research hypothesis.

- A **Type II error** occurs when a null hypothesis that should be rejected is accepted. If a null hypothesis is incorrectly rejected, this is a **Type I error.**
- Researchers control the risk of making a Type I error by establishing a **level of significance** (or **alpha** level), which specifies the probability that such an error will occur. The .05 level means that in only 5 of 100 samples would the null hypothesis be rejected when it should have been accepted.
- Results from hypothesis tests are either significant or nonsignificant; statistically significant means that the obtained results are not likely to be due to chance fluctuations at a given probability level (**p level**).
- **Parametric statistical tests** involve the estimation of at least one parameter, the use of interval- or ratio-level data, and assumptions of normally distributed variables; nonparametric tests are used when the data are nominal or ordinal and the normality of the distribution cannot be assumed.
- Two common statistical tests are the **t-test** and **analysis of variance (ANOVA)**, both of which can be used to test the significance of the difference between group means; ANOVA is used when there are more than two groups.
- The most frequently used nonparametric test is the **chi-squared test,** which is used to test hypotheses relating to differences in proportions.
- Pearson's r can be used to test whether a correlation is significantly different from zero.
- **Multivariate statistical procedures** are increasingly being used in nursing research to untangle complex relationships among three or more variables.
- **Multiple regression,** or **multiple correlation,** is a method for understanding the effects of two or more independent variables on a dependent variable. The **multiple correlation coefficient (R),** can be squared to estimate the proportion of variability in the dependent variable accounted for by the independent variables.
- **Analysis of covariance (ANCOVA)** permits the researcher to control extraneous variables (called **covariates**) before determining whether group differences are statistically significant.
- Other multivariate procedures used by nurse researchers include **discriminant function analysis, logistic regression, factor analysis, multivariate analysis of variance (MANOVA), multivariate analysis of covariance (MANCOVA), path analysis,** and **LISREL.**

➤➤➤➤ *CRITICAL THINKING ACTIVITIES*

Chapter 13 of the accompanying *Study Guide to Accompany Essentials of Nursing Research,* 5th edition, offers various exercises and study suggestions for reinforcing the concepts presented in this chapter. In addition, you can address the following:

1. Read the method section from the quantitative research study in the Appendix of this book, and then answer the questions in Box 13-2.

2. What is the level of measurement of the two variables in Table 13-6?

3. Write a paragraph summarizing the main features of the correlation matrix in Table 13-7.

For additional review, see questions 172–197 on the study CD provided with Polit: Study Guide to Accompany Essentials of Nursing Research.

SUGGESTED READINGS

Methodologic References

Jaccard, J., & Becker, M.A. (2001). *Statistics for the behavioral sciences* (4th ed.). Belmont, CA: Wadsworth.

McCall, R. B. (2000). *Fundamental statistics for behavioral sciences* (8th ed.). Belmont, CA: Wadsworth.

Polit, D. F. (1996). *Data analysis and statistics for nursing research.* Stamford, CT: Appleton & Lange.

Welkowitz, J., Ewen, R. B., & Cohen, J. (2000). *Introductory statistics for the behavioral sciences* (5th ed.). New York: Harcourt College Publishers.

Substantive References

Bell, L., St-Cyr-Tribble, D., & Paul, D. (2001). Le point sur l'allaitement maternel en Estrie. *L'infirmière du Québec, 9,* 12–22.

Bottorff, J. L., Ratner, P. A., Balneaves, L. G., Richardson, C. G., McCullum, M., Hack, T., Chalmers, K., & Buxton, J. (2002). Women's interest in genetic testing for breast cancer risk: The influence of sociodemographics and knowledge. *Cancer Epidemiology, Biomarkers & Prevention, 11,* 89–95.

Davies, B. L. & Hodnett, E. (2002). Labor support: Nurses' self-efficacy and views about factors influencing implementation. *Journal of Obstetric, Gynecologic, and Neonatal Nursing, 31,* 48–56.

Duncan, S. M., Hyndman, K., Estabrooks, C. A., Hesketh, K., Humphrey, C. K., Wong, J. S. et al. (2001). Nurses' experience of violence in Alberta and British Columbia hospitals. *Canadian Journal of Nursing Research, 32,* 57–78.

Forchuk, C., Norman, R., Malla, A., Martin, M. L., McLean, T., Cheng, S., Diaz, K., McIntosh, E., Rickwood, A., Vos, S., & Gibney, C. (2002). Schizophrenia and the motivation for smoking. *Perspectives in Psychiatric Care, 38,* 41–49.

Gibbins, S., Stevens, B., Hodnett, E., Pinelli, J., Ohlsson, A., & Darlington, G. (2002). Efficacy and safety of sucrose for procedural pain relief in preterm and term neonates. *Nursing Research, 51,* 375–382

Gold, N., Issenman, R., Roberts, J., & Watt, S. (2000). Well-adjusted children: An alternate view of children with inflammatory bowel disease and functional gastrointestinal complaints. *Inflammatory Bowel Diseases, 6,* 1–7.

Goulet, C., Gevry, H., Gauthier, R.J., Lepage, L., Fraser, W., & Aita, M. (2001). A controlled clinical trial of home care management versus hospital care management for preterm labour. *International Journal of Nursing Studies, 38,* 259–269.

Johnson, J. L., Budz, B., Mackay, M., & Miller, C. (1999). Evaluation of a nurse-delivered smoking cessation intervention for hospitalized patients with cardiac disease. *Heart & Lung, 28,* 55–64.

Johnston, C.C., Stevens, B., Pinelli, J., Gibbins, S., Filion, F., Jack, A., Steele, S., Boyer,

K., Veilleux, A. (In press). Kangaroo care is effective in diminishing pain response in preterm neonates. *Archives of Pediatrics & Adolescent Medicine.*

King, K. M. (2000). Gender and short-term recovery from cardiac surgery. *Nursing Research, 49,* 29–36.

Kodis, J., Smith, K. M., Arthur, H. M., Daniels, C., Suskin, N., & McKelvie, R. S. (2001). Changes in exercise capacity and lipids after clinic versus home-based aerobic training in coronary artery bypass graft surgery patients. *Journal of Cardiopulmonary Rehabilitation, 21,* 31–36.

Lobchuk, M. M., & Degner, L. F. (2002). Symptom experiences: Perceptual accuracy between advanced-stage cancer patients and family caregivers in the home care setting. *Journal of Clinical Oncology, 20,* 3495–3507.

O'Neill, A. L., & Duffey, M. A. (2000). Communication of research and practice knowledge in nursing literature. *Nursing Research, 49,* 224–230.

Rosberger, Z., Edgar, L., Collet, J-P., & Fournier, M. A. (2002). Patterns of coping in women completing treatment for breast cancer: A randomized controlled trial of Nucare, a brief psychoeducation workshop. *Journal of Psychosocial Oncology, 20*(3), 19–37.

Ross, M. M., Carswell, A., & and Dalziel, W. B. (2001). Family caregiving in long-term care facilities. *Clinical Nursing Research, 10,* 347–363.

Tourangeau, A. E., Giovannetti, P., Tu, J. V., & Wood, M. (2002). Nursing-related determinants of 30-day mortality for hospitalized patients. *Canadian Journal of Nursing Research, 33,* 71–88.

Wilson, D. M. (2002). The duration and degree of end-of-life dependency of home care clients and hospital inpatients. *Applied Nursing Research, 15,* 81–86.

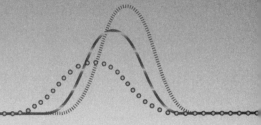

Analyzing Qualitative Data

INTRODUCTION TO QUALITATIVE ANALYSIS
Qualitative Analysis: General Considerations
Analysis Styles
The Qualitative Analysis Process
QUALITATIVE DATA MANAGEMENT AND ORGANIZATION
Developing a Categorization Scheme
Coding Qualitative Data
Manual Methods of Organizing Qualitative Data
Computer Programs for Managing Qualitative Data
ANALYTIC PROCEDURES
A General Analytic Overview
Grounded Theory Analysis
Phenomenological Analysis

CRITIQUING QUALITATIVE ANALYSES
RESEARCH EXAMPLES
Research Example of a Grounded Theory Analysis
Research Example of an Analysis for an Ethnographic Study
Research Example of a Phenomenological Analysis
SUMMARY POINTS
CRITICAL THINKING ACTIVITIES
SUGGESTED READINGS
Methodologic References
Substantive References

Student Objectives

On completion of this chapter, the student will be able to:

○ distinguish four prototypical qualitative analysis styles
○ describe the four intellectual processes that typically play a role in qualitative analysis
○ describe activities that qualitative researchers perform to manage and organize their data
○ discuss the procedures used to analyze qualitative data, including both general procedures and those used in the grounded theory approach
○ assess the adequacy of the researcher's description of the steps used to analyze the data
○ evaluate the steps a qualitative analyst took to validate the understandings gleaned from thematic analysis
○ define new terms in the chapter

New Terms

Basic social process (BSP)	Qualitative content analysis
Categorization scheme	Quasi-statistical analysis style
Conceptual files	Quasi-statistics
Constant comparison	Recontextualization
Core variable	Selective approach to analysis
Detailed approach to analysis	Selective coding
Editing analysis style	Substantive coding
Holistic approach to analysis	Template
Immersion/crystallization analysis style	Template analysis style
Manifest content analysis	Theme
Memos	Theoretical coding
Open coding	

Qualitative data take the form of loosely structured, narrative materials, such as verbatim transcripts from an in-depth interview, field notes from participant observation, or personal diaries. This chapter describes methods for analyzing such qualitative data.

INTRODUCTION TO QUALITATIVE ANALYSIS

Qualitative analysis is a labour-intensive activity that requires creativity, conceptual sensitivity, and sheer hard work. Qualitative analysis does not proceed in a linear fashion and is more complex and difficult than quantitative analysis because it is less formulaic. In this section, we discuss some general considerations relating to qualitative analysis.

Qualitative Analysis: General Considerations

The purpose of data analysis, regardless of the type of data or the underlying research tradition, is to organize, provide structure to, and elicit meaning from research data. The data analysis task is particularly challenging for qualitative researchers, for three major reasons. First, there are no systematic rules for analyzing and presenting qualitative data. The absence of systematic analytic procedures makes it difficult to present findings in such a way that their validity is patently clear. Some of the procedures described in Chapter 12 (*e.g.,* member checking and investigator triangulation) are important tools for enhancing the trustworthiness not only of the data themselves but also of the analyses and interpretation of those data.

The second challenge of qualitative analysis is the enormous amount of work required. The qualitative analyst must organize and make sense of pages and pages of narrative materials. In a recent multimethod study where one of the Canadian authors (Profetto-McGrath) served as a research associate, the qualitative data consisted of field notes written by six research associates during 6 months of fieldwork as participant observers in a study about nurses' research utilization within the context of pain management. The typed field notes ranged from 3 to 40 pages in length, resulting in approximately 2000 pages that needed to be read, reread, coded, and analyzed.

The final challenge comes in reducing the data for reporting purposes. Quantitative results can often be summarized in two or three tables. However, if a researcher summarized the findings of a qualitative analysis without including numerous supporting excerpts from the narrative materials, the richness of the original data would disappear—and readers would have no basis for challenging the researcher's interpretation. As a consequence, it is sometimes difficult to do a thorough presentation of the results of qualitative research in a format that is compatible with space limitations in professional journals.

CONSUMER TIP

Qualitative analyses are often more difficult to do than quantitative ones, but qualitative findings are usually easier to understand than quantitative findings because the stories are often told in everyday language. The readability of the qualitative reports is usually enhanced by the inclusion of verbatim excerpts taken directly from the narrative data. However, qualitative analyses are often harder to evaluate critically than quantitative analyses because the person reading the report cannot know first-hand whether the researcher adequately captured thematic patterns in the data. ∎

Analysis Styles

Crabtree and Miller (1992) observed that there are nearly as many qualitative analysis strategies as there are qualitative researchers. However, they have identified four major analysis styles or patterns that fall along a continuum. At one extreme is a style that is more objective, systematic, and standardized, and at the other extreme is a style that is more intuitive, subjective, and interpretive. The four prototypical styles they described are as follows:

- **Quasi-statistical analysis style.** The researcher using a quasi-statistical style typically begins with some preconceived ideas about the analysis and uses those ideas to sort the data. This approach is sometimes referred to as **manifest content analysis**—the researcher reviews the content of the narrative data, searching for particular words or themes that have been specified in advance. The result of the search is information that can be analyzed statistically, and hence the name **quasi-statistics.** For example, the analyst can count the frequency of occurrence of specific themes or can cross-tabulate the occurrence of certain words.

- **Template analysis style.** In this style, the researcher develops a **template** or analysis guide to which the narrative data are applied. The units for the template are typically behaviours, events, or linguistic expressions (*e.g.,* words). A template is more adaptable than a codebook in the quasi-statistical style. Although the researcher may begin with a rudimentary template before collecting any data, it undergoes constant revision as more data are gathered. The analysis of the resulting data, once sorted according to the template, is interpretive and not statistical. This type of style is most likely to be adopted by researchers whose research tradition is ethnography, ethology, discourse analysis, or ethnoscience.

- **Editing analysis style.** The researcher using the editing style acts as an interpreter who reads through the data in search of meaningful segments. Once segments are identified and reviewed, the interpreter develops a **categorization scheme** and corresponding codes that can be used to sort and organize the data. The researcher then searches for the patterns and structure that connect the thematic categories. The grounded theory approach typically incorporates this type of style. Researchers whose research tradition is phenomenology, hermeneutics, or ethnomethodology use procedures that fall within the editing analysis pattern.

- **Immersion/crystallization analysis style.** This style involves the analyst's total immersion in and reflection of the text materials, resulting in an intuitive crystallization of the data. This interpretive and subjective style is exemplified in personal case reports of a semianecdotal nature and is less frequently encountered in the nursing research literature than the other three styles.

Nurse researchers are especially likely to use an analytic strategy that can best be characterized as an editing style. Most of the remainder of this chapter describes analytic activities that are consistent with that style.

 CONSUMER TIP

In an actual research report, the researcher is unlikely to use terms like template analysis style or editing style; these terms are post hoc characterizations of styles that are often adopted. However, if a study was done within a qualitative research tradition such as ethnography or grounded theory, this fact is likely to be reported, thereby providing readers with a sense of the overall analytic strategy. ■

The Qualitative Analysis Process

The analysis of qualitative data typically is an active and interactive process. Qualitative researchers typically scrutinize their data carefully and deliberatively. Insights and theories cannot spring forth from the data unless the researcher is completely familiar with those data. Qualitative researchers often read their narrative data over and over in search of meaning and deeper understandings. Morse and Field (1995) note that qualitative analysis is "a process of fitting data together, of making the invisible obvious, of linking and attributing consequences to antecedents. It is a process of conjecture and verification, of correction and modification, of suggestion and defense" (p. 126). Morse and Field identified four intellectual processes that play a role in qualitative analysis:

- *Comprehending.* Early in the analytic process, qualitative researchers strive to make sense of the data and to learn "what is going on." When comprehension is achieved, the researcher is able to prepare a thorough and rich description of the phenomenon under study, and new data do not add much to that description. Thus, comprehension is completed when saturation has been attained.
- *Synthesizing.* Synthesizing involves a "sifting" of the data and putting pieces together. At this stage, the researcher gets a sense of what is typical with regard to the phenomenon and of what variation is like. At the end of the synthesis process, the researcher can make some generalized statements about the phenomenon and about the study participants.
- *Theorizing.* Theorizing involves a systematic sorting of the data. During the theorizing process, the researcher develops alternative explanations of the phenomenon under study and then holds these explanations up to determine their "fit" with the data. The theorizing process continues to evolve until the best and most parsimonious explanation is obtained.
- *Recontextualizing.* The process of **recontextualization** involves the further development of the theory such that its applicability to other settings or groups is explored. In qualitative inquiries whose ultimate goal is theory development, it is the theory that must be recontextualized and generalized.

Although the intellectual processes in qualitative analysis are not linear in the same sense that quantitative analysis is, it is nevertheless true that these four processes follow a rough progression over the course of the study. Comprehension occurs primarily while in the field. Synthesis begins in the field but may continue well after the fieldwork has been completed. Theorizing and recontextualizing are processes that are difficult to undertake before synthesis has been completed.

QUALITATIVE DATA MANAGEMENT AND ORGANIZATION

The intellectual processes of qualitative analysis are supported and facilitated by tasks that help to organize and manage the masses of narrative data.

Developing a Categorization Scheme

The first step in analyzing qualitative data is to organize them, and the main organizational task is developing a method to classify and index the materials. The researcher must design a mechanism for gaining access to parts of the data, without having to repeatedly reread the data set in its entirety. This phase of data analysis is essentially reductionist—data must be converted to smaller, more manageable units that can be retrieved and reviewed.

The most widely used procedure is to develop a categorization scheme and to then code the data according to the categories. A categorization system is sometimes prepared (at least in a preliminary version) before data collection, but more typically the qualitative analyst develops categories based on a scrutiny of the actual data.

There are, unfortunately, no straightforward or easy guidelines for this task. The development of a high-quality categorization scheme for qualitative data involves a careful reading of the data, with an eye to identifying underlying concepts and clusters of concepts. Depending on the aims of the study, the nature of the categories may vary in level of detail or specificity as well as in level of abstraction.

Researchers whose aims are primarily descriptive tend to use concrete categories. For example, the category scheme may focus on actions or events or on different phases in a chronological unfolding of an experience. In developing a category scheme, related concepts are often grouped together to facilitate the coding process.

Example of developing a category scheme:
The coding scheme used by Polit et al. (2000) to categorize data relating to food insecurity and hunger in low-income families (Fig. 14–1) is an example of a category system that is fairly concrete and descriptive. For example, it allows the coders to code discussions about the use of specific resources and food assistance programs. The coding system involved four major category clusters, each with subcodes. For example, an excerpt that described a mother's purchase of day-old bread would be coded under category C.4.

Studies designed to develop a theory are more likely to develop abstract and conceptual categories. In designing conceptual categories, the researcher must break the data into segments, closely examine them, and compare them with other segments for similarities and dissimilarities to determine what type of phenomena are reflected in them and what the meaning of those phenomena are. (This is part of the process referred to as **constant comparison**

A. Use of Food Services/Programs 　1. Food stamps 　2. WIC 　3. Food pantries 　4. Soup kitchens 　5. Free lunch programs **B. Food Inadequacy** 　1. Problems feeding family, having 　　enough food 　2. Having to eat undesirable food 　3. Hunger	**C. Strategies to Avoid Hunger** 　1. Bargain shopping 　2. Borrowing money 　3. Getting food from friends, relatives 　4. Eating old or unsafe food 　5. Doubling up to share food costs 　6. Stretching food, smaller portions 　7. Smoking in lieu of eating 　8. Illegal activities, fraud **D. Special Issues** 　1. Mothers sacrificing for children 　2. Effects of welfare reform on hunger 　3. Stigma

FIGURE 14-1. Polit et al.'s (2000) coding scheme for food insecurity and hunger in low-income families.

by grounded theory researchers.) The researcher asks questions about discrete events, incidents, or thoughts that are indicated in an observation or statement, such as the following:

> What is this?
> What is going on?
> What does it stand for?
> What else is like this?
> What is this distinct from?

Important concepts that emerge from close examination of the data are then given a label that forms the basis for a categorization scheme. These category names are necessarily abstractions, but the labels are usually sufficiently graphic that the nature of the material to which it refers is clear—and often provocative. Strauss and Corbin (1990) advise qualitative researchers as follows: "The important thing is to name a category, so that you can remember it, think about it, and most of all begin to develop it analytically" (pp. 67–68).

CONSUMER TIP

A good category scheme is crucial to the analysis of qualitative data. Without a comprehensive category system, the researcher cannot retrieve the narrative information that has been collected. Unfortunately, research reports rarely present the category scheme for readers to review. However, the researcher may provide information about the development of the category system, which can help you evaluate its adequacy (*e.g.*, the researcher may say that the scheme was reviewed by peers or developed collaboratively by two or more researchers). ■

Coding Qualitative Data

Once a categorization scheme has been developed, all of the data are then reviewed for content and coded for correspondence to or exemplification of the identified categories. The process of coding qualitative material is seldom easy, for several reasons. First, the researcher may have difficulty in deciding which code is most appropriate or may not fully comprehend the underlying meaning of some aspect of the data. It may take a second or third reading of the material to grasp its nuances.

Second, the researcher often discovers in going through the data that the initial category system was incomplete or inadequate. It is not unusual for some themes to emerge that were not initially conceptualized. When this happens, it is risky to assume that the topic failed to appear in previously coded materials. That is, a concept might not be identified as salient until it has emerged three or four times in the data. In such a case, it would be necessary to reread all previously coded material to have a truly complete grasp of that category.

Another issue is that narrative materials are usually not linear. For example, paragraphs from transcribed interviews may contain elements relating to three or four different categories, embedded in a complex fashion.

Example of coding qualitative data:

An example of a multitopic segment of an interview by Polit et al. (2000) in their study of hunger in low-income families is shown in Figure 14–2. The codes in the margin represent codes from the scheme presented in Figure 14–1.

Manual Methods of Organizing Qualitative Data

A variety of procedures have traditionally been used to organize and manage qualitative data. Before the advent of computer programs for managing qualitative data, the most usual procedure was the development of **conceptual files.** In this approach, a physical file is developed for each category, and all of the materials relating to that topic, based on the codes, are cut out and inserted into the file. In this fashion, all of the content on a particular topic can be retrieved by going to the applicable file folder.

The creation of such conceptual files is clearly a cumbersome and labour-intensive task. This is particularly true when segments of the narrative materials have multiple codes (*e.g.,* the excerpt shown in Fig. 14–2). In such a situation, there would need to be six copies of the paragraph—one for each file corresponding to the six codes. The researcher must also be sensitive to the need to provide enough context that the cut-up material can be understood. Thus, it might be necessary to include material preceding or following the directly relevant materials.

Computer Programs for Managing Qualitative Data

The traditional manual methods of organizing qualitative data have a long and respected history, but sophisticated computer programs for managing qualitative data are now widely used. These programs permit the entire data file to be

B1	I hate being on welfare, it is a pain in the butt. I don't need their cash, but the food stamps, they help a lot because it is hard, it is really hard. I got to live day by day for food for my kids. I have to call down to the shelter to get them to send you food, and you hate doing that because it is embarrassing, but I have to live day by day. I have to do things so my kids can eat. I don't worry about me, just for my kids because I can go a day without eating, but as long as my kids eat.
D1	But I never have to worry about my kids starving because I have family.

with codes **A1**, **A3**, **D3**, **C3** in right margin.

FIGURE 14-2. Coded excerpt from study by Polit et al. (2000).

entered onto the computer, each portion of an interview or observational record coded, and then portions of the text corresponding to specified codes retrieved and printed (or shown on a screen) for analysis. The current generation of programs also has features that go beyond simple indexing and retrieval—they offer possibilities for actual analysis and integration of the data.

Computer programs remove the drudgery of cutting and pasting pages and pages of narrative material. However, some people prefer manual indexing because it allows the researcher to get closer to the data. Others have raised concerns about using programs for the analysis of qualitative data, objecting to having a process that is basically cognitive turned into an activity that is mechanical and technical. Despite these issues, many qualitative researchers have switched to computerized data management because it frees up their time and permits them to pay greater attention to more important conceptual issues.

CONSUMER TIP

A good coding system is of little utility if the actual coding is not done with care. There is, of course, no way for you as a reader to know whether coding was diligently performed. However, you can have more confidence if the report mentions that two or more people were involved in coding the data, or at least portions of it, to ensure intercoder reliability. ■

ANALYTIC PROCEDURES

Data *management* tasks in qualitative research are typically reductionist in nature because they convert large masses of data into smaller, more manageable segments. By contrast, qualitative data *analysis* tasks are constructionist; they involve putting segments together into a meaningful conceptual pattern. Although there are several approaches to qualitative data analysis, some elements are common to several of them. We provide some general guidelines, followed by a description of the procedures used by grounded theory researchers and phenomenologists.

> ### ✍ CONSUMER TIP
>
> Research reports vary in the amount of detail provided about qualitative analytic procedures. At one extreme are researchers who say little more than that their data were analyzed qualitatively. At the other extreme are researchers who describe the steps they took to analyze their data and validate the emerging themes. Most studies fall between the two extremes, but limited detail is more prevalent than abundant detail. ■

A General Analytic Overview

The analysis of qualitative materials usually begins with a search for **themes** or recurring regularities. Themes often develop within categories of data (*i.e.,* within categories of the coding scheme used for indexing materials) but sometimes cut across them. For example, in the study by Polit and colleagues (2000; see Fig. 14–1), one theme that emerged was that the mothers took tremendous pride in their ability to provide food for their families, including their resourcefulness in accessing food services (A codes) and in using a variety of strategies to avoid hunger (C codes).

The search for themes involves not only the discovery of commonalities across participants but also a search for natural variation. Themes that emerge are never universal. The researcher must attend not only to what themes arise but also to how they are patterned. Does the theme apply only to certain subgroups? In certain types of communities or organizations? In certain contexts? At certain periods? What are the conditions that precede the observed phenomenon, and what are the apparent consequences of it? In other words, the qualitative analyst must be sensitive to *relationships* within the data.

> ### ✍ CONSUMER TIP
>
> Major themes are often the subheadings used by qualitative researchers in the results section of their reports. For example, LeClerc et al. (2002) studied the everyday issues, challenges, struggles, and needs of community-dwelling elderly women in the first weeks after hospital discharge. They identified the following five themes, which were used to organize their results section: "Struggling with intense physical and emotional needs as one gradually recovers," "Changing one's usual lifestyle to cope with struggles," "Relying on family and friends to meet the needs not addressed by home care givers," "Experiencing anxiety related to struggles that were not anticipated while in the hospital" and "Accepting one's situation because of a reluctance to complain." ■

A further step involves validation—that is, whether the themes inferred are an accurate representation of the phenomenon. Several validation procedures can be used, as discussed in Chapter 12. If more than one researcher is working on the study, sessions in which the themes are reviewed and specific cases discussed can be highly productive. Investigator triangulation cannot ensure thematic validity, but it can minimize idiosyncratic biases. It is also useful to undertake member checks—that is, to present the preliminary thematic analysis to some informants, who can be encouraged to offer comments to support or contradict the analysis.

At this point, some researchers introduce quasi-statistics—a tabulation of the frequency with which certain themes, relations, or insights are supported by the data. The frequencies cannot be interpreted in the same way as frequencies generated in survey studies because of imprecision in the sampling of cases and enumeration of the themes. Nevertheless, as Becker (1970) pointed out:

> Quasi-statistics may allow the investigator to dispose of certain troublesome null hypotheses. A simple frequency count of the number of times a given phenomenon appears may make untenable the null hypothesis that the phenomenon is infrequent. A comparison of the number of such instances with the number of negative cases—instances in which some alternative phenomenon that would not be predicted by his theory appears—may make possible a stronger conclusion, especially if the theory was developed early enough in the observational period to allow a systematic search for negative cases. (p. 81)

Example of tabulating qualitative data:

Boughn and Holdom (2002) conducted semistructured interviews with 44 women with trichotillomania (a compulsion to pull out one's hair). In analyzing the women's beliefs about the effectiveness of treatments they had used, the researchers quantified their data. They found, for example, that 21 of the women had used Prozac, but none had found this to have long-term effectiveness.

In the final analysis stage, the researcher strives to weave the thematic pieces together into an integrated whole. The various themes need to be interrelated to provide an overall structure (such as a theory or integrated description) to the data. The integration task is difficult because it demands creativity and intellectual rigor if it is to be successful.

Grounded Theory Analysis

The general analytic procedures just described provide an overview of how qualitative researchers make sense of their data and distill from them insights into processes and behaviours operating in naturalistic settings. However, variations in the goals and philosophies of qualitative researchers also lead to variations in analytic strategies. A widely used analytic approach among nurse researchers is Glaser and Strauss' (1967) grounded theory method of generating theories from data. Because of its popularity, we describe here some of the specific analytic techniques of grounded theory.

Grounded theory uses the constant comparative method of data analysis. With this method, the researcher simultaneously collects, codes, and analyzes data. Coding is a process used to conceptualize data into patterns or concepts. The empirical substance of the topic being studied is conceptualized by **substantive codes,** whereas **theoretical codes** conceptualize how the substantive codes relate to each other.

There are two kinds of substantive codes: open and selective. **Open coding** is used in the first stage of the constant comparative analysis to capture what is going on in the data. Open codes may be the actual words used by the participants. Through open coding, data are broken down into incidents, and their similarities and differences are examined. When coding at this level, the researcher asks, "What category or property of a category does this incident indicate?" (Glaser, 1978, p. 57). Open coding ends when the core variable is discovered, and then selective coding begins.

The **core variable** is a pattern of behaviour that is relevant or problematic for study participants. In **selective coding,** the researcher codes only those variables that are related to the core variable. One kind of core variable can be a **basic social process (BSP),** which evolves over time in two or more phases. All BSPs are core variables, but not all core variables have to be BSPs.

Theoretical codes help the grounded theorist to weave the broken pieces of data back together again. Glaser (1978) identified 18 families of theoretical codes that researchers can use to help determine how the substantive codes relate to each other. Examples of these coding families are as follows:

- Cutting point family includes boundaries, critical junctures
- Strategy family focuses on tactics, strategies, and techniques

Throughout the coding and analysis process, grounded theory analysts document their ideas about the data, themes, and the emerging conceptual scheme in the form of memos. **Memos** preserve ideas that may initially not seem productive but may later prove valuable once further developed. Memos also encourage the researcher to reflect on and describe patterns in the data, relationships between categories, and emergent conceptualizations.

The grounded theory method is concerned with the generation of categories, properties, and hypotheses rather than testing them. The product of the typical grounded theory analysis is a conceptual or theoretical model that endeavors to explain a pattern of behaviour that is both relevant and problematic for the people in the study. Once the basic problem emerges, the grounded theorist then goes on to discover the process these participants go through to cope or resolve this problem.

Example of grounded theory analysis:

Wuest and Merritt-Gray (2001) developed a grounded theory of the process of leaving an abusive male partner. The researchers discovered the basic social process of *reclaiming self,* in which the women voyaged through four stages: counteracting abuse, breaking free, not going back, and moving on.

Phenomenological Analysis

Schools of phenomenology have developed different approaches for data analysis. In nursing, three frequently used methods of data analysis for descriptive phenomenology are the methods of Colaizzi (1978), Giorgi (1985), and Van Kaam (1966), all of whom are from the Duquesne school of phenomenology, based on Husserl's philosophy. Table 14-1 presents a compari-

TABLE 14-1. Comparison of Three Phenomenological Methods

COLAIZZI (1978)	GIORGI (1985)	VAN KAAM (1966)
1. Read all protocols to acquire a feeling for them.	1. Read the entire set of protocols to get a sense of the whole.	1. List and group preliminarily the descriptive expressions that must be agreed on by expert judges. Final listing presents percentages of these categories in that particular sample.
2. Review each protocol and extract significant statements.	2. Discriminate units from participants' description of phenomenon being studied.	2. Reduce the concrete, vague, and overlapping expressions of the participants to more descriptive terms. (Intersubjective agreement among judges needed.)
3. Spell out of the meaning of each significant statement (*i.e.*, formulate meanings).	3. Articulate the psychological insight in each of the meaning units.	3. Eliminate elements not inherent in the phenomenon being studied or that represent blending of two related phenomena.
4. Organize the formulated meanings into clusters of themes. a. Refer these clusters back to the original protocols to validate them. b. Note discrepancies among and/or between the various clusters, avoiding temptation of ignoring data or themes that do not fit.	4. Synthesize all of the transformed meaning units into a consistent statement regarding participants' experiences (referred to as the "structure of the experience"); can be expressed on a specific or general level.	4. Write a hypothetical identification and description of the phenomenon being studied.
5. Integrate results into an exhaustive description of the phenomenon under study.		5. Apply hypothetical description to randomly selected cases from the sample. If necessary, revise the hypothesized description, which must then be tested again on a new sample.
6. Formulate an exhaustive description of the phenomenon under study in as unequivocal a statement of identification as possible.		6. Consider the hypothesized identification as a valid identification and description once preceding operations have been carried out successfully.
7. Ask participants about the findings thus far as a final validating step.		

son of the steps involved in these three methods of analysis. The basic outcome of all three methods is the description of the meaning of an experience, often through the identification of essential themes. The phenomenologist searches for common patterns shared by particular instances. However, there are some important differences among these three approaches. Colaizzi's method, for example, is the only one that calls for a final validation of the results by returning to study participants. Giorgi's analysis relies solely on the researcher. His view is that it is inappropriate to either return to the participants to validate the findings or to use external judges to review the analysis. Van Kaam's method requires that intersubjective agreement be reached with other expert judges.

A second school of phenomenolgy is the Utrecht School. Phenomenologists using this Dutch approach combine characteristics of descriptive and interpretive phenomenology. Van Manen's (1990) method is an example of this combined approach in which the researcher tries to grasp the essential meaning of the experience being studied. In reflecting on lived experience, the researcher analyzes the thematic aspects of that experience. According to Van Manen, themes can be uncovered or isolated from participants' descriptions of an experience by three different means: (1) the holistic approach, (2) the selective or highlighting approach, and the (3) detailed or line-by-line approach. In the **holistic approach,** the researcher views the text as a whole and tries to capture its meanings. In the **selective approach,** the researcher underlines, highlights, or pulls out statements or phrases that seem essential to the experience under study. In the **detailed approach,** the researcher analyzes every sentence. Once the themes have been identified, they become the objects of reflecting and interpreting through follow-up interviews with participants. Through this process, the essential themes are discovered.

A third school of phenomenology is an interpretive approach called Heideggerian hermeneutics. Diekelmann and colleagues (1989) have described a seven-stage process of data analysis. Its outcome is to describe shared practices and common meanings. Diekelmann and colleagues' stages include the following:

1. Reading of all the interviews or texts for an overall understanding
2. Preparation of interpretive summaries of each interview
3. Analysis of selected transcribed interviews or texts by a team of researchers
4. Resolution of any disagreements on interpretation by going back to the text
5. Identification of common meaning by comparing and contrasting the text's shared practices
6. Emergence of relationships among themes
7. Presentation of a draft of the themes, along with exemplars from texts, to the team; responses and suggestions incorporated into the final draft

CONSUMER TIP

Qualitative researchers who conduct studies that are not based in a formal research tradition often say that a content analysis was performed. **Qualitative content analysis** is the analysis of the content of narrative data to identify prominent themes and patterns among the themes—primarily using an analysis style that can be characterized as either template analysis or editing analysis. ∎

CRITIQUING QUALITATIVE ANALYSES

The task of evaluating a qualitative analysis is not easy, even for researchers with experience in doing qualitative research. The problem stems, in part, from the lack of standardized procedures for data analysis, but the difficulty lies mainly in the fact that readers must accept largely on faith that the researcher exercised good judgment and critical insight in coding the narrative materials, developing a thematic analysis, and integrating the materials into a meaningful whole. This is because the researcher is seldom able to include more than a handful of examples of actual data in a research report published in a journal and because the process of inductively abstracting meaning from the data is difficult to describe.

In quantitative analysis, the research can be evaluated in terms of the adequacy of specific analytic decisions (*e.g.,* did the researcher use the appropriate statistical test?). In a critique of qualitative analysis, however, the primary task is usually determining whether the researcher took sufficient steps to validate inferences and conclusions. A major focus of a critique of qualitative analyses, then, is whether the researcher has adequately documented the analytic process. Some guidelines that may be helpful in evaluating qualitative analyses are presented in Box 14-1.

RESEARCH EXAMPLES

The number of qualitative studies that have been published in nursing journals during the past decade has risen dramatically. Three research examples are described below.

Research Example of a Grounded Theory Analysis

Research Summary
Beck (2002) undertook a grounded theory study of mothering twins during the first year of life. Figure 14–3 presents her model, which was developed using Glaser and Strauss' constant comparative method. Data for this study consisted of transcripts from 16 in-depth interviews, and 14 months of field notes from participant observation in mothers' homes and during support

---

BOX 14-1 ## GUIDELINES FOR CRITIQUING QUALITATIVE ANALYSES

1. Based on information in the report regarding either the analyses strategy or the research tradition, what type of analysis style appears to have been used?

2. Is the initial categorization scheme described? If so, does the scheme appear logical and complete? Was the scheme validated in any way (*e.g.,* did more than one person develop it collaboratively?

3. Who coded the data—the researcher or assistants? Did the report indicate that efforts were made to determine interrator reliability of the coding?

4. Does the report describe the process by which an integrated thematic analysis was performed? What major themes emerged? If excerpts from the data are provided, do the themes appear to capture the meaning of the narratives (*i.e.,* does it appear that the researcher adequately interpreted the data and conceptualized the themes)?

5. Is the analysis parsimonious—could two or more themes be collapsed into a broader and perhaps more useful conceptualization?

6. What evidence does the report provide that the researcher's analysis is accurate and replicable?

7. Were data displayed in a manner that allows you to verify the researcher's conclusions? Was a conceptual map, model, or diagram effectively displayed to communicate important processes?

8. Was the context of the phenomenon adequately described? Does the report give you a clear picture of the social or emotional world of the study participants?

9. If the result of the study is an emergent theory or conceptualization, does it seem trivial or obvious? Does the scheme yield a meaningful and insightful picture of the phenomenon under study?

---

group meetings for parents of multiples. *Life on Hold* was identified as the basic social psychological problem of mothering twins. As one mother expressed, "I would say that my life is on hold since the twins were born. It is a rare occasion when I can undo the pause button."

Coding continued until the basic social process, also the core variable, was discovered. *Releasing the Pause Button* was the process mothers progressed through as they attempted to resume their lives. Once this core variable was discovered, Beck shifted from open coding to selective coding. The core variable consisted of the four phases of (1) draining power, (2) pausing own life, (3) striving to reset, and (4) resuming own life.

To help make the wealth of data more manageable, Beck collapsed substantive codes into broader, more abstract categories. An example of this process involved collapsing five substantive codes (enjoying the twins, feeling blessed, getting attention, amazing, and twin bonding) into the category of

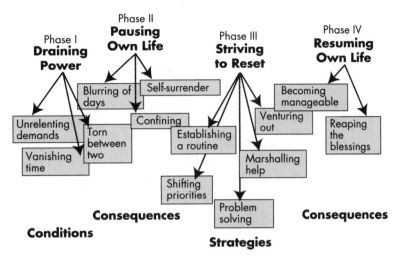

FIGURE 14-3. Life on hold: Releasing the pause button.

Reaping the Blessings. Next, Beck collapsed the categories of *Reaping the Blessings* and *Becoming Manageable* into the more abstract category of *Resuming Own Life.* She used 10 of Glaser's (1978) 18 coding families in her theoretical coding for the process of *Releasing the Pause Button,* included the "strategy" and "cutting point" families. The family "cutting point" provides an illustration of a theoretical code. Three months seemed to be the cutting or turning point for mothers when life started to become more manageable. The following are a few excerpts from transcripts of interviews that Beck coded as cutting points: "I just pushed through the first 3 months, then it got easier and I felt like I would survive." "Three months came around and the twins sort of slept through the night and it made a huge, huge difference." "The first 3 months definitely were the hardest. It wasn't very rewarding. It was like being a servant to two demanding people. They really weren't giving anything back."

Clinical Relevance

The current explosion of multiple births presents nursing with the challenge of providing optimal care for these high-risk families. Depression and anxiety disorders can affect more than 25% of multiple birth parents. Beck's (2002) grounded theory can help to educate clinicians about the differences in the multiple birth experience so they can provide realistic and knowledgeable guidance to these parents. Clinicians can use this four-phase process of *Releasing the Pause Button* to identify where in this process mothers of multiples are. Specific nursing interventions can then be designed to target the different phases in this process of mothers resuming their own life. For example, the most vulnerable time for mothers of twins was found to be the first 3 months after delivery. Telephone communication with nurses can be lifelines for mothers of multiples before they start to venture out with their twins. Support groups for mothers of multiples need to be in place to support women through this vulnerable period. Due to Beck's attention to the details of Glaser and Strauss's grounded theory approach, such as theoretical coding and the constant comparative method of data analysis, the credibility of her findings for clinicians is increased.

Research Example of an Analysis for an Ethnographic Study

Research Summary

Browne and Fiske (2001) conducted an ethnographic study to explore First Nation (Aboriginal) women's experiences with mainstream health care services. The study sought to understand how First Nations women perceived their encounters with local mainstream health care services, and how those encounters were shaped by social, political, and economic factors.

The research was conducted in a First Nations reserve community with a population of 600 in a rural area of northwest Canada. Using input from community leaders, the researchers selected 10 women to participate in two rounds of interviews. Participants were asked to describe both positive encounters (model cases) and negative encounters (contrary cases) with the health care establishment.

An interpretive thematic analysis was conducted in stages, based on transcripts from these interviews. The narratives first were reviewed as a whole by the research team for an overall understanding of the main issues. Then the text was read and reread repeatedly to identify patterns of regularities and recurring ideas. During this process, categories and conceptual themes were formulated and reformulated. Critical examination of and reflection on theoretical perspectives led to further development and refinement of the emerging conceptual themes. To ensure that the emergent analysis was credible and congruent with what the women had intended, study participants were asked to critique and validate the themes and interpretations. Finally, the conceptual themes were refined and synthesized into a coherent account of participants' health care encounters.

The narratives revealed that the "women's encounters were shaped by racism, discrimination, and structural inequalities that continue to marginalize and disadvantage First Nations women" (p. 126). Participants described situations in which their health concerns or reported symptoms were not taken seriously or were trivialized. Encounters that revealed health care workers' discriminatory attitudes and behaviours were found to be pervasive.

Clinical Relevance

Aboriginal women, although relatively small in number, represent a vibrant and varied segment of Canada's population who share a common legacy of marginalization and oppression. Aboriginal women face a variety of problems and challenges, especially in the areas of health and healing and violence and abuse, but these problems are not adequately addressed in the research literature. Understanding the unique challenges that confront Aboriginal women, especially in the health care environment, is vital to strengthening Aboriginal women and the communities in which they live.

Browne and Fiske, through their research with First Nations women, have contributed to heath care providers' understanding about these women's personal experiences when they enter the health care system. Drawing on the work of other researchers, they point out that the middle-class orientation of Western nurses and doctors can potentially create culturally unsafe clinical encounters. As Browne and Fiske also indicate, the attitutes and behaviours of health care providers such as nurses can begin to change only when the providers consider and situate the complexities of the encounters involving First Nations women. Viewing these encounters from a cultural safety standpoint could help to reduce racism, inequity, and marginalization.

Research Example of a Phenomenological Analysis

Research Summary

Anderson and Spencer (2002) conducted a phenomenological study to describe AIDS patients' cognitive representation of their illness. The purposive sample consisted of 58 men and women with a diagnosis of AIDS. In-depth interviews, conducted over an 18-month period, posed such questions as: "What meaning does it [AIDS] have in your life?" (p. 1342). All interviews were audiotaped and transcribed verbatim.

Colaizzi's method was used to analyze the verbatim transcripts. After reading the transcripts several times, the researchers identified significant phrases or sentences that pertained directly to the lived experience of AIDS, and then formulated meanings from them. The researchers provided several examples of this process, such as the following:

> Significant statement: "AIDS is a disease that has no cure. Meaning of dread and doom and you got to fight it the best way you can. You got to fight it with everything you can to keep going."
>
> Formulated meaning: "AIDS is a dangerous disease that requires every fiber of your being to fight so you can live" (p. 1343).

The formulated meanings were then clustered into themes, and the results were integrated into an in-depth, exhaustive description of the phenomenon that was validated by some of the participants who took part in the study.

Data analysis yielded 175 significant statements describing the individuals' cognitive representation of their illness. These significant statements were organized into the following eleven themes:

1. *Inescapable death*—reflected participants' focus on the negative consequences associated with AIDS.
2. *Dreaded bodily destruction*—captured respondents' descriptions of physical changes related to their illness.
3. *Devouring life*—individuals grieved for the life they had.

4. *Hoping for the right drug*—theme related to participants' focus on pharmacologic treatment/cure for AIDS.
5. *Caring for oneself*—encompassed their attempt to manage the disease's progress through self-care activities.
6. *Just a disease*—these theme represented the respondents' images as to how they viewed AIDS.
7. *Holding a wildcat*—participants reflected on their watchfulness and alertness toward the disease.
8. *Magic of not thinking*—captures how participants endeavoured to block out their disease and/or requirement for treatment.
9. *Accepting AIDS*—theme centres on respondents' common acceptance of the diagnosis of AIDS.
10. *Turning to a higher power*—the cognitive representation associated with this theme was linked to "God," "prayer," "church," and "spirituality."
11. *Recouping with time*—centres on the notion that as time progressed, time became a healer.

Clinical Relevance

Implications for nursing practice with patients diagnosed with AIDS can be derived from each of these 11 themes. For example, based on theme 4 and 11, the importance of maintaining a sense of hope would be a crucial nursing intervention to help enhance the effects of positive thinking. As another example, a nursing intervention that could be derived from theme 5 could focus on positive actions that patients considered important to maintaining life (*i.e.*, taking medications, eating nutritious food). Another example of a nursing intervention that can be based on the findings of this study comes from theme 8. To assist individuals in focusing their thoughts to other areas of their lives, nurses can suggest activities of interest to them such as music therapy that can be soothing in nature and serve as a diversion therapy.

● ● ● ● ● **SUMMARY POINTS**

- Qualitative analysis is a challenging, labour-intensive activity—and one that is guided by few standardized rules.
- Although there are no universal strategies for qualitative analysis, four prototypical styles have been identified: (1) a **quasi-statistical style** that begins with pre-established themes and that lends itself to basic descriptive statistical analysis; (2) a **template analysis style** that involves the development of an analysis guide (**template**) to sort the data; (3) an **editing analysis style** that involves an interpretation of the data on which a **categorization scheme** is based; and (4) an **immersion/crystallization style** that is characterized by the analyst's total immersion in and reflection of text materials.
- Qualitative analysis typically involves four types of intellectual processes: comprehending, synthesizing, theorizing, and **recontextualizing** (ex-

ploration of the developed theory in terms of its applicability to other settings or groups).

- The first major step in analyzing qualitative data is to organize and index the materials for easy retrieval, typically by coding the content of the data according to a categorization scheme.
- Traditionally, researchers have organized their data by developing **conceptual files,** which are physical files in which coded excerpts of data relevant to specific categories are placed. However, computer programs are now available that perform basic indexing functions and also offer various enhancements that facilitate data analysis.
- The actual analysis of data begins with a search for **themes,** which involves the discovery of commonalities across subjects as well as natural variation in the data.
- The next analytic step usually involves a validation of the thematic analysis. Some researchers use **quasi-statistics,** which involves a tabulation of the frequency with which certain themes or relations are supported by the data.
- In a final analytic step, the analyst tries to weave the thematic strands together into an integrated picture of the phenomenon under investigation.
- Grounded theory uses the constant comparative method of data analysis.
- There are two broad types of codes in grounded theory: **substantive codes** (in which the empirical substance of the topic is conceptualized) and **theoretical codes** (in which the relationships among the substantive codes are conceptualized).
- Substantive coding involves **open coding** to capture what is going on in the data, and then **selective coding,** in which only variables relating to a core variable are coded. The **core variable,** a behaviour pattern that has relevance for participants, is sometimes a **basic social process** (BSP) that involves an evolutionary process of coping or adaptation.
- There are numerous different approaches to phenomenological analysis, including the descriptive methods of Colaizzi, Giorgi, and Van Kaam, in which the goal is to find common patterns of experiences shared by particular instances.
- In Van Manen's approach, which involves efforts to grasp the essential meaning of the experience being studied, the researcher searches for themes, using either a **holistic approach** (viewing text as a whole), **selective approach** (pulling out key statements and phrases), or **detailed approach** (analyzing every sentence).
- Some researchers identify neither a specific approach nor a specific research tradition; rather, they might say that they used **qualitative content analysis** as their analytic method.

➤ ➤ ➤ ➤ *CRITICAL THINKING ACTIVITIES*

Chapter 14 of the accompanying *Study Guide to Accompany Essentials of Nursing Research,* 5th edition, offers various exercises and study suggestions for reinforcing the concepts presented in this chapter. In addition, you can address the following:

1. Read the method section from the qualitative research study in the Appendix of this book, and then answer the questions in Box 14-1.

2. What is the basic social process that was identified in Small's study of parents and their adolescents (the research example described in Chapter 9)? The citation is: Small, S. P., Brennan-Hunter, A. L.., Best, D. G., & Solberg, S. M. (2002). Struggling to understand: The experience of nonsmoking parents with adolescents who smoke. *Qualitative Health Research, 12,* 1202–1219.

For additional review, see questions 198–205 on the study CD provided with Polit: Study Guide to Accompany Essentials of Nursing Research.

SUGGESTED READINGS

Methodologic References

Beck, C. T. (1994). Reliability and validity issues in phenomenology. *Western Journal of Nursing Research, 16,* 254–267.

Beck, C. T. (1999). Grounded theory. In J. Fain (Ed.), *Reading, understanding, and applying nursing research* (pp. 205–225). Philadelphia: F. A. Davis.

Becker, H. S. (1970). *Sociological work.* Chicago: Aldine.

Colaizzi, P. (1978). Psychological research as the phenomenologist views it. In R. Valle & M. King (Eds.), *Existential phenomenological alternatives for psychology.* New York: Oxford University Press.

Crabtree, B. F., & Miller, W. L. (Eds.). (1992). *Doing qualitative research.* Newbury Park, CA: Sage.

Diekelmann, N., Allen, D., & Tanner, C. (1989). *The NLN criteria for appraisal of baccalaureate programs: A critical hermeneutic analysis.* New York: NLN Press.

Giorgi, A. (1985). *Phenomenology and psychological research.* Pittsburgh, PA: Duquesne University Press.

Glaser, B. G. (1978). *Theoretical sensitivity: Advances in the methodology of grounded theory.* Mill Valley, CA: Sociology Press.

Glaser, B. G., & Strauss, A. L. (1967). *The discovery of grounded theory: Strategies for qualitative research.* Chicago: Aldine.

Miles, M. B., & Huberman, A. M. (1994). *Qualitative data analysis* (2nd ed.). Beverly Hills, CA: Sage.

Morse, J. M., & Field, P. A. (1995). *Qualitative research methods for health professionals* (2nd ed.). Thousand Oaks, CA: Sage.

Strauss, A., & Corbin, J. (1990). *Basics of qualitative research.* Newbury Park, CA: Sage.

Van Kaam, A. (1966). *Existential foundations of psychology.* Pittsburgh, PA: Duquesne University Press.

Van Manen, M. (1990). *Researching lived experience.* New York: State University of New York.

Substantive References

Anderson, E. H., & Spencer, H. M. (2002). Cognitive representations of AIDS: A phenomenological study. *Qualitative Health Research, 12*(10), 1338–1352.

Beck, C. T. (2002). Releasing the pause button: Mothering twins during the first year of life. *Qualitative Health Research, 12,* 593–608.

Boughn, S., & Holdom, J. (2002). Trichotillomania: Women's reports of treatment efficacy. *Research in Nursing & Health, 25,* 135–144.

Browne, A. J., & Fiske, J. (2001). First Nations women's encounters with mainstream health care services. *Western Journal of Nursing Research, 23,* 126–147.

LeClerc, C. M., Wells, D. L., Craig, D., & Wilson, J. L. (2002). Falling short of the mark. *Clinical Nursing Research, 11,* 242–263.

Morris, M. (2002, March). Violence against women and girls—Fact sheet. *Canadian Research Institute for the Advancement of Women.* Retrieved from http://www.criaw-icref.ca/Violence fact_sheet_a.htm.

Myrick, F. (2002). Preceptorship and critical thinking in nursing education. *Journal of Nursing Education, 41*(4), 154–164.

Polit, D. F., London, A., & Martinez (2000). *Food security and hunger in poor, mother-headed families in four U.S. cities.* New York: MDRC.

Wuest, J., & Merritt-Gray, M. (2001). Beyond survival: reclaiming self after leaving an abusive male partner. *Canadian Journal of Nursing Research, 32*(4), 79–94.

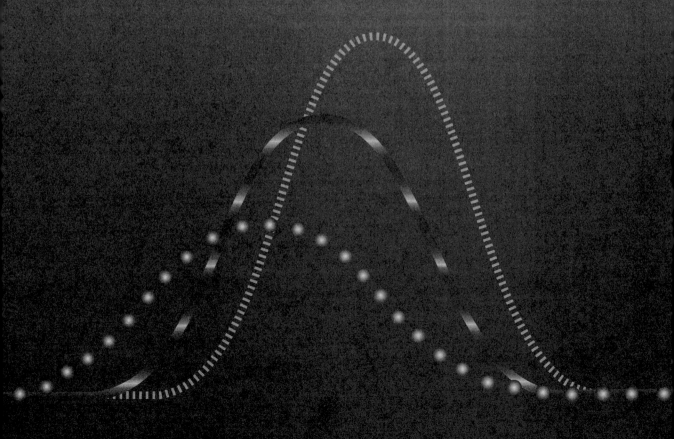

PART VI

CRITICAL APPRAISAL AND UTILIZATION OF NURSING RESEARCH

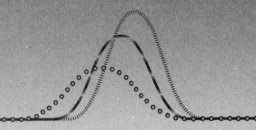

Critiquing Research Reports

INTERPRETING STUDY RESULTS
Interpreting Quantitative Results
Interpreting Qualitative Results
RESEARCH CRITIQUE
Critiquing Research Decisions
Purposes of a Research Critique
ELEMENTS OF A RESEARCH CRITIQUE
Substantive and Theoretical Dimensions
Methodologic Dimensions
Ethical Dimensions
Interpretive Dimensions
Presentation and Stylistic Dimensions

RESEARCH EXAMPLES
Research Example of a Quantitative Report
and Critical Comments
Research Example of a Qualitative Report
and Critical Comments
SUMMARY POINTS
CRITICAL THINKING ACTIVITIES
SUGGESTED READINGS
Substantive References
Methodologic References

Student Objectives

On completion of this chapter, the student will be able to:

○ describe aspects of a study's findings important to consider in developing an interpretation of quantitative and qualitative studies
○ describe strategies for interpreting hypothesized, unhypothesized, or mixed results in quantitative studies
○ distinguish practical and statistical significance
○ describe the purpose, features, and dimensions of a research critique
○ evaluate the substantive, methodologic, and ethical dimensions of a study
○ evaluate a researcher's interpretation of his or her results
○ define new terms in the chapter

New Terms

Critique   Mixed results
Interpretation   Results
Methodologic decisions   Unhypothesized results

Throughout this book, we have provided guidelines for critiquing various aspects of nursing research projects reported in the nursing literature. This chapter describes the purposes of a research critique and offers some further tips on how to evaluate research reports. One important aspect of a research critique involves the reviewer's interpretation of the study findings. Therefore, we begin this chapter by offering some suggestions on interpreting research results.

INTERPRETING STUDY RESULTS

The analysis of research data provides the **results** of the study. These results need to be evaluated and interpreted, which is often a challenging task. **Interpretation** should take into consideration the study's aims, its theoretical underpinnings, the existing body of related research knowledge, and the limitations of the adopted research methods. The interpretive task involves a consideration of the following aspects of the study findings:

- The credibility and accuracy of the results
- The meaning of the results
- The importance of the results

- The extent to which the results can be generalized or have potential for use in other contexts
- The implications for practice, theory, or research

In this section, we review issues relating to these interpretive aspects for quantitative and qualitative research reports.

Interpreting Quantitative Results

Quantitative research results often offer the consumer more interpretive opportunities than qualitative ones—in large part, because a quantitative report can summarize much of the study data, whereas qualitative reports contain only illustrative examples of the data. Readers of quantitative reports need to give careful thought to the possible meaning behind the numbers.

The Credibility of Quantitative Results

One of the first tasks you will face in interpreting quantitative results is assessing how accurate and believable they are. A thorough assessment of the accuracy of the results relies on your critical thinking skills and on your understanding of research methods. The evaluation should be based on an analysis of evidence, not on personal opinions and "gut feelings." Both external and internal evidence can be brought to bear. External evidence comes primarily from the body of prior research. If the results are consistent, the credibility of the findings is enhanced. If the results are inconsistent with prior research, possible reasons for the discrepancy should be sought. What was different about the way the data were collected, the sample was selected, key variables were operationalized, extraneous variables were controlled, and so on?

Internal evidence for the accuracy of the findings comes from an evaluation of the methods used. You will need to evaluate carefully all the major methodologic decisions made in planning and executing the study to determine whether alternative decisions might have yielded different results. This issue is discussed in greater detail later in this chapter.

A critical analysis of the research methods and conceptualization, and an examination of various types of external and internal evidence, almost inevitably indicates some limitations. These limitations must be taken into account in interpreting the results.

The Meaning of Quantitative Results

In quantitative studies, the results are usually in the form of test statistical values and probability levels, which do not in and of themselves confer meaning. The statistical results must be translated conceptually and interpreted. In this section, we discuss the interpretation of various types of research outcomes within a statistical hypothesis testing context.

> **CONSUMER TIP**
>
> Many research reports do not formally specify the hypotheses that are being tested, but rather present research questions or a statement of purpose (see Chap. 5). However, every time researchers use an inferential statistic such as a *t*-test, ANOVA, chi-squared test, and so on, they are using statistics to test a hypothesis. The hypothesis being tested is that, in the population, the groups being compared are different, or that there are true, reliable relationships between variables. When hypotheses are not stated but statistical tests are performed, you may have to infer the hypotheses. ∎

Interpreting Hypothesized Significant Results. When statistical tests support the researcher's hypotheses, the task of interpreting the results may be straightforward because the rationale for the hypotheses presumably offers an explanation of what the findings mean. However, hypotheses can be correct even when the researcher's explanation of what is going on is not. As a reviewer, you will need to be sure that the researcher does not go beyond the data in interpreting the results. For example, suppose a nurse researcher hypothesized that a relationship exists between a pregnant woman's level of anxiety about the labour and delivery experience and the number of children she has already borne. The data reveal that a negative relationship between anxiety levels and parity does exist ($r = -.40$; $p < .05$). The researcher concludes that childbirth experience reduces anxiety. Is this conclusion supported by the data? The conclusion seems logical, but, in fact, there is nothing within the data that leads to this interpretation. An important, indeed critical, research precept is: correlation does not prove causation. The finding that two variables are related offers no evidence about which of the two variables—if either—caused the other. Alternative explanations for the findings should always be considered. If competing interpretations can be excluded on the basis of the data or previous research findings, so much the better, but interpretations should always be given adequate competition. Throughout the interpretation process, you should bear in mind that the support of research hypotheses through statistical testing never constitutes proof of their veracity. Hypothesis testing is probabilistic, and it is always possible that obtained relationships were due to chance. Also, if there are reasons to question the study's credibility, there may also be reasons to challenge the findings.

> **Example of corroboration of a hypothesis:**
>
> Robertson and Kayhko (2001) used an experimental design to test the hypothesis that a home follow-up intervention for post-myocardial infarction patients would lower rates of rehospitalization and associated health care costs. Their hypothesis was fully supported.

Interpreting Nonsignificant Results. Nonsignificant results pose interpretive problems. Standard statistical procedures are geared toward disconfirmation of the null hypothesis. Failure to reject a null hypothesis (*i.e.,* obtaining results indicating no relationship between the independent and dependent variables) could occur for either of two reasons: (1) because the null hypothesis is true (*i.e.,* there really is no relationship among research variables), or (2) because the null hypothesis is false (*i.e.,* a true relationship exists but the data failed to reveal it). Neither you nor the researcher knows which of these situations prevails. In the first situation, the problem is likely to be in the logical reasoning or the conceptualization that led the researcher to the stated hypotheses. The second situation (a false null hypothesis), by contrast, generally reflects methodologic limitations, such as internal validity problems, a small or atypical sample, or a weak statistical procedure. These limitations should previously have been identified in assessing the credibility of the results. Thus, the interpretation must consider both substantive and methodologic reasons for nonsignificant results. Whatever the underlying cause, there is never justification for interpreting a retained null hypothesis as proof of a lack of relationship among variables. The safest interpretation is that nonsignificant findings represent a lack of evidence for either truth or falsity of the hypothesis.

Note, however, that there is a decided bias against publishing the results of studies in which the results are nonsignificant. This may reflect reviewers' beliefs that nonsignificant results are likely to reflect methodologic limitations.

Example of nonsignificant results:

Hodnett et al. (2002) compared women who received continuous labour support by a specially trained nurse and women receiving usual care during labour in terms of a range of maternal, perinatal, and neonatal outcomes. There were no significant differences between the two groups on any of the outcomes.

Interpreting Unhypothesized Significant Results. Although this does not happen frequently, there are situations in which the researcher obtains significant results that are the opposite of the research hypothesis; these are referred to as **unhypothesized results.** For example, a researcher might predict a negative relationship between patient satisfaction with nursing care and the length of stay in the hospital, but a significant positive relationship might be found. In such cases, it is less likely that the methods are flawed than that the reasoning or theory is incorrect. In attempting to explain such findings, you should pay particular attention to the results of previous research and alternative theories. It is also useful, however, to consider whether there is anything unusual about the sample that might lead its members to behave or respond atypically.

Example of unhypothesized significant results:

Carpenter et al. (2002) conducted a randomized pilot study to evaluate the effectiveness and acceptability of magnetic therapy for hot flashes among breast cancer survivors. Contrary to expectations, the placebo treatment was more effective than magnets in decreasing hot-flash frequency, bother, interference with daily activities, and overall quality of life.

Interpreting Mixed Results.   The interpretive process is often confounded by **mixed results:** some hypotheses are supported by the data, whereas others are not. Or a hypothesis may be accepted when one measure of the dependent variable is used but rejected with a different measure. When only some results run counter to a theoretical position or conceptual scheme, the research methods are the first aspect of the study deserving critical scrutiny. Differences in the validity and reliability of the various measures may account for such discrepancies, for example. On the other hand, mixed results may suggest that a theory needs to be qualified or that certain constructs within the theory need to be reconceptualized.

Example of mixed results:

McCusker et al. (2001) tested the effect of a rapid emergency department intervention for older adults on functional status, depressive symptoms, caregiver health status, and satisfaction with care. As expected, the intervention was associated with a significantly reduced rate of functional decline at 4 months after intervention. However, the intervention had no effect on patient depressive symptoms, caregiver outcomes, or satisfaction with care.

The Importance of Quantitative Results

In quantitative studies, results supporting the hypotheses are described as being significant. A careful analysis of study results involves an evaluation of whether, in addition to being statistically significant, they are important.

The fact that statistical significance was attained in testing the hypothesis does not necessarily mean the results were of value. Statistical significance indicates that the results were unlikely to be a function of chance. This means that the observed group differences or observed relationships were probably real—but not necessarily important. With large samples, even modest relationships are statistically significant. For instance, with a sample of 500 participants, a correlation coefficient of .10 is significant at the .05 level, but a relationship of this magnitude might have little practical value. As a reviewer, therefore, you should pay attention to the numeric values obtained in an analysis group (*e.g.,* means) in addition to the significance level when assessing the implications of the findings.

Conversely, the absence of statistically significant results does not mean that the results are unimportant—although, because of problems in interpreting nonsignificant results, the case is more complex. Suppose a study compared two alternatives for making a clinical assessment (*e.g.,* body temperature). Suppose that a researcher retained the null hypothesis (*i.e.,* found no statistically significant differences between the two methods). If the study involved a small sample, the nonsignificant results would be difficult to interpret. If a very large sample was used, however, there would be a low probability of a Type II error. In such a situation, it might reasonably be concluded that the two procedures yield equally accurate assessments. If one of these procedures were more efficient, less painful, or less costly than the other, the nonsignificant findings could, indeed, be clinically important.

Another criterion for assessing the importance of quantitative research results concerns whether the findings are trivial or obvious. If the findings do little more than confirm common sense, their contribution to knowledge is marginal.

The Generalizability of Quantitative Results
Another aspect of quantitative results that you should assess is their generalizability. Researchers are rarely interested in discovering relationships among variables for a specific group of people at a specific point in time. The aim of nursing research is to gain insights for the improvement of nursing practice. Therefore, an important interpretive question is whether the intervention will work or whether the relationships will hold in other settings, with other people. Part of the interpretive process involves asking the question: To what groups, environments, and conditions can the results of the study be applied?

The Implications of Quantitative Results
After you have formed conclusions about the accuracy, meaning, importance, and generalizability of the results, you are ready to draw inferences about their implications. You might consider the implications of the findings with respect to future research (What should other researchers working in this area do?) or theory development (What are the implications for nursing theory?). However, you are most likely to consider the implications for nursing practice (How, if at all, should the results be used by other nurses in their practice—or by me in my own role as a nurse?). Of course, if you have reached the conclusion that the results have limited credibility or importance, they may be of little utility to your practice.

Interpreting Qualitative Results

It is usually difficult for a reviewer to interpret qualitative findings thoroughly because the researcher is selective in the amount and types of data included in the report for a reviewer's perusal. Nevertheless, you should strive to consider the same five interpretive dimensions for a qualitative study as for a quantitative one.

The Credibility of Qualitative Results
As with the case of quantitative reports, you should question whether the results of a qualitative inquiry are believable. It is reasonable to expect authors of qualitative reports to provide evidence of the credibility of the findings, as

described in Chapter 12—although this does not always happen. Because readers of qualitative reports are exposed to only a portion of the data, they must rely on the researcher's efforts to corroborate the findings through such mechanisms as peer debriefings, member checks, audits, and triangulation.

CONSUMER TIP

Even when peer debriefings or member checks have been undertaken, you should realize that they do not unequivocally establish proof that the results are believable. For example, member checks may not always be effective in illuminating flaws. Perhaps some participants are too polite to disagree with the researcher's interpretations. Or perhaps they become intrigued with a conceptualization they themselves would never have developed on their own—a conceptualization that is not necessarily accurate. ■

In thinking about the believability of qualitative results—as with quantitative results—it is advisable to adopt the posture of a person who needs to be persuaded and to expect the researcher to marshal solid evidence with which to persuade you.

The Meaning of Qualitative Results

In qualitative studies, explication and analysis of the data often occur simultaneously. That is, the researchers make sense of the data as they are coding it, developing a thematic analysis and integrating the themes into a unified whole. Efforts to validate the qualitative analysis are necessarily efforts to validate the thematic or interpretive development as well. Thus, in a qualitative study, the meaning of the data flows from the analysis, and it is seldom necessary to puzzle through the findings in search of a deeper meaning. Moreover, the qualitative researcher rarely establishes *a priori* hypotheses, and thus the task of gleaning meaning does not involve elucidating unhypothesized or mixed results.

The Importance of Qualitative Results

Qualitative research is especially productive when it is used to describe and explain poorly understood phenomena. But the amount of prior research on a topic is not a sufficient barometer for deciding whether the findings can make a contribution to nursing knowledge. The phenomenon must be one that merits rigourous scrutiny. For example, some people prefer the colour green and others like red. Colour preference may not, however, be a sufficiently important topic for an in-depth inquiry. Thus, you must judge whether the topic under study is important or trivial.

In a critical evaluation of a study's importance, you should also consider whether the findings themselves are trivial. Perhaps the topic is worthwhile, but you may feel after reading the report that nothing new has been learned—which can result when the data are too "thin" or when the conceptualization is shallow. Qualitative researchers often attach catchy labels to their themes and processes, but you should ask yourself whether the labels have really captured an insightful construct that goes beyond common knowledge.

The Transferability of Qualitative Results

Although qualitative researchers do not strive for generalizability, the application of the results to other settings and contexts must be considered. If the findings are only relevant to the study participants, they cannot be useful to nursing practice. Thus, in interpreting qualitative results, you should consider how transferable the findings are. In what other types of settings and contexts would you expect the phenomena under study to be manifested in a similar fashion? Of course, to make such an assessment, the author of the report must have described in sufficient detail the context in which the data were collected. Because qualitative studies are context bound, it is only through a careful analysis of the key parameters of the study context that the transferability of results can be assessed.

The Implications of Qualitative Results

If the findings are judged to be believable and important, and if you are satisfied with your interpretation of the meaning of the results, you can begin to consider what the implications of the findings might be. As with quantitative studies, the implications can be multidimensional. First, you can consider the implications for further research: Should a similar study be undertaken in a new setting? Can the study be expanded (or circumscribed) in meaningful or productive ways? Do the results suggest that an important construct has been identified that merits the development of a formal measuring instrument? Does the emerging theory suggest hypotheses that could be tested through controlled quantitative research? Second, do the findings have implications for nursing practice? For example, could the health care needs of a subculture (*e.g.*, the homeless) be identified and addressed more effectively as a result of the study? Finally, do the findings shed light on fundamental processes that are incorporated into nursing theory?

RESEARCH CRITIQUE

If nursing practice is to be based on scientific knowledge, the worth of studies appearing in the nursing literature must be critically appraised. Sometimes, consumers mistakenly believe that if a research report was accepted for publication, the study must be sound. Unfortunately, this is not necessarily the case. Indeed, most research has limitations and weaknesses, and, for this reason, no single study can provide unchallengeable answers to research questions. Nevertheless, the methods of disciplined inquiry continue to provide us with the best possible means of answering certain questions. Knowledge is accumulated not by an individual researcher conducting a single, isolated study but rather through the conduct of several studies addressing the same or similar research questions and through the subsequent critical appraisal of these studies by others. Thus, consumers who can thoughtfully critique research reports also play a role in the advancement of nursing knowledge.

Critiquing Research Decisions

The quality of a study depends on the decisions the researcher made in conceptualizing, designing, and executing the study and in interpreting and communicating the study results. Each study tends to have its own peculiar flaws because each researcher, in addressing the same or a similar research question, makes different decisions about how the study should be done. It is not uncommon for researchers who have made different **methodologic decisions** to arrive at different answers to the same research question. It is precisely for this reason that consumers must be knowledgeable about research methods. You must be able to evaluate research decisions so that you can determine how much faith should be put in the conclusions. You must ask: What other approaches could have been used to study this research problem? and, If another approach had been used, would the results have been more reliable, credible, or replicable? In other words, you need to evaluate the impact of the researcher's decisions on the study's ability to reveal the truth.

Much of this book has been designed to acquaint you with a range of methodologic options for the conduct of research—options on how to design a study, measure variables, select a sample, analyze data, and so on. We hope a familiarity with these options will provide you with the tools to challenge a researcher's decisions when it is appropriate to do so.

Purposes of a Research Critique

A research **critique** is not just a summary of a study but rather a careful appraisal of its merits and flaws. A critique can vary in scope and length, depending on its intended purpose. As a student, you may be asked to prepare a thorough and comprehensive critique of a research report. The purpose of such a critique is to cultivate critical thinking, to induce you to use newly acquired skills in research methods, and to obtain documentation of those skills. Comprehensive critiques are also sometimes prepared by researchers writing commentaries for publication or by discussants at research conferences.

Critiques are often prepared by scholars and researchers to help journal editors in making publication decisions and to offer guidance to researchers on how their research reports could be effectively revised. These critiques typically are not long and generally focus primarily on key substantive and methodologic issues. These critiques may be written in narrative, essay form or may take the form of a bulleted list of the study's strengths and weaknesses.

Practicing nurses also critique research reports—sometimes in writing and sometimes orally in discussion groups or journal clubs. These critiques, which are especially important in relation to the utilization of research results (see Chap. 16), tend to focus on the scientific merit of the study and on its implications for nursing practice. Their purpose is to help practicing nurses think about how study findings can be used and, sometimes, actually to plan a utilization project.

Regardless of the scope of a critique, its function is not to hunt dogmatically for and expose mistakes. A good critique objectively identifies areas of adequacy and inadequacy, virtues as well as faults. Sometimes, the need for this balance is obscured by the terms *critique* and *critical appraisal,* which connote unfavourable observations. The merits of a study are as important as its limitations in coming to conclusions about the worth of its findings. Therefore, the research critique should reflect a thoughtful, objective, and balanced consideration of the study's validity and significance.

Each chapter in this text has offered guidelines for evaluating various research decisions as well as various aspects of written research reports. In preparing a written critique, these guidelines should be reviewed. Box 15-1 presents some further, more general tips for those preparing a formal research critique.

ELEMENTS OF A RESEARCH CRITIQUE

Each research report has several important dimensions that should be considered in a comprehensive critical evaluation of the study's worth (although some dimensions may be given limited consideration in targeted critiques).

BOX 15-1 **GUIDELINES FOR THE CONDUCT OF A WRITTEN RESEARCH CRITIQUE**

1. Be sure to comment on the study's strengths as well as its limitations. The critique should be a balanced consideration of the worth of the research. Each research report has *some* positive features. Be sure to find them and note them.

2. Give specific examples of the study's strengths and limitations. Avoid vague generalizations of praise and fault finding.

3. Try to justify your criticisms. Offer a rationale for how a different approach would have solved a problem that the researcher failed to address.

4. Be as objective as possible. Try to avoid being overly critical of a study because you are not particularly interested in a topic or because you have a world view that is inconsistent with the underlying paradigm.

5. Be sensitive in handling negative comments. Try to put yourself in the shoes of the researcher receiving the critical appraisal. Do not be condescending or sarcastic.

6. Suggest realistic alternatives that the researcher (or future researchers) might want to consider. Do not just identify problems—offer some recommended solutions, making sure that the recommendations are practical ones.

7. Evaluate all aspects of the study—its substantive, theoretical, methodologic, ethical, interpretive, and presentational dimensions.

The aspects we review here include the substantive and theoretical, methodologic, ethical, interpretive, and presentation and stylistic aspects.

Substantive and Theoretical Dimensions

In preparing a critique, you need to determine whether the study was important in terms of the significance of the problem, the soundness of the conceptualizations, the appropriateness of the theoretical framework, and the insightfulness of the analysis and interpretation. The research problem should have obvious relevance to some aspect of nursing. It is not enough that a problem be interesting if it offers no possibility of contributing to nursing knowledge or improving nursing practice.

Many problems that are relevant to nursing are still not necessarily worthwhile substantively. You may need to ask a question such as, "Given what we know about this topic, is this research the right next step?" Knowledge tends to be incremental. Researchers must consider how to advance knowledge on a topic in the most beneficial way. They should avoid unnecessary replications of a study once a body of research clearly points to an answer, but they also should not leap several steps ahead when there is an insecure foundation. Sometimes, replication is exactly what is needed to enhance the credibility or generalizability of earlier findings. Thus, the study problem must be considered in terms of the existing body of research.

Another issue that has both substantive and methodologic implications is the congruence between the study question and the methods used to address it. There must be a good fit between the research problem on the one hand and the overall study design, data collection methods, and analytic approach on the other. Questions that deal with poorly understood phenomena, with processes, with the dynamics of a situation, or with in-depth description, for example, are usually best addressed with flexible designs, unstructured methods of data collection, and qualitative analysis. Questions that involve the measurement of well-defined variables, cause-and-effect relationships, or the effectiveness of some specific intervention, however, are usually better suited to more structured, quantitative approaches using designs that maximize research control.

A final issue to consider is whether the researcher has appropriately placed the research problem into a larger theoretical context. As we stressed in Chapter 7, a researcher does little to enhance the value of the study if the connection between the research problem and a conceptual framework is contrived. But a research problem that is genuinely framed as a part of a larger intellectual problem usually can go farther in advancing knowledge than a problem that ignores its theoretical underpinnings.

Methodologic Dimensions

Researchers make a number of important decisions regarding how best to answer their research questions or test their research hypotheses. It is your job as consumer to evaluate critically the consequences of those decisions. In fact, the heart of the research critique lies in the appraisal of the researcher's methodologic decisions.

Although the researcher makes hundreds of decisions about the methods for conducting a study, some are more consequential than others. In a quantitative study, you should focus critical attention on the following four major decisions:

- *Decision 1, Research Design:* What design will yield the most unambiguous and meaningful (internally valid) results about the relationship between the independent and dependent variables, or the most valid descriptions of the concepts under study?
- *Decision 2, Research Sample:* Who should participate in the study? What are the characteristics of the population to which the findings should be generalized? How large should the sample be, from where should participants be recruited, and what sampling approach should be used to select the sample?
- *Decision 3, Data Collection:* How should the research data be gathered? How can the variables be operationalized and reliably and validly measured?
- *Decision 4, Data Analysis:* What statistical analyses will provide the most appropriate tests of the research hypotheses or answers to the research questions?

In a quantitative study, these methodologic decisions are typically made up-front, and the researcher then executes the prespecified plan. In a qualitative study, by contrast, the researcher makes ongoing methodologic decisions while in the process of collecting and analyzing data—after the very important decisions about the research setting and research tradition have been made. In a qualitative study, the major methodologic decisions you should consider in your critique are as follows:

- *Decision 1, Setting:* Where should the study take place? What setting will yield the richest information about the phenomenon under study?
- *Decision 2, Data Collection:* What should the data sources be, and how should the data be gathered? Should multiple sources of data (*e.g.,* unstructured interviews and observations) be used to achieve method triangulation?
- *Decision 3, Sample:* Who should participate in the study? How can participants be selected to enhance the theoretical richness of the study? How many participants will be needed to achieve data saturation? How much time should be spent in the field to achieve "prolonged engagement"?
- *Decision 4, Data Quality:* What types of evidence can be obtained to support the credibility, transferability, dependability, and confirmability of the data, the analysis, and the interpretation?

Because of practical constraints, research studies almost always involve making compromises between what is ideal and what is feasible. For example, a quantitative researcher might ideally like to work with a sample of 500 participants, but because of limited resources, may have to be content with a sample of 200 participants. A qualitative researcher might realize that 3 years of fieldwork would yield an especially rich and deep understanding of the culture or group under study, but cannot afford to devote this much time to the effort. The person doing a research critique cannot realistically demand that researchers attain these methodologic ideals but must be prepared to evaluate how much damage has been done by failure to achieve them.

Ethical Dimensions

In performing a comprehensive critique, you should consider whether there is evidence of ethical violations. If there are any potential ethical problems, you will need to consider the impact of those problems on the scientific merit of the study as well as on the participants' well-being.

There are two main types of ethical transgressions in research studies. The first class consists of inadvertent actions or activities that the researcher did not foresee as creating an ethical dilemma. For example, in one study that examined married couples' experiences with sexually transmitted diseases, the researcher asked the husband and wife each to complete, privately, a self-administered questionnaire. The researcher offered to mail back copies of the questionnaires to couples who wanted an opportunity to discuss their responses. This offer was intended as a means of enhancing couple communication. However, some participants may have felt compelled to say, under spousal pressure, that they wanted to have a copy of their responses returned in the mail, when, in fact, they did not. The use of the mail to return these sensitive completed questionnaires was also questionable. In this case, the ethical problem was inadvertent and could easily be resolved (*e.g.*, the researcher could give out blank copies of the questionnaire for the couples to go over together).

In other cases, the researcher is aware of potential ethical problems, but consciously decides that the violation is minor in relation to the knowledge gain. For example, the researcher may decide not to obtain informed consent from the parents of minor children attending a family planning clinic because such consent might discourage participation in the study and lead to a biased sample of clinic users; it could also violate the minors' right to confidential treatment at the clinic. When the researcher knowingly elects not to follow the ethical principles outlined in Chapter 4, both the decision and the researcher's rationale should be evaluated.

Interpretive Dimensions

Research reports almost always conclude with a discussion, conclusions, or implications section. In this final section, the researcher offers an interpretation of the findings, considers whether the findings support a theoretical framework, and discusses what the findings might imply for nursing.

As a reviewer, you should be somewhat wary if the discussion section fails to point out any limitations. The researcher is in the best position to detect and assess the impact of sampling deficiencies, practical constraints, data quality problems, and so on, and it is a professional responsibility to alert readers to these difficulties. Moreover, when a researcher notes methodologic shortcomings, readers know that these limitations were taken into account in the interpretation of results. As an example, Carty and coworkers (1996) conducted a study of women's perceptions of fatigue during pregnancy and postpartum. Women who were discharged within 3 days of delivery were compared with women who were discharged after 3 days with respect to fatigue levels. The researchers found few differences between the two groups with regard to hours slept, perceptions of tiredness, and impact of tiredness on daily life. However, the researchers included a word of caution in their discussion section:

> The following limitations should be considered when interpreting the findings: The women in this study chose their discharge time, those who went home early had significant follow-up by nurses, and the questionnaire developed for this study does not have established reliability (p. 77).

Of course, researchers are unlikely to note all relevant shortcomings of their own work. For instance, in the above example, the authors failed to point out that the absence of significant group differences could have resulted from the use of a relatively small sample. Thus, the inclusion of comments about study limitations in the discussion section, although important, does not relieve you of the responsibility of appraising methodologic decisions.

Your task as reviewer is to contrast your own interpretation with that of the researcher and to challenge conclusions that do not appear to be warranted by the results. If your objective evaluation of the research methods and findings leads to an interpretation notably different from that of the researcher, the interpretive dimension of the study merits critical commentary.

In addition to contrasting your interpretation with that of the researchers, your critique should also draw conclusions about the stated implications of the study. Some researchers make grandiose claims or offer unfounded recommendations on the basis of modest results. Some guidelines for evaluating the researcher's interpretation and implications are offered in Box 15-2.

Presentation and Stylistic Dimensions

Although the worth of the study is primarily reflected in the dimensions discussed thus far, the manner in which the information is communicated in the research report is also fair game in a comprehensive critical appraisal. Box 15-3 summarizes the major points that should be considered in evaluating the presentation of a research report.

An important consideration is whether the research report has provided sufficient information for a thoughtful critique of the other dimensions. For

BOX 15-2

GUIDELINES FOR CRITIQUING THE INTERPRETATIVE DIMENSIONS OF A RESEARCH REPORT

1. Does the discussion section offer conclusions or interpretations for all the important results?

2. Are the interpretations consistent with the results? Do the interpretations give due consideration to the limitations of the research methods?

3. What types of evidence in support of the interpretation does the researcher offer? Is that evidence persuasive? Are the results interpreted in light of findings from other studies?

4. Are alternative explanations for the findings mentioned, and is the rationale for their rejection presented?

5. In quantitative studies, does the interpretation distinguish between practical and statistical significance?

6. Are generalizations made that are not warranted on the basis of the sample used?

7. Does the researcher offer implications of the research for nursing practice, nursing theory, or nursing research? Are the implications appropriate, given the study's limitations?

8. Are specific recommendations for practice or future studies made? Are the recommendations consistent with the findings and consistent with the body of knowledge on the topic?

example, if the report does not describe how participants were selected, the reviewer cannot comment on the adequacy of the sample, but can criticize the researcher's failure to include information on sampling. When vital pieces of information are missing, the researcher leaves the reader little choice but to assume the worst because this would lead to the most cautious interpretation of the results.

The writing in a research report, as in any published document, should be clear, grammatical, concise, and well organized. Unnecessary jargon should be minimized, but colloquialisms generally should be avoided. Inadequate organization is another presentation flaw in some research reports. Continuity and logical thematic development are critical to good communication of scientific information, but these qualities are often difficult to attain.

Styles of writing do differ for qualitative and quantitative reports, and it is unreasonable to apply the standards considered appropriate for one paradigm to the other. Quantitative research reports are typically written in a more formal, impersonal fashion, using either the third person or passive voice to connote objectivity. Qualitative studies are likely to be written in a more literary style, using the first or second person and active voice to connote proximity and inti-

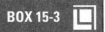

GUIDELINES FOR CRITIQUING THE PRESENTATION OF A RESEARCH REPORT

1. Does the report include a sufficient amount of detail to permit a thorough critique of the study's purpose, conceptual framework, design and methods, handling of critical ethical issues, analysis of data, and interpretation?

2. Is the report well written and grammatical? Are pretentious words or jargon used when a simpler wording would have been possible?

3. Is the report well organized, or is the presentation confusing? Is there an orderly, logical presentation of ideas? Are transitions smooth, and is the report characterized by continuity of thought and expression?

4. Is the report sufficiently concise, or does the author include a lot of irrelevant detail? Are important details omitted?

5. Does the report suggest overt biases?

6. Is the report written using tentative language as befits the nature of the disciplined inquiry, or does the author talk about what the study did or did not "prove"?

7. Is sexist language avoided?

8. Does the title of the report adequately capture the key concepts and the population under investigation? Does the abstract (if any) adequately summarize the research problem, study methods, and important findings?

macy with the data and the phenomenon under study. Regardless of style, however, as a reviewer you should be alert to indications of overt biases, unwarranted exaggerations, emotionally laden comments, or melodramatic language.

In summary, the research report is meant to be an account of how and why a problem was studied and what results were obtained. The report should be accurate, clearly written, cogent, and concise. It should reflect scholarship, but not pedantry, and it should be written in a manner that piques the reader's interest and curiosity.

RESEARCH EXAMPLES

The appendix offers two research reports—one qualitative and the other quantitative—in their entirety. The guidelines in this chapter and throughout the book can be used to conduct a critical appraisal of these studies. (In addition, there are two complete research reports in the accompanying *Study Guide for Essentials of Nursing Research,* 5th edition.

In this section, we describe two studies by nurse researchers and present excerpts from published written critiques. Note that these comments are not comprehensive—they do not cover all the dimensions of a research critique as described in this chapter. However, the excerpts should provide a flavor for the kinds of things that are noted in a critique.

Research Example of a Quantitative Report and Critical Comments

Ross, Carswell, and Dalziel (2001) investigated family caregiving within institutional settings. Their published report was accompanied by a commentary by one reviewer.

Research Summary

Ross and her colleagues addressed several questions in their descriptive study of family caregiving to relatives within long-term care facilities, including the following: (1) How frequently do families visit following the admission of a relative? (2) What care-related activities do families carry out for their institutionalized relative? and (3) What are their care-related learning needs and resources?

Nineteen long-term care facilities in the Ottawa-Carleton region were identified, 9 of which were invited to participate in the study. Facilities were chosen to reflect diversity in size, urban/rural location, language, and type of ownership. Staff in these facilities identified family members who were personally involved with their relative, and 194 of those identified were randomly selected to be participants. Questionnaires that included both closed-ended and open-ended questions were mailed to selected family members, and a total of 122 completed questionnaires were returned.

Descriptive statistics (mostly percentages and means) were used to analyze the data. The findings indicated that families visited their institutionalized relatives frequently. While visiting, family members generally provided both direct care (*e.g.,* grooming) and, especially, indirect care (*e.g.,* communicating with staff). The majority of family members indicated an interest in learning to provide better emotional support. On the basis of their findings, the researchers made several recommendations for policy and practice, such as the development of mechanisms to facilitate the visiting experience and creating a comfortable environment.

Commentary

Penrod (2001) prepared a commentary that was published in the same issue as the Ross and colleagues study. Penrod had many favourable comments about the study and its purpose. For example, she noted the following:

> . . . These authors cogently argue that we know little about what the visiting experience is like for family members. Observation of visible task perfor-

mance provides a superficial glimpse of what is going on during these visits, but understanding these actions from the perspectives of the family members falls woefully short." (p. 364)

Penrod did, however, express concerns about some methodologic aspects of the study. One concern focused on the sampling plan. Noting that the initial pool of eligibles had been identified by facility staff members, she commented that the researchers had not provided information about what selection criteria staff used. Moreover, by seeking residents whose family members were personally involved with their relative, there was a risk that results would be biased. Penrod concluded that ". . . further clarification of sampling and selection would strengthen the study" (p. 365).

A more general concern related to the cross-sectional nature of the design. Penrod noted that caregivers' views and experiences are dynamic and change over time. This is of particular concern because the residents had lived in the facility for an average of 3.5 years, and presumably the range of time institutionalized varied widely. Penrod asked the following questions, which could best be answered by a longitudinal design, but which also could have been explored with the existing data but were not:

> "Did the caregivers' perceptions of frequency, duration, and reasons for visiting change over time? Did their views on task performance shift between direct and indirect care activities over this time? . . . And was there any evidence of more dynamic learning needs as the caregivers lived through the initial admission and orientation processes followed by the deteriorating health status of their loved ones?" (p. 365).

Penrod concluded by praising the contribution that the study made to an understanding of caregiving *postplacement,* but also commented that "the time has come to advance science beyond description of what is to begin exploring what can be done to maximize potential contributions of caregivers" (p. 367).

Clinical Relevance

The study by Ross and colleagues addresses a clinical issue that has yet to be fully described: the needs and contributions of family members in terms of caring for an institutionalized relative in long-term care. Their study shows that family caregiving does not end with institutionalization. In fact, families remain involved and continue to participate in both direct and indirect caregiving. These findings serve to broaden our view of family caregiving within institutions and also underscore the importance, for nurses, of providing support to family members involved in the care of their elderly relative. Three strategies were suggested by the authors for supporting family caregiving: (1) facilitating the visiting experience, (2) strengthening support for the provision of family care, and (3) creating a comfortable environment. This does not suggest that increased responsibility for care should be placed on families, but rather that they should be supported in the care they are able and willing to provide.

Research Example of a Qualitative Report and Critical Comments

Butler, Banfield, Sveinson, and Allen (1998) conducted a qualitative study to describe women's experiences with changes in sexual function following treatment for gynecologic cancer. Their research report, which appeared in *Western Journal of Nursing Research,* was followed by commentaries by two reviewers.

Research Summary

Butler and her colleagues conducted a multimethod study that explored issues of sexual health for women with cervical and endometrial cancer. The qualitative portion of their study involved in-depth interviews with a sample of 17 women, using a semistructured interview guide. The questions were designed to stimulate discussion about the effects of cancer and its treatment on how the participants viewed themselves as women, as partners, and as mothers. The interviews, which were taped and transcribed, lasted about 90 minutes. Content analysis was used for data analysis. Three of the investigators independently coded the data; intercoder agreement was high.

Although the study's purpose was to pursue issues relating to sexual functioning, the women described a broader concept of sexual health in which functioning was only one aspect contributing to the view of self as a sexual being. The analysis revealed multiple components that need to be considered in developing a conceptual model of sexual health.

One of the central categories the women discussed was the effect of relationships—with health care personnel, family, friends, and partners—on their sexual well-being. The absence of discussions about sexual health by nurses and physicians suggested to the women that their sexuality was not really a medical concern. This interpretation was shared with their partners, resulting in couples making efforts to adjust with little information or support. The authors concluded that health care professionals should examine their own values and beliefs about sexuality and assess their knowledge and comfort level about these topics.

Critical Commentary and Response

Downe-Wamboldt (1998) praised Butler and her colleagues for undertaking an interesting study on an important topic and encouraged them to continue with research in this area: "The important topic of sexual health in the context of cancer care has received little attention from researchers, and this article makes a valuable contribution to the nursing literature" (p. 700).

Downe-Wamboldt did not offer any criticism of the actual study, except to note its limited generalizability, but made some suggestions about improving the report itself:

> To more meaningfully interpret the findings, it would have been helpful to have a description of the specific questions that were asked that provided

the data for the study. Were there any questions that the women found too sensitive or were not comfortable to answer? The identified themes and relevant quotations generally provided a clear picture of how the themes emerged from the data. One notable exception is the theme of sexual health influenced by the environment. It is difficult to assess the validity of this theme based on the quality and quantity of quotations provided. (pp. 700–701)

Alteneder (1998), who wrote a second commentary, also expressed a desire for more information than was provided in the report:

The authors said that nurses rarely discussed sexual functioning; however, it would be of interest to the reader what the nurses did cover when they spoke on this topic. . . . Because 6 of the participants had no longer continued to be sexually active post-treatment, information about why they were no longer active would have added to the description of the women. (p. 702)

This second commentator further suggested that the researchers could have improved the study by interviewing the women's partners; she also expressed some misgivings about the data collection:

I have some concern about the use of the semistructured interview guide, which was reviewed for content and face validity by three oncology nurses and one physician. I feel that this type of study should be open to learn from the participants, and the restricting structure might inhibit the type of information received by the investigator. (p. 702)

In their response, Butler and her colleagues provided the commentators with some of the information they were seeking (*e.g.*, the six women's reasons for not being sexually active). They acknowledged the need for replication of the study and also commented on data quality issues:

The purpose statement may not have adequately reflected the depth of exploration provided by the semistructured interview guide. . . . The study participants did not appear to have any difficulty with questions asked during the interview and openly described how the cancer affected their well-being. (p. 704)

Clinical Relevance

In her critical commentary, Downe-Wamboldt (1998) noted that Butler and colleagues' study addressed an important gap in nursing knowledge and makes a valuable contribution to the nursing literature. Minimal research has been conducted on sexual health in cancer care. After treatment for gynecologic cancer, many women try to cope with changes in their sexual health with insufficient help from clinicians.

Some methodologic concerns raised by the two reviewers have implications for the credibility of this study's findings, such as the restrictive nature of the semistructured interview. This type of interview may have hindered the emergence of flow of rich data. Another limitation was the limited data supporting the theme of sexual health influenced by the environment.

Despite these limitations, the study has made a valuable contribution to health professionals' understanding of key issues for women who have undergone treatment for gynecologic cancer. Alteneder (1998) noted that sexuality has not been a concern of health professionals when they are establishing priorities for treating cancer. The findings suggest that nurses should examine their beliefs, knowledge, and attitudes regarding sexuality to facilitate their comfort in discussing sensitive sexual health issues with their female patients and partners. Open discussions with women who have had gynecologic cancer treatment are critical to help foster their sexual expression, communication, and intimacy.

● ● ● ● ● *SUMMARY POINTS*

- The **interpretation** of research findings is a search for the broader meaning and implications of the results of an investigation.
- Interpretation of both qualitative and quantitative results typically involves five steps: (1) analyzing the credibility of the results; (2) determining their meaning; (3) considering their importance; (4) determining the generalizability or transferability of the findings; and (5) assessing the implications in regard to theory, nursing practice, and future research.
- A research **critique** is a careful, critical appraisal of the strengths and limitations of a study.
- A reviewer preparing a comprehensive review should consider five major dimensions of the study: the substantive and theoretical, methodologic, ethical, interpretive, and presentation and stylistic dimensions. Many critiques focus primarily on the methodologic dimension.
- Researchers designing a study must make a number of important **methodologic decisions** that affect the quality and integrity of the research. Consumers preparing a critique must evaluate the decisions the researchers made to determine how much faith can be placed in the results.

➤ ➤ ➤ ➤ *CRITICAL THINKING ACTIVITIES*

Chapter 15 of the accompanying *Study Guide to Accompany Essentials of Nursing Research*, 5th edition, offers various exercises and study suggestions for reinforcing the concepts presented in this chapter. In addition, you can address the following:

1. Prepare a written critique of one of the two studies that appear in the Appendix.

2. Read one or both of the studies that appear as research examples in this chapter, together with the two commentaries. To what degree do you agree with the commentaries? What additional comments would you have to offer the researchers? To what extent did the researchers' responses address the concerns of the commentators?

For additional review, see questions 206–215 on the study CD provided with Polit: Study Guide to Accompany Essentials of Nursing Research.

SUGGESTED READINGS

Methodologic References

Beck, C. T. (1990). The research critique: General criteria for evaluating a research report. *Journal of Obstetric, Gynecologic, and Neonatal Nursing, 19,* 18–22.

Beck, C. T. (1993). Qualitative research: The evaluation of its credibility, fittingness, and auditability. *Western Journal of Nursing Research, 15,* 263–266.

Burns, N. (1989). Standards for qualitative research. *Nursing Science Quarterly, 2,* 254–260.

Evertz, J. (2001). Evaluating qualitative research. In P.L. Munhall (Ed.), *Nursing research: A qualitative perspective* (pp.599–612). New York: NLN.

Giuffre, M. (1998). Critiquing a research article. *Journal of Perianesthesia Nursing, 13,* 104–108.

Rasmussen, L., O'Conner, M., Shinkle, S., & Thomas, M. K. (2000). The basic research review checklist. *Journal of Continuing Education in Nursing, 31*(1), 13–18.

Ryan-Wenger, N. M. (1992). Guidelines for critique of a research report. *Heart & Lung, 21,* 394–401.

Substantive References

Alteneder, R. A. (1998). Commentary. *Western Journal of Nursing Research, 20,* 701–703.

Butler, L., Banfield, V., Sveinson, T., & Allen, K. (1998). Conceptualizing sexual health in cancer care. *Western Journal of Nursing Research, 20,* 683–699.

Carpenter, J.S., Wells, N., Lambert, B., Watson, P., Slayton, T., Chak, B., Hepworth, J.T., & Worthington, W. B. (2002) A pilot study of magnetic therapy for hot flashes after breast cancer. *Cancer Nursing, 25,* 104–109.

Carty, E. M., Bradley, C., & Winslow, W. (1996). Women's perceptions of fatigue during pregnancy and postpartum. *Clinical Nursing Research, 5,* 67–80.

Downe-Wamboldt, B. (1998). Commentary. *Western Journal of Nursing Research, 20,* 700–701.

Hodnett, E. D., Lowe, N. K., Hannah, M. E., Willan, A. R., Stevens, B., Weston, J. A., Ohlsson, A. Gafni, A., Muir, H., Myhr, T. L., & Stremler, R. (2002). Effectiveness of nurses as providers of birth labor support in North American hospitals. *JAMA, 288,* 1373–1381.

McCusker, J., Verdon, J., Tousignant, P. Poulin De Courval, L., Dendukuri, N., & Belzile, E. (2001). Rapid emergency department intervention for older people reduces risk of functional decline: Results of a multicenter randomized trial. *Journal of the American Geriatric Society, 49,* 1272–1281.

Penrod, J. (2001). Commentary on "Family caregiving in long-term care facilities." *Clinical Nursing Research, 10,* 364–368.

Robertson. K. A., & Kayhko, K. (2001). Cost analysis of an intensive home follow-up program for first-time post-myocardial infarction patients and their families. *Dynamics, 12,* 25–31.

Ross, M. M., Carswell, A., & Dalziel, W. B. (2001). Family caregiving in long-term care facilities. *Clinical Nursing Research, 10,* 347–363.

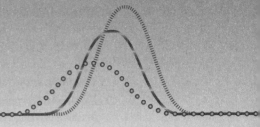

CHAPTER 16

Using Research Findings in Nursing Practice

RESEARCH UTILIZATION AND EVIDENCE-BASED PRACTICE IN NURSING
  The Utilization of Nursing Research
  Evidence-Based Nursing Practice
BARRIERS TO UTILIZING NURSING RESEARCH AND RELATED STRATEGIES TO ENHANCE UTILIZATION
  Research-Related Barriers
  Nurse-Related Barriers
  Organizational Barriers
  Nursing Profession-Related Barriers

THE PROCESS OF USING RESEARCH IN NURSING PRACTICE
  Models for Evidence-Based Nursing Practice
  Steps in Using Research in Nursing Practice
  Other Utilization Approaches
RESEARCH EXAMPLE
SUMMARY POINTS
CRITICAL THINKING ACTIVITIES
WORLD WIDE WEBSITES
SUGGESTED READINGS
  Methodologic References
  Substantive References

Student Objectives

On completion of this chapter, the student will be able to:

○ distinguish research utilization (RU) and evidence-based practice (EBP) and describe the history of both within nursing
○ describe a continuum along which RU can occur
○ discuss the current status of RU and EBP within nursing
○ identify barriers to utilizing nursing research and strategies for improving utilization and EBP
○ identify several models or theories that have relevance for RU and EBP
○ describe the general steps in RU/EBP projects
○ describe the role that integrative reviews play in EBP
○ evaluate the extent to which a nurse researcher adequately addresses the issue of utilization in the discussion section of a research report
○ define new terms in the chapter

New Terms

Cochrane Collaboration
Conceptual utilization
Cost–benefit assessment
CURN project
Decision accretion
Direct research utilization
Evidence-based practice
Evidence hierarchy
Evidence report
Implementation potential
Indirect research utilization

Instrumental utilization
Integrative reviews
Iowa Model
Knowledge creep
Knowledge-focused triggers
Ottawa Model of Research Use (OMRU)
Persuasive utilization
Problem-focused triggers
Research utilization
Stetler Model

Most nurse researchers would like to have their findings incorporated into nursing protocols, decisions, and curricula. In addition, most nurses working in clinical settings are aware of the benefits of research-based practice. That is, there is a growing interest in developing a practice in which there is solid evidence from disciplined research that specific nursing actions are clinically appropriate and cost-effective and result in positive outcomes for patients. In this chapter, we discuss various aspects of using nursing research to support an evidence-based practice.

RESEARCH UTILIZATION AND EVIDENCE-BASED PRACTICE

The term **research utilization (RU)** is sometimes used synonymously with **evidence-based practice (EBP).** Although there is an overlap between the two concepts, they are, in fact, distinct. EBP, the broader of the two terms, involves making clinical decisions on the basis of the best possible evidence. Usually, the best evidence comes from rigorous research, but EBP also uses other sources of credible information. A basic feature of EBP is that it de-emphasizes decision making based on custom, authority opinion, or ritual. Rather, the emphasis is on identifying the best available research evidence and *integrating* it with clinical expertise, patient input, and existing resources.

Broadly speaking, RU refers to the use of the findings from a disciplined study or set of studies in a practical application that is unrelated to the original research. In projects that have had RU as a goal, the emphasis is on translating empirically derived knowledge into real-world applications. Figure 16–1 provides a basic schema of how RU and EBP are interrelated. This section further explores and distinguishes the two concepts.

The Utilization of Nursing Research

During the 1980s and early 1990s, RU became an important buzz word, and several changes in nursing education and nursing research were prompted by the desire to develop a knowledge base for nursing practice. In education, nursing schools increasingly began to include courses on research methods so that students would become intelligent research consumers. In the research arena, there was a shift in focus toward clinical nursing problems. These changes, coupled with the completion of several large RU projects, played a role in sensitizing the nursing community to the desirability of using research as a basis for practice; they were not enough, however, to lead to widespread

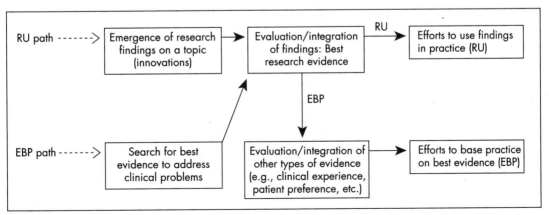

FIGURE 16-1. Research utilization (RU) and evidence-based practice (EBP).

integration of research findings into the delivery of nursing care. RU, as the nursing community has come to recognize, is a complex and nonlinear phenomenon that poses professional challenges.

The Research Utilization Continuum

As Figure 16–1 indicates, the start point of RU is the emergence of new knowledge and new ideas. Research is conducted and, over time, knowledge on a topic accumulates. In turn, knowledge works its way into use, to varying degrees and at differing rates. Theorists who have studied the phenomenon of knowledge development and the diffusion of ideas typically recognize a continuum in terms of the specificity of the use to which research findings are put. At one end of the continuum are discrete, clearly identifiable attempts to base specific actions on research findings. For example, a series of studies in the 1960s and 1970s demonstrated that the optimal placement time of a glass thermometer for accurate oral temperature determination is 9 minutes (*e.g.*, Nichols & Verhonick, 1968). When nurses specifically altered their behaviour from shorter placement times to the empirically based recommendation of 9 minutes, this constituted an instance of RU at this end of the continuum. This type of utilization has been referred to as **instrumental utilization** (Caplan & Rich, 1975).

Research findings can, however, be used in a more diffuse manner—in a way that promotes cumulative awareness, understanding, or enlightenment. Caplan and Rich (1975) refer to this end of the utilization continuum as **conceptual utilization.** Thus, a practicing nurse may read a qualitative research report describing *courage* among individuals with long-term health problems as a dynamic process that includes efforts to fully accept reality and to develop problem-solving skills. The nurse may be reluctant to alter his or her own behaviour or suggest an intervention based on the results, but the study may make the nurse more observant in working with patients with long-term illnesses; it may also lead to informal efforts to promote problem-solving skills. Conceptual utilization, then, refers to situations in which users are influenced in their thinking about an issue based on their knowledge of studies but do not put this knowledge to any specific, documentable use.

The middle ground of this continuum involves the partial impact of research findings on nursing activities. This middle ground frequently is the result of a slow evolutionary process that does not reflect a conscious decision to use an innovative procedure but rather reflects what Weiss (1980) has termed knowledge creep and decision accretion. **Knowledge creep** refers to an evolving "percolation" of research ideas and findings. **Decision accretion** refers to the manner in which momentum for a decision builds over a period of time based on accumulated information gained through readings, informal discussions, meetings, and so on. Increasingly, however, nurses *are* making conscious decisions to use research in their clinical practice, and the EBP movement has contributed to this change.

Estabrooks (1999) recently studied research utilization by collecting survey data from 600 nurses in Canada. She found evidence to support three distinct types of research utilization: (1) **indirect research utilization,** involving changes in nurses' thinking and therefore analogous to conceptual utilization; (2) **direct research utilization,** involving the direct use of findings in giving patient care and therefore analogous to instrumental utilization; and (3) **persuasive utilization,** involving the use of findings to persuade others (typically those in decision-making positions) to make changes in policies or practices relevant to nursing care.

These varying ways of thinking about RU clearly suggest that both qualitative and quantitative research can play key roles in guiding and improving nursing practice. Indeed, Estabrooks (2001) argues that the process of implementing research findings into practice is essentially the same for both quantitative and qualitative research. What differentiates qualitative research, however, is its form. Because qualitative findings are presented in narrative form, Estabrooks claims that this type of research may have a privileged position in RU. Clinicians do not need a strong background in statistics to understand qualitative research, and thus one less step is required of readers of qualitative research. It is not necessary to translate the results into everyday language before the findings can be used conceptually.

Research Utilization in Nursing Practice

During the 1980s and 1990s, there was considerable concern that nurses had failed to use research findings as a basis for making decisions and for developing nursing interventions. This concern was based on some studies suggesting that nurses were not always aware of research results or did not incorporate results into their practice. In one such study, Ketefian (1975) reported on the oral temperature determination practices of 87 registered nurses. As indicated earlier, the results of several studies had clearly demonstrated that the optimal placement time for oral temperature determination using glass thermometers is 9 minutes. Ketefian's study was designed to learn what "happens to research findings relative to nursing practice after five or ten years of dissemination in the nursing literature" (p. 90). In Ketefian's study, only 1 of 87 nurses reported the correct placement time, suggesting that these practicing nurses were unaware of or ignored the research findings about optimal placement time. Other studies in the 1980s (Kirchhoff,1982), were similarly discouraging.

Coyle and Sokop (1990) investigated practicing nurses' adoption of 14 nursing innovations that had been reported in the nursing research literature, replicating a study by Brett (1987). The 14 innovations were selected according to the following criteria: the scientific merit of the study, the significance of the findings for practice, and the suitability of the findings for application to practice. A sample of 113 nurses practicing in 10 hospitals (randomly selected from the medium-sized hospitals in North Carolina) completed questionnaires that measured the nurses' awareness and use of the study findings. The results indicated much variation across the 14 innovations, with awareness of them ranging from 34% at one extreme to 94% at the other. Coyle and Sokop used a scheme to categorize each innovation according to its stage of adoption: awareness (indicating knowledge of the innovation); persuasion (indicating the nurses' belief that nurses should use the innovation in practice); occasional use in practice; and regular use in practice. Only 1 of the 14 studies was at the regular-use stage of adoption. Six studies were in the persuasion stage, indicating that the nurses knew of the innovation and thought it *should* be incorporated into nursing practice but were not basing their own nursing decisions on it.

More recently, a Canadian study by Varcoe and Hilton (1995) with 183 nurses found that 9 of the 10 research-based practices investigated were used by 50% or more of the acute care nurses at least sometime. Rutledge and coworkers (1996) studied the extent to which oncology staff nurses adopted eight research-based practices. The researchers found that awareness levels were high in their sample of over 1000 nurses, with between 53% and 96% of them reporting awareness of the eight practices. Moreover, almost 90% of aware nurses used seven of the practices at least some of the time. Similar results have been reported in a recent survey of nearly 1000 nurses in Scotland (Rodgers, 2000). Table 16–1 describes 5 of the 14 nursing innovations included in Rodgers' study (2000) and shows the stage of adoption of these innovations among nurses who participated in the study.

The results of the recent studies are more encouraging than the studies by Ketefian and Kirchhoff because they suggest that, on average, practicing nurses are aware of many innovations based on research results, are persuaded that the innovations should be used, and are beginning to use them on occasion.

Efforts to Improve Utilization of Nursing Research

The need to reduce the gap between nursing research and nursing practice has been hotly discussed and has led to numerous formal attempts to bridge the gap. In this section, we briefly describe a few of these projects.

The best-known of several early nursing research utilization projects is the **Conduct and Utilization of Research in Nursing (CURN) project,** a 5-year development project awarded to the Michigan Nurses' Association by the Division of Nursing in the 1970s. The major objective of the CURN project was to increase the use of research findings in the daily practice of RNs by disseminating current research findings, facilitating organizational changes needed to implement innovations, and encouraging collaborative clinical research. One CURN activity was to stimulate the conduct of research in clinical settings. The CURN project also focused on helping nurses to use research findings in their practice. The CURN project staff saw RU as primarily an organizational process, with the commitment of organizations that employ nurses as essential to the RU process (Horsley, Crane, & Bingle, 1978). The CURN project team concluded that RU by practicing nurses is feasible, but only if the research is relevant to practice and if the results are broadly disseminated. The CURN project generated considerable international interest. For example, the Cross Cancer Institute in Edmonton, Alberta used the CURN model as a framework to integrate research findings into nursing practice (Alberta Association of Registered Nurses, 1997).

TABLE 16-1. Extent of Adoption of Five Nursing Practices*

NURSING INNOVATION	NOT AWARE (%)	AWARE (%)	PERSUADED (%)	USE SOMETIMES (%)	USE ALWAYS (%)	N
Any type of antiseptic causes damage to the tissues and is not effective in reducing contamination. In general wards, it is recommended that all wounds are cleansed with normasol or normal saline 0.9%	16	0	2	8	74	676
Completing a pain assessment chart enables nurses to assess a patient's pain more accurately and so provide more appropriate pain relief.	16	7	22	43	12	674
There are several stages that dying patients may experience, for example, denial, anger. A knowledge of these can help the nurse understand a patient's behaviour and feelings.	3	0	2	23	72	663
Maintaining a closed drainage system for urinary catheters is one of the most important steps in the prevention of urinary tract infections in patients with indwelling catheters.	4	<1	1	10	85	674
The use of deliberative touch by nurses for therapeutic means (*e.g.,* holding of hands or hugging) has been shown to promote psychological well-being in some patients.	16	<1	5	51	28	680

*Based on findings reported in Rodgers, S. E. (2000). The extent of nursing research utilization in general medical and surgical wards. *Journal of Advanced Nursing, 32*, 182–193. The sample consisted of 936 nurses from 25 hospitals using a random two-stage stratified sampling.

During the 1980s and 1990s, utilization projects were undertaken by a growing number of hospitals and organizations, and descriptions of these projects began to appear regularly in the nursing research literature. These projects were generally institutional attempts to implement a change in nursing practice on the basis of research findings and to evaluate the effects of the innovation. Two examples of broadly focused projects are cited here to illustrate approaches that have been used to close the research–practice gap.

A project in California focused on building organizational capacity as a tool for increasing RU (Rutledge & Donaldson, 1995). The Orange County Research

Utilization in Nursing (OCRUN) project developed a regional network of 20 nursing service organizations and 6 academic institutions. During a 3-year period, nearly 400 nurses participated in continuing education courses that focused on the development of RU competency. The project influenced nurse executives' perceptions of organizational readiness for change and ultimately influenced participating organizations' utilization processes.

Logan and coworkers (1999) described a project implemented at three Ottawa health care settings during a time of multiple restructuring changes. The **Ottawa Model of Research Use (ORMU),** which we describe in a later section, was applied in an effort to increase evidence-based decision making in the three project sites. The 3-year initiative, funded by the Ontario Ministry of Health, was a component of a provincial demonstration project to expand centres of nursing excellence. A major goal of the project was to improve continuity of care across the health continuum. Multiple approaches aimed at research transfer were used, with a major emphasis on educational activities such as workshops.

Evidence-Based Nursing Practice

During the 1990s, the call for RU began to be superceded by the push for EBP. The RU process begins with an empirically based innovation or new idea that gets scrutinized for possible adoption in practice settings. EBP, by contrast, begins with a search for information about how best to solve specific practice problems (see Fig. 16–1). Findings from rigourous research are considered the best possible source of information, but EBP also draws on other sources. A basic feature of EBP is that it de-emphasizes decision making based on custom, authority opinion, or ritual. Rather, the emphasis is on identifying the best available research evidence and *integrating* it with clinical expertise, patient input, and existing resources.

The EBP movement has given rise to considerable debate, with both staunch, zealous advocates and skeptics who urge caution and a balanced approach to health care practice. Supporters argue that EBP offers a solution to sustaining high health care quality in our current cost-constrained environment. Their position is that a rational approach is needed to provide the best possible care to the most people, with the most cost-effective use of resources. Critics worry that the advantages of EBP are exaggerated and that individual clinical judgments and patient inputs are being devalued. Although there is a need for close scrutiny of how the EBP journey unfolds, it seems likely that the EBP path is one that health care professions are likely to follow in the early 21st century.

Overview of the Evidence-Based Practice Movement

One of the cornerstones of the EBP movement is the Cochrane Collaboration, which was based on the work of British epidemiologist Archie Cochrane. Cochrane published an influential book in the early 1970s that drew attention to the dearth of solid evidence about the effects of health care. He called for efforts to make research summaries available to health care decision makers. This eventually led to the development of the Cochrane Centre in Oxford in 1992, and an international collaboration called the **Cochrane Collaboration,** with centres established in 15 locations throughout the world. The aim of the collaboration is to help people make good decisions about health care by preparing, maintaining, and disseminating systematic reviews of the effects of health care interventions.

At about the same time as the Cochrane Collaboration got underway, a group from McMaster Medical School developed a clinical learning strategy they called evidence-based medicine. Dr. David Sackett, a pioneer of evidence-based medicine at McMaster, defined evidence-based medicine as "the conscientious, explicit, and judicious use of current best evidence in making decisions about the care of individual patients. The practice of evidence-based medicine means integrating individual clinical expertise with the best available external evidence from systematic research" (Sackett et al., 1996, p. 71). The evidence-based medicine movement has shifted over time to a broader conception of using best evidence by all health care practitioners (not just doctors) in a multidisciplinary team. EBP has been considered a major paradigm shift for health care education and practice.

Types of Evidence and Evidence Hierarchies

There is no consensus about what constitutes usable evidence for EBP, but there is general agreement that findings from rigourous studies are paramount. In the initial phases of the EBP movement, there was a definite bias toward reliance on information from randomized clinical trials (RCTs). This bias, in turn, led to some resistance to EBP by nurses who felt that evidence from qualitative and non-RCT studies would be ignored. As Closs and Cheater (1999) have noted, "Some antagonism towards EBN seems to derive from viewing it as an unwelcome extension of the positivist tradition" (p. 13).

Positions about what constitutes useful evidence have loosened, but there have nevertheless been efforts to develop **evidence hierarchies** that rank studies according to the strength of evidence they provide. Several such hierarchies have been developed, many based on the one proposed by Archie Cochrane. Most hierarchies put meta-analyses of RCT studies at the pinnacle and other types of nonresearch evidence (*e.g.,* clinical expertise) at the base. As one example, Stetler and her colleagues (1998) developed a six-level evidence hierarchy that also assigns grades on study quality (from A to D) within each of the six levels. The levels (from strongest to weakest) are as follows: (I) meta-analyses of RCTs; (II) individual experimental studies; (III) quasi-experimental studies or matched case-control studies; (IV) nonexperimental studies (*e.g.,* correlational studies, qualitative studies); (V) RU studies, quality improvement projects, case reports; and (VI) opinions of respected authorities and of expert committees.

To date, there have been relatively few published RCT studies (level II) in nursing and even fewer published meta-analyses of RCT nursing studies. Therefore, evidence from other types of research will play an important role in evidence-based nursing practice. Many clinical questions of importance to nurses can best be answered with rich descriptive and qualitative data from level IV and V studies. Another issue is that there continue to be clinical practice questions for which there are relatively little research data.

Thus, though EBP encompasses RU, both research and nonresearch sources of information play a role in EBP. Nurses and other health care professionals must be able to locate evidence, evaluate it, and integrate it with clinical judgment and patient preferences to determine the most clinically effective solutions to health problems. Note that an important feature of EBP is that it does not necessarily imply practice changes; the best evidence may confirm that existing practices are effective and cost-efficient.

BARRIERS TO USING RESEARCH IN NURSING PRACTICE AND RELATED STRATEGIES TO ENHANCE UTILIZATION

In the next section, we discuss some models for RU and EBP endeavours. First, however, we review some barriers to RU and EBP in nursing and present some strategies for addressing them. Several studies that have explored nurses' perception of barriers to RU have yielded remarkably similar results about constraints clinical nurses face (Dobbins et al., 2002; Estabrooks, Scott-Findlay, & Winther, in press; McCaughan et al., 2002; Oranta et al., 2002). These barriers can be broadly grouped into four categories—research characteristics, individual (nurse) characteristics, organizational characteristics, and characteristics attributed to the nursing profession.

Research-Related Barriers

For many nursing problems, the state of the art of research knowledge is at a fairly rudimentary level. Results reported in the literature often do not warrant their incorporation into practice if methodologic flaws are extensive. Methodologic flaws often raise questions about the soundness or generalizability of study findings. Thus, a major impediment to RU by practicing nurses is that, for many problems, an extensive base of valid and trustworthy study results has not been developed.

As we have repeatedly stressed, most studies have flaws of one type or another, and so if nurses were to wait for the perfect study before basing clinical decisions on research findings, they would have a very long wait indeed. It is precisely because of the limits of research methods that replication is essential. When repeated efforts to address a research question in different settings yield similar results, there can be greater confidence in the findings. Single studies rarely provide an adequate basis for making changes in nursing practice. Therefore, another utilization constraint is the dearth of published replications.

⟋⟋ **CONSUMER TIP**

Given these issues, some tips for researchers interested in promoting the use of research findings in clinical practice are as follows:

- *Collaborate with clinicians.* Practicing nurses will be more willing to use research findings if researchers address pressing clinical questions.
- *Do high-quality research.* The quality of nursing studies has improved dramatically in the past two decades, but progress remains to be made to ensure valid and transferable findings.
- *Replicate.* Use of research results can rarely be justified based on a single study, so researchers must make a real commitment to replicating studies and publishing the results.
- *Communicate clearly.* A general aim should be to write research reports that are user-friendly, with a minimum of research jargon.
- *Suggest clinical implications.* If an implications section with suggestions for clinical practice became a standard feature of research reports, then the burden of using research evidence would be lighter for nurse clinicians.
- *Disseminate aggressively.* If researchers fail to communicate the results of a study to other nurses, it is obvious that the results will never be used by practicing nurses.
- *Disseminate broadly.* It is especially important from a utilization standpoint for researchers to report their results in specialty journals, which are more likely to be read by practicing nurses than the nursing research journals. Researchers should also take steps to disseminate study findings at conferences, colloquia, and workshops attended by nurse clinicians.
- *Prepare integrative research reviews.* There is an urgent need for high-quality integrative reviews of research. Such reviews can play an invaluable role for practicing nurses, who generally do not have the time to do extensive literature reviews and who may have some difficulty in critically evaluating individual studies. Integrative reviews are a core feature of the EBP process.

As a consumer, you can and should evaluate the extent to which researchers have adopted these strategies to enhance RU and EBP. ■

Nurse-Related Barriers

Studies have found that many clinical nurses have characteristics that constrain the use of research evidence in practice. One issue concerns nurses' educational preparation and their research skills. Many have not received any formal instruction in research and may lack the skills to judge the merits of a study. Courses on research methodology are now typically offered in baccalaureate nursing programs, but the ability to critique a research report is not necessarily sufficient for effectively incorporating research results into daily decision making.

Nurses' attitudes toward research and their motivation to engage in EBP have repeatedly been identified as potential barriers. Studies have found that the more positive the attitude, the more likely is the nurse to use research in practice. Some nurses see RU and EBP as little more than a "necessary evil" (Thompson, 2001), but there has been a trend toward more positive attitudes.

Another characteristic is one that is common to most humans: people are often resistant to change. Change requires effort, retraining, and restructuring of work habits. Change may also be perceived as threatening (*e.g.,* changes may be perceived as affecting job security). Thus, there is likely to be some opposition to introducing innovations in the practice setting. However, evidence from a survey of more than 1200 nurses suggests that nurses value nursing research and want to be involved in research-related activities (Rizzuto, Bostrom, Suter, & Chenitz, 1994).

CONSUMER TIP

Every nurse can play a role in using research evidence. Here are some strategies:

- *Read widely and critically.* Professionally accountable nurses keep abreast of important developments and should read journals relating to their specialty, including research reports in them.
- *Attend professional conferences.* Many nursing conferences include presentations of studies that have clinical relevance. Conference attendees get opportunities to meet researchers and to explore practice implications.
- *Learn to expect evidence that a procedure is effective.* Every time nurses or nursing students are told about a nursing procedure, they have a right to ask the question: "Why?" Nurses need to develop expectations that the decisions they make in their clinical practice are based on sound rationales.
- *Become involved in a journal club.* Many organizations that employ nurses sponsor journal clubs that meet to review research articles that have potential relevance to practice.
- *Pursue and participate in RU/EBP projects.* Sometimes ideas for RU or EBP projects come from staff nurses (*e.g.,* ideas may emerge within a journal club). Several studies have found that nurses who are involved in research-related activities (*e.g.,* a utilization project or data collection activities) develop more positive attitudes toward research and better research skills. ■

Organizational Barriers

Many of the major impediments to using research in practice stem from the organizations that educate and employ nurses. Organizations, perhaps to an even greater degree than individuals, resist change unless there is a strong organizational perception that there is something fundamentally wrong with the status quo. To challenge tradition and accepted practices, a spirit of intellectual curiosity and openess must prevail.

In many practice settings, administrators have established procedures to reward competence in nursing practice; however, few practice settings have established a system to reward nurses for critiquing nursing studies, for using research in practice, or for discussing research findings with patients. Thus, organizations have failed to motivate or reward nurses to seek ways to implement appropriate findings with patients. Research review and use are often considered appropriate activities only when time is available, but available time is generally limited. In several studies of barriers to RU, one of the greatest reported barriers to RU was "insufficient time on the job to implement new ideas."

Organizations may also be reluctant to expend resources for RU projects and EBP or for implementing changes to organizational policy. Resources may be required for the use of outside consultants, staff release time, library materials, and Internet access, evaluating the effects of an innovation, and so on. With the push toward cost containment in health care settings, resource constraints may pose a barrier to change—unless the project has cost containment as an explicit goal.

EBP will become part of organizational norms only if there is a commitment on the part of managers and adminstrators. Strong leadership in health care organizations is essential to making EBP happen.

CONSUMER TIP

To promote the use of research evidence, administrators can adopt the following strategies:

- *Foster a climate of intellectual curiosity.* Open communication is important in persuading staff nurses that their experiences and problems are important and that the administration is willing to consider innovative solutions.
- *Offer emotional or moral support.* Administrators need to make their support visible by informing staff and prospective staff of such support, by establishing RU or EBP committees, by helping to develop journal clubs, and by serving as role models for staff nurses.
- *Offer financial or resource support for utilization.* RU and EBP projects typically require some resources. If the administration expects nurses to engage in utilization activities on their own time and at their own expense, the message is that RU is unimportant to those managing the organization.
- *Reward efforts for utilization and EBP.* Administrators use various criteria to evaluate nursing performance. RU and EBP should not be a primary criterion for evaluating nurses' performance, but its inclusion as one of several important criteria is likely to have an impact on their behaviour.
- *Seek opportunities for institutional RU or EBP projects.* Organizational efforts and commitment are essential for the type of RU and EBP projects we discuss in the next section. ■

Nursing Profession-Related Barriers

Some impediments that contribute to the gap between research and practice are more global, reflecting the state of the nursing profession or, even more broadly, the state of Western society.

It has sometimes been difficult to encourage clinicians and researchers to interact and collaborate. They are generally in different settings and have many different professional concerns. Relatively few systematic attempts have been made to form collaborative arrangements, and to date, even fewer of these arrangements have been formalized as permanent entities.

Phillips (1986) also noted two other noteworthy barriers to bridging the research–practice gap. One is the shortage of appropriate role models—nurses who can be emulated for their success in using or promoting the use of research in clinical practice. The other barrier is the historical "baggage" that has defined nursing in such a way that practicing nurses may not typically perceive themselves as independent professionals capable of recommending changes based on research results. If practicing nurses believe that their role is to await direction from the medical community, and if they believe they have no power to be self-directed, then they will have difficulty in initiating innovations based on research findings. In the previously mentioned national survey, the barrier perceived by the largest percentage of nurses was the nurses' feeling that they did not have "enough authority to change patient care procedures" (Funk, Champagne, Wiese, & Tornquist, 1991). Fortunately, much progress has been made in our society and in the profession with regard to these two barriers. In particular, several professional nursing organizations have taken a strong stance to promote the use of research in practice.

Finally, some of the burden for changes in the profession must rest with nursing educators. As Funk and colleagues (1995) note, "The valuing of nursing research as the *sine qua non* on which practice is based must be conveyed throughout baccalaureate, associate degree, and diploma programs. This is not teaching of the conduct of research, but rather the valuing it as a way of knowing and as the foundation on which practice is based" (p. 400).

THE PROCESS OF USING RESEARCH IN NURSING PRACTICE

In the years ahead, many of you are likely to be engaged in individual and institutional efforts to use research as a basis for clinical decisions. This section describes how that might be accomplished. We begin with an overview of some RU and EBP models developed by nurses. A number of different models of RU have been developed by nurse researchers in Canada, the United States, and the United Kingdom during the past few decades. These models offer guidelines for designing and implementing utilization projects in practice settings. Some models focus on the use of research from the perspective of an individual clinician, some focus on utilization from an organizational perspective, whereas others concentrate on multiple perspectives. This section discusses mechanisms for applying research findings to nursing practice.

Models for Evidence-Based Nursing Practice

During the past two decades, several models of RU have been developed. These include: the Registered Nurses Association of British Columbia Model (RNABC, 1991), the Horn Model of Research Utilization (Goode & Bulechek, 1992), the Stetler Model of Research Utilization (Stetler 1994, 2001), the Iowa Model of Research in Practice (Titler et al., 1994, 2001), the Collaborative Research Model (Dufault, 1995), the Ottawa Model of Research Use (Logan &

Graham, 1998), Kitson and coworkers' Multidimensional Framework of Research Utilization (Kitson, Harvey, & McCormack, 1998), the Evidence-Based Multidisciplinary Practice Model (Goode & Piedalue, 1999), the Model for Change to Evidence-Based Practice (Rosswurm & Larabee, 1999), the Center for Advanced Nursing Practice Model (Soukop, 2000), and A Framework for the Dissemination and Utilization of Research for Health-Care Policy and Practice (Dobbins et al., 2002).

The most prominent of these models have been the Stetler and Iowa Models. These two models have been updated to incorporate EBP processes, rather than RU processes alone.

Stetler Model of Research Utilization

This model was first developed in 1976 with Marram and refined in 1994. The **Stetler Model** (1994) was designed with the assumption that RU could be undertaken not only by organizations, but also by individual clinicians and managers. It was a model designed to promote and facilitate ciritical thinking about the application of research findings in practice. The updated and refined models is based on many of the same assumptions and strategies as the original, but provides "an enhanced approach to the overall application of research in the service setting" (Stetler, 2001, p. 273). Stetler's model involves five sequential phases that are designed to "facilitate critical thinking about the pragmatic application of research findings" (Stetler, 2001, p. 275):

1. *Preparation.* In this phase, nurses would define the underlying purpose and outcomes of the project; search, sort, and select sources of research evidence; consider external factors that can influence potential application and internal factors that can diminish objectivity; and affirm the priority of the perceived problem.
2. *Validation.* This phase involves a utilization-focused critique of each source of evidence, focusing in particular on whether it is sufficiently sound for potential application in practice. (The process stops at this point if the evidence sources are rejected.)
3. *Comparative Evaluation and Decision Making.* This phase involves a synthesis of findings and the application of four criteria that, taken together, are used tò determine the desirability and feasibility of applying findings from validated sources to nursing practice. These criteria (fit of setting, feasibility, current practice, and substantive evidence) are summarized in Table 16-2. The end result of the comparative evaluation is to make a decision about using study findings. If the decision is a rejection, no further steps are necessary.
4. *Translation/Application.* This phase involves activities to (a) confirm how the findings will be used (*e.g.*, formally or informally) and (b) spell out the operational details of the application, and implementing them. The latter might involve the development of a guideline, detailed procedure, or plan of action, possibly including plans for formal organizational change.

TABLE 16-2. Criteria for Comparative Evaluation Phase of the Stetler Model of Research Utilization*

1. Fit of Setting
   Similarity of characteristics of sample to your client population
   Similarity of study's environment to the one in which you work
2. Feasibility
   Potential risks of implementation to patients, staff, and the organization
   Readiness for change among those who would be involved in a change in practice
   Resource requirements and availability
3. Current Practice
   Congruency of the study with your theoretical basis for current practice behavior
4. Substantiating Evidence
   Availability of confirming evidence from other studies
   Availability of confirming evidence from a meta-analysis or integrative review

*Adapted from Stetler, C. B. (1994). Refinement of the Stetler/Marram model for application of research findings to practice. *Nursing Outlook, 42,* 15–25.

---

5. *Evaluation.* In the final phase, the application would be evaluated. Informal use of the innovation versus formal use would lead to different evaluative strategies.

Although the Stetler Model was designed as a tool for individual practitioners, it has also been the basis of formal RU and EBP projects by groups of nurses.

Example of an application of the Stetler Model:
Bauer et al. (2002) applied the five phases of the Stetler Model to pressure ulcer prevention and care project by groups of nurses in home health care environments.

Iowa Model

Efforts to use research evidence to improve nursing practice are often addressed by groups of nurses interested in the same practice issue. Formal RU and EBP projects typically have followed systematic procedures using one of several models that have been developed, such as the Iowa Model of Research in Practice (Titler et al., 1994). This model, like the Stetler Model, was revised recently, and renamed the **Iowa Model of Evidence-Based Practice to Promote Quality Care** (Titler et al., 2001). The current version of the Iowa Model, shown in Figure 16–2, acknowledges that a formal RU or EBP project begins with a *trigger*—an impetus to explore possible changes to practice. The start point can be either (1) a **knowledge-focused trigger** that emerges from awareness of innovative research findings (and thus follows a more traditional RU path, as in the top panel of Figure 16–1); or (2) a **problem-focused trigger** that has its roots in a clinical or organizational problem

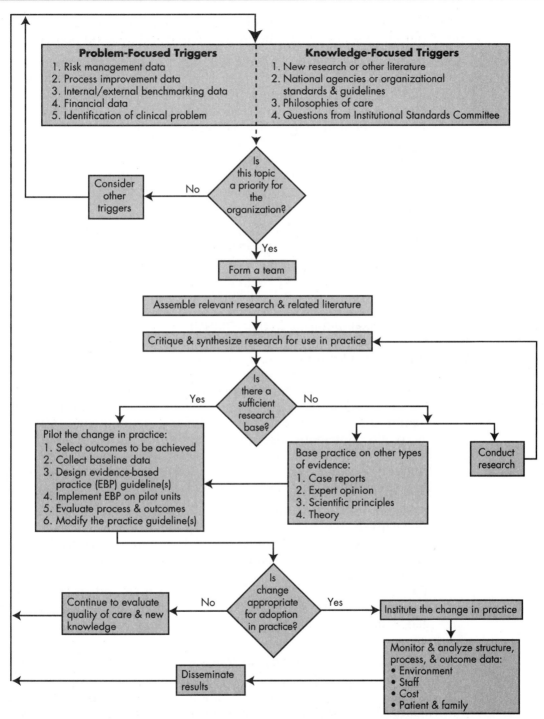

FIGURE 16-2. Iowa Model of Evidence-Based Practice to Promote Quality Care (Adapted from Titler, et al. (2001). The Iowa Model of Evidence-Based Practice to Promote Quality Care. *Critical Care Nursing Clinics of North America, 13,* 497–509.)

(and thus following a path that more closely resembles an EBP path). The model outlines a series of activities with three critical decision points:

1. Deciding whether the problem is a sufficient priority for the organization exploring possible changes; if yes, a team is formed to proceed with the project and, if no, a new trigger would be sought.
2. Deciding whether there is a sufficient research base; if yes, the innovation is piloted in the practice setting and, if no, the team would either search for other sources of evidence or conduct its own research.
3. Deciding whether the change is appropriate for adoption in practice; if yes, a change would be instituted and monitored and, if no, the team would continue to evaluate quality of care and search for new knowledge.

Example of an application of the Iowa Model:

Montgomery et al. (1999) used the Iowa Model to develop a guideline for intravenous infiltration in pediatric patients.

The Ottawa Model of Research Use (OMRU)

The OMRU, developed by Logan and Graham (1998) consists of six key components interrelated through the process of evaluation. The six components deal with "the practice environment, the potential research adopter (administrators and clinical staff), the evidence-based innovation (the research intented for use in practice), strategies for transfering the innovation into practice, adoption/use of the evidence, and health and other outcomes" (Logan et al., 1999, p. 39). Systematic assessment, monitoring, and evaluation (AME) are central to the OMRU and are applied to each of the six components discussed above before, during, and after any effort to transfer research findings. The data gathered through AME serves several purposes:

- To determine potential barriers to and supports for research use associated with the practice environment
- To offer direction for choosing and tailoring transfer strategies to surmount the recognized barriers and enhance strategies that were deemed supportive
- To evaluate the evidence-based innovation used and the influence it had on the results of interest (Logan & Graham as summarized by Logan, et al, 1999, p. 39)

Example of an application of the Ottawa Model:

Logan et al. (1999) used the Ottawa Model at four sites in Ontario as part of the Province-Wide Nursing Project (PWNP) focusing on pressure-ulcer practice. The PWNP focused on four pillars of nursing practice: clinical decision making, EBP, continous quality improvement, and primary nursing. Since the initiation of this project, the researchers noted significant change in "attitudes and organizational culture to support the use of evidence at both the practitioner and organizational levels" (p. 48).

Steps in Using Research in Nursing Practice

Using research to improve nursing practice involves a series of activities and decisions. The Stetler, Iowa, and OMRU models (as well as others) are used as a basis for discussing major activities to support RU and EBP.

Selecting a Topic or Problem

The Iowa Model acknowledges that there are two types of stimulus for an EBP or RU endeavour—identification of a clinical practice problem in need of solution, or through reading in the research literature. Problem-focused triggers may arise in the normal course of clinical practice or in the context of quality assessment or quality improvement efforts. This problem identification approach is likely to have staff support if the selected problem is one that numerous nurses have encountered, and is likely to have considerable clinical relevance because a specific clinical situation generated interest in the problem in the first place.

Gennaro (2001) advises nurses following this approach to begin by clarifying the practice problem that needs to be solved and framing it as a question. The goal can be finding the best way to anticipate a problem (how to diagnose it) or how best to solve a problem (how to intervene). Clinical practice questions may well take the form of "What is the best way to . . ."; for example, "What is the best way to encourage women to do breast self-examinations regularly?"

CONSUMER TIP

Several websites may be helpful in framing a clinical practice question for EBP. For example, the University of Alberta offers an "Evidence-Based Medicine Tool Kit" that provides such assistance (www.med.ualberta.ca/ebm/ebm.htm). ∎

A second catalyst for an RU or EBP project begins with the research literature—corresponding to the knowledge-focused triggers identified in the Iowa Model. This approach could occur if, for example, a utilization project emerged as a result of discussions within a journal club. In this approach, a preliminary assessment would need to be made of the clinical relevance of the research. The central issue here is whether a problem of significance to nurses will be solved by making some change or introducing a new intervention. Five questions relating to clinical relevance (Box 16-1) can be applied to a research report or set of related reports. If the answer is yes to any of these questions, the next step in the process can be pursued, but if it is determined that the research base is not clinically relevant, it would be necessary to start all over.

BOX 16-1 ⊡ **CRITERIA FOR EVALUATING THE CLINICAL RELEVANCE OF A BODY OF RESEARCH**

1. Does the research have the potential to help solve a problem faced by practicing nurses?

2. Does the research have the potential to help with clinical decision making with regard to (1) making appropriate observations, (2) identifying client risks or complications, or (3) selecting an appropriate intervention?

3. Are clinically relevant theoretical propositions tested by the research?

4. If the research involves an intervention, does the intervention have potential for use in clinical settings?

5. Can the data collection measures used in the research be applied to clinical practice?

With both types of triggers, it is important to ensure that there is a general consensus about the importance of the problem and the need for improving practice. Titler and colleagues (2001) include as the first decision point in their revised Iowa Model the determination of whether the topic is a priority for the organization considering practice changes. They advise that the following issues be taken into account when finalizing a topic for an EBP project: the topic's fit with the organization's strategic plan, the magnitude of the problem, the number of people invested in the problem, support of nurse leaders and of those in other disciplines, costs, and possible barriers to change. Rosenfeld and colleagues (2000) present a model for examining and prioritizing practice problems as perceived by staff nurses.

⚡ CONSUMER TIP

The method of selecting a topic does not appear to have any bearing on the success of an RU/EBP project. What is important, however, is that the nursing staff who will implement an innovation are involved in the topic selection and that key stakeholders are "on board." ■

Assembling and Evaluating Evidence

Once a clinical practice question has been selected and a team has been formed to work on the project, the next step is to search for and assemble research evidence (and other relevant evidence) on the topic. Chapter 6 provided information about locating research information, but some additional issues are relevant.

In doing a literature review as background for a new study, the central goal is to discover where the gaps are and how best to advance knowledge. For EBP or RU projects, which typically have as end products prescriptive practice protocols or clinical guidelines, literature reviews are typically much more rigourous and formalized. The emphasis is on gathering comprehensive information on the topic, weighing pieces of evidence, and integrating information to draw conclusions about the state of knowledge. Commentators have noted that **integrative reviews** have become a cornerstone of EBP (Jennings, 2000; Stevens, 2001). If practitioners are to glean best practices from research findings, they must take into account as much of the evidence as possible, organized and synthesized in a rigorous manner.

An integrative review is not just a literature review—it is in itself a systematic inquiry that follows many of the same rules as those described in this book for primary studies. In other words, those doing an integrative review develop research questions or hypotheses, devise a sampling plan and data collection strategy, collect the relevant data, and analyze and interpret those data.

Integrative reviews can take various forms. Until recently, the most common type of integrative review was narrative (qualitative) integration that used various nonstatistical methods to merge and synthesize research findings. More recently, meta-analytic techniques that use a common metric for combining studies statistically have been increasingly used to integrate quantitative findings. (The reviews in the Cochrane Collaboration are meta-analyses.) Among qualitative researchers, the technique of metasynthesis has been developed to integrate and compare findings from qualitative studies.

High-quality integrative reviews represent a critical tool for RU/EBP, and if the assembled team has the skills to complete one, this is clearly advantageous. It is, however, unlikely that every clinical organization will be able to assemble the skills needed to accomplish a high-quality critical review of the research literature on the chosen topic. Moreover, as Funk and her co-authors (1995) have noted, cost efficiencies make this impractical: "With the shrinking health care dollar, we can no longer afford to have nurses in practice settings throughout the nation duplicating the work of searching for the most up-to-date literature, evaluating it, synthesizing it, and drawing practice conclusions" (p. 403).

Fortunately, many researchers and organizations have taken on the responsibility of preparing integrative reviews and making them available for EBP in professional journals and on the Internet. Cochrane reviews are an especially important resource. These reports describe the background and objectives of the review, the methods used to search for, select, and evaluate studies, the main results, and, importantly, the reviewers' conclusions. Cochrane reviews are checked and updated regularly.

Example of Cochrane review conclusions:

One Cochrane review that examined interventions for promoting smoking cessation during pregnancy came to the following conclusions: "Smoking cessation programs in pregnancy appear to reduce smoking, low birthweight and preterm birth, but no effect was detected for very low birthweight or perinatal mortality."

Another critical resource for those wishing to use available integrative reviews is the Agency for Healthcare Research and Quality (AHRQ). This agency awarded 12 5-year contracts in 1997 to establish EBP centres at institutions in the United States and Canada (*e.g.,* at Johns Hopkins University, McMaster University) and new 5-year contracts were awarded in 2002. Each centre issues **evidence reports** that are based on rigourous integrative reviews of relevant scientific literature; dozens of these reports are now available to help "improve the quality, effectiveness, and appropriateness of clinical care" (AHRQ website, May, 2002, www.ahrq.gov).

Example of evidence reports from AHRQ EBP centers:

The titles of two evidence reports prepared by EBP Centres in 2002 are: *Utility of Blood Pressure Monitoring Outside of the Clinic Setting* and *Management of Prolonged Pregnancy.*

Many other resources are available for locating integrative reviews. One particularly useful website at the University of Sheffield in the United Kingdom is referred to as "Netting the Web" (www.shef.ac.uk/uni/academic/R-Z/scharr/ir/netting.html). This site offers a comprehensive listing of other websites devoted to providing evidence for practice. Another useful website, also based in the United Kingdom, is the University of York's Centre for Evidence-Based Nursing (www.york.ac.uk/depts/hstd/centres/evidence/cebn.htm).

If an integrative review has been prepared by experts, it is possible that a formal evidence-based clinical guideline has been developed and can be used directly in an RU/EBP project. AHRQ, for example, has developed such guidelines on pain management, continence, and other problems of relevance to nurses. AHRQ no longer develops guidelines but helps to support the National Guideline Clearinghouse (www.guidelines.gov), which provides a comprehensive database of such guidelines. Nursing organizations (*e.g.,* Association of Women's Health, Obstetrics, and Neonatal Nurses) have also developed clinical practice guidelines on several topics.

Of course, there are many clinical practice questions for which integrative reviews and clinical guidelines are not available. This may mean that an integrative review or synthesis of the research literature relating to the selected clinical question will need to be prepared.

CONSUMER TIP

If an integrative review already exists, it is wise to make sure that it is as up-to-date as possible and that new findings published after the review are taken into account. Moreover, even a published integrative review needs to be critiqued and the validity of its conclusions assessed. Stetler and her colleagues (1998) offer a form for evaluating integrative reviews. ■

The review, evaluation, and synthesis of research evidence ideally would allow the RU or EBP team to draw conclusions about the sufficiency of the research base for guiding clinical practice. Adequacy of research evidence depends on such factors as the consistency of findings across studies, the quality and rigour of the studies, the strength of any observed effect, the transferability of the findings to clinical settings, and cost-effectiveness.

Coming to conclusions about the body of evidence can result in several possible outcomes and thus to different decisions for further action. First, if the research base is weak—or if there is a strong base with ambiguous conclusions—the team could opt to pursue one of three courses. The first is to go back to the beginning to pursue a new topic. A second option (preferable in the EBP environment) is to assemble other types of nonresearch evidence (*e.g.,* through consultation with experts, surveys of patients, and so on) and assess whether that evidence suggests a practice change. Finally, another possibility is to pursue an original clinical study to directly address the practice question, thereby gathering new evidence and contributing to the base of practice knowledge. This last course of action may well be impractical for many nurses and would clearly result in years of delay before any further conclusions could be drawn.

If, on the other hand, there is a solid research base, the evidence could point in different directions. One possibility is that the evidence would support existing practices (which might lead to an analysis of why the clinical practice question emerged and what might make existing practices work more effectively). Another possibility is that there would be clearcut and compelling evidence that a clinical change is warranted, which would lead to the next set of activities.

Assessing Implementation Potential

Some models of RU/EBP move directly from the conclusion that evidence supports a change in practice to the pilot testing of the innovation. Others include steps to first evaluate the appropriateness of innovation within the specific organizational context; in some cases, such an assessment (or aspects of it) may be warranted even before embarking on efforts to assemble best evidence. Other models suggest evaluating issues of fit *after* the practice change has been implemented. We think a preliminary assessment of the **implementation potential** of an innovation is often sensible, although there may be situations with little need for such a formal assessment.

In determining the implementation potential of an innovation in a particular setting several issues should be considered, particularly the transferability of the innovation, the feasibility of implementating it, and the cost–benefit ratio. Box 16-2 presents some assessment questions for these categories.

- *Transferability.* The main issue in the transferability of findings question is whether it makes good sense to implement the innovation in the new practice setting. If some aspect of the practice setting is fundamentally incongruent with the innovation in terms of its philosophy,

BOX 16-2

CRITERIA FOR EVALUATING THE IMPLEMENTATION POTENTIAL OF AN INNOVATION

Transferability of the Findings

1. Will the innovation "fit" in the proposed new setting?

2. How similar are the target populations in the research and in the new setting?

3. Is the philosophy of care underlying the innovation compatible with the philosophy prevailing in the new setting?

4. Is there a sufficiently large number of patients in the new setting who could benefit from the innovation?

Feasibility

1. Will nurses have the authority to carry out the innovation and to terminate it if it is considered undesirable?

2. Is there reasonable consensus among staff, administrators, and medical personnel that the innovation should be tested? Are there major pockets of resistance that could undermine efforts to implement and evaluate the innovation fairly?

3. Are the skills needed to carry out the utilization project—both the implementation and the clinical evaluation—available within the nursing staff? If not, are there avenues to collaborate with others with the necessary skills?

4. Does the organization have the equipment and facilities necessary for the innovation? If not, is there a way to obtain needed resources?

5. If nursing staff need to be released from other practice activities to learn about and implement the innovation, what is the likelihood that this could happen?

Cost–Benefit Ratio

1. What are the risks to which patients would be exposed during the implementation of the innovation? What are the potential benefits?

2. What are the risks of maintaining current practices (*i.e.,* the cost of *not* trying the innovation)? What are the benefits?

3. What are the short-term and long-term material costs of implementing the innovation?

4. What are the material costs of *not* implementing the innovation (*i.e.,* could the new procedure result in some efficiencies that could lower the cost of providing care)?

5. What are the potential nonmaterial costs of implementing the innovation to the organization (*e.g.,* lower staff morale, staff turnover, absenteeism)?

6. What are the potential nonmaterial benefits of implementing the innovation (*e.g.,* improved staff morale, improved staff recruitment, positive community publicity)?

types of patients it serves, personnel, or financial or administrative structure, it makes little sense to try to adopt the innovation, even if it has been shown to be clinically effective in other contexts.

- *Feasibility.* The feasibility questions in Box 16-2 address various practical concerns about the availability of staff and resources, the organizational climate, the need for and availability of external assistance, and the potential for clinical evaluation. An important issue here is whether nurses will have (or share) control over the innovation. When nurses do not have full control over the new procedure, it is important to recognize the interdependent nature of the project and to proceed as early as possible to establish necessary cooperative arrangements.
- *Cost–Benefit Ratio.* A critical part of any decision to proceed with an RU or EBP project is a careful assessment of the costs and benefits of the innovation. The **cost–benefit assessment** should encompass likely costs and benefits to various groups, including patients, staff, and the overall organization. Clearly, the most important factor is the patient. If the degree of risk in introducing a new procedure is high, then the potential benefits must be great and the knowledge base must be extremely sound. A cost–benefit assessment should consider the opposite side of the coin as well: the costs and benefits of *not* implementing the innovation. It is sometimes easy to forget that the status quo bears its own risks and that failure to change, especially when such change is based on a firm knowledge base, is costly to patients, to organizations, and to the entire nursing community.

If the implementation assessment suggests that there might be problems in testing the innovation within that particular practice setting, the team can either identify a new problem and begin the process anew or consider adopting a plan to improve the implementation potential (*e.g.,* seeking external resources if costs were the inhibiting factor).

CONSUMER TIP

Documentation of the implementation potential of an innovation is highly recommended. Committing ideas to writing is useful because it can help to resolve ambiguities, can serve as a problem-solving tool if there are barriers to implementation, and can also be used to persuade others of the value of the project. ■

Developing, Implementing, and Evaluating the Innovation

If the implementation criteria are met, the team can then proceed to design the protocol for the innovation. Building on the Iowa Model, this phase of the project would involve the following activities:

- Developing an evaluation plan (*e.g.,* identifying outcomes to be achieved, determining how many patients to involve in the pilot, deciding when and how often to take measurements and so on)

- Collecting baseline data relating to those outcomes, to develop a comparison against which the outcomes of the innovation would be assessed
- Developing a written EBP guideline based on the synthesis of the evidence, preferably a guideline that is clear and user friendly, and that uses such devices as flow charts and decision trees
- Training relevant staff in the use of the new guideline and, if necessary "marketing" the innovation to users so that it is given a fair test
- Trying the guideline out on one or more units or with a sample of patients
- Evaluating the pilot project, in terms of both process (*e.g.,* how was the innovation received, to what extent were the guidelines actually followed, what implementation problems were encountered?) and outcomes (in terms of patient outcomes and cost-effectiveness)

Evaluation data should be gathered over a sufficiently long period (typically 6–12 months) to allow for a true test of a "mature" innovation. The end result of this process is a decision about whether to adopt the innovation, to modify it for ongoing use, or to revert to prior practices.

CONSUMER TIP

A final optional step, but one that is highly advisable, is the dissemination of the results of the utilization project so that other practicing nurses can benefit. ■

Other Utilization Approaches

Research can be incorporated into nursing practice even without undertaking a formal RU or EBP project. Increasingly, research-based nursing protocols are being published in the literature and are essentially ready for adoption—although it is wise to undertake an implementation assessment to determine whether the adoption of a new protocol is sensible. If the publication of the protocol is not recent, it is also prudent to ensure that current research and theory on the topic remain consistent with the protocol.

The Registered Nurses Association of Ontario (RNAO), for example, launched its Nursing Best Practice Guidelines (NBPG) project in November 1999. Funded as a multiyear project by the Ontario Ministry of Health and Long Term Care, the project team has developed 11 guidelines to date and are available for downloading on the RNAO Best Practice Guidelines microsite at www.rnao.org/bestpractices (Grinspun, Virani, & Bajnok, 2001–2002; MacLeod, Harrison, & Graham, 2002). An additional six guidelines are in progress.

Example of research-based nursing protocols:

Two examples of published reports with full research-based protocols include McDonald (2001), who developed a protocol for clean intermittent catheterization, and Larsen and Thurston (1997), who developed a procedure for the care of patients for central venous catheters.

RESEARCH EXAMPLE

Many utilization projects have been undertaken by nurses in practice settings, and many of these projects were described in the nursing literature. Table 16-3 provides examples of several RU and EBP projects. Another project, described in greater detail below, illustrates the potential of such projects to result in improved nursing care.

Research Summary

The Association of Women's Health, Obstetric, and Neonatal Nurses (AWHONN) has conducted three major research utilization projects. One recent project focused on urinary incontinence in women (Samselle et al., 2000a, 2000b). Using the guidelines prepared by the Agency for Health Care Policy and Research (the agency that was renamed AHRQ) as a starting point, AWHONN initiated a project with the aim of developing an evidence-based protocol for urinary incontinence in women and designing procedures to facilitate the protocol's implementation into clinical practice.

The project consisted of three 1-year phases that began in 1995. Phase I (Planning) involved the development of the evidence-based protocol by a team of nurses. The end product was a protocol that provided step-by-step procedures for (1) assessing all women for urinary incontinence; (2) conducting a baseline evaluation of symptomatic women; (3) giving behavioural instruction for bladder training and pelvic floor muscle training; and (4) when indicated, referring women for specialized care. During the planning phase, the project's advisory team also developed data management forms.

The second phase involved the implementation of the protocols. Clinical sites (general ambulatory women's health care settings) were recruited through

TABLE 16-3. Examples of Research Utilization and Evidence-Based Projects

INNOVATION	RESULTS OF UTILIZATION PROJECTS	CITATION
Use of clean technique for intermittent catheterization (IC)	Took nearly a year before technique became firmly rooted in daily practice	McDonald, 2001
Improving and developing services for women with serious mental health problems	Successfully set up the women's network. Women staff from residential, day care, and community services collaborated to provide a safe meeting place for a group of women users	Owen & Milburn, 2001
Use of standardized protocol to identify delirium in elderly hospital patients	Continued use of assessment protocol on all newly admitted patients aged 75 years and older	Lacko, Bryan, Dellasega, & Salerno, 1999
Structured support for breastfeeding mothers	Adoption as part of quality improvement efforts, change in awareness of and attitude toward RU	Janken, Blythe, Campbell, & Carter, 1999

mailings to AWHONN membership. Of those responding, 36 sites from across the United States were selected to participate (21 ultimately did participate). Coordinators from each site were brought together for a training session on the use of and rationale for the protocol. Each site was asked to administer screening questions to the first 100 nonpregnant female clients seen at the site and to follow the protocol's procedures.

Phase III of the project, Evaluation, involved an assessment of the outcomes. The evaluation addressed two broad questions:

1. Did change occur in clinical practice after clinicians were trained to identify urinary incontinence and to intervene using an evidence-based protocol?
2. Were patient outcomes positively affected after the protocol was instituted in the clinical setting?

The protocol was implemented in the 21 sites, and the process had a number of positive aspects. Participating nurses reported increased respect for the importance of evidence-based practice as well as greater professional satisfaction. A negative outcome concerned the increased demands on the clinicians' time and the problems arising from billing practices that made it difficult to justify the time required.

Nevertheless, the findings indicated that a substantially higher percentage of women screened positive for urinary incontinence using the protocol (57%) than has been reported in the literature (38% to 41%), suggesting that the screening was successful in identifying women in need of intervention. It was discovered that women who had had a hysterectomy were at significantly higher risk of incontinence than other women, indicating the need for heightened vigilance when assessing this group.

Patient outcomes were studied using a one-group before–after design. Women who were exposed to the protocol's treatment (pelvic floor muscle and bladder training) and who provided feedback at a 4-month follow-up had significant improvements in the frequency of incontinent episodes, volume of leakage per episode, perceptions of "bother," and avoidance of activities due to incontinence.

The project team concluded that the results "demonstrate the effectiveness of the evidence-based protocol in actual clinical settings. The participating sites represented a wide range of practice settings, and the overall sample was reasonably diverse. . . . This supports an acceptable level of generalizability and warrants the implementation of the protocol in general ambulatory women's health care settings" (Samselle et al., 2000b, pp. 24–25.)

Clinical Relevance

As this project discovered, many women experience urinary incontinence, a problem that affects women's health and well-being. AWHONN selected an important topic that has a sound base of scientific knowledge.

A few barriers to implementing the protocol were identified, including cooperation by office staff in a few sites and billing practices. The team recommended examining the presence of financial disincentives for sites desiring to implement the protocol.

Despite some implementation problems, the findings suggest that there are clear benefits to incorporating the protocol into standard ambulatory practice. More women with incontinence were identified than has typically been reported, and women who provided feedback reported decreases in the frequency, volume, and life impact of incontinence after treatment.

However, as noted by the team, a high percentage of women identified as having an incontinence problem did not persist with treatment and provide follow-up information. Women who were least likely to continue treatment were younger, were black or Latina, and had lower severity of incontinence. Thus, further utilization research is needed to determine (1) what steps can be taken to prevent high attrition among these groups, and (2) whether the innovation is equally effective for these women. Additionally, information on net financial costs or savings would be extremely useful.

● ● ● ● ● *SUMMARY POINTS*

- **Research utilization (RU)** and **evidence-based practice (EBP)** are overlapping concepts that concern efforts to use research as a basis for clinical decisions. RU starts with a research-based innovation that gets evaluated for possible use in practice. EBP starts with a search for the best possible evidence for a clinical problem, with emphasis on research-based evidence.
- Research utilization exists on a continuum, with direct utilization of some specific innovation at one end (**instrumental utilization**) and more diffuse situations in which users are influenced in their thinking about an issue based on some research (**conceptual utilization**) at the other end.
- Several major utilization projects have been implemented (*e.g.*, the **Conduct and Utilization of Research in Nursing [CURN] projects**), which have demonstrated that research utilization can be increased but have also shed light on barriers to utilization.
- EBP, which de-emphasizes clinical decision-making based on custom or ritual, integrates the best available research evidence with other sources of data, including clinical expertise and patient preferences.
- In nursing, EBP and RU efforts often face a variety of barriers, including methodologically weak or unreplicated studies, nurses' limited training in research and EBP, resistance to change, lack of organizational support, resource constraints, and limited communication and collaboration between practiotioners and researchers.
- Many models of RU and EBP have been developed, including models for individual clinicians (*e.g.*, the **Stetler Model**) and models for organizations or groups of clinicians (*e.g.*, the **Iowa Model of Evidence-Based Practice to Promote Quality Care** and the **Ottawa Model of Research Use**).

- Most models of utilization involve the following steps: selecting a topic or problem; assembling and evaluating evidence; assessing the **implementation potential** of an evidence-based innovation; evaluating outcomes; and deciding whether to adopt or modify the innovation or revert to prior practices.
- Assessing implementation potential includes the dimensions of transferability of findings, feasibility of using the findings in the new setting, and the cost–benefit ratio of a new practice.
- EBP relies on rigorous integration of research evidence on a topic through integrative reviews, which are rigourous, systematic inquiries with many similarities to original primary studies.

➤ ➤ ➤ ➤ *CRITICAL THINKING ACTIVITIES*

Chapter 16 of the accompanying *Study Guide to Accompany Essentials of Nursing Research,* 5th edition, offers various exercises and study suggestions for reinforcing the concepts presented in this chapter. In addition, you can consider the following:

1. Find an article in a recent issue of a nursing research journal that does not discuss the implications of the study for nursing practice. Evaluate the study's relevance to nursing practice, and if appropriate, write one to two paragraphs summarizing the implications.

2. Consider your personal situation. What are the barriers that might inhibit your use of research findings?

WORLD WIDE WEBSITES

AHCPR/AHRQ Clinical Practice Guidelines: http://www.ahrq.gov and http://www.guidelines.gov

BMJ Journals "Evidence Based Nursing Journal": http://www.ebn.bmjjournals.com.com/cqi/etoc

The Cochrane Collaboration: (http://www.cochrane.org/)

E-watch on Innovation in Health Services: http://kucc.chair.ulaval.ca/english/master.php?url=bulletin.php

Knowledge Utilization Studies in Practice: http://www.nursing.ualberta.ca/estabrooks/kusp/

National Guidelines Clearinghouse: www.guideline.gov/asp/register.asp

New Zealand Evidence-Based Health Care Bulletin: http://www.nzgg.org.nz/bulletin/current.cfm

RNAO Best Practice Guidelines: http://www.rnao.org/bestpractices

SUGGESTED READINGS

Methodologic References

Alberta Association of Registered Nurses. (1997). Nursing research dissemination and utilization. Alberta Association of Registered Nurses Website (*www.nurses.ab.ca*)

Canadian Nurses Association. (2002, November). *Evidence-based decision-making and nursing practice–position statement.* Ottawa, ON: Author.

Caplan, N., & Rich, R. F. (1975). *The use of social science knowledge in policy decisions at the national level.* Ann Arbor, MI: Institute for Social Research, University of Michigan.

Closs, S. J., & Cheater, F. M. (1999). Evidence for nursing practice: A clarification of the issues. *Journal of Advanced Nursing, 30,* 10–17.

Denis, J-L., Hebert, Y., Langley, A., Lozeau, D., & Trottier, L-H. (2002). Explaining diffusion patterns for complex health care innovations. *Health Care Management Review, 27,* 60–73.

Dufault, M. (1995). A collaborative model for research development and utilization: process, structure, and outcomes. *Journal for Nursing Staff Development, 11,* 139–144.

Dufault, M. A., Bielecki, C., Collins, E., & Willey, C. (1995). Changing nurses' pain assessment practice: A collaborative research utilization approach. *Journal of Advanced Nursing, 21,* 634–645.

Estabrooks, C. E. (2001). Research utilization and qualitative research. In J. M. Morse, J. M. Swanson, & A.J. Kuzel (Eds.), *The nature of qualitative evidence* (pp. 275–298). Thousand Oaks, CA: Sage.

Funk, S. G., Champagne, M. T., Wiese, R. A., & Tornquist, E. M. (1991). Barriers to using research findings in practice: The clinician's perspective. *Applied Nursing Research, 4,* 90–95.

Gennaro, S. (2001). Making evidence-based practice a reality in your institution. *MCN: The American Journal of Maternal/Child Nursing, 26,* 236–244.

Goode, C., & Bulechek, G. (1992). Research utilization: An organizational process that enhances quality of care. *Journal of Nursing Care Quality* (Suppl.), 27–35.

Goode, C., & Piedalue, F. (1999). Evidence based clinical practice. *Journal of Nursing Administration, 29,* 15–21.

Grinspun, D., Virani, T., & Bajnok, I. (2001–2002). Nursing best practice guidelines: The RNAO (Registered Nurses Association of Ontario) project. *Hospital Quaterly, 5,* 56–60.

Horsley, J. A., Crane, J., & Bingle, J. D. (1978). Research utilization as an organizational process. *Journal of Nursing Administration, 8,* 4–6.

Jennings, B. M. (2000). Evidence-based practice: The road best traveled. *Research in Nursing & Health, 23,* 343–345.

Kitson, A., Harvey, G., & McCormack, B. (1998). Enabling the implementation of evidence based practice: a conceptual framework. *Quality in Health Care. 7,* 149–158.

Logan, J., & Graham, I. (1998). Toward a comprehensive interdisciplinary model of health care research use. *Science Communication, 20,* 227–246.

MacLeod, F. E., Harrison, M. B., & Graham, I. D. (2002). The process of developing best practice guidelines for nurses in Ontario: Risk assessment and prevention of pressure ulcers. *Ostomy Wound Management, 48,* 34–38.

Phillips, L. R. F. (1986). *A clinician's guide to the critique and utilization of nursing research.* Norwalk, CT: Appleton-Century-Crofts.

Registered Nurses Association of British Columbia. (1991). Making a difference. From ritual to research-based nursing practice. Vancouver, BC: Author.

Rizzuto, C., Bostrom, J., Suter, W. N., & Chenitz, W. C. (1994). Predictors of nurses' involvement in research activities. *Western Journal of Nursing Research, 16,* 193–204.

Rogers, E. M. (1995). *Diffusion of innovations* (4th ed.). New York: Free Press.

Rosenfeld, P., Duthie, E., Bier, J., Bower-Ferres, S., Fulmer, T., Iervolino, L., McClure, M., McGivern, D., & Roncoli, M. (2000). Engaging staff nurses in evidence-based research to identify nursing practice problems and solutions. *Applied Nursing Research, 13,* 197–203.

Rosswurm, M. A., & Larrabee, J. H. (1999). A model for change to evidence-based practice. *Image: Journal of Nursing Scholarship, 31,* 317–322.

Rutledge, D. N., & Donaldson, N. E. (1995). Building organization capacity to engage in research utilization. *Journal of Nursing Administration, 25,* 12–16.

Rutledge, D. N., Greene, P., Mooney, K., Nail, L. M., & Ropka, M. (1996). Use of research-based practices by oncology staff nurses. *Oncology Nursing Forum, 23,* 1235–1244.

Sackett, D.L., Rosenberg, W., Muir Gray, J. A., Haynes, R., & Richardson, W. (1996). Evidence based medicine: What it is and what it isn't. *British Medical Journal, 312,* 71–72.

Soukoup, Sr. M. (2000). The Center for Advanced Nursing Practice Evidence-Based Practice Model: Promoting the scholarship of practice. *Nursing Clinics of North America, 5,* 301–309.

Stetler, C. B. (1994). Refinement of the Stetler/Marram model for application of research findings to practice. *Nursing Outlook, 42,* 15–25.

Stetler, C. B., Morsi, D., Rucki, S., Broughton, S., Corrigan, B., Fitzgerald, J., Giuliano, K., Havener, P., & Sheridan, E. A. (1998). Utilization-focused integrative reviews in a nursing service. *Applied Nursing Research, 11,* 195–206.

Stetler, C. B. (2001). Updating the Stetler Model of Research Utilization to facilitate evidence-based practice. *Nursing Outlook, 49,* 272–279.

Stevens, K. R. (2001). Systematic reviews: The heart of evidence-based practice. *AACN Clinical Issues, 12,* 529–538.

Thompson, C. J. (2001). The meaning of research utilization: A preliminary typology. *Critical Care Nursing Clinics of North America, 13,* 475–485.

Tibbles, L., & Sanford, R., (1994). The research journal club: A mechanism for research utilization. *Clinical Nurse Specialist, 8,* 23–26.

Titler, M. G., Kleiber, C., Steelman, V., Goode, C., Rakel, B., Barry-Walker, J., & Small, S. (1994). Infusing research into practice to promote quality care. *Nursing Research, 43,* 307–313.

Titler, M. G., Kleiber, C., Steelman, V., Rakel, B., Budreau, G., Everett, L., Buckwalter, K., Tripp-Reimer, T., & Goode, C. (2001). The Iowa Model of Evidence-Based Practice to Promote Quality Care. *Critical Care Nursing Clinics of North America, 13,* 497–509.

Weiss, C. (1980). Knowledge creep and decision accretion. *Knowledge: Creation, Diffusion, Utilization, 1,* 381–404.

Substantive References

Bauer, N., Bushey, F., & Amaros, D. (2002). Diffusion of responsibility and pressure ulcers. *World Council of Enterostomal Therapist Journal, 22,* 9–18.

Beyea, S. C., & Nicoll, L. H. (1995). Administration of medication via the intramuscular route: An integrative review of the literature and research-based protocol for the procedure. *Applied Nursing Research, 8,* 28–29.

Brett, J. L. L. (1987). Use of nursing practice research findings. *Nursing Research, 36,* 344–349.

Coyle, L. A., & Sokop, A. G. (1990). Innovation adoption behavior among nurses. *Nursing Research, 9,* 176–180.

Dobbins, M., Ciliska, D., Cockerill, R., Barnsley, J., & DiCenso, A. (2002). A framework for the dissemination and utilization of research for health-care policy and practice. *The Online Journal of Knowledge Synthesis for Nursing, 9,* 1–15.

Estabrooks, C. A. (1999). The conceptual structure of research utilization. *Research in Nursing & Health, 22,* 203–216.

Estabrooks, C. E., Scott-Findlay, S., & Winther, C. (in press). Knowledge utilization in nursing and the allied health sciences. In F.Champagne & L. Lemieux-Charles (Eds.), *Multidisciplinary perspectives on evidence-based decision-making in health care.*

Funk, S. G., Champagne, M. T., Wiese, R. A., & Tornquist, E. M. (1991). Barriers to using research findings in practice: The clinician's perspective. *Applied Nursing Research, 4,* 90–95.

Funk, S. G., Tornquist, E. M., & Champagne, M. T. (1995). Barriers and facilitators of research utilization: An integrative review. *Nursing Clinics of North America, 30,* 395–407.

Janken, J. K., Blythe, G., Campbell, P. T., & Carter, R. H. (1999). Changing nursing practice through research utilization: Consistent support for breastfeeding mothers. *Applied Nursing Research, 12,* 22–29.

Ketefian, S. (1975). Application of selected nursing research findings into nursing practice. *Nursing Research, 24,* 89–92.

Kirchhoff, K. T. (1982). A diffusion survey of coronary precautions. *Nursing Research, 31,* 196–201.

Lacko, L., Bryan, Y., Dellasega, C., & Salerno, F. (1999). Changing clinical practice through research: The case of delirium. *Clinical Nursing Research, 8,* 235–250.

Larsen, L. L., & Thurston, N. E. (1997). Research utilization: development of a central venous catheter procedure. *Applied Nursing Research, 10,* 44–51.

Logan, J., Harrison, M. B., Graham, I. D., Dunn, K., & Bissonnette, J. (1999). Evidence-based pressure-ulcer practice: The Ottawa Model of Research Use. *Canadian Journal of Nursing Research, 31,* 37–52.

McDonald, H. (2001). Changing practice: Modified clean technique for intermittent catheterization. *SCI Nursing, 18,* 30–33.

McCaughan, D., Thompson, C., Cullum, N., Sheldon, T. A., & Thompson, D. R. (2002). Acute care nurses' perceptions of barriers to using research information in clinical decision-making. *Journal of Advanced Nursing, 39,* 46–60.

Medoff-Cooper, B. (1994). Transition of the preterm infant to an open crib. *Journal of Obstetric, Gynecologic, and Neonatal Nursing, 23,* 329–335.

Montgomery, L., Hanrahan, K., Kottman, K., Otto, A., Barrett, T., & Hermington, B. (1999). Guideline for i.v. infiltration in pediatric patients. *Pediatric Nursing, 25,* 167–169.

Nichols, G. A., & Verhonick, P. J. (1968). Placement times for oral temperatures: A nursing study replication. *Nursing Research, 17,* 159–161.

Oranta O, Routasalo P, Hupli M. (2002). Barriers to and facilitators of research utilization among Finnish registered nurses. *Journal of Clinical Nursing 11,* 205–213.

Owen, S., & Millburn, C. (2001). Implementing research findings into practice: Improving and developing services for women with serious and enduring mental health problems. *Journal of Psychiatric and Mental Health Nursing, 8,* 221–231.

Rizzuto, C., Bostrom, J., Suter, W. N., & Chenitz, W. C. (1994). Predictors of nurses' involvement in research activities. *Western Journal of Nursing Research, 16,* 193–204.

Rodgers, S. E. (2000). The extent of nursing research utilization in general medical and surgical wards. *Journal of Advanced Nursing, 32,* 182–193.

Rosenfeld, P., Duthie, E., Bier, J., Bower-Ferres, S., Fulmer, T., Iervolino, L., McClure, M., McGivern, D., & Roncoli, M. (2000). Engaging staff nurses in evidence-based research to identify nursing practice problems and solutions. *Applied Nursing Research, 13,* 197–203.

Rutledge, D. N., Greene, P., Mooney, K., Nail, L. M., & Ropka, M. (1996). Use of research-based practices by oncology staff nurses. *Oncology Nursing Forum, 23,* 1235–1244.

Samselle, C. M., Wyman, J. F., Thomas, K. K., Newman, D. K., Gray, M., Dougherty, M., & Burns, P. A. (2000a). Continence for women: A test of AWHONN's evidence-based practice protocol in clinical practice. *Journal of Obstetric, Gynecologic, and Neonatal Nursing, 29,* 18–26.

Samselle, C. M., Wyman, J. F., Thomas, K. K., Newman, D. K., Gray, M., Dougherty, M., & Burns, P. A. (2000b). Continence for women: Evaluation of AWHONN's third research utilization project. *Journal of Obstetric, Gynecologic, and Neonatal Nursing, 29,* 9–17.

Varcoe, C., & Hilton, A. (1995). Factors affecting acute-care nurses' use of research findings. *Canadian Journal of Nursing Research, 27,* 51–71.

Glossary

abstract A brief description of a completed or proposed study; in research journals, usually located at the beginning of the journal article.

accessible population The population of people available for a particular study; often a nonrandom subset of the target population.

accidental sampling Selection of the most readily available persons (or units) as participants in a study; also known as *convenience sampling*.

acquiescence response set A bias in self-report instruments, especially in social psychological scales, created when study participants characteristically agree with statements ("yea-say") independent of their content.

after-only design An experimental design in which data are collected from subjects only after the experimental intervention has been introduced.

alpha (α) (1) In tests of statistical significance, the level designating the probability of committing a Type I error; (2) in estimates of internal consistency, a reliability coefficient, as in Cronbach's alpha.

analysis A process of organizing and synthesizing data so as to answer research questions and test hypotheses.

analysis of covariance (ANCOVA) A statistical procedure used to test mean differences among groups on a dependent variable, while controlling for one or more extraneous variables (covariates).

analysis of variance (ANOVA) A statistical procedure for testing mean differences among three or more groups by comparing the variability between the groups to the variability within them.

anonymity Protection of participants in a study such that even the researcher cannot link individuals with the information provided.

applied research Research that concentrates on finding a solution to a practical problem.

assumptions Basic principles that are accepted as being true on the basis of logic or reason, without proof or verification.

attrition The loss of participants during the course of a study (usually a longitudinal study), which can create bias.

audit trail The systematic collection and documentation of materials that allow an independent auditor in an inquiry audit of qualitative data to draw conclusions about the data.

baseline measure A measure of the dependent variable prior to the introduction of an experimental intervention.

basic research Research designed to extend the base of knowledge in a discipline for the sake of knowledge or theory construction, rather than for solving an immediate problem.

basic social process (BSP) The central social process emerging through an analysis of grounded theory data.

before–after design An experimental design in which data are collected from research subjects both before and after the introduction of the experimental intervention.

beneficence A fundamental ethical principle that seeks to prevent harm and exploitation of, and maximize benefits for, study participants.

between-subjects design A research design in which there are separate groups of people being compared (*e.g.,* smokers and nonsmokers).

bias Any influence that produces a distortion in the results of a study.

bimodal distribution A distribution of data values with two peaks (high frequencies).

bivariate statistics Statistics derived from the analysis of two variables simultaneously, for the purpose of assessing the empirical relationship between them.

"blind" review The review of a manuscript or proposal such that neither the author nor the reviewer is identified to the other party.

borrowed theory A theory borrowed from another discipline or field to guide nursing practice or research.

bracketing In phenomenological inquiries, the process of identifying and holding in abeyance any preconceived beliefs and opinions about the phenomena under study.

bricolage The tendency in qualitative research to derive a complex array of data from a variety of sources, using a variety of methods.

case-control study A research design, typically found in retrospective ex post facto research, that involves the comparison of a "case" (*i.e.,* a person with the condition under scrutiny, such as lung cancer) and a matched control (a similar person without the condition).

categorical variable A variable with discrete values rather than values incrementally placed along a continuum (*e.g.,* a person's marital status).

category system In observational studies, the pre-specified plan for organizing and recording the behaviours and events under observation.

causal modeling The development and statistical testing of an explanatory model of hypothesized causal relationships among phenomena.

causal relationship A relationship between two variables such that the presence of one variable (the "cause") affects the presence or value of the other (the "effect").

cell (1) The intersection of a row and column in a table with two or more dimensions; (2) in an experimental design, a cell is the representation of an experimental condition in a schematic diagram.

central tendency A statistical index of the "typicalness" of a set of scores that comes from the centre of the distribution of scores; the three most common indices of central tendency are the mode, the median, and the mean.

chi-squared test A nonparametric test of statistical significance used to assess whether a relationship exists between two categorical variables; symbolized as χ^2.

clinical relevance The degree to which a study addresses a problem of significance to the practice of nursing.

clinical research Research designed to generate knowledge to guide nursing practice.

clinical trial An experiment involving a test of the effectiveness of a clinical treatment, generally involving a large and heterogeneous sample of subjects.

closed-ended question A question that offers respondents a set of mutually exclusive and jointly exhaustive alternative replies, from which the best or most accurate answer must be chosen.

cluster sampling A form of sampling in which large groupings ("clusters") are selected first (*e.g.,* nursing schools), with successive subsampling of smaller units (*e.g.,* nursing students).

code of ethics The fundamental ethical principles that are established by a discipline or institution to guide researchers' conduct in research with human (or animal) subjects.

coding The process of transforming raw data into standardized form for data processing and analysis; in quantitative research, the process of attaching numbers to categories; in qualitative research, the process of identifying recurring words, themes, or concepts within the data.

coefficient alpha (Cronbach's alpha) A reliability index that estimates the internal consistency or homogeneity of a measure composed of several items or subparts.

coercion In a research context, the explicit or implicit use of threats (or excessive rewards) to get people to agree to participate in a study.

comparison group A group of subjects whose scores on a dependent variable are used as a basis for evaluating the scores of the group of primary interest (*e.g.,* nonsmokers as compared to smokers); term used in lieu of control group in studies not using a true experimental design.

concealment A tactic involving the unobtrusive collection of research data without the participants' knowledge or consent, used as a means of obtaining an accurate view of naturalistic behaviour when the known presence of an observer would distort the behaviour of interest.

concept An abstraction based on observations of certain behaviours or characteristics (*e.g.,* stress, pain).

conceptual model Interrelated concepts or abstractions that are assembled together in a rational scheme by virtue of their relevance to a common theme; sometimes referred to as *conceptual framework*.

conceptual utilization The use of research findings in a general, conceptual way to broaden one's thinking about an issue, although the knowledge is not put to any specific use.

concurrent validity The degree to which scores on an instrument are correlated with an external criterion, measured at the same time.

confidentiality Protection of participants in a study such that their individual identities will not be linked to the information they provide and will never be publicly divulged.

confirmability The objectivity or neutrality of qualitative data once they are obtained; a criterion for evaluating data quality.

consent form A written agreement signed by a study participant and a researcher concerning the terms and conditions of a participant's voluntary participation in a study.

constant comparison A procedure often used in a grounded theory analysis wherein newly collected data are compared in an ongoing fashion with data obtained earlier, to refine theoretically relevant categories.

construct An abstraction or concept that is deliberately invented (constructed) by researchers for a scientific purpose.

construct validity The degree to which an instrument measures the construct under investigation.

consumer An individual who reads, reviews, and critiques research findings and who attempts to use and apply the findings in practice.

content analysis The process of organizing and integrating narrative, qualitative information according to emerging themes and concepts; classically, a procedure for analyzing written or verbal communications in a systematic fashion, typically with the goal of quantitatively measuring variables.

content validity The degree to which the items in an instrument adequately represent the universe of content.

contingency table A two-dimensional table that permits a cross-tabulation of the frequencies of two categorical variables.

continuous variable A variable that can take on an infinite range of values along a specified continuum (*e.g.*, height).

control The process of holding constant possible influences on the dependent variable under investigation.

control group Subjects in an experiment who do not receive the experimental treatment and whose performance provides a baseline against which the effects of the treatment can be measured (see also *comparison group*).

convenience sampling Selection of the most readily available people as participants in a study; also known as *accidental sampling*.

core variable In a grounded theory study, a central phenomenon or pattern of behaviour relevant to study participants, and used to integrate all categories of the data.

correlation A tendency for variation in one variable to be related to variation in another variable.

correlation coefficient An index that summarizes the degree of relationship between two variables. Correlation coefficients typically range from +1.00 (for a perfect positive relationship) through 0.0 (for no relationship) to −1.00 (for a perfect negative relationship).

correlation matrix A two-dimensional display showing the correlation coefficients between all combinations of variables.

correlational research Research that explores the interrelationships among variables of interest without any active intervention on the part of the researcher.

cost–benefit analysis An evaluation of the financial costs of a program or intervention relative to the financial gains attributable to it.

cost–benefit assessment The assessment of relative costs and benefits, to individuals, organizations, and society, of implementing an innovation.

covariate A variable that is statistically controlled (held constant) in analysis of covariance. The covariate is typically an extraneous, confounding influence on the dependent variable or a baseline measure of the dependent variable.

covert data collection The collection of information in a study without the participant's knowledge.

credibility A criterion for evaluating data quality in qualitative studies, referring to confidence in the truth value of the qualitative data.

criterion-related validity The degree to which scores on an instrument are correlated with an external criterion.

critique An objective, critical, and balanced appraisal of a research report.

Cronbach's alpha A widely-used reliability index that estimates the internal consistency or homogeneity of a measure composed of several subparts; also referred to as *coefficient alpha*.

crossover design See *repeated measures design*.

cross-sectional study A study based on observations of different age or developmental groups at a single point in time for the purpose of inferring trends over time.

cross-tabulation A determination of the number of cases occurring when two variables are considered simultaneously (*e.g.,* gender—male/female—crosstabulated with smoking status—smoker/nonsmoker). The results are typically presented in a table with rows and columns divided according to the values of the variables.

data The pieces of information obtained in the course of a study (singular is *datum*).

data analysis The systematic organization and synthesis of research data, and the testing of research hypotheses using those data.

data collection The gathering of information needed to address a research problem.

data saturation See *saturation*.

debriefing Communication with study participants, generally after their participation has been completed, regarding various aspects of the study.

deductive reasoning The process of developing specific predictions from general principles (see also *inductive reasoning*).

degrees of freedom (*df*) A concept used in conjunction with statistical tests, referring to the number of sample values that are free to vary (*e.g.*, with a given sample mean, all but one value would be free to vary); degrees of freedom is often $N-1$, but different formulas are relevant for different tests.

dependability A criterion for evaluating data quality in qualitative data, referring to the stability of data over time and over conditions.

dependent variable The outcome variable of interest; the variable that is hypothesized to depend on or be caused by the *independent variable*.

descriptive correlational study A study in which the researcher is primarily interested in describing relationships among variables, without seeking to establish a causal connection.

descriptive research Research studies that have as their main objective the accurate portrayal of the characteristics of persons, situations, or groups, and/or the frequency with which certain phenomena occur.

descriptive statistics Statistics that describe and summarize data (*e.g.*, mean, standard deviation).

descriptive theory A broad characterization that thoroughly accounts for a single phenomenon.

determinism The belief that phenomena are not haphazard or random, but rather have antecedent causes; an assumption in the positivist paradigm.

directional hypothesis A hypothesis that makes a specific prediction about the direction and nature of the relationship between two variables.

discriminant function analysis A statistical procedure used to predict group membership— or status on a categorical (nominal level) variable— on the basis of two or more independent variables.

disproportionate sample A sample that results when the researcher samples differing proportions of study participants from different strata in the population to ensure adequate representation of strata that are comparatively smaller.

double-blind experiment An experiment in which neither the subjects nor those who administer the treatment know who is in the experimental or control group.

electronic database Bibliographic files that can be accessed by computer for the purpose of conducting a literature review.

element The most basic unit of a population, from which a sample will be drawn; in nursing research, the element is typically humans.

eligibility criteria The criteria used by a researcher to designate the specific attributes of the target population, and by which participants are selected for participation in a study.

emergent design A design that unfolds in the course of a qualitative study as the researcher makes ongoing design decisions reflecting what has already been learned.

emic perspective A term used by ethnographers to refer to the way members of a culture themselves view their world; the "insider's view."

empirical evidence Evidence that is rooted in objective reality, based on the collection of data using one's senses.

equivalence The degree of similarity between alternate forms of a measuring instrument.

error of measurement The deviation between true scores and obtained scores of a measured characteristic.

ethics A system of moral values that is concerned with the degree to which research procedures adhere to professional, legal, and social obligations to the study participants.

ethnography A branch of human inquiry, associated with the field of anthropology, that focuses on the culture of a group of people, with an effort to understand the world view of those under study.

ethnomethodology A branch of human inquiry, associated with sociology, that focuses on the way in which people make sense of their everyday activities and come to behave in socially acceptable ways.

ethnonursing research The study of human cultures, with a focus on a group's beliefs and practices relating to nursing care and related health behaviours.

etic perspective A term used by ethnographers to refer to the "outsider's" view of the experiences of a cultural group.

evaluation A type of research designed to determine the effectiveness of a program, treatment, practice, or policy.

event sampling In observational studies, a sampling plan that involves the selection of integral behaviours or events.

evidence-based practice Nursing practice that uses research findings as a basis for nurses' decisions, actions, and interactions with clients.

***ex post facto* research** Research conducted after the variations in the independent variable have occurred in the natural course of events; a form of nonexperimental research in which causal explanations are inferred "after the fact."

experiment A research study in which the investigator controls (manipulates) the independent variable and randomly assigns subjects to different conditions.

experimental group The subjects who receive the experimental treatment or intervention.

experimental intervention (experimental treatment) See *intervention; treatment.*

external validity The degree to which the results of a study can be generalized to settings or samples other than the ones studied.

extraneous variable A variable that confounds the relationship between the independent and dependent variables and that needs to be controlled either in the research design or through statistical procedures.

extreme case sampling A sampling approach used by qualitative researchers that involves the purposeful selection of the most extreme or unusual cases.

extreme response set A bias in self-report instruments, especially in social psychological scales, created when participants express their opinions in terms of extreme response alternatives (*e.g.*, "strongly agree") independent of the question's content.

***F*-ratio** The statistic obtained in several statistical tests (*e.g.*, ANOVA) in which variation attributable to different sources (*e.g.*, between groups and within groups) is compared.

face validity The extent to which a measuring instrument looks as though it is measuring what it purports to measure.

factor analysis A statistical procedure for reducing a large set of variables into a smaller set of variables by identifying underlying dimensions.

factorial design An experimental design in which two or more independent variables are simultaneously manipulated; this design permits analysis of the main effects of the independent variables, plus interaction effects.

field notes The notes taken by researchers describing the unstructured observations they have made in the field, and their interpretation of those observations.

field research Research in which the data are collected "in the field" from individuals in their normal roles, with the aim of understanding the practices, behaviours, and beliefs of individuals or groups as they normally function in real life.

findings The results of the analyses of the research data that address the research questions or hypothesis.

fixed alternative question A question that offers respondents a set of pre-specified responses, from which the respondent must choose the alternative that is the most appropriate or accurate response.

focus group interview An interview with a group of individuals assembled to answer and discuss questions on a given topic.

focused interview A loosely structured interview in which the interviewer guides the respondent through a set of questions using a topic guide.

follow-up study A study undertaken to determine the outcomes of people with a specified condition or who have received a specified treatment.

framework The conceptual underpinnings of a study; often referred to as a *theoretical framework* in studies based on a theory, or as a *conceptual framework* in studies that have roots in a specific conceptual model.

frequency distribution A systematic array of numeric values from the lowest to the highest, together with a count of the number of times each value was obtained.

frequency polygon Graphic display of a frequency distribution depicting the number of times a score value occurs in a set of data.

full disclosure The communication of complete information to potential study participants regarding the nature of the research, the person's right to refuse participation, and the likely risks and benefits that would be incurred.

functional relationship An association between two variables wherein it cannot be assumed that one variable caused the other, but values for variable *X* change as a function of changes in variable *Y*.

gaining entrée The process of gaining access to study participants in qualitative field studies through the cooperation of key actors in the selected site.

generalizability The degree to which it can be inferred that the findings can be generalized from a sample to a population.

grand theory A theory aimed at describing large segments of the physical, social, or behavioural world; also referred to as a *macro-theory*.

grand tour question A broad question asked in an unstructured interview to gain a general overview of a phenomenon, on the basis of which more focused questions are subsequently asked.

grounded theory An approach to collecting and analyzing qualitative data with the aim of developing theories and theoretical propositions grounded in real-world observations.

Hawthorne effect The effect on the dependent variable resulting from subjects' awareness that they are participants under study.

hermeneutics A qualitative research tradition, drawing on interpretive phenomenology, that focuses on the lived experiences of humans, and on how they interpret those experiences.

heterogeneity The degree to which objects are dissimilar (*i.e.,* characterized by high variability) with respect to some attribute.

histogram A graphic presentation of frequency distribution data.

historical research Systematic studies designed to establish facts and relationships about past events.

history threat A threat to the internal validity of a study; refers to the occurrence of events external to the intervention, but concurrent with it, that can affect the dependent variable of interest.

homogeneity (1) In terms of the reliability of an instrument, the degree to which the subparts are internally consistent (*i.e.,* are measuring the same critical attribute). (2) More generally, the degree to which objects are similar (*i.e.,* characterized by low variability).

hypothesis A prediction about relationships between variables.

impact analysis An evaluation of the effects of an intervention on outcomes of interest, net of other factors influencing those outcomes.

implementation analysis An evaluation that describes the process by which a program or intervention was implemented in practice.

implementation potential The extent to which an innovation is amenable to implementation in a new setting, an assessment of which is made in a research utilization or evidence-based practice project.

independent variable The variable that is believed to cause or influence the dependent variable; in experimental research, the manipulated (treatment) variable.

inductive reasoning The process of reasoning from specific observations to more general conceptualizations (see also *deductive reasoning*).

inferential statistics Statistics that permit inferences on whether relationships observed in a sample are likely to occur in a population.

informant A term used to refer to those individuals who provide information to researchers about a phenomenon under study, often used in qualitative studies.

informed consent An ethical principle that requires researchers to obtain the voluntary participation of subjects, after informing them of possible risks and benefits.

inquiry audit An independent scrutiny of qualitative data and relevant supporting documents by an external reviewer, a method used to determine the dependability and confirmability of qualitative data.

instrument The device that a researcher uses to collect data (*e.g.,* questionnaires, scales, observation schedules, etc.).

instrumental utilization Clearly identifiable attempts to base a specific action or intervention on research findings.

integrated research design A research design that integrates qualitative and quantitative methodologies and data.

interaction effect The effect of two or more independent variables acting in combination (interactively) on a dependent variable rather than as unconnected factors.

internal consistency The degree to which the subparts of an instrument are all measuring the same attribute or dimension, as an index of the instrument's reliability.

internal validity The degree to which it can be inferred that the independent variable, rather than uncontrolled, extraneous factors, is responsible for observed effects on the dependent variable.

interrater (interobserver) reliability The degree to which two raters or observers, operating independently, assign the same values for an attribute being measured or observed.

interval measure A level of measurement in which an attribute of a variable is rank-ordered on a scale that has equal distances between points on that scale (*e.g.,* Centigrade degrees).

intervention In experimental research, the experimental treatment or manipulation.

interview schedule The formal instrument, used in structured self-report studies, that specifies the wording of all questions to be asked of respondents.

inverse relationship A negative correlation between two variables; *i.e.,* a relationship characterized by the tendency of high values on one variable to be associated with low values on the second variable.

item A single question on a test or questionnaire, or a single statement on a scale (*e.g.,* a final examination might consist of 100 items).

journal article A report that summarizes an investigation in a professional journal.

journal club A group that meets regularly (often in clinical settings) to discuss and critique research reports appearing in research journals, often with the goal of assessing the utilization potential of the findings.

judgmental sampling A nonprobability sampling method in which the researcher selects study participants on the basis of personal judgment about which ones will be most representative or productive; also referred to as *purposive sampling.*

known-groups technique A technique for estimating the construct validity of an instrument through an analysis of the degree to which the instrument separates groups that are predicted to differ on the basis of known characteristics or a theory.

level of measurement A system of classifying measurements according to the nature of the measurement and the type of mathematical operations to which they are amenable; the four levels are nominal, ordinal, interval, and ratio.

level of significance The risk of making a Type I error, established by the researcher before statistical analysis (*e.g.,* the .05 level).

life history A narrative self-report about a person's life experiences vis-à-vis a theme of interest to the researcher.

Likert scale A composite measure of attitudes that involves summation of scores on a set of items (statements) to which respondents are asked to indicate their degree of agreement or disagreement.

LISREL The widely-used acronym for linear structural relation analysis, typically used for testing causal models.

literature review A critical summary of research on a topic of interest, often prepared to put a research problem in context or as the basis for a utilization project.

log In participant observation studies, the observer's daily record of events and conversations.

logical positivism The philosophy underlying the traditional scientific approach; see also *positivist paradigm.*

logistic regression A multivariate regression procedure that analyzes relationships between multiple independent variables and categorical dependent variables; also referred to as *logit analysis.*

longitudinal study A study designed to collect data at more than one point in time, in contrast to a cross-sectional study.

macro-theory A theory aimed at describing large segments of the physical, social, or behavioural world; also referred to as a *grand theory.*

main effects In a study with multiple independent variables, the effects of a single independent variable on the dependent variable.

manipulation An intervention or treatment introduced by the researcher in an experimental or quasi-experimental study; the researcher manipulates the independent variable to assess its impact on the dependent variable.

matching The pairing of subjects in one group with those in another group based on their similarity on one or more dimension, done to enhance the comparability of groups.

maturation threat A threat to the internal validity of a study that occurs when changes to the outcome measure (dependent variable) result from the passage of time.

maximum variation sampling A sampling approach used by qualitative researchers that involves the purposeful selection of cases with a wide range of variation.

mean A descriptive statistic that is a measure of central tendency, computed by summing all scores and dividing by the number of subjects.

measurement The assignment of numbers to objects according to specified rules to characterize quantities of an attribute.

median A descriptive statistic that is a measure of central tendency, representing the exact middle score in a distribution of scores; the median is the value above and below which 50 percent of the scores lie.

mediating variable A variable that mediates or acts like a "go-between" in a chain linking two other variables (*e.g.,* coping skills mediate the relationship between stressful events and anxiety).

member check A method of validating the credibility of qualitative data through debriefings and discussions with informants.

meta-analysis A technique for quantitatively combining and thus integrating the results of multiple studies on a given topic.

methodologic notes In observational field studies, the notes kept by the researcher regarding the methods used in collecting the data.

methods (research) The steps, procedures, and strategies for gathering and analyzing the data in a research investigation.

middle-range theory A theory that focuses on only a piece of reality or human experience, involving a selected number of concepts (*e.g.,* theories of stress).

modality A characteristic of a frequency distribution describing the number of peaks; that is, values with high frequencies.

mode A descriptive statistic that is a measure of central tendency; the score or value that occurs most frequently in a distribution of scores.

model A symbolic representation of concepts or variables, and interrelationships among them.

mortality threat A threat to the internal validity of a study, referring to the differential loss of participants (attrition) from different groups.

multimethod research Generally, research in which multiple approaches are used to address a research problem; often used to designate research in which both qualitative and quantitative data are collected and analyzed.

multimodal distribution A distribution of values with more than one peak (high frequency).

multiple comparison procedures Statistical tests, normally applied after an ANOVA indicates statistically significant group differences, that compare different pairs of groups; also referred to as *post hoc tests.*

multiple correlation coefficient An index that summarizes the degree of relationship between two or more independent variables and a dependent variable; symbolized as *R.*

multiple regression analysis A statistical procedure for understanding the simultaneous effects of two or more independent (predictor) variables on a dependent variable.

multi-stage sampling A sampling strategy that proceeds through a set of stages from larger to smaller sampling units (e.g., from states, to nursing schools, to faculty members).

multivariate analysis of variance (MANOVA) A statistical procedure used to test the significance of differences between the means of two or more groups on two or more dependent variables, considered simultaneously.

multivariate statistics Statistical procedures designed to analyze the relationships among three or more variables; commonly used multivariate statistics include multiple regression, analysis of covariance, and factor analysis.

N Often used to designate the total number of study participants (e.g., "the total N was 500").

n Often used to designate the number of participants in a subgroup or in a cell of a study (e.g., "each of the four groups had an n of 125, for a total N of 500").

naturalistic paradigm An alternative paradigm to the traditional positivist paradigm that holds that there are multiple interpretations of reality, and that the goal of research is to understand how individuals construct reality within their context; often associated with qualitative research.

naturalistic setting A setting for the collection of research data that is natural to those being studied (e.g., homes, places of work, and so on).

negative case analysis A method used in a qualitative study to extend the understanding of the findings by searching for exceptions that will increase variation in the data.

negative relationship A relationship between two variables in which there is a tendency for higher values on one variable to be associated with lower values on the other (e.g., as temperature increases, people's productivity may decrease); also referred to as an *inverse relationship.*

negative results Research results that fail to support the researcher's hypotheses.

negatively skewed distribution An asymmetric distribution of data values, with a disproportionately high number of cases having high values—i.e., falling at the upper end of the distribution; when displayed graphically, the tail points to the left.

net effects The impacts of an intervention, over and above what would have occurred in its absence.

network sampling The sampling of participants based on referrals from others already in the sample, sometimes referred to as *snowball sampling.*

nominal measure The lowest level of measurement that involves the assignment of characteristics into categories (e.g., males, category 1; females, category 2).

nondirectional hypothesis A research hypothesis that does not stipulate in advance the expected direction of the relationship between variables.

nonequivalent control group design A quasi-experimental design involving a comparison group that was not developed on the basis of random assignment, but from whom preintervention data are obtained to assess the initial equivalence of the groups.

nonexperimental research Studies in which the researcher collects data without introducing any treatment.

nonparametric statistics A general class of inferential statistics that does not involve rigorous assumptions about the distribution of the critical variables; most often used when the data are measured on the nominal or ordinal scales.

nonprobability sampling The selection of participants or sampling units from a population using nonrandom procedures; examples include convenience, purposive, and quota sampling.

nonresponse bias A bias that can result when a nonrandom subset of people invited to participate in a study fail to do so.

nonsignificant result The result of a statistical test indicating that a relationship between variables could have occurred as a result of chance, at a given level of significance; sometimes abbreviated as *NS* in research journals.

normal distribution A distribution that is bell-shaped and symmetrical; also referred to as a *normal curve*.

null hypothesis The hypothesis that states there is no relationship between the variables under study; used with tests of statistical significance as the hypothesis to be rejected.

objectivity The extent to which two independent researchers would arrive at similar judgments or conclusions (*i.e.*, judgments not biased by personal values or beliefs).

observational methods Techniques for acquiring data through the direct observation of phenomena.

observational notes In field studies, the observer's descriptions of observed events and conversations.

observational research Studies in which the data are collected by observing and recording behaviours or activities of interest.

obtained (observed) score The actual score or numerical value assigned to a person on a measure.

open-ended question A question in an interview or questionnaire that does not restrict the respondents' answers to preestablished alternatives.

open coding The first level of coding in a grounded theory study, used to capture what is going on in the data.

operational definition The definition of a concept or variable in terms of the operations or procedures by which it is to be measured.

ordinal measure A level of measurement that yields rank orders of a variable along some dimension.

outcome analysis An evaluation of what happens with respect to outcomes of interest after implementing a program, without use of an experimental design to assess net effects; see also *impact analysis*.

outcome variable A term sometimes used to refer to the dependent variable in experimental research, *i.e.,* the measure that captures the outcome of the intervention.

outcomes research Research designed to document the effectiveness of health care services and the end results of patient care.

***p* value** In statistical testing, the probability that the obtained results are due to chance alone; the probability of committing a Type I error.

panel study A type of longitudinal study in which data are collected from the same people at two or more points in time.

paradigm A way of looking at natural phenomena that encompasses a set of philosophical assumptions and that guides one's approach to inquiry.

parameter A characteristic of a population (*e.g.,* the mean age of all Canadian citizens).

parametric statistics A class of inferential statistics that involves (a) assumptions about the distribution of the variables, (b) the estimation of a parameter, and (c) the use of interval or ratio measures.

participant See *study participant.*

participant observation A method of collecting data through the observation of a group or organization in which the researcher participates as a member.

path analysis A regression-based procedure for testing causal models, typically using nonexperimental data.

Pearson's *r* The most widely-used correlation coefficient, designating the magnitude of relationship between two variables measured on at least an interval scale; also referred to as the *product–moment correlation.*

peer debriefing In qualitative research, a session held with objective peers to review various aspects of the inquiry as a means of strengthening the trustworthiness of the data.

peer reviewer A person who reviews and critiques a research report, who himself/herself is a researcher (usually working on similar research problems as those under review), and who makes a recommendation about publishing the research.

perfect relationship A correlation between two variables such that the values of one variable permit perfect prediction of the values of the other; designated as 1.00 or -1.00.

personal interview A face-to-face interview between an interviewer and a respondent.

personal notes In field studies, written comments about the observer's own feelings during the research process.

phenomenon The abstract entity or concept under investigation in a study, most often used by qualitative researchers in lieu of the term "variable."

phenomenology A qualitative research tradition, with roots in philosophy, that focuses on the lived experience of humans.

pilot study A small scale version, or trial run, done in preparation for a major study.

population The entire set of individuals (or objects) having some common characteristics (*e.g.,* all RNs in Alberta); sometimes referred to as *universe.*

positive relationship A relationship between two variables in which there is a tendency for high values on one variable to be associated with high values on the other (*e.g.,* as physical activity increases, pulse rate also increases).

positive results Research results that are consistent with the researcher's hypotheses.

positively skewed distribution An asymmetric distribution of values, with a disproportionately high number of cases having low values—*i.e.,* falling at the lower end of the distribution; when displayed graphically, the tail points to the right.

positivist paradigm The traditional paradigm underlying the scientific approach, which assumes that there is a fixed, orderly reality that can be objectively studied; often associated with quantitative research.

***post hoc* test** A test for comparing all possible pairs of groups following a significant test of overall group differences (*e.g.,* in an ANOVA).

poster session A session at a professional conference in which several researchers simultaneously present visual displays summarizing their studies, while conference attendees circulate around the room perusing the displays.

posttest The collection of data after the introduction of an experimental intervention.

posttest-only design An experimental design in which data are collected from subjects only after an intervention has been introduced; also referred to as an *after-only design.*

power analysis A procedure for estimating (a) the likelihood of committing a Type II error, or (b) sample size requirements.

predictive validity The degree to which an instrument can predict a criterion observed at a future time.

pre-experimental design A research design that does not include mechanisms to compensate for the absence of either randomization or a control group.

pretest (1) The collection of data prior to the experimental intervention; sometimes referred to as *baseline data.* (2) The trial administration of a newly developed instrument to identify flaws or assess time requirements.

pretest—posttest design An experimental design in which data are collected from subjects both before and after the introduction of an intervention; also referred to as a *before-after design.*

primary source First-hand reports of facts, findings or events; in terms of research, the primary source is the original research report prepared by the investigator who conducted the study.

probability sampling The selection of participants or sampling units from a population using random procedures; examples include simple random sampling, cluster sampling, and systematic sampling.

problem statement The statement of the research problem, sometimes phrased in the form of a research question.

process analysis An evaluation focusing on the process by which a program or intervention gets implemented and used in practice.

process consent In a qualitative study, an ongoing, transactional process of negotiating consent with study participants, allowing them to play a collaborative role in the decision-making regarding their continued participation.

product–moment correlation coefficient (*r*) The most widely-used correlation coefficient, designating the magnitude of relationship between two variables measured on at least an interval scale; also referred to as *Pearson's r*.

projective techniques Methods for measuring psychological attributes (values, attitudes, personality) by providing respondents with unstructured stimuli to which to respond.

prolonged engagement In qualitative research, the investment of sufficient time in the collection of data to have an in-depth understanding of the group under study; a mechanism for achieving data credibility.

proportionate sample A sample that results when the researcher samples from different strata of the population in direct proportion to their representation in the population.

prospective study A study that begins with an examination of presumed causes (*e.g.,* cigarette smoking) and then goes forward in time to observe presumed effects (*e.g.,* lung cancer).

psychometric evaluation An assessment of the quality of an instrument, based primarily on evidence of its reliability and validity.

purposive (purposeful) sampling A nonprobability sampling method in which the researcher selects study participants on the basis of personal judgment about which ones will be most representative or productive; also referred to as *judgmental sampling*.

Q sort A data collection method in which the participant sorts statements into a number of piles (usually 9 or 11) according to some bipolar dimension (e.g., most like me/least like me).

qualitative analysis The organization and interpretation of nonnumerical data for the purpose of discovering important underlying dimensions and patterns of relationships.

qualitative data Information collected in narrative (nonnumerical) form, such as the transcript of an unstructured interview.

qualitative research The investigation of phenomena, typically in an in-depth and holistic fashion, through the collection of rich narrative materials using a flexible research design.

quantitative analysis The manipulation of numeric data through statistical procedures for the purpose of describing phenomena or assessing the magnitude and reliability of relationships among them.

quantitative data Information collected in a numeric form.

quantitative research The study of phenomena that lend themselves to precise measurement and quantification, often involving a rigorous and controlled design.

quasi-experiment A study in which subjects are not randomly assigned to treatment conditions, but the researcher does manipulate the independent variable and exercises certain controls to enhance the internal validity of the results.

quasi-statistics An "accounting" system used to assess the validity of conclusions derived from qualitative analysis.

questionnaire A method of gathering self-report information from respondents through administration of questions in a paper-and-pencil format.

quota sampling The nonrandom selection of participants in which the researcher pre-specifies characteristics of the sample, to increase its representativeness.

r The symbol used to designate a bivariate correlation coefficient, summarizing the magnitude and direction of a relationship between two variables.

R The symbol used to designate the multiple correlation coefficient, indicating the magnitude (but not direction) of the relationship between the dependent variable and multiple independent variables, taken together.

R^2 The squared multiple correlation coefficient, indicating the proportion of variance in the dependent variable accounted for or explained by a group of independent variables.

random assignment The assignment of subjects to treatment conditions in a random manner (*i.e.,* in a manner determined by chance alone); also known as *randomization*.

random sampling The selection of a sample such that each member of a population has an equal probability of being included.

randomization See *random assignment.*

range A measure of variability, consisting of the difference between the highest and lowest values in a distribution of scores.

ratio measure A level of measurement in which there are equal distances between score units, and that has a true meaningful zero point (*e.g.,* weight).

raw data Data that are in the exact form in which they were collected.

reactivity A measurement distortion arising from the study participant's awareness of being observed, or, more generally, from the effect of the measurement procedure itself.

relationship A bond or association between two or more variables.

reliability The degree of consistency or accuracy with which an instrument measures the attribute it is designed to measure.

reliability coefficient A quantitative index, usually ranging in value from .00 to 1.00, that provides an estimate of how reliable an instrument is.

repeated-measures design An experimental design in which one group of subjects is exposed to more than one condition or treatment in random order; sometimes referred to as a *crossover design.*

replication The deliberate repetition of research procedures in a second investigation for the purpose of determining if earlier results can be repeated.

representative sample A sample whose characteristics are highly similar to those of the population from which it is drawn.

research Systematic inquiry that uses orderly, disciplined methods to answer questions or solve problems.

research-based practice See *evidence-based practice.*

research control See *control*.

research design The overall plan for addressing a research question, including specifications for enhancing the integrity of the study.

research problem A situation involving an enigmatic, perplexing, or conflictful condition that can be investigated through disciplined inquiry.

research question A statement of the specific query the investigator wants to answer through research.

research report A document that summarizes the main features of a study, including the research question, the methods used to address it, the findings, and the interpretation and implications of the findings.

research utilization The use of some aspect of a scientific investigation in an application unrelated to the original research.

respondent In a self-report study, the participant who responds to questions posed by the researcher.

response rate The rate of participation in a study, calculated by dividing the number of people participating by the number of people sampled.

response set bias The measurement error introduced by the tendency of some individuals to respond to items in characteristic ways (*e.g.*, always agreeing), independently of the item's content.

results The answers to research questions, obtained through an analysis of the collected data; in a quantitative study, the information obtained through statistical tests.

retrospective study A study that begins with the occurrence of the dependent variable in the present (*e.g.*, lung cancer) and then links this effect to some presumed cause occurring in the past (*e.g.*, cigarette smoking).

risk–benefit ratio The relative costs and benefits, to an individual subject and to society at large, of participation in a study; also, the relative costs and benefits of implementing an innovation.

rival hypothesis An alternative explanation, competing with the researcher's hypothesis, for understanding the results of a study.

sample A subset of a population selected to participate in a study.

sample size The number of study participants in a sample.

sampling The process of selecting a portion of the population to represent the entire population.

sampling bias Distortions that arise when a sample is not representative of the population from which it was drawn.

sampling distribution A theoretical distribution of a statistic, using the values of the statistic computed from an infinite number of samples as the data points in the distribution.

sampling error The fluctuation of the value of a statistic from one sample to another drawn from the same population.

sampling frame A list of all the elements in the population, from which the sample is drawn.

sampling plan In a quantitative study, the pre-specified plan that indicates in advance what the eligibility criteria are, how the sample will be selected, and how many subjects there will be.

saturation The process of collecting data in a grounded theory study to the point where a sense of closure is attained because new data yield redundant information.

scale A composite measure of an attribute, involving the combination of several items that have a logical and empirical relationship to each other, resulting in the assignment of a score to place people on a continuum with respect to the attribute.

scientific approach A set of orderly, systematic, controlled procedures for acquiring dependable, empirical—and typically quantitative—information; the methodologic approach associated with the positivist paradigm.

scientific merit The degree to which a study is methodologically and conceptually sound.

secondary source Second-hand accounts of events or facts; in a research context, a description of a study or studies prepared by someone other than the original researcher.

selection threat (self-selection) A threat to the internal validity of the study resulting from pre-existing differences between the groups under study; the differences affect the dependent variable in ways extraneous to the effect of the independent variable.

selective coding The type of substantive coding in a grounded theory study that involves the coding of only those variables that are related to the core variable.

self-report Any procedure for collecting data that involves a direct report of information by the person who is being studied (*e.g.,* by interview or questionnaire).

self selection A bias that can occur when the members of groups being studied are in the groups, in part, because they differentially possess traits or characteristics extraneous to the research problem, characteristics that possibly influence or are otherwise related to the research variables.

semantic differential A technique used to measure attitudes that asks respondents to rate a concept of interest on a series of bipolar rating scales.

setting The physical location and conditions in which data collection takes place in a study.

significance level The probability that an observed relationship could be caused by chance (*i.e.,* as a result of sampling error); significance at the .05 level indicates the probability that a relationship of the observed magnitude would be found by chance only 5 times out of 100.

simple random sampling The most basic type of probability sampling, wherein a sampling frame is created by enumerating all members of a population of interest, and then selecting a sample from the sampling frame through completely random procedures.

skewed distribution The asymmetric distribution of a set of data values around a central point.

snowball sampling The selection of participants by means of referrals from earlier participants; also referred to as *network sampling*.

social desirability response set A bias in self-report instruments created when participants have a tendency to misrepresent their opinions in the direction of answers consistent with prevailing social norms.

Spearman's rank-order correlation (Spearman's rho) A correlation coefficient indicating the magnitude of a relationship between variables measured on the ordinal scale.

split-half technique A method for estimating the internal consistency reliability of an instrument by correlating scores on half of the measure with scores on the other half.

standard deviation The most frequently used statistic for measuring the degree of variability in a set of scores.

standard error The standard deviation of a sampling distribution, such as the sampling distribution of means.

statement of purpose A broad declarative statement of the goals of a research project.

statistic An estimate of a parameter, calculated from sample data.

statistical analysis The organization and analysis of quantitative data using statistical procedures, including both descriptive and inferential statistics.

statistical inference The process of inferring attributes about the population based on information from a sample, using laws of probability.

statistical significance A term indicating that the results obtained in an analysis of sample data are unlikely to have been caused by chance, at some specified level of probability.

statistical test An analytic procedure that allows a researcher to determine the probability that obtained results from a sample reflect true population results.

stipend A monetary payment to individuals participating in a study to serve as an incentive for participation and/or to compensate for time and expenses.

strata Subdivisions of the population according to some characteristic (*e.g.*, males and females); singular is *stratum.*

stratified random sampling The random selection of study participants from two or more strata of the population independently.

structured data collection An approach to collecting information from participants, either through self-report or observations, wherein the researcher determines in advance the variables and categories of interest.

structured observation A procedure for collecting observational data in which the nature of the observations to be made are pre-specified, and a procedure for sampling observational units has been designated.

structured self-report A procedure for collecting data that involves asking a pre-specified set of questions in a pre-specified order, usually with a preponderance of closed-ended questions.

study participant An individual who participates and provides information in a research investigation.

subject An individual who participates and provides data in a study; term used primarily in quantitative research.

summated rating scale See *Likert scale.*

survey research Nonexperimental research that focuses on obtaining information regarding the activities, beliefs, preferences, and attitudes of people via direct questioning of a sample of respondents.

symmetric distribution A distribution of values that has two halves that are mirror images of each other; a distribution that is not skewed.

systematic sampling The selection of study participants such that every kth (*e.g.*, every tenth) person (or element) in a sampling frame or list is chosen.

target population The entire population in which the researcher is interested and to which he or she would like to generalize the results of a study.

test statistic A statistic used to test for the statistical significance of relationships between variables; the sampling distributions of test statistics are known for circumstances in which the null hypothesis is true; examples include chi-squared, F-ratio, t, and Pearson's r.

test–retest reliability Assessment of the stability of an instrument by correlating the scores obtained on repeated administrations.

theme A recurring regularity emerging from an analysis of qualitative data.

theoretical notes In field studies, notes detailing the researcher's interpretations of observed behaviour.

theoretical sampling In qualitative studies (especially in grounded theory studies), the selection of sample members based on emerging findings/theory to ensure adequate representation and full variation of important themes.

theory An abstract generalization that presents a systematic explanation about the relationships among phenomena.

thick description A rich and thorough description of the research context in a qualitative study.

time sampling In observational research, the selection of time periods during which observations will take place.

time series design A quasi-experimental design that involves the collection of information over an extended time period, with multiple data collection points prior to and after the introduction of a treatment.

topic guide A list of broad question areas to be covered in a semi-structured interview or focus group interview.

transferability (1) A criterion for evaluating the quality of qualitative data, referring to the extent to which the findings from the data can be transferred to other settings or groups—analogous to generalizability; (2) also, a criterion used in an implementation assessment of a utilization project.

treatment The experimental intervention under study; the condition being manipulated.

trend study A form of longitudinal study in which different samples from a population are studied over time with respect to some phenomenon (*e.g.*, annual Gallup polls on abortion attitudes).

triangulation The use of multiple methods or perspectives to collect and interpret data about a phenomenon, to converge on an accurate representation of reality.

true score A hypothetical score that would be obtained if a measure were infallible; the portion of the observed score not due to random error or measurement bias.

trustworthiness A term used in the evaluation of qualitative data, assessed using the criteria of credibility, transferability, dependability, and confirmability.

t-test A parametric statistical test used for analyzing the difference between two means.

Type I error An error created by rejecting the null hypothesis when it is true (*i.e.,* the researcher concludes that a relationship exists when in fact it does not).

Type II error An error created by accepting the null hypothesis when it is false (*i.e.,* the researcher concludes that *no* relationship exists when in fact it does).

unimodal distribution A distribution of values with one peak (high frequency).

univariate descriptive study A study that gathers information on the occurrence, frequency of occurrence, or average value of the variables of interest, one variable at a time, without focusing on interrelationships among variables.

univariate statistics Statistical procedures for analyzing a single variable for purposes of description.

unstructured interview An oral self-report in which the researcher asks questions without having a predetermined plan regarding the specific content or flow of information to be gathered.

unstructured observation The collection of descriptive information through direct observation, whereby the observer is guided by some general research questions but does not follow a prespecified plan for observing, enumerating, or recording the information.

validity The degree to which an instrument measures what it is intended to measure.

validity coefficient A quantitative index, usually ranging in value from .00 to 1.00, that provides an estimate of how valid an instrument is; usually computed in conjunction with the criterion-related approach to validating an instrument.

variability The degree to which values on a set of scores are widely different or dispersed.

variable An attribute of a person or object that varies, that is, takes on different values (*e.g.,* body temperature, age, heart rate).

variance A measure of variability or dispersion, equal to the standard deviation squared.

vignette A brief description of an event, person, or situation to which respondents are asked to react and to describe their reactions.

visual analog scale A scaling procedure used to measure clinical symptoms (*e.g.,* pain, fatigue) by having people indicate on a straight line the intensity of the attribute being measured.

vulnerable subjects Special groups of people whose rights in studies need special protection because of their inability to provide meaningful informed consent or because their circumstances place them at higher-than-average-risk of adverse effects; examples include young children, the mentally retarded, and unconscious patients.

weighting A correction procedure used to arrive at population values when a disproportionate sampling design has been used.

within-subjects design A research design in which a single group of subjects is compared under different conditions or at different points in time (*e.g.,* before and after surgery).

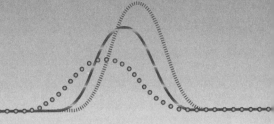

Quantitative Study
Preventing Smoking Relapse In Postpartum Women

JOY L. JOHNSON, PAMELA A. RATNER, JOAN L. BOTTORFF, WENDY HALL,
AND SUSAN DAHINTEN

- **Background:** Although many women quit smoking during pregnancy, the majority resume smoking shortly after giving birth.
- **Objectives:** To test a program to prevent smoking relapse in the postpartum period by comparing the rates of continuous smoking abstinence, daily smoking, and smoking cessation self-efficacy in treatment and control groups.
- **Methods:** In a randomized clinical trial, nurses provided face-to-face, in-hospital counseling sessions at birth, followed by telephone counseling. The target population included women who quit smoking during pregnancy and who gave birth at one of five hospitals. The 254 participating women were interviewed 6 months after delivery and assessed biochemically to determine smoking status.
- **Results:** The 6-month continuous smoking abstinence rate was 38% in the treatment group and 27% in the control group (odds ratio [OR] = 1.63, 95% confidence interval [CI] = .96–2.78). Significantly more control (48%) than treatment (34%) group participants reported smoking daily (OR = 1.80, 95% CI = 1.08–2.99). Smoking cessation self-efficacy did not vary significantly between the groups.
- **Conclusions:** Smoking cessation interventions focusing on the prenatal period have failed to achieve long-term abstinence. Interventions can be strengthened if they are extended into the postpartum period.
- **Key Words:** smoking cessation • postnatal care • telephone counseling

Since the 1960s, there has been minimal reduction in the proportion of Canadian women who smoke. Up to 15,000 Canadian women die annually from diseases attributable to smoking, and the rate of lung cancer among women is rising (Canadian Cancer Society, 1997; Ellison, Mao, & Gibbons, 1995). When women smoke during pregnancy and after childbirth, they put the fetus, neonate, and growing child at risk for several health problems (Charlton, 1994; U.S. Department of Health and Human Services, 1989).

The effects of smoking during pregnancy are well known and provide a strong inducement for many women to quit. Half of women quit smoking during pregnancy and remain abstinent for 4 to 9 months (O'Campo, Faden, Brown, & Gielen, 1992; Secker-Walker et al., 1995). However, studies have revealed that approximately 70% of these women resume smoking shortly after giving birth (Fingerhut, Kleinman, & Kendrick, 1990; Mullen, Richardson, Quinn, & Ershoff, 1997; Sexton, Hebel, & Fox, 1987). Although these rates of relapse are comparable with the rates among quitters in the general population (Brandon, Tiffany, Obremski, & Baker, 1990), many pregnant women experience prolonged abstinence before relapse. These women may be unaware of the risks of smoking for their infants and themselves, or more likely they lack the support, skills, or commitment required to maintain long-term abstinence.

The purpose of this study was to test an intervention to help postpartum women to avoid or manage smoking lapses, thereby enhancing their likelihood of maintaining continuous smoking abstinence and reducing their risk of daily smoking after the birth of their babies. Three hypotheses were tested:

Hypothesis 1: The rate of continuous smoking abstinence at 6 months postpartum, based on self-report and biochemical validation, will be significantly higher in the treatment group than in the control group.

Hypothesis 2: The rate of daily smoking at 6 months postpartum will be significantly lower in the treatment group than in the control group.

Hypothesis 3: Smoking cessation self-efficacy at 6 months postpartum will be significantly higher in the treatment group than in the control group.

RELEVANT LITERATURE

It has been recognized that smoking cessation is not a binary event in which people shift from being smokers to nonsmokers (Prochaska & DiClemente, 1983; Prochaska, DiClemente, & Norcross, 1992). Accordingly, research attention has turned to understanding the factors that cause lapses and to developing interventions that prevent relapse. The work of Marlatt (1985, 1996) and Marlatt and Gordon (1985) addresses relapse after behavior change and focuses on events surrounding the initial use of the undesired substance during the postcessation period. The author conceptualizes relapse as a process influenced by cognitive and behavioral mechanisms rather than a discrete, irreversible event, and distinguishes between lapse (initial use of a substance) and complete relapse (full return to regular use of the substance). This model, widely used in relapse prevention, has been supported by empirical evidence (Baer, Holt, & Lichtenstein, 1986; Cohen & Lichtenstein, 1990; Curry et al., 1993).

The precipitants of relapse in the postpartum period include demographic and contextual variables such as contact with other smokers, parity, sociodemographic variables, amount smoked before pregnancy, and whether women quit early or late in pregnancy (Fingerhut et al., 1990; McBride, Pirie, & Curry, 1992; O'Campo et al., 1992). Greater self-efficacy and some types of coping strategies have been demonstrated to reduce the probability of postpartum relapse (McBride et al., 1992). Women require coping strategies relevant to their particular circumstances, and the coping strategies used during pregnancy may not be effective in the postpartum period (McBride et al., 1992).

Marlatt's relapse model is the cornerstone of a group of interventions referred to as "relapse prevention training" (RPT), which includes skills training to anticipate and resist lapsing in high-risk situations and cognitive restructuring to deal with self-defeating attributions after a lapse. Although not a panacea, RPT is a promising approach for the prevention of relapse. Studies in which RPT was used generally have rendered positive results, particularly with women and light smokers (Curry, Marlatt, Gordon, & Baer, 1988; Hall, Rugg, Tunstall, & Jones, 1984). Exposure to RPT has been found to be associated with long-term abstinence (Davis, Faust, & Ordentlich, 1984; Stevens & Hollis, 1989). In contrast to these positive outcomes, others have reported no effect when self-help RPT was used, perhaps because they did not incorporate tailored approaches or sufficient counseling support (Curry et al., 1988; Killen, Fortmann, Newman, & Varady, 1990; Omenn et al., 1988).

A number of studies have investigated smoking-cessation interventions with pregnant women, but few have extended their interventions to the early postpartum period (Petersen, Handel, Kotch, Podedworny, & Rosen, 1992; Secker-Walker et al., 1995). Although possibly the result of Type II error, with 175 women assigned to two study groups, Secker-Walker et al. (1995) failed to affect early postpartum relapse rates when they augmented antenatal smoking-cessation counseling with a single postpartum visit. Petersen et al. (1992) tested several interventions based on self-help materials and professional counseling during the antenatal period and the first month postpartum. The most intensive intervention, including regular counseling, significantly increased the proportion of women who remained abstinent at 8 weeks postpartum. The longer-term benefits of such interventions remain unknown.

The value of pregnancy as an intervention point for smoking cessation is being undermined by high relapse rates in the postpartum period. If abstinence during pregnancy is to result in long-term smoking cessation, more attention must be given to developing interventions to prevent and manage relapse. This experimental, pretest–posttest control group study aimed to evaluate the effectiveness of an intervention for postpartum women who quit smoking during pregnancy. Because continuous abstinence may not be a realistic goal for many individuals engaged in the smoking cessation process, the outcome measures of continuous abstinence and resumption of daily smoking were the variables of interest.

METHODS

Sample

The target population consisted of all the women who gave birth at one of five hospitals during a 7-month period and who met the following criteria: (a) identified herself as a smoker before pregnancy; (b) quit smoking once aware of pregnancy or in attempting to become pregnant; (c) ceased smoking for at least 6 weeks before delivery; (d) if smoking occurred in the 6-week period immediately before delivery, smoked on fewer than six occasions; (e) gave birth to a healthy infant not requiring hospitalization beyond discharge of the mother; (f) planned to remain in hospital for at least 24 hours; (g) was able to read and comprehend English; and (h) could be contacted by telephone.

Of the 8,837 women admitted for labor and delivery over the course of the recruitment period, 8,290 were screened. The 547 unscreened women were missed because they were discharged within a few hours of delivery (519), because they would not discuss eligibility (22), or because of another reason (6). Of 416 eligible women, 254 agreed to participate and gave their informed consent, resulting in a participation rate of 61.1%. Three of the consenting subjects were excluded from analysis: One was randomly assigned as a control participant but was inadvertently given the intervention, and two were assigned to the treatment group but did not receive any telephone contacts. The final sample was 251 women: 125 in the treatment group and 126 in the control group.

Measures

Smoking status was measured using self-report items, including those related to frequency of smoking and amount smoked. Because reports of smoking status may be unreliable (Apseloff, Ashton, Friedman, & Gerber, 1994), biochemical assessments were completed with Bedfont EC50 Smokerlyzers. Carbon monoxide (CO) readings of 10 or more parts per million (ppm) were concluded to be indicative of recent smoking. Biochemical measures such as CO readings not only validate self-reports, but also enhance the validity of self-reports, especially because the participants were uninformed about the sensitivity of the measure (Patrick et al., 1994).

When participants denied smoking but obtained CO readings of 10 ppm or more, or when they admitted to smoking but obtained CO readings of less than 10 ppm, perhaps because they smoked irregularly, they were classified as not being continuously abstinent. Self-reports were used for participants who were unable to provide a CO reading because the follow-up evaluation was conducted by telephone. Continuous abstinence referred to the complete avoidance of smoking during the entire 6-month period. Daily smoking was measured by self-reports at follow-up of one or more cigarettes typically smoked per day. Validation of participants' self-reports of daily smoking was not possible with CO monitoring because single measures of CO levels are not indicative of smoking frequency.

Smoking cessation self-efficacy was measured with the Smoking Abstinence Self-Efficacy Scale (SASE; DiClemente, 1981; Prochaska, DiClemente, Velicer, Ginpil, & Norcross, 1985), an instrument designed to assess smokers' level of confidence that they will not smoke in 20 challenging situations. The instrument consists of three subscales: (a) the negative/affective subscale measuring the degree of confidence when frustrated or facing conflict or emotional distress; (b) the habit/addictive subscale measuring the degree of confidence when the urge to smoke is felt; and (c) the positive/social subscale measuring confidence in resisting temptation in social or celebratory situations. Of the 20 items, 17 are scored with a range from 0% (not at all confident) to 100% (completely confident) (Velicer, DiClemente, Rossi, & Prochaska, 1990).

The SASE has demonstrated acceptable construct and predictive validity and acceptable internal consistency, with a Cronbach's alpha ranging from .88 to .92 (DiClemente, 1981; Prochaska et al., 1985; Velicer et al., 1990). Each subscale has demonstrated internal consistency (.92–.95), and the responses are not associated with social desirability. The data obtained in this study were subjected to factor analysis with maximum likelihood extraction and varimax rotation, which confirmed the presence of three factors. The alpha coefficients for the three subscales ranged from .80 to .88.

A number of covariates were assessed because they have been found associated with smoking and relapse. Demographic items were included to measure age, income, education, employment status, marital status, and parity. The demographic items were adapted from well-established surveys such as Canada's Health Promotion Survey (Stephens & Graham, 1993) and have undergone rigorous pretesting.

Participants were asked on a scale from 1 (not at all likely) to 10 (extremely likely) whether they expected to return to their desired weight within 6 months. Items that measured smoking history, number of cigarettes smoked daily, number of years smoked, number of prior quit attempts, and longest period of abstinence were included. Items that measured partners' smoking histories focused on smoking patterns during the pregnancy.

Social support for smoking cessation was determined by asking each woman how much encouragement from family and friends she expected to receive for her efforts to remain abstinent. The response categories were as follows: no encouragement at all, hardly any encouragement, some encouragement, and a great deal of encouragement. This item was used by Strecher, Becker, Kirscht, Eraker, and Graham-Tomasi (1985), who argued that the concept of encouragement traverses key elements of social support.

Because it has been argued that stress can interfere with the ability to make and maintain behavior changes, and that depressive moods can place people at higher risk for relapse, mental health was measured by five items taken from Canada's Health Promotion Survey (Stephens & Graham, 1993).

One item measured overall happiness. The remaining items were used to create a composite scale of mental health status. The items included respondents' reported frequency of feeling "cheerful and lighthearted," "loved and wanted," "downhearted and blue," and "lonely." On factor analysis, these four items were found to measure a single factor or dimension. The smallest factor loading was .45 (59.1% of the variance was explained). The internal consistency (Cronbach's alpha) for these four items was .76. Consequently, a mental health status scale was created by taking the average of these four items (range = 1–4). Larger values were indicative of better mental health.

Physical (physiologic) dependence on nicotine or addiction was measured with the 10-item Revised Fagerstrom Tolerance Questionnaire (RTQ), which accounts for amount smoked, patterns of smoking, and ability to refrain from smoking (e.g., in banned areas and when sick) (Fagerstrom, 1978; Tate & Schmitz, 1993). Five-point Likert scales were used to score each item. Reported scores were averaged across the 10 items, with lower scores indicating relatively weaker dependence.

The RTQ has demonstrated concurrent validity with various withdrawal responses, including body temperature and heart rate elevation. Tate and Schmitz (1993) tested the RTQ with four samples of smokers and reported reliability coefficients ranging from .72 to .85. Test–retest reliability over 1 to 1.5 months duration was .88. Factor analysis identified one common factor (40% of total-item variance explained). In the current study, the questions were posed retrospectively to capture physical dependence before cessation.

Intervention

A postpartum counseling intervention was designed to prevent or interrupt the relapse process by teaching skills to deal with high-risk situations and cognitive restructuring techniques to deal with lapses. The intervention was based on the following principles derived from Marlatt's relapse model (Marlatt, 1985; Marlatt & Gordon, 1980, 1985): (a) Smoking cessation is a process, and relapse is not an irrevocable state; (b) smoking cessation is influenced by cognitive and behavioral mechanisms; (c) maintaining abstinence requires a sense of control and self-efficacy; (d) lapses are most likely to occur in high-risk situations; (e) it is possible to prevent lapses from leading to complete relapse by helping individuals cognitively to restructure lapse events; and (f) cessation efforts need to be reinforced with long-term follow-up sessions.

Nurses were hired and trained to provide the one-to-one counseling intervention. The in-hospital component consisted of sharing information and beginning skill building. The nurse began by learning about the woman's smoking experiences and the context of the smoking cessation effort. After advising about the importance of remaining a nonsmoker, the nurse reviewed potential effects of smoking on the health of the newborn, the family, and the woman herself. The skill-building component focused on teaching the woman to recognize high-risk situations in which she may be tempted to smoke, and to problem solve about how to manage those situations. The nurse reviewed cognitive strategies for dealing with lapses and modeled them using situations provided by the woman. When feasible, the woman was encouraged to role-play the strategy.

The counseling was augmented with materials developed for the study and tailored to the particular circumstances of postpartum women including (a) a pamphlet outlining the risk of smoking during the postpartum period, with strategies to deal with cravings, and a pamphlet focusing on the effects of secondhand smoke on children; (b) a two-sided "self-help" card directed toward problem solving for high-risk situations and cognitively restructuring lapses; and (c) materials to facilitate the maintenance of smoke-free environments, including signs to place on coffee tables, on doors, and in automobiles.

Eight subsequent at-home telephone counseling sessions were provided by the nurse who initially enrolled the participant. These sessions focused on efforts to maintain smoking cessation, review of high-risk situations and their management, possible lapses, guidance in problem solving, and support and encouragement. The telephone sessions were held weekly during the first month postpartum and biweekly during the second and third months. The telephone contacts ranged from 1 to 20 minutes ($M = 4.5$, $SD = 1.5$). It was noted that the average duration of the telephone contacts increased progressively over time, with the first telephone contact lasting an average of 3.7 minutes ($SD = 1.8$) and the eighth contact lasting, on the average, 5.3 minutes ($SD = 2.7$). Although the treatment group participants were expected to receive all eight telephone contacts, it was difficult to meet the study design expectations because participants often were found to be too busy or not available. Only 24.8% of the participants received eight contacts: 42.4% missed one contact; 21.6% missed two; 8% missed three; and 3.2% missed four or five.

Procedure

Group assignment was random, with identification numbers randomly assigned to two groups, in blocks of 50, via a computer software package. The intervention was provided only to the women assigned to the treatment group. The control group received "usual care," which did not include any information about the effects of smoking or prevention of smoking relapse. In the hospital, all participants were administered a baseline questionnaire, and two breath samples were collected to measure CO in expired air. At 6 months after delivery, all participants were interviewed in their homes by research assistants who had not delivered the intervention, and who were blind to group assignment. Carbon monoxide in expired air also was determined.

RESULTS

Participants ($N = 251$) ranged in age from 15 to 40 years ($M = 27.6$, $SD = 5.5$) with educational attainment ranging from some elementary school to earned postgraduate degrees (Mdn = completed technical/trade school). Their total annual household income, before deductions and taxes, ranged from less than $9,000 to more than $150,000 ($Mdn$ = $40,000-$49,999). The majority (60.6%) usually worked for pay on a full-time basis, and 19.9% worked part-time. Most participants (60.2%) were married and living with a spouse; 23.9% lived with a common-law partner, 14.7% were single (never married), and the rest were either separated or divorced. The current birth was the first child for the majority of participants (74.1%). Three quarters of the participants (74.9%) were born in Canada, and the remainder were born in 40 different countries. Similarly, 75.3% reported that English was their first language. The demographics of the study groups differed only regarding their country of origin: The treatment group was more likely to have been born outside Canada (Table A-1).

Baseline Data

Almost all of the participants (94.4%) intended to breast-feed, and expected to do so for 2 weeks to 2 years (34.1% expected to breast-feed for more than 6 months). The mean score for perceived likelihood of achieving desired weight within 6 months was 7.5 (SD = 2.3), suggesting that the majority were confident of weight loss. Two thirds of the participants (68.1%) were reportedly "very happy," 30.3% "pretty happy," and 1.6% "not too happy." The mean score on the composite mental health scale was 3.1 (SD = 0.6). The two study groups differed statistically only with respect to their mental health: The treatment group reported slightly better mental health (Table A-1).

The participants reported that 4 to 52 weeks had elapsed since they quit smoking (M = 32.9, SD = 7.1). Only 10 of the participants (4%) reported smoking in the week immediately preceding the baseline interview, and all had smoked five or fewer cigarettes during that week. Seven of those 10 participants were assigned to the treatment group. As reported, 22 of the participants (8.8%) had smoked during the 6 weeks immediately before baseline data collection (5.6% of the control group and 12% of the treatment group): χ^2 (1, N = 251) = 2.50 with Yates' Continuity Correction; p = .11. The self-reports of recent smoking were consistent with the two CO breathalyzers, except for those of two participants who obtained CO readings slightly above 10 ppm while reporting complete abstinence for at least 6 weeks.

Almost all of the respondents (93.6%) reported that the primary reason why they quit smoking was concern for the health of their unborn baby. Other reasons for quitting included (a) concern for their own health (3.2%), (b) nausea too great to smoke (2.8%), and (c) recognition that it was a good opportunity to quit (.4%). Almost all (90.8%) reported that they intended to remain nonsmokers postpartum. A small percentage of the participants (15.5%) had made no other smoking cessation attempts (defined as lasting more than 24 hours). Almost one half of the participants (45.8%) had made one or two previous attempts to quit; 30.8% had made 3 to 10 previous attempts; and the remaining 8% reported 11 or more attempts.

TABLE 1. Comparisons of Control and Treatment Groups by Demographic and Personal Characteristics (at Baseline)

VARIABLES	CONTROL ($n = 126$)	TREATMENT ($n = 125$)	STATISTICS t	STATISTICS χ^2
Age (mean, years)	27.4	27.8	−0.54	
Education level (%)				
Less than high school	17.5	14.4		
High school or equivalent	23.0	28.8		
Some/completed trade/community college	33.3	40.0		
Some/completed university	26.2	16.8		4.51
Annual household income (%)[a]				
≤$29,999	29.8	24.8		
$30,000–$49,999	23.7	28.3		
$50,000–$69,999	21.1	18.6		
$70,000+	25.4	28.3		1.35
Marital status (%)				
Married and living with spouse	62.7	57.6		
Common-law/live-in relationship	22.2	25.6		
Separated/divorced/widowed/single	15.1	16.8		0.69
First child (%)				
Yes	69.8	78.4		
No	30.2	21.6		1.97[b]
Employment status (%)				
Does not work for pay	21.4	17.6		
Works part-time	20.6	19.2		
Works full-time	57.9	63.2		0.82
Born in Canada (%)				
Yes	82.5	67.2		
No	17.5	32.8		7.06[b,c]
First language spoken (%)				
English	80.2	70.4		
Other	19.8	29.6		2.71[b]
Intention to breast-feed (%)				
Yes	96.0	92.8		
No	4.0	7.2		0.71[b]
Expected duration of breast-feeding (mean, weeks)	30.6	32.7	−0.90	
Desired weight achieved within 6 months (mean)	7.4	7.6	−0.81	
Happiness (%)				
Very happy	67.5	68.8		
Not too or pretty happy	32.5	31.2		0.01[b]
Mental health (mean)	3.0	3.1	−2.0[c]	

[a] $n = 227$ (9.6% missing cases).
[b] Yates' Continuity Correction used.
[c] $p < .05$.

Before quitting, the participants reported smoking less than 1 to as many as 38 cigarettes daily (M = 10.4, SD = 7.2). Averaged scores on the 10-item RTQ ranged from 1.6 to 4.5 (M = 2.7, SD = .6), indicating low to moderate physical dependence. Participants were fairly confident that they could resist the urge to smoke in various situations. Their average SASE scores on the negative/affective, habit/addictive, and positive/social subscales were: 67.1% (SD = 26.2%), 87.3% (SD = 15%), and 73.1% (SD = 21.8%), respectively.

Among the 234 women with partners, 47.4% of the partners were smokers at baseline; 15% quit along with the woman; 26.5% never smoked; and 11.1% had quit at some time in the past. Approximately one third of the participants (29.6%) reported that all or most of the people with whom they spent their time smoked; 30.4% reported that some of their social contacts smoked; and the remaining 40% reported that very few if any of the people with whom they had contact smoked. Most participants (72.5%) expected to receive a great deal of encouragement from their family and friends to help them remain nonsmokers. Among all the smoking-related variables, no statistically significant differences were noted between the control and treatment groups (Table A-2).

Data From 6-Month Follow-Up Interview

Some participants were difficult to locate, so the follow-up interviews occurred between 24.1 and 50 weeks after baseline data collection (M = 28.1, SD = 3.1). Eleven of the interviews (4.6%) were conducted at locations other than the participants' homes (e.g., restaurants, shopping malls), and 19 (7.9%) were conducted over the telephone (as a result, the breathalyzer was not completed). Ten participants (4%) either refused to participate or could not be located (six from the control group and four from the treatment group). These women were included in the analyses, where possible, and coded as failing to maintain continuous abstinence and as daily smokers. Self-efficacy scores were not imputed for these women.

Hypothesis 1. At 6 months postpartum, the rate of continuous smoking abstinence was higher in the treatment (37.6%) than the control (27%) group, although the difference did not achieve statistical significance: χ^2 (1, N = 251) = 2.8, p = .10 with Yates' continuity correction; OR = 1.63; 95% CI = .96–2.78.

Hypothesis 2. Significantly more participants in the control group than in the treatment group reported smoking daily: 47.6% vs. 33.6%, χ^2 (1, N = 251) = 4.6, p = .03 with Yates' continuity correction; OR = 1.80; 95% CI = 1.08–2.99.

Hypothesis 3. The 6-month smoking cessation self-efficacy scores for each subscale were subjected to between-groups analysis of covariance. The independent variables were group assignment and baseline scores for the respective self-efficacy subscale. After adjustment for baseline scores, self-efficacy did not vary significantly on any of the three subscales.

			STATISTICS	
VARIABLES	**CONTROL** ($n = 126$)	**TREATMENT** ($n = 125$)	*t*	χ^2
Time elapsed since quit date (at birth; mean, weeks)	33.0	32.8	0.31	
Reason for smoking cessation (%)				
Health of unborn	96.0	91.2		
Other	4.0	8.8		1.71[a]
Intend to remain nonsmoking postpartum (%)				
Yes	91.3	90.4		
No/don't know	8.7	9.6		0.00[a]
Number of previous quit attempts (mean)	2.8	3.2	−1.01	
Number of cigarettes/day while smoking (mean)	10.4	10.5	−0.05	
Revised Fagerstrom tolerance (RTQ; mean)	2.6	2.7	−0.91	
Smoking abstinence self-efficacy (SASE)				
Negative/affective subscale	67.3	66.9	0.12	
Habit/addictive subscale	86.9	87.7	−0.40	
Positive/social subscale	73.7	72.5	0.45	
Husband/partner's smoking status (%)[b]				
Never smoked	26.3	26.7		
Quit for the pregnancy	11.9	18.1		
Quite before pregnancy	11.9	10.3		
Current smoker	50.0	44.8		1.98
Social contacts who smoke (%)				
All or most	32.0	27.2		
Some	24.8	36.0		
Very few or none	43.2	36.8		3.71
Expected encouragement for nonsmoking from family and friends (%)				
None/hardly any	8.9	8.9		
Some	20.2	17.1		
A great deal	71.0	74.0		0.39

TABLE 2. Comparisons of Control and Treatment Groups by Smoking-Related Factors (at Baseline)

Note: $p < .05$.
[a]Yates' Continuity Correction used.
[b]$n = 234$ (6.8% reported no partner).

Multivariate Analysis. The rejection of Hypothesis 3 led to the question of how the intervention successfully reduced daily smoking among the treatment group. To explore possible answers to this question, a stepwise multiple logistic regression analysis was conducted to identify predictors of daily smoking, including variables that may have confounded or interacted with the intervention. No demographic variables were found to be significant. Only two smoking-related variables were associated with daily smoking at 6 months (Table A-3). Participants having relatively strong negative/affective self-efficacy or relatively high mental health scores at baseline were less likely

TABLE 3. Mixed Effects Logistic Regression Model of Daily Smoking

VARIABLES	OR	95% CI
Group assignment		
Treatment	.56[c]	.32–.98
Control[a]	1.00	
Negative/affective self-efficacy (at baseline)[b]	.82[c]	.73–.91
Mental health (at baseline)	.44[c]	.27–.74

[a]Reference group.
[b]Variable scaled to 10% unit increments.
[c]$p < .05$.
OR = odds ratio; CI = confidence interval.

to smoke daily. Neither of these variables was found to confound or interact with the intervention.

DISCUSSION

Although the intervention did not prove effective in ensuring continuous smoking abstinence, the control group, as compared with the treatment group, was almost twice as likely to resume daily smoking. These findings are encouraging because they suggest that nurses can successfully intervene and help women in their commitment to achieve smoking cessation. Although continuous abstinence is the desired long-term goal, this rigid outcome measure of smoking status contradicts current thinking about the process of smoking cessation. Theorists have recommended that smoking behavior not be conceptualized as a binary event (Marlatt, 1985, 1996; Miller, 1996; Prochaska & DiClemente, 1983). Prochaska and DiClemente's (1983) model of behavior change acknowledges that those in the process of cessation may smoke at times. The question for researchers is this: "At what point is smoking a normal part of the cessation process rather than an indication of complete relapse?"

An appropriate set of outcome criteria for research purposes, sensitive to the process of change, must be identified. Donovan (1996) described five definitions of relapse in the addiction literature: (a) a gradual and insidious process, (b) a discrete event of substance use (lapse), (c) a return to original patterns of substance use (amount and frequency, relapse), (d) daily use for a specified time period, and (e) substance use that requires treatment. Collectively, these definitions point to the complex and dynamic nature of the relapse process. Miller (1996) went so far as to suggest that we should abandon the concept of relapse and preferably identify terms that describe the "normal" resolution process for addictive behaviors such as smoking.

The intervention was effective in preventing the resumption of daily smoking regardless of individual differences in self-efficacy and mental health.

Apart from the group differences in resumption of daily smoking, the identified covariates suggest that those with relatively better mental health and stronger negative/affective self-efficacy (i.e., degree of confidence in resisting urges to smoke when frustrated, facing conflict, or undergoing emotional distress) at the outset are likely to avoid relapsing to daily smoking. However, the intervention did not affect self-efficacy. Participants with relatively strong baseline negative/affective self-efficacy scores were more successful in avoiding daily smoking, but overall, the self-efficacy scores were not improved in the intervention group. Indeed, the baseline self-efficacy scores were somewhat higher, on the average, than the 6-month scores, in both groups.

Why did the intervention not operate through self-efficacy, as hypothesized, and why then was it effective at all? It may be that the measure of self-efficacy used in this study, the SASE, was not appropriate for this particular population. The SASE focuses on common high-risk situations (e.g., being at a bar or cocktail lounge having a drink) and asks respondents to assess their confidence in abstaining from smoking. At baseline, many of the situations described in the SASE were not relevant to the participants' cessation experiences (e.g., while pregnant they avoided alcohol consumption). Women who have just given birth and are facing "new terrain" may be unable realistically to predict their ability to resist the temptation to smoke.

Stotts, DiClemente, Carbonari, and Mullen (1996) noted that the process of smoking cessation for pregnant women is somewhat different than for nonpregnant female smokers. Cessation during pregnancy was observed to be relatively easy, to require minimal use of coping strategies, and to result in high self-efficacy. The researchers speculated that this putative success results from specific factors that typically promote smoking cessation among pregnant women (e.g., social stigma, concern for baby's health, nausea). They therefore argue that abstinence may be better conceived as "stopping" rather than "quitting" smoking. Women who stop smoking for pregnancy may not have gone through the experiential and behavioral processes usually associated with the action phase of smoking cessation. In addition, new mothers (74.1% were primiparas in the current study) may not anticipate that the challenges in the postpartum period are different, and possibly more difficult, than those faced while pregnant.

Rather than by strengthening self-efficacy, the intervention may have been effective because of the social support provided during the initial 3-month postpartum period. Unlike other intervention studies, this study focused on the provision of sustained support, specifically targeted toward the maintenance of smoking cessation during a critical period when smoking relapse is likely.

Paradoxically, whereas the strength of the intervention may have rested on meeting the particular needs of the participants, such an approach poses a threat to research design validity. Tailoring interventions to respond to individual need may make it more difficult to ensure that the same intervention at the same dose is provided to all subjects. Fluctuations in delivery of the intervention may account for the weaker than anticipated effect. A limitation related to external validity is the 39% refusal rate among eligible women. It may have been that women with particular characteristics were attracted to receiving assistance with their smoking cessation maintenance.

Although current smoking cessation interventions for childbearing women tend to focus on the prenatal period, entry into the difficult action phase of smoking cessation may commence in the postpartum period. Smoking cessation programs designed to take advantage of the "window of opportunity" provided by pregnancy can be strengthened if interventions are extended into the postpartum period, focusing on the action phase of the smoking cessation process as well as relapse prevention.

Accepted for publication July 8, 1998.

This project was funded by the Tobacco Demand Reduction Strategy of Health Canada through a grant provided by the National Health Research and Development Program. Pilot work funding was provided by the British Columbia Medical Services Foundation. In-kind support was provided by the Nursing Consortium of the British Columbia Research Institute in Child and Family Health. Ms. Hall acknowledges the Social Sciences and Humanities Research Council provision of a doctoral fellowship and the British Commonwealth for a scholar award. Ms. Dahinten acknowledges the British Columbia Health Research Foundation's provision of a doctoral studentship.

Address reprint requests to Joy L. Johnson, PhD, RN, School of Nursing, University of British Columbia, T201–2211 Wesbrook Mall, Vancouver, BC V6T 2B5 Canada;

E-mail: *johnson@nursing.ubc.ca.*

Joy L. Johnson, PhD, RN, is Associate Professor and National Health Research and Development Program Health Research Scholar, School of Nursing, University of British Columbia, Vancouver, Canada.

Pamela A. Ratner, PhD, RN, is an Assistant Professor, School of Nursing, and Assistant Director, Institute of Health Promotion Research, University of British Columbia, Vancouver, Canada.

Joan L. Bottorff, PhD, RN, is the Associate Director of Research, an Associate Professor, and a National Health Research and Development Program Health Research Scholar, School of Nursing, University of British Columbia, Vancouver, Canada.

Wendy Hall, PhD, RN, is an Associate Professor and Doctoral Candidate, School of Nursing, University of British Columbia, Vancouver, Canada.

Susan Dahinten, MSN, RN, is a Doctoral Candidate, School of Nursing, University of British Columbia, Vancouver, Canada, and an Assistant Professor, Faculty of Nursing, University of Brunswick, Fredericton, Canada.

REFERENCES

Apseloff, G., Ashton, H. M., Friedman, H., & Gerber, N. (1994). The importance of measuring cotinine levels to identify smokers in clinical trials. *Clinical Pharmacology and Therapeutics, 56,* 460–462.

Baer, J. S., Holt, C. S., & Lichtenstein, E. (1986). Self-efficacy and smoking reexamined: Construct validity and clinical utility. *Journal of Consulting and Clinical Psychology, 54,* 846–852.

Brandon, T. H., Tiffany, S. T., Obremski, K. M., & Baker, T. B. (1990). Postcessation cigarette use: The process of relapse. *Addictive Behaviors, 15,* 105–114.

Canadian Cancer Society. (1997). Canadian cancer statistics 1997. Toronto: Author.

Charlton, A. (1994). Children and passive smoking: A review. *Journal of Family Practice, 38,* 267–277.

Cohen, S., & Lichtenstein, E. (1990). Perceived stress, quitting smoking, and smoking relapse. *Health Psychology, 9,* 466–478.

Curry, S. J., Marlatt, G. A., Gordon, J., & Baer, J. S. (1988). A comparison of alternative theoretical approaches to smoking cessation and relapse. *Health Psychology, 7,* 545–556.

Curry, S. J., Wagner, E. H., Cheadle, A., Diehr, P., Koepsell, T., Psaty, B., & McBride, C. (1993). Assessment of community-level influences on individuals' attitudes about cigarette smoking, alcohol use, and consumption of dietary fat. *American Journal of Preventive Medicine, 9,* 78–84.

Davis, A. L., Faust, R., & Ordentlich, M. (1984). Self-help smoking cessation and maintenance programs: A comparative study with 12-month follow-up by the American Lung Association. *American Journal of Public Health, 74,* 1212–1217.

DiClemente, C. C. (1981). Self-efficacy and smoking cessation maintenance: A preliminary report. *Cognitive Therapy and Research, 5,* 175–187.

Donovan, D. M. (1996). Assessment issues and domains in the prediction of relapse. *Addiction, 91,* S29-S36.

Ellison, L. F., Mao, Y., & Gibbons, L. (1995). Projected smoking-attributable mortality in Canada, 1991–2000. *Chronic Diseases in Canada, 16*(2), 84–89.

Fagerstrom, K. O. (1978). Measuring degree of physical dependence to tobacco smoking with reference to individualization of treatment. *Addictive Behaviors, 3,* 235–241.

Fingerhut, L. A., Kleinman, J. C., & Kendrick, J. S. (1990). Smoking before, during, and after pregnancy. *American Journal of Public Health, 80,* 541–544.

Hall, S. M., Rugg, D., Tunstall, C., & Jones, R. T. (1984). Preventing relapse to cigarette smoking by behavioral skill training. *Journal of Consulting and Clinical Psychology, 52,* 372–382.

Killen, J. D., Fortmann, S. P., Newman, B., & Varady, A. (1990). Evaluation of a treatment approach combining nicotine gum with self-guided behavioral treatments for smoking relapse prevention. *Journal of Consulting and Clinical Psychology, 58,* 85–92.

Marlatt, G. A. (1985). Relapse prevention: Theoretical rationale and overview of the model. In G. A. Marlatt & J. R. Gordon (Eds.), *Relapse prevention: Maintenance strategies in the treatment of addictive behaviors* (pp. 3–70). New York: Guilford Press.

Marlatt, G. A. (1996). Taxonomy of high-risk situations for alcohol relapse: Evolution and development of a cognitive-behavioral model. *Addiction, 91,* S37-S49.

Marlatt, G. A., & Gordon, J. R. (1980). Determinants of relapse: Implications for the maintenance of behavior change. In P. O. Davidson & S. M. Davidson (Eds.), *Behavioral medicine: Changing health lifestyles* (pp. 191–215). New York: Brunner/Mazel.

Marlatt, G. A., & Gordon, J. R. (Eds.). (1985). *Relapse prevention: Maintenance strategies in the treatment of addictive behaviors.* New York: Guilford Press.

McBride, C. M., Pirie, P. L., & Curry, S. J. (1992). Postpartum relapse to smoking: A prospective study. *Health Education Research, 7,* 381–390.

Miller, W. R. (1996). What is a relapse? Fifty ways to leave the wagon. *Addiction, 91,* S15-S27.

Mullen, P. D., Richardson, M. A., Quinn, V. P., & Ershoff, D. H. (1997). Postpartum return to smoking: Who is at risk and when. *American Journal of Health Promotion, 11,* 323–330.

O'Campo, P., Faden, R. R., Brown, H., & Gielen, A. C. (1992). The impact of pregnancy on women's prenatal and postpartum smoking behavior. *American Journal of Preventive Medicine, 8,* 8–13.

Omenn, G. S., Thompson, B., Sexton, M., Hessol, N., Breitenstein, B., Curry, S., Michnich, M., & Peterson, A. (1988). A randomized comparison of worksite-sponsored smoking cessation programs. *American Journal of Preventive Medicine, 4,* 261–267.

Patrick, D. L., Cheadle, A., Thompson, D. C., Diehr, P., Koepsell, T., & Kinne, S. (1994). The validity of self-reported smoking: A review and meta-analysis. *American Journal of Public Health, 84,* 1086–1093.

Petersen, L., Handel, J., Kotch, J., Podedworny, T., & Rosen, A. (1992). Smoking reduction during pregnancy by a program of self-help and clinical support. *Obstetrics and Gynecology, 79,* 924–930.

Prochaska, J. O., & DiClemente, C. C. (1983). Stages and processes of self-change of smoking: Toward an integrative model of change. *Journal of Consulting and Clinical Psychology, 51,* 390–395.

Prochaska, J. O., DiClemente, C. C., & Norcross, J. C. (1992). In search of how people change: Applications to addictive behaviors. *American Psychologist, 47,* 1102–1114.

Prochaska, J. O., DiClemente, C. C., Velicer, W. F., Ginpil, S., & Norcross, J. C. (1985). Predicting change in smoking status for self-changers. *Addictive Behaviors, 10,* 395–406.

Secker-Walker, R. H., Solomon, L. J., Flynn, B. S., Skelly, J. M., Lepage, S. S., Goodwin, G. D., & Mead, P. B. (1995). Smoking relapse prevention counseling during prenatal and early postnatal care. *American Journal of Preventive Medicine, 11,* 86–93.

Sexton, M., Hebel, R., & Fox, N. L. (1987). Postpartum smoking. In M. J. Rosenberg (Ed.), *Smoking and reproductive health* (pp. 222–226). Littleton, MA: PSG Publishing.

Stephens, T., & Graham, D. F. (Eds.). (1993). *Canada's health promotion survey 1990: Technical report.* Ottawa: Minister of Supply and Services.

Stevens, V. J., & Hollis, J. F. (1989). Preventing smoking relapse, using an individually tailored skills-training technique. *Journal of Consulting and Clinical Psychology, 57,* 420–424.

Stotts, A. L., DiClemente, C. C., Carbonari, J. P., & Mullen, P. D. (1996). Pregnancy smoking cessation: A case of mistaken identity. *Addictive Behaviors, 21,* 459–471.

Strecher, V. J., Becker, M. H., Kirscht, J. P., Eraker, S. A., & Graham-Tomasi, R. P. (1985). Evaluation of a minimal-contact smoking cessation program in a health care setting. *Patient Education and Counseling, 7,* 395–407.

Tate, J. C., & Schmitz, J. M. (1993). A proposed revision of the Fagerstrom Tolerance Questionnaire. *Addictive Behaviors, 18,* 135–143.

U.S. Department of Health and Human Services. (1989). *Reducing the health consequences of smoking: 25 years of progress: A report of the Surgeon General.* Superintendent of Documents (DHHS Publication No. CDC 90–8411). Washington, DC: Author.

Velicer, W. F., DiClemente, C. C., Rossi, J. S., & Prochaska, J. O. (1990). Relapse situations and self-efficacy: An integrative model. *Addictive Behaviors, 15,* 271–283.

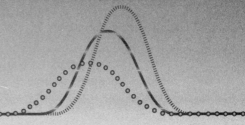

Qualitative Study
Redefining Parental Identity: Caregiving and Schizophrenia

P. JANE MILLIKEN, HERBERT C. NORTHCOTT

When parents try to assume responsibility for an ill adult-child with schizophrenia, the law, mental health practitioners, and often the ill person reject their right to do so. Consequently, these parents regard themselves as disenfranchised, i.e., lacking the rights required to care properly for their loved ones. Redefining Parental Identity, a grounded theory of caregiving and schizophrenia, traces changes in a parent's identity and caregiving during the erratic course of the child's mental illness. Participants were a purposive sample of 29 parent caregivers from 19 families in British Columbia, Canada, caring for 20 adult children. This understanding of their experience will be helpful to parents of people with schizophrenia, professional practitioners, and those involved in mental health care reform.

Schizophrenia causes disability in the form of impaired social functioning that lasts for a protracted period, often the rest of the individual's life. Community care for the mentally ill has proven effective where there is appropriate discharge planning, coordinated case management, and the necessary social supports, both formal and informal, for patients and their families (Stein & Test, 1980: Reynolds & Hoult, 1984). Unfortunately, reports of patients' "falling through the cracks" of the mental health care system (Isaac & Armat, 1990; Torrey, 1995, 1997) remain prevalent. The consequences of this include homelessness or inadequate housing (Mechanic & Rochefort, 1990; Torrey, 1988), poverty (Lurigio & Lewis, 1989), victimization, and/or criminalization of the mentally ill (French, 1987), as well as a "revolving door" cycle of hospital admission-discharge-readmission (Geller, 1992). In the process of dein-

Reprinted with permission from QUALITATIVE HEALTH RESEARCH, Vol. 13 No. 1, January 2003 100–113. © 2003 Sage Publications.

stitutionalization, a significant amount of care has been transferred from professionals to inadequately prepared lay people—frequently the ill person's family. Consequently, with schizophrenia having its onset in adolescence or young adulthood, the burden of providing consistent care generally falls by default to the individual's parents.

Studies of family care for mentally ill persons are, for the most part, either descriptive or focused on identifying the tasks required to provide technical aspects of care (see, for example, Hatfield & Lefley, 1987; Thornton & Seeman, 1991; Torrey, 1995). Theoretical models of caregiving generally follow the stress paradigm (Biegel, Sales, & Schulz, 1991; Maurin & Boyd, 1990) and emphasize both ongoing family disruption (Terkelsen, 1987) and the endless duration of caregiving (Howard, 1994). Many researchers have measured caregiver burden (Pickett, Cook, & Solomon, 1995; Wright, 1994) or the degree of expressed emotion in the family as a risk factor for the sufferer's relapse (Brooker, 1990; Hogarty, 1985).[1]

Research employing interpretive methodologies is less common. Tuck, du-Mont, Evans, and Shupe (1997) outline the phenomenological transformations in family life and the grief suffered by parents when an adult-child has schizophrenia. They note that these parents must reformulate what it means to be a parent to their changed relative. The present study revealed parents undergoing this reformulation sporadically in response to the erratic course of their adult-child's illness. Chesla (1991) identified a typology of four approaches to parental caregiving for schizophrenia: engaged care, conflicted care, managed care, and distanced care. We agree with Chesla's conclusion that conventional research into caregiver burden misses the distinctions among these groups of parents; however, we suggest that by grouping parents' caring practices in this way, we can describe a particular family only at a given point in time. Over the course of the illness, parents are likely to vary their caring practices in response to the adult-child's illness trajectory and the involvement of mental health professionals. Consequently, we saw the need for a grounded theory study to explain the subjective and emotional experience of parental caregiving in schizophrenia. As an exploratory method, grounded theory, with its emphasis on social interaction, is "the method of choice when we want to learn how people manage their lives in the context of existing or potential health challenges" (Schreiber & Stern, 2001, p. xvii).

Due to the unforeseen but often tragic consequences of deinstitutionalization, health care professionals and policy makers need a more thorough understanding of caregiving for people with serious mental illnesses. Knowledge of the consequences of caring for a mentally ill family member is essential in planning for better psychosocial rehabilitation services. To this end, the Canadian Alliance for Research on Schizophrenia called for psychosocial research "to evaluate the concrete and complex interactions of specific families in order to identify positive attributes which could, in turn, predict improved outcome" (1994, p. 14). This study directly addresses these points, to help us understand the challenges of schizophrenia for families and to inform mental health researchers with interests in grief, caregiver burden, and quality of life.

METHOD

Following university research ethics approval, we recruited participants through the newsletters of the British Columbia Schizophrenia Society and the Caregivers Association of British Columbia. Others were recruited through snowballing or, in one case, after the study was mentioned on a local radio program. We interviewed 29 parents from 19 middle- or working-class families, many of whom were retired (mean age = 62)—both parents in 10 families, the mother in 6 families, and the father in the remaining 3.

In total, the interviewed parents had 6 daughters and 14 sons afflicted with schizophrenia, two of whom had died in the 5 years prior to the study. Of the remaining 18, daughters averaged almost 30 years of age (range = 21–38), having been diagnosed on average at just over age 20, whereas the sons averaged 32 years (range = 23–42) and were diagnosed about 6 months earlier on average than the daughters (mean = 19.6). None of these young adults had ever been married and none were employed at the time of the interview. Most had lived with their parents for extended periods during their illness, but only four did so at the time of the study. The rest were about equally divided between group homes and semi-independent or independent apartments. In total, these parents had been caregiving for schizophrenia for an average of 11.5 years (range = 0.5–23 years) after their child's diagnosis; however, many of these children were also ill for a lengthy period before being diagnosed.

If roughly one third of people with schizophrenia recover, one third have a variable disease course, and one third remain chronically ill (Walsh, 1985), this group is more chronic than average. Nevertheless, this study examines a wide variation in parental experience. The grounded theory of redefining parental identity that emerged from this study illustrates their diverse caregiving experiences and should help us understand caregiving by other parents in similar circumstances.

In-depth, audiotaped interviews of approximately 1.5 to 2 hours were held in a private setting chosen by each participant. This was generally the parents' home. Couples, except for one, were interviewed separately. We guaranteed confidentiality and anonymity, and informed participants of their right to withdraw at any point. Near the end of the project, several participants had follow-up interviews, which were aimed at theoretical elaboration, saturation of incomplete categories, and verification of the theory. The final tally was 32 interviews, for a total of 53 hours. The interviews were transcribed verbatim to preserve the richness of the data.

Initially, we asked participants broad, open-ended questions to elicit both the positive and negative consequences of caring for a family member with schizophrenia. In keeping with the constant comparative method of grounded theory, data collection and analysis proceeded concurrently. We coded transcripts phrase by phrase and collapsed similar codes into increasingly broad categories. Over time, the interview questions changed as analytic categories became saturated or participants introduced new categories that generated new hypotheses to be explored during further data collection. As the theory developed, we validated the emerging concepts against the stories of new interviewees and in follow-up interviews with selected respondents, using theoretical sampling. Data collection ended when the interviews produced no new categories and the analysis revealed the basic social problem experienced by these parents and the ways in which they work through it.

A GROUNDED THEORY OF REDEFINING PARENTAL IDENTITY

In general, a grounded theory serves to explain the process through which a social problem common to the participant group is resolved. The basic social problem identified in this study is that parents believe they have the right and responsibility to care for, protect, and make decisions for children whom they do not see as capable of caring for and protecting themselves or making appropriate decisions in their own best interests. However, when a child is deemed an adult, this belief is not sanctioned by society, which denies parents that right. In response, parents whose adult-children suffer from schizophrenia engage in the basic social process (BSP) of redefining their parental identity and thus adapting their caregiving.

The socially prescribed change in parental caregiving for teens and young adults is toward freedom from management and direction. Parents are expected to socialize their children toward independence, and as this happens, parents anticipate that their own responsibilities will decrease accordingly. Ultimately, parents expect to be emancipated from active parenting.

After a child is diagnosed with schizophrenia, the parents' identity shifts. Initially, they find themselves disenfranchised from the role they expected to fulfill; then, they find new ways to exert their rights and responsibilities, thus establishing a new parental role. We have identified four parental identities, and the transitions between them, that constitute seven stages of a BSP called Redefining Parental Identity. The stages, parent of a teen or young adult, becoming marginalized, the disenfranchised parent, embracing the collective, the reenfranchised parent, evaluating my life, and the emancipated parent, are summarized in the following sections of this article.

Parent of a Teen or Young Adult

Adolescence, characterized by young people's testing the limits of their independence, can be challenging for both parents and teenagers. Parents need to find a comfortable balance between granting freedom and providing supervision, with a gradual increase in freedom and a corresponding decrease in supervision, until the child achieves independent adult status. Accordingly, parents expect that the adolescent period will be time limited and that eventually they will be able to invest more time and effort on their personal interests and adult relationships. This anticipation of freedom from the constraints of parenting is rooted in the promise of their children's aspirations and remembrance of their children's early achievements, behavior, and personality. Thus, parents of teens and young adults can be described as *anticipating liberty*[2] *while tolerating adolescent challenges*. Participants in this study described their children's early development as normal, with positive traits outweighing negative qualities and lacking any indication of impending mental illness. None of these parents was overly surprised when grades began to slip and/or behavior deteriorated during adolescence, and only two of the parents suspected antisocial attributes as signaling mental health problems. Eventually, however, all of these parents found that they could no longer view their son's or daughter's conduct as normal teenage behavior.

Becoming Marginalized

This initial status passage,[3] or transition, for these parents involves *becoming alarmed* and *assuming responsibility* for the child, but also *encountering barriers*. Parents in all but four of these families[4] reached a crisis point when the child's personality, behavior, and relationships with family and friends became so disruptive, bizarre, or dangerous that the changes could no longer be disregarded. Their children became excessively angry, depressed, anxious, isolated, or preoccupied, and family relationships suffered. Insomnia and street drug use were common, as was an attraction to nonmainstream religious groups and a propensity to disappear abruptly, often to live on the streets. When contacted by the child for money or by the police or social workers, parents willingly rescued their children and brought them home, often at considerable expense.

Rising concern compelled the parents to assert more control and assume responsibility for helping and protecting their child. Reluctantly, parents admitted to suspicions of mental illness and consulted a doctor or mental health professional, often taking the young person involuntarily to the hospital, sometimes with the help of the police. Still, a diagnosis and treatment were not always obtained. Some of the young people, fearing hospitalization, were able to cover up their symptoms long enough to fool the authorities. For example, the police released one daughter, who immediately disappeared again and was returned much later by an elderly couple who found her wandering on the beach. At home, after being revived from the cold, she

> became completely hysterical, throwing herself on the floor, hiding from monsters, and just totally disorganized, [with] paranoid delusions. She was again convinced that Michael the archangel was after her and was going to gouge out her eyes. She thought that I had murdered her brother and chopped him up and buried him in the backyard, that I had murdered Teresa[5] [her mother] and replaced her with an android. I went downstairs . . . and phoned the police again. They came with two cars, four officers, and an ambulance. They took her to the hospital. This time they realized that she was ill and she was admitted. (Bruce)

Once the diagnosis of schizophrenia was made, parents found that their influence on their children's care was severely limited. These "children" had reached the age of majority or were otherwise deemed to be responsible for their own decisions. Parents learned that even when a psychotic person loses the right to self-determination, professional caregivers, rather than parents, have the authority to direct care. Although parents believe they know their child better than anyone else, psychiatrists and other professionals seldom consulted or even listened to them. Yet, paradoxically, the young person was often discharged to the parents' home and care. The majority of these parents discovered that their ability to take responsibility for their child was effectively blocked by the law, by mental health professionals, and often by their own child. When these parents realized that they had no formally recognized right to assume that responsibility, they had, indeed, become marginalized and, consequently, they assumed a new parental identity. They now saw themselves as disenfranchised.

The Disenfranchised Parent

Parents felt obliged to safeguard their loved one's health and welfare and to ensure that professional help was obtained early to avoid another crisis. Nevertheless, they continually met obstructions whenever they tried to intercede on their child's behalf. At this stage, they described a miserable existence composed of *maintaining vigilance, grieving alone,* and *grasping at straws.* One father observed,

> The only thing that keeps her alive during those periods is our resourcefulness. You know, our vigilance. So even though she is an intelligent 26-year-old woman, it is still as though you have a 2-year-old you're worried is going to run out in front of a car, because she does do things like that. (Bruce)

Life revolved around constant surveillance, watching carefully for signs that the hallucinations, delusions, and bizarre behavior that characterize schizophrenia were returning or worsening. Watching a loved one deteriorate and feeling powerless to intervene is painful for parents, who see a young person becoming increasingly socially withdrawn, emotionally deprived, and lacking in motivation. A mother whose son committed suicide after a decade of illness said,

> As he got sicker and sicker his personal hygiene went down the drain. He frequently smelled bad the last few years of his life because I guess he just didn't have energy to shower. One of the people that came to his memorial service was the barber. The barber was a big deal in our life because when we could get him to agree to go to the barber, quite often he went to the barber's home so he wouldn't have to meet other people, and this man was very understanding. (Sue)

Parents watched over their child's psychiatric treatment, trying to ensure compliance with medication and keeping track of developing side effects. In an underfunded system, many parents become, by default, their child's case manager. Although a few were able to establish communication with practitioners, most either lacked access to health care providers or perceived that practitioners did not respect their opinions. Gwen knew the pattern of her son's illness well. When he stopped taking his medication, fired his psychiatrist, and switched to a psychologist, she tried to avert a relapse:

> I had phoned his counselor who actually had an MA in psychology, and I said to him, "You know, Colin was definitely becoming ill again, heading for a breakdown. I don't know if you realize this because he is very clever at concealing it." And he said, "Oh well, what makes you think he is?" And I said, "Well, one of the things is that he is reading the Bible constantly and this has always been one of the early symptoms." So he said in a very sarcastic voice, "Oh, I see. Because your son is reading the Bible, you think he should be on medication?" (Gwen)

A parent's vigilance is also motivated by fear: fear of schizophrenia, fear for the ill child's safety and future, and sometimes fear of his or her violent behavior. Parents feared that they would be unable to cope or that they might provoke a relapse, that their child would never recover, and that another child or grandchild would also become ill. The unpredictability of schizophrenia was particularly difficult, as one mother's story illustrates:

> I've realized that it's not so much the things that happen, though a lot of really painful disturbing instances have happened, but they are quite short, the instances in themselves. It's the fear in between. It's the remembering and the anticipation and the wondering if you can cope with it. It's like waiting for the other shoe to fall all the time. If you could just get that under control, you would be stronger to deal with the instance and you would recover from them more quickly because you wouldn't be anticipating the next one. (Maggie)

Initially, most parents learn about schizophrenia from the media, where violent behavior is often emphasized. In these families, violence was relatively infrequent and seldom reached the severity found in the press. Still, several of these parents were attacked by their offspring—one mother fatally. More commonly, violent acts were directed at property or themselves. Eight of these young people had attempted suicide—one successfully.

Furthermore, especially when they stopped taking medication, the ill persons' lifestyle made them vulnerable to victimization. Many of these young people ran away from home, took illegal drugs, and lived on the streets for months at a time. Three of these young people were beaten up in major cities far from home. Several had money and belongings stolen. Parents worried about their child contracting sexually transmitted diseases. Even those living semi-independently or in apartments were easy targets for burglary.

Not surprisingly, these parents reported high levels of stress, born out of feelings of frustration, powerlessness, and poor self-esteem:

> Elaine and I watched the powerlessness that we sensed, that grew in over the 2-year period. You know how sometimes you have a gut feeling you are in a losing situation? That's how I felt the entire time. Every time we'd lose something. (Fred)

Extra expenses, such as supplementing their child's limited social assistance, airline tickets to bring a runaway home, replacing damaged belongings, and moving expenses following eviction, add financial strain. Frequent crises, coupled with their determination not to give up and to try to normalize life for the rest of their family, only add to the pressure.

From the diagnosis of their child's schizophrenia onward, these parents experienced emotions that are associated with grief, as described below:

> What I grieve every day is [her lack of a] functional life. I grieve that every day, for Anne. Every day. Anne is never out of my thoughts and I say, "How could that happen?" How could that happen to others too? Not just Anne, but how could the illness be so cruel? Cruel, right in the bloom days, that's when it flares up. Anne will never see those years again. (Teresa)

Disenfranchised in their caregiving, their grief is also disenfranchised (Doka, 1989). This child is not dead but instead has become like a stranger.[6] Although parents grieve for the child that they once had, our society provides only rituals to help ease grief following physical death. In addition, totally preoccupied with caring for their ill child, many parents become socially quite isolated. Consequently, although they grieve for the person their child once was and for the life that they hoped their adult-child would have, they have little opportunity to communicate or share their grief with others. They grieve alone.

At this point, parents will grasp at any straw, looking for answers and, especially, for a cure. They desperately seek out second opinions, new and experimental treatments, and more knowledge about schizophrenia. Whether these parents learned anything about schizophrenia from their child's psychiatrist was a matter of luck. Some had doctors who were helpful and forthright in giving them information and describing the possibilities in terms of prognosis. Others—like Gwen and Irwin, who were told only to prepare for a "bumpy ride"—were given the diagnosis and nothing else. Information gleaned from various sources was often conflicting or overly technical. Instead, these parents needed practical advice from others in similar circumstances. Reaching out for that kind of help signaled a redefinition of parental identity beyond being disenfranchised.

Embracing the Collective

Requiring practical information about caring for someone with schizophrenia and an opportunity to communicate with people who understand their plight leads many parents to a support group. In British Columbia, the B.C. Schizophrenia Society usually provides this service. By *connecting with others*, they quickly learn that they no longer face mental illness alone. They find empathic people with whom they can speak honestly. In addition, they learn useful ways to approach people, either personal acquaintances or mental health service providers, who are less understanding. The Schizophrenia Society also offers a library of books and videotapes, organized educational programs, and monthly meetings with knowledgeable guest speakers. As a bonus, they make new friends.

> If you want to get on top of the disease, you have to get access to that information, and experience, and counseling, and support. And the monthly meetings for some people are tremendous. Right off the bat they can unburden themselves and people will just understand and they will say, "Well, when you do so and so", "If you try such and such" or "This piece of information will tell you how to access that". And that's when the support starts to roll out. [long pause] That's the one piece of advice that just stands a mile high in my view. [You need to] talk to people that have been there. (Michael)

In time, these new friends become their primary reference group, which leads parents to *redefining their child.* Having been blocked so often in their attempts to help their own ill child and to influence his or her care, these parents began working for the betterment of all those who suffer from this devastating illness. They realized that helping everyone with schizophrenia in turn benefits their own child. Thus, they appear to have expanded the scope of their parenting and to have symbolically redefined their "child" as the community of people affected by schizophrenia, both patients and other families. Once they have fully embraced the collective, they have entered the next identity, the Reenfranchised Parent.

The Reenfranchised Parent

The identity of Reenfranchised Parent allows these parents to regain their parental rights and responsibilities by *taking on the "system"* through doing volunteer work, advocating for the mentally ill, and providing public education about schizophrenia. These parents develop and apply their personal skills and efforts toward mental health care reform, improving community services, raising public awareness about schizophrenia, and trying to reduce the stigma against mental illness. For example, they advocate for low-cost housing that supports varying degrees of independence; culturally appropriate care for ethnic minorities; family services, including respite care; and the promotion of research. Because of their efforts, parents (and other family members) are increasingly being included in treatment planning:

> When I spoke to the staff at [the psychiatric hospital], I said that finally family members are being included in a discussion and a treatment plan and, I said, it's a little bit like women getting the vote, that it was something they had to fight for, and it should have been a natural process. And so I say the whole question of including family in the treatment and discussion isn't something that should have been fought for. It should have been there from day one. (Willow)[7]

Although parents approach their volunteering and advocacy with enthusiasm, change is not easily won and the difficulties inherent in taking on an entrenched bureaucracy soon become apparent. *Being disillusioned* with the system centers around three broadly defined problem areas. First, parents observe limited funding for mental health services in comparison to the technologically exciting fields of health care. They also perceive poor accountability in the mental health system when policy makers, program directors, and individual therapists make promises that they fail to deliver. Finally, they observe the political maneuvering involved in health care reform and become discouraged when changes in mental health programming appear to be based on either political pressure or economic restraints rather than clear scientific evidence of efficacy. As Teresa wryly noted, politicians can afford to ignore the mentally ill because few psychiatric patients vote.

On a positive note, parents no longer have to grieve alone; instead, they are *mourning together.* The work that they do is valued and shared by others in the Schizophrenia Society and represents an acceptable public expression of their loss, at last allowing them to accept their situation and come to terms with their grief. According to Michael, acceptance means that you might still experience sadness and discouragement, but you never return to really deep despair.

With time, often many years, the ill son or daughter improves somewhat, and perhaps benefits from supportive housing and community services. The parents are older. Although their volunteer activity was satisfying, they become tired. Many have developed their own health problems, some of which might be stress related. Confronting their aging, they begin to reassess how they wish to spend their remaining years.

Evaluating My Life

At this time, parents engage in two evaluative processes: *acknowledging realities* and *identifying their personal needs.* Realistic expectations for their child's future evolve from their recognition of the ill person's social functioning and the acceptance of the chronic nature of schizophrenia. In essence, the parents adopt the stranger but continue to hope for a better future; however, these more limited hopes center on their child's achieving contentment and what Margaret referred to as "reasonable times of happiness." After years of being preoccupied by their child's illness, they can begin to focus more on themselves on or other long-ignored interests and move toward the status of the Emancipated Parent.

The Emancipated Parent

How parents periodically reconstruct their parental identity can be interpreted as a journey toward the ideal type of the Emancipated Parent, when parents expect to maintain a relationship with their children but withdraw from direct control and decision-making. They anticipate eventually enjoying the successes of their self-sufficient offspring, content in a significant amount of well-earned mutual independence. When a child is ill, the parents' journey toward emancipation is delayed, and their position depends on the location of the child on his or her individual illness trajectory (Strauss, 1975). Although the lives of all of the parents who participated in this study and their ill children improved, mutual independence was an unattainable goal.

Once a child's diagnosis is confirmed, the specter of schizophrenia never completely disappears. Evelyn stated it in this way:

> I guess for every person, you bring the baby home from the hospital and you teach them to be independent and you look forward to the wedding day when they are totally off your hands, and yet if you have a child who is affected with an illness, a chronic illness like schizophrenia, the pattern is going to be slightly different. In a sense, you are never totally the emancipated parent.

For these parents, the end point was a hybrid identity combining (in various degrees) The Reenfranchised Parent and movement toward Emancipation. Indeed, parental emancipation can be a relative thing for all parents, and complete independence is a myth that occurs only in what Willow called the "airy fairy TV family." Perhaps no parent ever truly gets there, whether the children are healthy or not. Still, for parents of children with schizophrenia, emancipation remains more elusive than it is for many others.

DISCUSSION AND CONCLUSION

Although the above overview describes Redefining Parental Identity as a linear process, it seldom (if ever) is. The self-identities of these parents respond to the fluctuating course of the child's schizophrenia illness trajectory. With each relapse, parents tend to regress toward disenfranchisement; with improvement, they once again move forward.

Although the terms *caring* and *caregiving* are often used interchangeably in the caregiving literature, some authors draw a distinction that is important for this grounded theory. For example, Fisher and Tronto (1990) define four interconnected components of caring: caring about, taking care of, caregiving, and care-receiving. *Caring about* involves paying attention to a person's needs. *Taking care* of implies assuming responsibility for those needs, whereas caregiving is "the hands-on work of maintenance and repair" (p. 40). *Care-receiving* is the child's response to *caregiving* and is influenced by the extent to which the caregiver and receiver agree about what is required.

For these families, the connections among the four components of caring were disrupted, and conflicts arose among parents, the ill adult-child, and other caregivers. Parents cared about their loved one and tried to take care of and provide caregiving to the adult-child. Unfortunately, they frequently lacked basic resources, including time, knowledge, and the necessary skills. More fundamentally, they lacked legal and societal permission to do so. Thus, the vital "taking care of" link between parents' caring about and their caregiving was disrupted. Their lack of authority blocked the connection between their moral and legal responsibilities for caring.

Fisher and Tronto (1990) state, "One of the most pervasive contradictions involved in taking care of concerns the asymmetry between responsibility and power" (p. 43). They contend that bureaucratic requirements for a division of labor, a hierarchy of power and authority, and the standardization of routines and policies cause contradictions and poor integration among the phases of caring. Such features are characteristic of the mental health system. In Fisher and Tronto's estimation, resolving these conflicts requires us to consider caring to be a contextual process. The immediate context of schizophrenia is the family within which it occurs and, to address the contradictions that exist among the components of caring, care for people with schizophrenia must incorporate the needs of their families.

Instead, the tendency has been to disregard and silence families. Feminists explain that oppression hinges on the silencing of women and other marginalized groups by those with power (Belenky, Clinchy, Goldberger, & Tarule, 1986; Gilligan, 1993). A parallel can be drawn to the experience of these parents whose voices are silenced when professional caregivers decline to consult, inform, or even listen to them in regard to their child's illness, treatment, and prognosis. As a result, these parents are similar to other oppressed and marginalized groups. At the same time, like women more generally in our society, they are expected to care for their ill children. Even if not overtly asked to do so, they are driven to assume that responsibility when no one else takes a perpetual interest in the child's well-being.

The concept of disenfranchisement of rights is important in conceptualization and measurement of caregiver burden. Statistical models of caregiver burden should incorporate a measure of powerlessness or, alternatively, mastery—something that few researchers besides Noh and his associates have done (Noh & Avison, 1988; Noh & Turner, 1987). Similarly, the suggestion by Reinhard (1991) to include grief in any study of caregiver burden is supported here. Finally, caregiving for someone with schizophrenia lasts for a protracted period, often decades. Most studies of caregiver burden provide us with a snapshot understanding of subjective and objective burden measured once, usually relatively soon after the patient has left the hospital. Only Pai and Kapur (1982) measured burden over time and then for only 6 months. If burden and mastery are assessed later in the proves, when a caregiving parent has reached the stage of The Reenfranchised Parent, mastery will likely have increased and burden will have decreased. Thus, there is a need for long-term studies of caregiving to track the changes in burden over time.

One means of testing and refining a grounded theory is to investigate how well the theory can be extended to other groups with similar experiences. Changes in parental identity might help explain caregiving for parents' adult children who are disabled by other mental illnesses like bipolar illness, by catastrophic accidents causing quadriplegia or brain injury, or by drug or alcohol addiction. The theory may also extend to sibling caregivers, who must redefine their identity as brothers and sisters. As well, the applicability of the model to parent caregivers from diverse cultural backgrounds should be assessed.

In addition to the above implications for research, the study highlights a number of issues for mental health care reform. Professional caregivers must recognize the contribution that families make to the patient's therapy but also accept professional responsibility to provide care for family caregivers. Respect, compassion, and education for family members, including practical advice about how to interact and communicate with a psychotic person, should be included in the treatment plan, not left for family members to obtain on an ad hoc basis. Case management and assertive community treatment are the cornerstones of a safe and comprehensive community program rather than the responsibility of parents. Care must come to the ill person and his or her family, not the other way around. To accomplish this, community programs must be staffed sufficiently well to ensure that caseloads are manageable.

Finally, in-patient treatment should be readily available whenever a mentally ill person is psychotic, to ensure that parents are not forced to try to manage a son or daughter who has been turned away from the emergency department. Parents told me that policy makers must address how the legal system defines "danger to oneself and others" and institute a more liberal application of commitment to psychiatric care. Refusal of treatment combined with an inability to provide an appropriate level of self-care should be considered as dangerous to self. Although such measures might be perceived by some as patriarchal and an infringement of patients' rights, they are necessary to achieve more humane treatment of the mentally ill and vital for countering the disenfranchisement of caregiving parents. With mental health care improvements that more fully incorporate the needs of families, parents who might never become emancipated from caregiving would at least be less disenfranchised.

NOTES

1. Milliken (2001) describes selected characteristics of this caregiving experience that are particularly difficult for mothers.
2. Within each state of this BSP are secondary social processes that define the parent's activities in that stage. Throughout this article, italics are used to identify these subprocesses.
3. The final phase of the constant comparative method is to link a new grounded theory with the relevant literature. In doing so, we discovered that Redefining Parental Identity is an empirical example of the formal grounded theory of status passage (Glaser & Strauss, 1971). According to Glaser and Straus, status passage involves a change from one social status to another with "a loss or gain of privilege, influence or power, and a changed identity and sense of self, as well as changed behavior" (p. 2).
4. Four of the ill adolescents accessed medical help before their parents recognized the need, one of them following a suicide attempt. One young woman was successful in hiding her delusions and hallucinations from her family until her psychiatrist admitted her to the hospital. In the other three cases, the parents were preoccupied with additional family problems. For example, the father in one family was terminally ill.
5. Pseudonyms have been used to ensure anonymity of participants and their family members.

6. All parents talked of how their son or daughter had changed since becoming ill and about how difficult it was to know how to react to or talk to this new person. Seven parents used the term "stranger" or said that someone else had taken over their child's body. Other authors have also used the same term when referring to how a family member with schizophrenia has changed (Hatfield, 1978, p. 358; Tuck, du-Mont, Evans, & Shupe, 1997, p. 118).

7. To emphasize Willow's point, we originally called this identity Parental Suffrage, to underscore the parents' own suffering, their tolerance of others, and their engagement in a cooperative and political process aimed at obtaining better understanding and treatment of people affected by schizophrenia. Ultimately, enhancing these collective rights introduces opportunities for parents to reclaim some individual rights and responsibilities with regard to their adult offspring.

REFERENCES

Belenky, M.F., Clinchy, M.F., Goldberger, N.R., & Tarule, J.M. (1986). *Women's ways of knowing*. New York: Basic Books.

Biegel, D.E., Sales, E., & Schulz, R. (1991). *Family caregiving in chronic illness: Alzheimer's disease, cancer, heart disease, mental illness, and stroke*. Newbury Park, CA: Sage.

Brooker, C. (1990). Expressed emotion and psychosocial intervention: A review. *International Journal of Nursing Studies, 27*(3), 267–276.

Canadian Alliance for Research on Schizophrenia. (1994). A national strategy for research on schizophrenia. *Journal of Psychiatry and Neuroscience, 19*(5, Suppl. 1), 3–49.

Chesla, C.A. (1991). Parents' caring practices with schizophrenic offspring. *Qualitative Health Research, 1,* 416–468.

Doka, K.J. (1989). Disenfranchised grief. In K.J. Doka (Ed.), *Disenfranchised grief: Recognizing hidden sorrow* (pp. 3–11). Lexington, MA: Lexington Books.

Fisher, B. & Tronto, J. (1990). Toward a feminist theory of caring. In E.K. Abel & M.K. Nelson (Eds.). *Circles of care: Work and identity in women's lives* (pp. 35–62). Albany: State University of New York Press.

French, L. (1987). Victimization of the mentally ill: An unintended consequence of deinstitutionalization. *Social Work, 32,* 502–505.

Geller, J.L. (1992). A historical perspective on the role of state hospitals viewed from the era of the "revolving door". *American Journal of Psychiatry, 149*(11), 1526–1532.

Gilligan, C. (1993). *In a different voice: Psychological theory and women's development*. Cambridge, MA: Harvard University Press.

Glaser, B.G., & Strauss, A.L. (1971). *Status passage*. Chicago: Aldine.

Hatfield, A.B. (1978). Psychological costs of schizophrenia to the family. *Social Work, 23,* 355–359.

Hatfield, A.B., & Lefley, H.P. (Eds.). (1987). *Families of the mentally ill: Coping and adaptation*. New York: Guilford.

Hogarty, G.E. (1985). Expressed emotion and schizophrenic relapse: Implications from the Pittsburgh study. In M. Alpert (Ed.), *Controversies in schizophrenia* (pp.354–365). New York: Guilford.

Howard, P.B. (1994). Lifelong maternal caregiving for children with schizophrenia. *Archives of Psychiatric Nursing, 8*(2), 107–114.

Isaac, R.J., & Armat, V.C. (1990). *Madness in the streets: How psychiatry and the law abandoned the mentally ill*. New York: Free Press.

Lurigio, A.J., & Lewis, D.A. (1989). Worlds that fail: A longitudinal study of urban mental patients. *Journal of Social Issues, 45*(3), 79–90.

Maurin, J.T., & Boyd, C.B. (1990). Burden of mental illness on the family: A critical review. *Archives of Psychiatric Nursing, 4*(2), 99–107.

Mechanic, D., & Rochefort, D.A. (1990). Deinstitutionalization: An appraisal of reform. *Annual Review of Sociology, 16,* 301–327.

Milliken, P.J. (2001). Disenfranchised mothers: Caring for an adult child with schizophrenia. *Health Care for Women International, 22*(1–2), 149–166.

Noh, S., & Avison, W.R. (1988). Spouses of discharged psychiatric patients: Factors associated with their experience of burden. *Journal of Marriage and the Family, 50,* 377–389.

Noh, S., & Turner, R.J. (1987). Living with psychiatric patients: Implications for the mental health of family members. *Social Science & Medicine, 25*(3), 263–271.

Pai, S., & Kapur, R.L. (1982). Impact of treatment intervention on the relationship between dimensions of clinical psychopathology, social dysfunction and burden on the family of psychiatric patients. *Psychological Medicine, 12,* 651–658.

Pickett, S.A., Cook, J.S., & Solomon, M.L. (1995). Dealing with daughters' difficulties: Caregiving burden experienced by parents of female offspring with severe mental illness. *Research in Community and Mental Health, 8,* 125–153.

Reinhard, S.C. (1991). Living with mental illness: Effects of professional contacts and personal control on caregiver burden (Doctoral dissertation, Rutgers University, 1991). Dissertation Abstracts International, 50/07, 2717.

Reynolds, I., & Hoult, J.E. (1984). The relatives of the mentally ill: A comparative trial of community-oriented and hospital-oriented psychiatric care. *Journal of Nervous and Mental Disease, 172*(8), 480–489.

Schreiber, R.S., & Stern, P.N. (2001). *Using grounded theory in nursing.* New York: Springer.

Stein, L.I., & Test, M.A. (1980). Alternative to mental hospital treatment: I. Conceptual model, treatment program, and clinical evaluation. *Archives of General Psychiatry, 37,* 392–397.

Strauss, A. (1975). *Chronic illness and the quality of life.* St. Louis: C.V., Mosby.

Terkelsen, K.G. (1987). The meaning of mental illness to the family. In A.B. Hatfield & H.P. Lefley (Eds.). *Families of the mentally ill: Coping and adaptation* (pp.128–150). New York: Guilford.

Thornton, J.F. & Seeman, M.V. (1991). *Schizophrenia simplified.* Toronto, Canada: Hogrefe & Huber.

Torrey, E.F. (1988). *Nowhere to go.* New York: Harper and Row.

Torrey, E.F. (1995). *Surviving schizophrenia* (3rd ed.). New York: HarperCollins.

Torrey, E.F. (1997). *Out of the shadows: Confronting America's mental health crisis.* New York: John Wiley.

Tuck, I. du-Mont, P., Evans, G., & Shupe, J. (1997). The experience of caring for an adult child with schizophrenia. *Archives of Psychiatric Nursing, 11*(3), 118–125.

Walsh, M. (1985). *Schizophrenia: Straight talk for family and friends.* New York: William Morrow.

Wright, E.R. (1994). Caring for those who "can't": Gender, network structure, and the burden of caring for people with mental illness. (Doctoral Dissertation, Indiana University, 1994). Dissertation Abstracts International, 55/02, 380.

P. Jane Milliken, R.N., Ph.D., is an assistant professor in the School of Nursing, University of Victoria, British Columbia, Canada.

Herbert C. Northcott, Ph.D., is a professor in the Department of Sociology, University of Alberta, Edmonton, Canada.

Index

Page numbers in bold indicate glossary entries.

A

Absolute value, 344
Abstract, **465**
 in the research literature, 129
 in research reports, 54, 55
Abstract journal, 129
Accessible population, 236, **465**
Accidental (convenience) sampling, 238, **465**
Acquiescence response set bias, 276, **465**
Active reading, 62–63
Adaptation Model (Roy), 151, 153
Advances in Nursing Science, 8
After-only (posttest-only) design, 173, **465**
Agency for Healthcare Research and Quality (AHRQ), 452
AIDSLINE database, 125
Aim, research, 99
Allen's McGill Model of Nursing, 152, 157–158
Alpha (α), **465**
 reliability (Cronbach's alpha), 309, **467**
 significance level, 350, 371
American Nurses Association (ANA), 8
Analysis, **465**. *See also* Data analysis; Qualitative analysis; Quantitative analysis
 computers and, 353, 388–389
 content, 384, 395, **468**
 cost–benefit, 188, **469**

data, 42, **469**. *See also* Data analysis
 discourse, 213, 214
 discrimination function, 365, **470**
 factor, 313, 366, 368, **472**
 impact, 188, **473**
 implementation, 188, **473**
 linear structural relations (LIS-REL), 367, **475**
 logit, 365–366
 meta-analysis, 136, **476**
 multiple regression, 362, **477**. *See also* Multiple regression
 negative case, 316, **477**
 outcome, 188, **478**
 path, 367, **479**
 power, 246, 350, **480**
 process, 188, **480**
 qualitative, 44, 382–395, **481**. *See also* Qualitative analysis
 quantitative, 42, 331–378, **481**. *See also* Quantitative analysis
 secondary, 264
 statistical, 42, 331–378, **485**. *See also* Quantitative analysis; Statistics
 styles of, qualitative, 383–384
 unit of, 136
Analysis of covariance (ANCOVA), 193–194, 363–365, 368, 373, **465**
Analysis of variance (ANOVA), 356–358, 361, **465**

 multivariate (MANOVA), 366–368, **477**
 repeated measures, 357, 361
Analysis styles, qualitative, 383–384
Analytic phase of quantitative research, 42
ANCOVA. *See* Analysis of covariance (ANCOVA)
Anecdotes, literature reviews and, 131
Animal subjects, 290
Annual Review of Nursing Research, 8
Anonymity, 81, 271, **465**
ANOVA. *See* Analysis of variance (ANOVA)
Applied Nursing Research, 8
Applied research, 22, **465**
Assessment, psychometric, 311
Associative relationships, 38
Assumptions, 13, **465**
 inferential statistics and, 352
 paradigms and, 14
 of scientific approach, 13
Asymmetric distribution, 334
Attitudes, measurement of, 272–273
Attrition, 186, 195, **466**
Audit, inquiry, 317, **474**
Audit trail, 318, **466**
Authorities, as knowledge source, 11
Author search, literature search and, 126
Average, 336

Axiologic question, paradigms and, 14
Azjen & Fishbein's Theory of Reasoned Action, 154

B

Back-stage knowledge, 283
Baseline date, 173, **466**
Basic research, 22, **466**
Basic social process (BSP), 392, **466**
Becker's Health Belief Model, 154
Before-after (pretest-posttest) design, 172, **466**
Being-in-the-world, 217
Bell-shaped curve (normal distribution), 336. *See also* Normal distribution
Beneficence, 84–85, **466**
Beta (β), 371
Between-subjects design, 171, 175, **466**
Bias, 173, **466**
  attrition and, 196
  control and, 14
  data collection and, 294
  full disclosure and, 78
  interviewer, 271
  nonresponse, 251, **478**
  observational bias, 288
  publication, 411
  research design and, 197
  response set, 275–276, 306, **483**
  sampling, 237, 238, 246–247, 251, **483**
  selection, 182, 195, **484**
  self-reports and, 278
  social desirability, 276, **484–485**
  statistical analysis of, 367
  systemic, 173
  threats to internal validity, 195
Bimodal distribution, 336, **466**
Biophysiologic measures, 265, 289–293
  critique of, 293
  evaluation of, 292
  types of, 291–292
  uses of, 290–291
Bipolar scale, 274, 277–278
Bivariate statistics, **466**
  descriptive, 341–345

inferential, 353–360. *See also* Inferential statistics
Black box question, 223
Blended methods, 219. *See also* Integration of qualitative and quantitative designs
"Blind" review, 53, **466**
Borrowed theory, 154, **466**
Bournes & Mitchell's conceptual model of waiting, 158–160
Bracketing, 217, 249
Bricolage, 209, **466**

C

Cafeteria question, 270
Canadian Health Services Foundation (CHSF), 9
Canadian Institute of Health Research (CIHR), 9
Canadian Journal of Nursing Research, 8
Canadian Nurses Association (CNA), 75
CancerLit database, 125
Carry-over effects, repeated measures design, 175
Case-control design, 181, **466**
Categorical variable, 32, **466**
Categorization scheme, qualitative data and, 384, 386–387
Category system, observational, 285, **466**
Causal (cause-and-effect) relationship, 38, **466–467**. *See also* Causality; Causal modeling
  criteria for, 176
  experimental research and, 176
  multimethod research and, 221–222
  nonexperimental research and, 182–183
  quasi-experimental research and, 180
Causality. *See also* Causal (cause-and-effect) relationship
  correlation and, 410
  determinism and, 13
  integrated analysis and, 221–222
  quantitative research and, 33
  research design and, 176

Causal modeling, 367, **466**
Cause-and-effect relationship. *See* Causal (cause-and-effect) relationship
Causes. *See also* Causal (cause-and-effect) relationship
  independent variables and, 33
  multiple, 33–34
CD-ROM, 124
Cell, **467**
  contingency tables and, 342–343, 359
  experimental design and, 174
Center for Research in Nursing, 8
Central tendency, 336–338, **467.** *See also* Mean
Change, resistance to and research utilization, 442
Checklist, observational research, 286
Chemical measures, 291–292
CHID database, 125
Children, as research subjects, 79–80
Chi-squared (χ^2) test, 358–359, 361, **467**
CINAHL database, 125–127
Clinical Effectiveness in Nursing, 9
Clinical Nursing Research, 9
Clinical relevance, 65, 449–450, **467**
Clinical research, 5, **467**. *See also* Nursing research
Clinical trial, 175–176, **467**
  randomized, 175, 439–440
Closed-ended question, 269, 280, **467**
Cluster (multistage) sampling, 244, **467**
Cochrane Collaboration, 438–439
Codebook, 384
Code of ethics, 74–75, **467**
Coding, **467**
  open, 392, **478**
  qualitative data and, 387–389
  quantitative data and, 42
  selective, 392, **484**
Coefficient
  alpha (Cronbach's alpha), 309, **467**
  correlation (Pearson's *r*), 344, 359–360, **469**
  of determination (R^2), 371

multiple correlation *(R)*, 362, 371, **476**
phi, 361
regression*(b)*, 371
reliability, 307, **482**
validity, 312, **487**
Coercion, 76, **467**
Cognitive anthropology, 213
Collaborative research, 436, 441
Communication
 constancy of, 191
 measurement and, 306
 of research problems, 102–106
 of research results, 42–43. *See also* Research report
Comparison
 constant, 218, 386–387, **468**
 multiple, 357, **476**
 qualitative studies and, 211
 research design and, 169–170, 172, 184
Comparison group, 178, **467**
Completely unstructured interview, 266
Complex hypotheses, 109
Composite scale, 272–273. *See also* Scale
Computer
 analysis of qualitative data and, 388–389
 analysis of quantitative data and, 353
 electronic literature searches and, 124
 Internet, 10, 124–125, 142, 460
 observations and, 281, 285
Concealment, 78–79, **467**
Concept, 31, **468**
 as component of theories, 145
 construct validity and, 313
 measurement and, 305–307
 models of nursing and, 151
 vs. construct, 31–32
Conceptual definition, 146–148
Conceptual file, 388
Conceptual framework, 146–148. *See also* Conceptual model; Theory
Conceptual map, 146
Conceptual model, 32, 146, **468**. *See also* Theory
 models of nursing, 150–153
 non-nursing models, 154

Conceptual model of waiting, (Bournes & Mitchell), 158–160
Conceptual phase of research
 qualitative studies and, 43–44
 quantitative studies and, 39–40
Conceptual utilization, 434, **468**
Concurrent validity, 312, **468**
Conduct and Utilization in Nursing Research (CURN) Project, 436–438
Conference, professional
 attending, 6, 442
 presentation at, 52–53
Conference on Research Priorities (CORP), 9
Confidence interval (CI), 371
Confidentiality, 81–82, **468**
Confirmability, data, 318, **468**
Consent
 implied, 76
 informed, 76–78, **474**
 process, 78, **481**
Consent form, 76–77, **468**
Conservation model (Levine), 152
Constancy of conditions, 190–191
Constant, 32
Constant comparison, 218, 386–387, **468**
Construct, 31–32, **468**. *See also* Concept
Construct validity, 313, **468**
Consumer of nursing research, 6, **468**
Content analysis, 395, **468**
 manifest, 384
Content validity, 311–312, **468**
Contingency table, 342–343, **468**
 chi-squared test and, 358–359
Continuous variable, 32, **468**
Control, research, 14, 170, 189–194, **468**
 evaluation of methods for, 194
 experimental design and, 171
 of external extraneous factors, 190–191
 of intrinsic extraneous factors, 191–193
 as purpose of research, 19, 21

quasi-experiments and, 178
 in scientific research, 14
 statistical, 193, 363–365, 373
 time dimension and, 184
 validity and. *See* External validity; Internal validity
Control group, 172, **468**
 nonequivalent, 177–178, 363, **477–478**
Convenience (accidental) sampling, 238–239, 248, **468**
Core variable, 392, **468**
CORP (Conference on Research Priorities), 9
Correlation, 343–345, 359, **469**. *See also* Causal (cause-and-effect) relationship; Relationship
 causation and, 410. *See also* Causality
 multiple, 362. *See also* Multiple regression
Correlational research, 180–184, **469**. *See also* Ex post facto (correlational) research
Correlation coefficient, 343–344, 359–360, **469**
 multiple *(R)*, 362, **476**
 Pearson's product moment *(r)*, 344, **479**. *See also* Pearson's *r*
 Spearman's rank order (rho), 344, **469**
Correlation matrix, 345–346, **469**
Cost–benefit analysis, evaluation research and, 188, **469**
Cost–benefit assessment, research utilization and, 454–455, **469**
Costs
 health care, 5
 questionnaire *vs.* interview, 271
 sampling and, 241
 to study participants *vs.* benefits, 83–84
Counterbalancing, 276
Covariate, 364, **469**
Covert data collection, 78–79, **469**
Credibility, qualitative data and, 315–317, **469**
Criterion-related validity, 312, **469**

Critique, research, 63, 65–66, 415–423, **469**
  ethical dimensions, 87–88, 420
  interpretive dimensions, 420–421
  literature reviews and, 137–138
  methodologic dimensions, 418–420
  presentation and stylistic dimensions, 421–423
  purpose of, 416–417
  research decisions and, 416
  substantive and theoretical dimensions, 418
Cronbach's alpha, 309, **469**
Crossover (repeated measures) design, 173
Cross-sectional study, 171, 185–186, **469**
  qualitative research and, 211
Cross-tabulation, 342, **469**
  chi-squared test and, 358–359
  contingency tables and, 342
  qualitative analysis and, 384
Cumulative Index to Nursing and Allied Health Literature (CINAHL), 129. *See also* CINAHL
CURN project, 436–438
Cytologic measures, 291–292

D

Data, 35–37, **469**. *See also* Qualitative data; Quantitative data
  analysis of. *See* Data analysis
  assessment of quality, 307–319. *See also* Data quality
  baseline, 173
  coding, 42, 387–388, 389
  collection of. *See* Data collection
  existing *vs.* new, 263–264
  posttest, 173
  pretest, 173
  qualitative, 36–37, **481**. *See also* Qualitative data
  quantitative, 36, **481**. *See also* Quantitative data
  raw, 45, **482**
  saturation of, 44, 249, **484**

  triangulation of, 315
  trustworthiness of, 314
Data analysis, **469**. *See also* Qualitative analysis; Quantitative analysis
  computers and, 353, 388–389
  descriptive statistics, 333–341. *See also* Descriptive statistics
  inferential statistics, bivariate, 345–353. *See also* Inferential statistics
  multivariate statistics, 360–367. *See also* Multivariate statistics
  preparation for, 42
  qualitative, 44. *See also* Qualitative analysis
  quantitative, 42. *See also* Quantitative analysis
Data collection, 42, 263–299, **469**. *See also* Measurement
  biophysiologic measures, 289–293
  covert, 78–79, **469**
  dimensions of, 264–265
  implementing plan for, 293–294
  measurement and. *See* Measurement
  observational methods, 281–289
  overview of methods, 263–265
  in research reports, 57
  scales, 272–276
  self-report methods, 266–280
  structured, 265, **485**
Data management, qualitative, 386–389
Data quality
  critiquing, 319–320
  measurement and, 306–307
  qualitative data and, 314–319
  quantitative data and, 307–314. *See also* Reliability; Validity
Data saturation, 44, 249, **484**
Data source triangulation, 315
Debriefing, **470**
  peer, 316, **479**
  study participant, 83, 85
Deception, 79
Decision accretion, 434
Decisions, methodologic, 170, 416

Declaration of Helsinki, 75
Deductive reasoning, 12, **470**
  theory testing and, 148, 149
Definition
  conceptual, 146–148
  operational, 34–35, **478**
Degrees of freedom *(df)*, 353, **470**
Dependability, qualitative data and, 317, **470**
Dependent groups *t*-test, 355, 361
Dependent variable, 33–34, **470**
  control and, 190
  experimental research and, 172, 176
  hypotheses and, 109, 111
  literature reviews and, 127
  qualitative research and, 212
  research questions and, 105
  statistical tests and, 361, 368
Description, as research approach, 18–19
Descriptive correlational study, 182, **470**
Descriptive phenomenology, 216
Descriptive research, 182, **470**
Descriptive statistics, 333–341, **470**
  bivariate, 341–345
  central tendency and, 336–338
  frequency distributions and, 334–336
  variability and, 338–341
Descriptive theory, 145, **470**
Design. *See* Research design
Design phase of quantitative research project, 40–41
Detailed approach, phenomenological analysis, 394
Determinism, 13, **470**
Deviation score *(x)*, 372
Diary, 268
Dichotomous question, 270
Dichotomous variable, 362, 366
Dilemma, ethical, 73–74
Directional hypotheses, 110, **470**
Direct research utilization, 435
Disabled people, as vulnerable subjects, 80
Disclosure, full, 76
Disconfirming evidence, 316
Discourse analysis, 213, 214
Discrimination function analysis, 365, 368, **470**

Discussion section, research report, 60–61
Dispersion. *See* Variability
Disproportionate sampling, 243, **470**
Dissemination of research results, 10. *See also* Research report
qualitative studies, 45
quantitative studies, 42–43
research utilization and, 441
Dissertations, 52
Distribution
asymmetric (skewed), 334
bimodal, 336, **466**
central tendency and, 336–337
frequency, 334–336, **472**. *See also* Frequency distribution
multimodal, 336, **476**
normal (bell-curve), 336, **478**. *See also* Normal distribution
sampling, 346–348, **483**
skewed, 334, **484**
symmetric, 334, **486**
theoretical, 346, 353
unimodal, 336, **487**
variability of, 338–341
Double-blind experiment, 177, **470**
Duquesne school of phenomenology, 393–394

E

Ecological psychology, 213, 214
Editing analysis style, 384
Electronic database, 124–127, **470**
CINAHL database, 125–127
Element sampling, 236, **470**
Eligibility criteria, 235, **470**
E-mail, 63
Embodiment, 217
Emergent design, 209, **470**
Emic perspective, 215, **470–471**
Empirical evidence, 14–15, 17, **471**
Empirical phase of quantitative research, 41–42
Environment
control of, 190–191
observation and, 281
Epistemologic question, paradigms and, 14

Equipment
biophysiologic measures, 291–292
data processing. *See* Computer
interviews and, 268
observational research and, 281
Equivalence, reliability and, 309, **471**
Error(s)
of measurement, 306–307, **471**
sampling, 245, 346, **483**
standard, of the mean, 346, **485**
Types I and Types II, 349–350, **487**
Essence, 216
Estimation procedures, 348
Eta-squared, 371
Ethical dilemma, 73–74
Ethical Guidelines for Nurses in Research Involving Human Participants, 75
Ethics, research, 17, 72–88, **471**
beneficence and, 84–85
code of ethics, 74–75
critiquing, 87–88, 420
experimental research and, 176
external reviews and, 86–87
harms and benefits, 83
historical background, 73
informed consent, 76–78
justice and, 82–83
need for guidelines and, 72–75
observational research and, 78–79, 281, 288
Research Ethics Boards (REBs), 86–87
respect for human dignity and, 75–81
respect for justice and inclusiveness, 82–83
respect for privacy and confidentiality, 81–82
risk/benefit ratio, 83–84
vulnerable subjects and, 79–81
Ethnography, 213, 215–216, **471**
Ethnomethodology, 213, 214, **471**
Ethnonursing research, 213, **471**
Ethnoscience, 213
Ethology, 213

Etic perspective, 215, **471**
Evaluation research, 188–189, **471**
Event sampling, 287, **471**
Evidence, types of, 439
Evidence-based practice, 5, 433, 438–440, **471**. *See also* Research utilization
barriers to, 440–444
implementation of, 455–456
implementation potential and, 453–455
literature review and, 450–451
models of, 444–449
overview, 438–439
randomized clinical trials and, 439–440
research utilization and, 433
topic selection, 449–450
types of evidence, 439–440
Evidence hierarchies, 439
Evidence reports, 452
Expected frequency, 359
Experiment, 171–177, **471**
advantages and disadvantages of, 176–177
causality and, 176
characteristics of, 172–173
control and, 194
designs for, 173–176
double-blind, 177, **470**
ethical constraints and, 176
integration of qualitative and quantitative data in, 223–224
internal validity and, 194–195
quasi-experiments and, 180
Experimental group, 172, **470**
Experimental intervention (treatment), 172, **474**
Explanation, as research purpose, 19, 20–21
Exploitation, freedom from, 85–86
Exploration, as research purpose, 19, 20
Exploratory research, 19, 20
Ex post facto (correlational) research, 180–181, **471**
advantages and disadvantages of, 182–184
causality and, 182
internal validity and, 194
interpretation and, 182–183
Expressive projective methods, 277

External review, ethical issues and, 86–87

External validity, 196–197, **470**

Extraneous variable, 170, **471.** *See also* Control, research analysis of covariance and, 363–365

controls for, 191–193

sampling design and, 250–251

statistical control and, 193, 363–365, 373

Extreme (deviant) case sampling, 249, **472**

Extreme response set bias, **472**

F

Face-to-face (personal) interview, 187–188, 272. *See also* Interview

Face validity, 311, **472**

Factor, in factorial designs, 174

Factor analysis, 313, 366, 368, **472**

Factorial design, 173–174, 357, **472**

Fair treatment, right to, 82–83

Feasibility, research utilization project and, 454–455

Field notes, 284–285, **472**

Field work, 16

embedding quantitative measures in, 223

ethnography and, 215–215

field research, **472**

File, conceptual, 388

Findings, research, 42, 45, 58, **472.** *See also* Results

Fixed alternative (closed-ended) question, 269, **472**

Flexible research design, 16, 209–210

Focus, research, 98

Focused interview, 267, **472**

Focus group interview, 267, **472**

Follow-up study, 187, **472**

Forced choice question, 270

Framework, 146–148, **472.** *See also* Conceptual model; Theoretical frameworks; Theory

F-ratio, **472**

in analysis of covariance, 365

in analysis of variance, 356–358, 361

in multiple regression, 362

Freedom

degrees of, 353

from exploitation, 85–86

from harm, 85–86

Frequency distribution, 334–336, **472.** *See also* Distribution

Frequency (*f*), 334

expected *vs.* observed, 359

qualitative analysis and, 391

Frequency polygon, 334, **472**

Friedman test, 361

Front-stage knowledge, 283

Full disclosure, 76, **472**

Functional relationship, 38, **473**

Funding of nursing research, 8, 41

G

Gaining entrée, 44, 210, 283, **473**

Gatekeeper, 210

Generalizability, 15, **473**

external validity and, 196

interpretation of results and, 413

in qualitative research, 16

in quantitative research, 15

sampling designs and, 196

transferability of data and, 318. *See also* Transferability

Goals, research, 17

Good Clinical Practice: Consolidated Guidelines, 75

Grand theory, 145, **473**

Grand tour question, 267, **473**

Grounded theory, **473**

data analysis and, 391–392

research traditions and, 213, 214, 218–219

samples and, 248

theory development and, 148

H

Harm, freedom from, 85–86

Harms and benefits of research, 83–86

Hawthorne effect, 177, **473**

Health as Expanding Consciousness (Newman), 152

Health Belief Model (Becker), 154

Health Canada, 75

Health Care Systems Model (Neuman), 151, 152

Health STAR database, 125

Hermeneutics, **473**

data analysis and, 394

research traditions and, 213, 216

Heterogeneity, 310, **473.** *See also* Homogeneity; Variability

Histologic measure, 291–292

Historical research, 214, 263–264, **473**

History threat, 194–195, **473**

Holism, qualitative research and, 14, 15–16, 209

Homogeneity, **473**

of measures (internal consistency), 308–309

research design and, 192

of sample and reliability, 310

sampling and, 237

Hospital Literature Index, 129

Human dignity, respect for, 75–81

Human rights, research subjects and. *See* Ethics, research

Hypothesis, 40, 99, 106–112, **473**

alternative (H_1), 371

characteristics of, 107–108

complex, 109

critique of, 112–114

directional, 110, **470**

formulating, 40

function of, 106–107

nondirectional, 110, **477**

null (statistical), 111, 349, **478**

proof and, 111–112

qualitative research and, 43, 45, 106

in research reports, 55

research (scientific, substantive), 111, 349

results and, 107

rival, 180, **483**

scientific (research), 349

simple, 109

testing of, 58, 108, 111–112. *See also* Hypothesis testing

theories and, 106–107, 110–111, 148, 149

wording of, 109–111

Hypothesis testing, 348–353. *See also* Inferential statistics; Statistics

interpretation of results and, 409–411

level of significance and, 350

null hypothesis and, 111, 349
overview of procedures for, 352–353
parametric and nonparametric tests and, 352
proof and, 134
tests of statistical significance and, 350–352
Type I and Type II errors and, 349–350

I

Identification, as research purpose, 18, 19
Identification (ID) number, 82
Immersion/crystallization analysis style, 384
Impact analysis, 188, **473**
Implementation analysis, 188, **473**
Implementation assessment, research utilization, 453–455
Implementation potential, 453–455
    research utilization, **473**
Implications of results, 61, 413, 415
    research problems and, 112–114
Implied consent, 76
Independent groups *t*-test, 355, 361
Independent variable, 33–34, **473**
    control over, 172, 211
    experimental research and, 172, 176
    hypotheses and, 109, 111
    literature reviews and, 127
    manipulation of, 172
    nonexperimental research and, 180
    qualitative research and, 211, 212
    quasi-experimental research and, 177
    research questions and, 105
    statistical tests and, 361, 368
Index, print, 129
Index Medicus, 129
Indirect research utilization, 435
Inductive reasoning, 12, **473**
    theory development and, 148
Inference
    observer, 286

statistical, 345, **485**
Inferential statistics, 345–353, **474.** *See also* Hypothesis testing; Multivariate statistics
    analysis of variance, 356–358
    assumptions and, 352
    chi-squared test, 358–359
    correlation coefficients, 359–360
    guide to bivariate tests, 361
    hypothesis testing and, 348–353. *See also* Hypothesis testing
    interpretation of, 409–413
    multivariate, 360–367. *See also* Multivariate statistics
    random sampling and, 346
    sampling distributions and, 346–348
    t-tests, 353–355
Informant, 31, **474.** *See also* Study participant; Subject
Informed consent, 76–78, **474**
Innovation, adoption of, 435–437
Inquiry audit, 317, **474**
Institutionalized people, vulnerability as subjects, 80
Institutional Review Board (IRB), **474**
Instrument, 268, **474.** *See also* Data collection; Measure; Measurement
    assessment of, 307–314. *See also* Data quality
    biophysiologic, 291, 292
    errors of measurement and, 306
    multimethod research and, 220
    psychometric evaluation of, 311
    researchers as, 215
Instrumental utilization, 434, **474**
Integration of qualitative and quantitative designs, 219–224, **474**
    applications, 220–222
    critique of, 224–225
    rationale for, 219–220
    strategies for, 222–224
Integrative reviews, 441, 451–452. *See also* Literature reviews

Interaction effect, 174, 357, **474**
Intercept constant *(a),* 371
Internal consistency reliability, 308–309, **474**
Internal validity, 194–196, **474**
    external validity and, 196–197
International Journal of Nursing Studies, 8
International Nursing Index, 129
Internet, 10, 124–125, 142, 460
Interobserver (interrater) reliability, 309, **474**
Interpretation of results, 42, 408–415. *See also* Results
    critique of, 420–421
    discussion section of report and, 61
    in qualitative research, 413–415
    in quantitative research, 42, 409–413
Interpretive phenomenology, 216
Interrater (interobserver) reliability, 309
Interval measurement, 332–333, **474**
Intervention, 169, 172, **474.** *See also* Experiment
Interview, 187–188. *See also* Self-reports
    completely unstructured, 266
    focused, 267, **472**
    focus group, 267, **472**
    personal (face-to-face), 187–188, **479**
    questionnaire *vs.,* 271–272
    structured, 268–269
    telephone, 187–188, 272
    unstructured, 266–268, **487**
Interviewer
    bias and, 271
    focus group, 267
    observations, 272
    structured interviews and, 272
    unstructured interviews and, 268
Interview schedule, 268, **474**
Introduction, research report, 54–56
Intuiting, 217
Intuition, knowledge and, 11–12
Inverse (negative) relationship, 344, **474**
Investigation, 31

Investigator, 31
Investigator triangulation, 315, 391
In vitro measure, 291–292
In vivo measure, 291
Iowa Model of Evidence-Based Practice, 446–448
Item(s), 272, **474**. *See also* Questions
  reversal of, 272
  sampling of, errors of measurement and, 306

J

Jargon, research, 30, 61, 63, 64
Journal, abstract, 129
Journal article, 53–61, **474**. *See also* Research report
  content of, 54–61
  literature reviews and, 135
  research utilization and, 441
  style of, 61–62
Journal club, 6, 442, **475**
Journal of Advanced Nursing, 8
Judgmental (purposive) sampling, 241, **475**
Justice, research ethics and, 82–83

K

Key words, literature search, 129
King's Model of Dynamic Interacting Systems, 151, 152
Knowledge
  back stage, 283
  extension of, 113
  front stage, 283
  of innovations, 435–437
  sources of, 11–12
  state-of-the-art, in literature reviews, 133
  tacit, 215
Knowledge creep, 434
Knowledge-focused trigger, 446–447
Known-groups technique, 313, **475**
Kruskal-Wallis test, 361

L

Laboratory analysis, 291–292
Laboratory setting, 171
Lambda (λ), 371

Lazarus and Folkman's Theory of Stress and Coping, 149–150, 154
Laws of probability, 345
Leininger's Theory of Culture Care Diversity and Universality, 152
Level, in factorial experiment, 174
Level of measurement, 331–333, **475**
  inferential statistics and, 361
  multivariate statistics and, 368
  parametric and nonparametric statistics and, 352
Level of significance, 59, 350, 353, **475**
Levine's Conversation Model, 152
Life history, 267, **475**
Likert scale, 272–273, **475**
Limitations
  discussion of, in research, 61
  of qualitative and quantitative studies, 219
  of the scientific approach, 15
  of a study, 61
Linear regression multiple, 362, 368
LISREL (linear structural relation analysis), 367, **475**
Literature reviews, 40, 122–142, **475**
  abstracting and recording notes for, 131
  content of, 133
  critiquing, 137–138
  electronic literature searches, 124–127
  in evidence-based practice, 450–451
  flow of tasks in, 130
  length of, 134
  locating sources for, 124–129
  organizing, 131–133
  print resources for, 127–128
  protocol for, 132
  purposes of, 122–124
  qualitative research and, 43, 123, 135
  reading and using, 135–138
  research reports and, 55–56
  as source of research problem, 100
  style of, 134, 135
  types of, 135–137

utilization and, 123
  writing, 129–135
Lived experience, 217
Log, observational, 284, **475**
Logical positivism, 12, **475**
Logical reasoning, 12. *See also* Reasoning
Logistic regression (logit analysis), 365–366, 368, **475**
Longitudinal study, 171, 186–187, **475**
  qualitative research and, 211

M

Macroethnography, 215
Macro-theory (grand theory), 145, **475**
Mailed questionnaire, 271
Main effect, 174, 357, **475**
MANCOVA, 367
Manifest content analysis, 384
Manipulation, 172, 475. *See also* Experiment; Intervention
Mann-Whitney U test, 361
MANOVA, 366–367
Map, conceptual, 146
Mapping, electronic searches and, 126
Matching (pair matching), 193, **475**
Matrix, correlation, 345–346, **469**
Maturation threat, 195, **476**
Maximum variation sampling, 249, **476**
McGill Model of Nursing (Allen), 152, 157–158
Mean, 338, **476**
  computation of, 338
  population (μ), 371
  sampling distribution of, 346
  standard deviation and, 338
  standard error of, 346
  testing differences between 3+ groups, 356–358
  testing differences between two groups, 354–355
Mean square *(MS)*, 371
Measure. *See also* Data collection; Instrument; Measurement
  assessment of, 305–314
  baseline, 173, **466**
  biophysiologic, 289–293
  observational, 281–289
  projective, 277

psychosocial scales, 272–276
self-report, 266–280
Measurement, 305–314, **476**. *See also* Data collection; Instrument; Measure
advantages of, 305–306
critique of, 319–320
errors of, 306–307
levels of, 331–333, **475**. *See also* Level of measurement
operational definitions and, 34–35
problems of, 15
reliability of instruments and, 307–308. *See also* Reliability
validity of, 310–314. *See also* Validity
Median, 338, **476**
Mediating variable, 190, **476**
Medical Research Council (MRC), 75
MEDLINE database, 125
Member check, 316, 391, **476**
Memos, in qualitative analysis, 392
Meta-analysis, 136, **476**
Metasynthesis, qualitative, 137
Methodologic decisions, 170, 416
Methodologic notes, 284, **476**
Methodologic questions, paradigms and, 14
Methods, research, 13–16, **476**. *See also* Data collection; Measurement; Qualitative analysis; Quantitative analysis; Research design; Sampling
Method section, research report, 56–58
Method slurring, 215
Method triangulation, 315
Microbiologic measures, 291–292
Microethnography, 215
Middle-range theory, 146, **476**
Mishel's Uncertainty in Illness Theory, 151, 153
Mixed method research, 219. *See also* Integration of qualitative and quantitative designs
Mixed results, 412
Mobile positioning, 284
Modality, **476**
Mode, 337–338, **476**
Model, 146, **476**

causal, 367, **466**
conceptual, 146, **468**. *See also* Conceptual model; Theory of research utilization/evidence-based practice, 444–449
schematic, 146
statistical, 146
Moderator, focus group, 267
Mortality threat, 195, **476**
Multimethod research, 219, **476**. *See also* Integration of qualitative and quantitative designs
Multimodal distribution, 336, **476**
Multiple-choice question, 270
Multiple comparison procedures, 357, **476**
Multiple correlation, 362, 368
Multiple correlation coefficient, 362, **476**
Multiple positioning, 284
Multiple regression, 362–363, 368, **477**
Multistage (cluster) sampling, 244, **477**
Multivariate analysis of covariance (MANCOVA), 367, 368
Multivariate analysis of variance (MANOVA), 366–368, **477**
Multivariate statistics, 360–367, **477**
analysis of covariance, 363–365. *See also* Analysis of covariance
causal modeling, 367
discrimination function analysis, 365
factor analysis, 313, 366
guide to, 368
LISREL, 367
logistic regression, 365–366
multiple regression, 362
multivariate analysis of covariance, 367
multivariate analysis of variance, 366–367
path analysis, 367

N

N, 334, 371, **477**
n, 371, **477**

Narrative data, 36–37. *See also* Qualitative data
Narrative literature review, 135–136
National Center for Nursing Research (NCNR), 8
National Institute of Health (NIH), 8
National Institute of Nursing Research (NINR), 9, 113
National Research Council of Canada, 75
Naturalistic methods, 15–16. *See also* Qualitative research
Naturalistic paradigm, 13, **477**
Naturalistic setting, 16, 171, **477**
Natural Sciences and Engineering Research Council (NSERC), 75
Nay-sayer, 276
Nazi experiments, 73
Negative case analysis, 316, **477**
Negative (inverse) relationship, 344, **477**
Negatively skewed distribution, 334, **477**
Negative result, 411, **477**
Net effect, 188, **477**
Network (snowball) sampling, 238, **477**
Neuman's Health Care Systems Model, 151, 152
Newman's Health as Expanding Consciousness Model, 152
NIH. *See* National Institute of Health (NIH)
NINR. *See* National Institute of Nursing Research (NINR)
Nominal measurement, 332, **477**
Nondirectional hypothesis, 110, **477**
Nonequivalent control-group design, 177–178, 363, **477–478**
Nonexperimental research, 171, 180–184, **478**. *See also Ex post facto* (correlational) research
Nonmaleficence, 85
Nonparametric statistics, 352, 361, **478**
Nonprobability sampling, 236, 238–242. *See also* Sample; Sampling

Nonprobability sampling
(*continued*)
convenience (accidental),
238, **468**
evaluation of, 241–242
purposive (judgmental), 241,
481
quota, 238–241, **482**
snowball (network), 238, 248,
484
theoretical, 248, **486**
Nonresponse bias, 251, 271,
478
Nonsignificant result, 41, 352,
353, **478**
Normal distribution (bell-shaped
curve), 336, **478**
assumption of, inferential statistics, 352
sampling distributions and,
346–347
standard deviations and,
339–341
Notes
field, 284–285, **472**
for literature reviews, 131
observational, 284, **478**
Null (statistical) hypothesis, 111,
349, 411, **478**. *See also* Hypothesis testing
Nuremberg Code, 74–75
Nurse(s)
as observers, 281
research utilization and,
441–442. *See also* Research
utilization
roles of in research, 6
Nursing. *See also* Nursing practice; Nursing research
conceptual models of,
151–153
importance of research in, 5.
See also Nursing research
Nursing Abstracts, 129
Nursing Best Practices Guidelines
(NBPG) project, 456
Nursing literature, 100, 122–124.
See also Literature reviews;
Research report
Nursing practice
research in, 5
research utilization and,
435–436. *See also* Evidence-
based practice; Research
utilization

as source of research problems, 100
Nursing research, 4–25. *See also*
Research
barriers to utilization of,
440–444
clinical, 5, 290
conceptual models for,
150–154. *See also* Conceptual model; Theory
consumer-producer contin-
uum, 6
funding for, 8, 41
future directions for, 10–11
historical evolution of, 7–9
importance of, 5
methods for, 13–16. *See also*
Methods, research
paradigms for, 12–13, 16–18
priorities for, 10–11
purposes of, 18–21
quantitative *vs.* qualitative,
14–16
roles of nurses in, 6
source of knowledge and,
11–12
utilization of, 6, 8, 10, 43,
433–438. *See also* Research
utilization
Nursing Research, 7, 54
Nursing Studies Index, 129

O

Objective, research, 98
Objectivity, 14, **478**
biophysiologic measures and,
292
confirmability of qualitative
data and, 318
data collection and, 265
measurement and, 305
paradigms and, 14
in research reports, 61–62
Observation, 265, 281–289, **478**
bias and, 288
critique of, 288–289
ethical issues and, 78–79, 281,
288
evaluation of, 287–288
interviewer, 272
participant, 282, **479**
sampling and, 287
self-reports *vs.,* 287
structured, 285–287, **485**

unstructured, 281–285, 288,
487
Observational notes, 284, **478**
Observed frequency, 359
Observed (obtained) source, 306,
478
Observer
bias, 288
interobserver reliability, 309
training of, 294
Odds, 366
Odds ratio, 366
One-group before-after design,
179
One-variable (univariate) statis-
tics, 333–341. *See also* De-
scriptive statistics
One-way analysis of variance,
356–357
On-line catalog system, 125
*Online Journal of Clinical Innova-
tion,* 10
On-line publishing, 10
On-line search, 124
Ontologic question, paradigms
and, 14
Open coding, 392, **478**
Open-ended question, 269, 270,
478
closed-ended *vs.,* 280
recording of responses for,
268
Open System Model (King), 152
Operational definition, 34–35,
478
Operationalization, 41. *See also*
Measurement
Orange County Research Utiliza-
tion in Nursing (OCRUN),
437–438
Ordinal measurement, 332, **478**
Orem's Self-Care model, 151,
152
Organizations, research utiliza-
tion and, 442–443
ORMU (Ottawa Model of Re-
search Use), 438, 448–449
Ottawa Model of Research Use
(ORMU), 438, 448–449
Outcome analysis, 188, **478**
Outcome variable (measure), 33,
478–479. *See also* Depen-
dent variable
Outcomes research, 10, 189,
479

P

Paired *t*-test, 355
Pair matching. *See* Matching
Panel study, 186, **479**
Paradigm, 12–18, **479**
    assumptions of, 14
    methods and, 13–16
    naturalistic, 13, **477**
    nursing research and, 16–18
    positivist, 12–13, **480**
    research problems and, 17–18,
        100, 113
Parameter, 333, **479**
    estimation of, 348
Parametric statistics, 352, **479**
    guide to, 361
Parse's Theory of Human Becom-
        ing, 148–149, 151, 153, 158
Participant. *See* Study participant
Participant observation, 282–283,
        479
Path analysis, 367, **479**
Pearson's *r*, **479**
    description of, 344
    inferential statistics and, 361,
        369–360
Peer debriefing, 316, **479**
Peer review, 53, 65, **479**
Pender's Health Promotion
        Model, 146, 147, 151
Percentage, 334
Perfect relationship, 343, **479**
Persistent observation, 315
Personal (face-to-face) interview,
        187–188, 479. *See also* In-
        terview; Self-reports
Personal notes, 284, **479**
Persuasive research utilization,
        435
Phases, of a quantitative research
        project, 39–43
Phenomenology, **479**
    data analysis for, 393–395
    research traditions and, 213,
        216–218
Phenomenon, 31, **479**
Phi coefficient, 361
Philosophical questions, para-
        digms and, 14
Physiologic measures. *See* Bio-
        physiologic measures
Pictorial projective technique,
        277
Pilot study, 41, **479**

Planning phase, research studies,
        40–41, 43–44
Population, 40, 235–236, **479.**
        See also Sampling
    accessible, 236, **465**
    homogeneity of, 237
    identifying, 40
    parameters and, 333
    target, 236, **486**
Positioning, in observational re-
        search, 284
Positively skewed distribution,
        334, **480**
Positive relationship, 344, **480**
Positive result, **480**
Positivist paradigm, 12–13, 14,
        480
Post hoc test, 357, **480**
Poster session, 53, **480**
Posttest data, 173, **480**
Posttest-only (after only) design,
        173, **480**
Power analysis, **480**
    sample size and, 246
    Type II errors and, 350
Prediction
    discriminant function analy-
        sis and, 365
    hypotheses and, 40, 98, 106
    multiple regression and,
        362–363
    as research purpose, 19, 21
Predictive validity, 312, **480**
Preexperimental design, 178,
        179, 196, **480**
Pregnant women, vulnerability
        as subjects, 80
Presentations, at conferences,
        52–53
Pretest, **480**
    preintervention measure, 173,
        178
    trial run of instrument, 269
Pretest-posttest (before-after) de-
        sign, 172, **480**
Primary source, 130, **480**
Print index, 129
Priorities for nursing research,
        10–12
Prisoners, as subjects, 80
Privacy, study participants and,
        81–82
Probability, laws of, 345
Probability level. *See* Level of sig-
        nificance

Probability sampling, 236,
        242–245, **480.** *See also*
        Sample; Sampling
    assumption of for inferential
        statistics, 346
    cluster (multistage), 244, **467**
    evaluation of, 245
    simple random, 242–243, **484**
    stratified random, 243–244,
        485
    systematic, 244–245, **486**
Problem, research. *See* Research
        problem
Problem-focused trigger, 446–447
Problem statement, 99, **480.** *See
        also* Hypothesis; Research
        problem
    critique of, 112–114
    wording of, 102–103
Process analysis, 188, **480**
Process consent, 78, **481**
Producer of nursing research, 6
Product-moment correlation co-
        efficient, 344, 359–360,
        361, **481**
Professional conference
    attending, 6, 442
    presentations at, 52–53
Professionalism, 5
Projective technique, 277, **481**
Prolonged engagement, 315, **481**
Proof
    hypothesis testing and,
        111–112, 134, 410
    theories and, 145
Proportionate sampling, 243, **481**
Proportion(s), chi-squared and,
        358–359, 361
Proposal, 41, 123
Prospective study, 171, 181, **481**
    qualitative research and, 212
Protocol
    for evidence-based practice,
        455–456
    literature review and, 132
    research, 191
Psychological Abstracts, 129
Psychometric evaluation, 311,
        481
Psychosocial scale. *See* Scale
PsycINFO database, 125
Publication. *See* Journal article;
        Research report
Purpose, statement of, 55, 99,
        103–104, **485**

Purposive (judgmental, purpose-ful) sampling, 241, 248, 481

p-value, 353, 369, **479**. *See also* Level of significance

Q

Q sort, 277–278, **481**

Qualitative analysis, 44, 382–395, **481**. *See also* Qualitative research
   analysis styles, 383–384
   analytic procedures, 389–395
   analytic process, 385
   computers and, 388–389
   critique of, 395–396
   data management and organi-zation, 386–389
   grounded theory methods in, 391–392
   interpretation and, 413–415
   phenomenological analysis, 393–395
   validation and, 391

Qualitative data, 36–37, **481**. *See also* Qualitative research
   analysis of. *See* Qualitative analysis
   assessment of data quality, 314–319
   coding of, 387–388
   observational methods and, 281–285
   organization of, 387–389
   self-reports and, 266–268

Qualitative Health Research, 9

Qualitative metasynthesis, 137

Qualitative research, 14, 15–16, **481**. *See also* Qualitative analysis; Qualitative data
   activities in, 43–45
   analysis and, 44, 382–395. *See also* Qualitative analysis; Qualitative data
   data collection and. *See* Un-structured data collection
   ethical issues and, 78, 82, 86
   guidelines for critiquing re-search designs, 225
   guidelines for critiquing sam-ple designs, 251
   guidelines for evaluation of data, 320
   hypotheses and, 43, 45, 106

   integration with quantitative research, 219–224
   interpretation of results and, 413–415
   literature reviews and, 43, 123, 135
   paradigms and, 14
   purposes of nursing research and, 18–21
   research design and, 208–219. *See also* Research design
   research problems and, 100
   research traditions in, 213–215
   research utilization and, 434
   sampling in, 248–250
   theory development and, 148

Quantifiability, 265

Quantification, 305. *See also* Mea-surement

Quantitative analysis, 42, 331–378, **481**. *See also* Hy-pothesis testing; Statistical tests; Statistics
   critique of, 370, 372–374
   descriptive statistics, 333–341. *See also* Descriptive statistics
   inferential statistics, 345–353. *See also* Inferential statistics
   interpretation of results and, 367, 369–370, 409–413. *See also* Results
   measurement levels and, 331–333
   multivariate statistics and, 360–367. *See also* Multi-variate statistics

Quantitative data, 36, **481**. *See also* Measurement; Quanti-tative analysis; Structured data collection

Quantitative research, 13–14, **481**. *See also* Quantitative analysis
   data collection and. *See* Struc-tured data collection
   guidelines for critiquing re-search designs, 198
   guidelines for critiquing sam-ple designs, 251
   guidelines for evaluation of data, 320
   integration with qualitative research, 219–224

   methodologic decisions and, 418–420
   phases in, 39–43
   positivist paradigm and, 13–14
   purposes of nursing research and, 18–21
   research designs and, 169–197. *See also* Research design
   research problems and, 100
   sampling and, 235–247
   scientific approach and, 14–15
   theories in, 149–150

Quasi-experiment, 171, 177–180, **481–482**
   advantages and disadvantages of, 180
   causality and, 180
   designs for, 177–179
   internal validity and, 194, 196

Quasi-statistical analysis style, 384

Quasi-statistics, 384, 391, **482**

Questionnaire, 268–272, **482**
   interview *vs.*, 271–272
   mailed, 271
   response rates and, 271
   surveys and, 187–188

Question(s). *See also specific ques-tion types*
   closed-ended (fixed-alternative), 269, 280, **467**
   grand tour, 266, **473**
   open-ended, 269, 280, **478**
   philosophical, paradigms and, 14
   purposes of nursing research and, 19
   research, 98–106, **483**
   types of, 270–271

Quota sampling, 238–241, **482**

R

r, 362–363, **482**

R, 344, 361, **482**

R^2, 363, **482**

Random assignment, 173, **482**. *See also* Randomization

Randomization, 173
   constraints on, 176, 194
   experimental designs and, 173

quasi-experimental designs and, 177
research control and, 191–192, 194
vs. random sampling, 242
Randomized clinical trials, 175
evidence-based practice and, 439–440
Random number table, 173
Random sampling, 242–245, **482.** *See also* Probability sampling
assumption of in inferential statistics, 346
randomization *vs.*, 242
Range, 339, **482**
Rank order question, 270
Rating question, 271
Rating scale, observational, 286
Ratio measurement, 333, **482**
Raw data, 45, **482**
Reactivity, 281, 288, **482**
Reading research reports, 63–64
Reasoning
deductive, 12, 148, 149, **470**
inductive, 12, 148, **473**
REBs (Research Ethics Boards), 86–87
Recontextualization, 385
Recording equipment
interviews and, 268
observations and, 281, 284–285
Records, as data source, 264
Reductionism, 15
References
in research report, 61
screening for literature review, 129–131
Registered Nurses Association of Ontario (RNAO), 456
Regression
logistic, 365–366, 368, **475**
multiple, 362–363, 368, **477**
Regression coefficient (*b*, β), 371
Reinforcement theory, 106, 145
Relationality, 217
Relationship, 37–38, **482.** *See also* Correlation
associative, 38
bivariate statistics and, 343–345
causal (cause-and-effect), 38, **466–467.** *See also* Causal

(cause-and-effect) relationship
functional, 38, **473**
hypotheses and, 106–112. *See also* Hypothesis
negative (inverse), 344, **477**
perfect, 343, **479**
positive, 344, **480**
qualitative research and, 38
theories and, 145
Reliability, 307–308, **482**
internal consistency, 308–309, **474**
interpretations of, 310
interrater (interobserver), 309, **474**
test-retest, 307, **486**
validity and, 310–311
Reliability coefficient, 307, **482**
Repeated measures ANOVA, 357, 361
Repeated measures (crossover) design, 174–175, 192, 194, 482
Replication, 10, **482**
research utilization and, 441
stepwise, data dependability and, 317
Report. *See* Research report
Representativeness of sample, 41, 236, 250–251, 346, **482**
Research, **482.** *See also* Nursing research; Research design
applied, 22, **465**
basic, 22, **466**
clinical, 5, 290, **467**
clinical relevance of, 449–450. *See also* Evidence-based practice
correlational, 180–181, **469**
descriptive, 182, **470**
ethical issues, 72–88. *See also* Ethics, research
ethnonursing, 216, **471**
evaluation, 188–189, **471**
experimental, 171–177. *See also* Experiment
exploratory, 19, 20
ex post facto, 180–181, **471**
field, **472.** *See also* Field work
historical, 214, 263–264, **473**
knowledge and, 11–12
multimethod, 219, **476.** *See also* Integration of qualita-

tive and quantitative designs
nonexperimental, 180–184, **478.** *See also* Nonexperimental research
nursing. *See* Nursing research
observational, 281–289, **478.** *See also* Observation
outcomes, 10, 189, **479**
preexperimental, 178, 196, **480**
purpose of, 18–21
qualitative, 14, 15–16, **481.** *See also* Qualitative research
quantitative, 13–14, **481.** *See also* Quantitative research
quasi-experiment, 177–180, **481–482.** *See also* Quasi-experiment
scientific, 14–15, **484**
survey, 187–188, **486**
terminology of, 30–38
theory and, 148
Research aim, 99
Research-based practice, 5. *See also* Research utilization
Research control. *See* Control, research
Research critique. *See* Critique
Research design, 40, 169–170, **483.** *See also* Research design, multimethod studies; Research design, qualitative studies; Research design, quantitative studies
communication with participants and, 191
controls for extraneous variables and, 170. *See also* Control, research
in research reports, 56
Research design, multimethod studies, 219–224
Research design, qualitative studies, 208–219
characteristics of, 209
critique of, 224–225
emergent design, 209, **470–471**
features of, 211–212
integration with quantitative approach, 219–224
phases of, 210
planning and, 209–210
research traditions and, 213–215

Research design, quantitative
studies, 40, 169–203. *See
also specific designs*
control and, 189–194. *See also*
Control, research
critique of, 197
experimental designs,
169–175
external validity and,
196–197
integration with qualitative
approach, 219–224
internal validity and, 194–196
nonexperimental designs,
180–184
purposes of, 169
quasi-experimental and preexperimental designs,
177–180
time dimension and, 184–187
Researcher, 31
credibility of, 317
as instrument, 215
obtrusiveness of, 265
research utilization and,
440–441
Research Ethics Boards (REBs),
86–87
Research findings, 42, 45, 58,
472. *See also* Implications
of results; Interpretation of
results; Results
Research hypothesis, 111. *See also*
Hypothesis
Research in Nursing & Health, 8
Research methods. *See* Methods,
research
Research personnel
interviewers, 268, 272
observers, 288
selection of for data collection, 294
training of, 294
Research problem, 98–106, **483**
communication of, 102–106
critique of, 112–114
development and refinement
of, 101–102
formulating, 39
paradigms and, 17–18, 100,
113
significance of, 112–114
sources of, 100–101
terms relating to, 98–100
theory and, 113

Research project, 31
Research proposal, 41, 123
Research protocol, 191
Research question, 17–18, 55,
98–106, **483.** *See also* Research problem
Research report, 42, **483**
critiquing, 63–66, 415–423.
See also Critique
journal articles, 53–61
locating, 124–129
overview of, 23, 45
presentation at conferences,
52, 53
reading, 62–63
as source of research questions, 100
theses and dissertations, 52
types of, 52–54
Research study, 31. *See also* Research
Research subject, 31. *See also*
Study participant
Research utilization, 6, 43,
432–456, **483.** *See also*
Evidence-based practice
barriers to, 440–444
conceptual, 434, **468**
continuum of, 434–435
critiques and, 416–417
direct, 435
efforts to improve, 436–438
evidence-based practice, 433,
438–440
indirect, 435
instrumental, 434, **474**
models of, 444–449
nurse-related barriers to,
441–442
in nursing, 6, 8, 10
nursing practice and, 435–436
nursing profession-related
barriers to, 443–444
organizational barriers to,
442–443
persuasive, 435
process of, 444–456
qualitative studies and, 434
relation to evidence-based
practice, 433
research-related barriers to,
440–441
Respect, human subjects and,
75–83
human dignity and, 75–81

informed consent and, 78–79
justice and, 82–83
privacy and, 81–82
right to full disclosure and, 76
right to self-determination
and, 75–76
vulnerable persons and, 79
Respondent, 31, **483.** *See also*
Study participant
Response alternatives, 269
Response bias, 275–276
Response rate, 251, 279, **483**
nonresponse bias and, 251
questionnaires *vs.* interviews,
271
Response set bias, 275–276, **483**
errors of measurement and,
306
Results, 408, **483**
credibility of, 409, 413–414
dissemination of, 42–43, 45.
See also Research report
generalizability of, 413. *See
also* Generalizability
hypothesized, 410
implications of, 413, 415
importance of, 412–413,
414–415
interpretation of, 408–415
meaning of, 409–411, 414
mixed, 412
negative, 411, **477**
nonsignificant, 352, 411, **478**
positive, **480**
qualitative, 413–415
quantitative, 42, 409–413
transferability of, 415
unhypothesized, 411–412
utilization of, 432–456. *See
also* Research utilization
Results section, research report,
58–60
Retrospective study, 171, 181,
483
qualitative research and, 212
Reversal, item, 272
Review
"blind," 53, **466**
ethical issues and, 86–87
literature, 39, 122–142, **475.**
See also Literature reviews
peer, 53, 65, **479**
of research reports, 45. *See
also* Critique, research
Rho, Spearman's, 344

Rights, human subject's. *See also* Ethics, research
  to fair treatment, 82–83
  to full disclosure, 76
  to privacy, 81–82
  to self-determination, 75
Risk–benefit ratio, 83–84, **483**
Risks, research participation and, 83–84
Rival hypothesis, 180, **483**
Rogers' Science of Unitary Human Beings, 148–149, 151, 153
Rorschach ink blot test, 277
Roy's Adaptation Model, 151, 153

S

Sample, 40–41, 236, **483**. *See also* Sample size; Sampling
  description in research reports, 56
  eligibility criteria and, 235
  representativeness of, 41, 236
Sample size, **483**
  power analysis and, 246
  qualitative studies and, 249–250
  quantitative studies and, 245–247
  standards errors and, 347–348
  Type II errors and, 349
Sampling, 234–256, **483**. *See also* Sample; Sample size; *specific types of sampling*
  basic concepts, 235–237
  critique of, 250–252
  design, 196
  external validity and, 196
  items, in measuring instruments, 306
  nonprobability, 238–242, 247–248, **478**. *See also* Nonprobability sampling
  observational, 287
  probability, 242–245, **480**. *See also* Probability sampling
  qualitative research and, 248–250
  rationale for, 237
  sample size and, 246
Sampling bias, 237, 246–247, 250–251, **483**
Sampling distribution, 346–348, **483**

Sampling error, 245, 346, **483**
Sampling frame, 242, **483**
Sampling interval, 244
Sampling plan, 41, 247, 250, **483**. *See also* Sampling
Saturation, data, 44, 249, **484**
Scale, 272–276, **484**
  Likert, 272–273, **475**
  rating, observational, 286
  response set bias and, 275–276
  semantic differential, 274–275, **484**
  summated rating, 273
  visual analogue, 274–275, **487–488**
Schematic model, 146
Science of Unitary Human Beings (Rogers), 151, 153
Scientific approach, 14–15, **484**. *See also* Quantitative research
Scientific merit, **484**
Scientific method. *See* Scientific approach
Scientific research. *See* Research; Scientific approach
Scientific (research) hypothesis, 111, 349. *See also* Hypothesis
Scientist, 31. *See also* Researcher
Score(s)
  obtained (observed), 306, **478**
  scales and, 274
  true, 306, **486–487**
Search, electronic literature, 124–127
Secondary analysis, 264
Secondary source, 130, **484**
Selection, random, 242
Selection threat (self-selection), 182, 195, **484**
Selective coding, 392, **484**
Self-administered questionnaire, 187–188. *See also* Questionnaire
Self-Care Model (Orem), 151, 152
Self-determination, 75–76
Self-report(s), 187, 265, 266–280, **484**. *See also* Interview; Questionnaire; Scale
  critique of, 279–280
  evaluation of method, 278–279
  observation *vs.*, 281
  projective techniques, 277

Q sorts, 277–278
  scales, 272
  structured, 268–272, **485**
  unstructured and semistructured, 266–268
  vignettes, 276, **487**
Self-selection, 182, 195, **484**
Semantic differential scale, 274–275, **484**
Semistructured (focused) interviews, 267
Setting, research, 44, **484**
  description of in research reports, 57
  laboratory, 171
  naturalistic, 171, **477**
  qualitative research and, 212
  quantitative research and, 170
Sigma, 372
Sigma Theta Tau International, 125
Significance
  clinical *vs.* statistical, 59, 412–413
  practical, 412–413
  of research problems, 56, 112–114
Significance level, 350, 353, **484**
Significance, statistical, 59, 352, **485**
  interpretation of results and, 410–412
  tests of, 350–352. *See also* Statistical tests
Simple hypothesis, 109
Simple random sampling, 242–243, **484**
Single positioning, 284
Site, 44
  multiple, 175
Situational contaminants, 306
Skewed distribution, 334, **484**
Snowball (network) sampling, 238, 248, **484**
Social desirability response bias, 276, **484–485**
Social Sciences and Humanities Research Council (SSHRC), 75
Source
  of data, 263–265
  of knowledge, 11–12
  primary, 130, **480**
  of research problems, 100–101
  secondary, 130, **484**

Spatiality, 217
Spearman's rank-order correlation (Spearman's rho), 344, 361, **485**
Split-half technique, 309, **485**
Stability, of measures, 307
Standard deviation *(SD)*, 339–341, **485**
Standard error of the mean (SEM), 346, 372, **485**
Standard *(z)* score, 372
Statement of purpose, 55, 103–104, **485**
Statistical analysis, 42, **485**. *See also* Quantitative analysis; Statistical tests; Statistic(s)
Statistical control, 193, 363–365, 372
Statistical inference, 345, **485**. *See also* Inferential statistics
Statistical model, 146
Statistical (null) hypothesis, 111. *See also* Null (statistical) hypothesis
Statistical significance, 59, 352, **485**
    clinical *vs.*, 59, 412–413
    level of, 59
    tests of, 350–352. *See also* Statistical tests
Statistical tests, 59–60, 350–352, **485**. *See also* Inferential statistics; Multivariate statistics; *specific tests*
    guide to bivariate tests, 361
    guide to multivariate tests, 368
Statistic(s), 333
    bivariate, 341–345, 361, **466**
    critique of, 370, 372–374
    descriptive, 333–341, **470**. *See also* Descriptive statistics
    inferential, 345–353, 361, **474**. *See also* Inferential statistics
    multivariate, 360–367, 368, **477**. *See also* Multivariate statistics
    nonparametric, 352, **478**
    parametric, 352, **479**
    quasi-statistics, 384, 391, **482**
    in research reports, 59–60
    tips on reading, 367, 369–370
    univariate, 334–341, **487**
Stepwise replication, 317

Stetler model of research utilization, 445–446
Stipend, 76, **485**
Strata, 237, 239, 243, **485**
Stratified random sampling, 243–244, **485**
Structured data collection, 265, **485**
    observation and, 285–287, **485**. *See also* Observation
    self-reports and, 268–272, 278–279, **485**. *See also* Self-reports
Study, 31. *See also* Research
Study participant, 31, **485**
    communication with, 191
    rights of, 76–79. *See also* Ethics, research
Style. *See* Analysis, styles of; Writing style
Subject, 31, **485**. *See also* Study participant
    description of in research reports, 56
    vulnerable, 79–81, **488**
Subjectivity, 13, 14, 16, 61. *See also* Objectivity
Subject search, literature search and, 126
Subject stipend, 76
Substantive codes, grounded theory, 391–392
Substantive hypothesis, 111. *See also* Hypothesis
Summated rating scale, 273
Sum of squares *(SS)*, 372
Survey research, 187–188, **486**. *See also* Self-reports
    integration of qualitative and quantitative approaches and, 222–223
Symbolic interaction, 218
Symmetric distribution, 334, **486**
Systematic bias, 173
Systematic sampling, 244–245, **486**

T

Table
    contingency, 342–343, **468**
    literature reviews and, 131
    statistical, 369–370, 372
    test statistics and, 353
Table of random numbers, 173
Tacit knowledge, 215

Target population, 236, **486**
Telephone interview, 187–188, 272
Template, 384
Template analysis style, 384
Temporality, 217
Terminology, basic research, 30–38
Test-retest reliability, 307–308, **486**
Test statistic, 350, 353, **486**. *See also* Statistical tests; Statistics
Textword search, literature search and, 126
Theme, in qualitative analysis, 60, 390, **486**
Theoretical code, grounded theory, 392
Theoretical distribution, 346, 353
Theoretical frameworks, 40, 146. *See also* Conceptual model; Theory
    critique of, 155–156, 418
    in research reports, 56
Theoretical notes, 284, **486**
Theoretical sampling, 248, **486**
Theory, 32, 144–160, **486**. *See also* Conceptual model
    borrowed, 154, **466**
    components of, 145
    construct validity and, 313
    critical, 12
    descriptive, 145, **470**
    development of, 113, 148–149
    grand (macro), 145, **473**
    grounded, 148, 218–219, 391–392, **473**. *See also* Grounded theory
    hypotheses and, 106–107, 110–111, 148, 149
    literature reviews and, 130
    middle-range, 146, **476**
    multimethod research, 222
    nursing research and, 150–154
    origin of, 145
    proof and, 145
    qualitative research and, 32
    quantitative research and, 32
    research and, 148
    as source of research problems, 100–101
    testing, 149–150
Theory of Caring (Watson), 153

Theory of Culture Care Diversity and Universality (Leininger), 152
Theory of Human Becoming (Parse), 151, 153, 158
Theory of Reasoned Action (Azjen-Fishbein), 154
Theory of Stress and Coping (Lararus & Folkman), 149–150, 154
Theory triangulation, 315
Theses, 52
Thick description, 318, **486**
Threat
    to external validity, 196–197
    to internal validity, 194–195
Time
    control of, 191
    research design and, 184–187, 211
Time sampling, 287, **486**
Time series design, 179, 187, **486**
Tool. *See* Instrument
Topic, research, 98, 100
Topic guide, 267, **486**
Tradition, knowledge source, 11
Transcription, interview, 266
Transferability, **486**
    of findings, utilization and, 453–455
    qualitative data and, 318, 415
Treatment, 172, **486**. *See also* Experiment; Quasi-experiment
Treatment group, 172
Trend study, 186, **486**
Trial and error, knowledge source, 11
Triangulation, 315, 391, **486**
Tri-Council Policy Statement: Ethical Conduct for Research Involving Humans, 75
True score, 306, **486–487**
Trustworthiness, qualitative data and, 44, 314–319, **487**
t-test, 353–355, 361, **487**
Tuskegee syphilis study, 73
Two-variable statistics. *See* Bivariate statistics
Two-way ANOVA, 357–358
Type I error, 349–350, **487**
Type II error, 349–350, 411, 412–413, **487**
    beta and, 371

power analysis and, 350
sample size and, 412–413
Typical case sampling, 249

U

Uncertainty in Illness Theory (Mishel), 151, 153
Unhypothesized results, 411–412
Unimodal distribution, 336, **487**
Unit of analysis, 136
Univariate descriptive statistics, 333–341, **487**
Univariate descriptive study, **487**
Unstructured data collection
    observations and, 281–285, 288, **487**
    self-reports and, 266–268, 279. *See also* Self-report
Unstructured interview, 266–268, **487**
U statistic, 361, 372
Utilization. *See* Research utilization
Utilization criteria, **487**. *See also* Research utilization
Utrecht school of phenomenology, 394

V

Validity, 310–311, **487**
    biophysiologic measures and, 292
    concurrent, 312, **468**
    construct, 313, **468**
    content, 311–312, **468**
    criterion-related, 312, **469**
    external, 196–197, **471**
    face, 311, **472**
    internal, 194–196, **474**
    interpretation of, 314
    multimethod approach and, 220, 221
    predictive, 312, **480**
    reliability and, 310–311
    self-reports and, 278–279
Validity coefficient, 312, **487**
Variability, 338–341, **487**. *See also* Heterogeneity; Homogeneity
Variable, 32–35, **487**
    categorical, 32, **466**
    continuous, 32, **468**
    core, 392, **468–469**
    dependent, 33–34, **470**. *See also* Dependent variable

dichotomous, 362, 366
extraneous, 146, **471**. *See also* Extraneous variable
independent, 33–34, **473**. *See also* Independent variable
measurement of, 41. *See also* Measurement
mediating, 190, **476**
operational definition of, 34–35
outcome, 33, **478–479**
Variance, 340, **487**
    analysis of variance (ANOVA), 356–358, 361, **465**
    multivariate analysis of variance (MANOVA), 366–368, **477**
    proportion accounted for, 362–363
VAS (visual analogue scale), 274–275, **487–488**
Verbal projective technique, 277
Vignettes, 276, **487**
Visual analogue scale, 274–275, **487–488**
Volunteer sample, 248
Vulnerable subjects, 79–81, **488**

W

Waiting, conceptual model of, (Bournes & Mitchell), 158–160
Watson's Theory of Caring, 153
Website, 27, 142, 460
Weighting, 243, **488**
Western Journal of Nursing Research, 8
Wilcoxon signed ranks test, 361
Wilks' lambda (λ), 371
Within-subjects design, 171, 175, **488**
Word association, 277
World Wide Web, 27, 142, 460
Writing style
    critiquing, 422–423
    of literature reviews, 134, 135
    of research reports, 61–62

Y

Yea-sayer, 276

Z

z (standard) score, 372